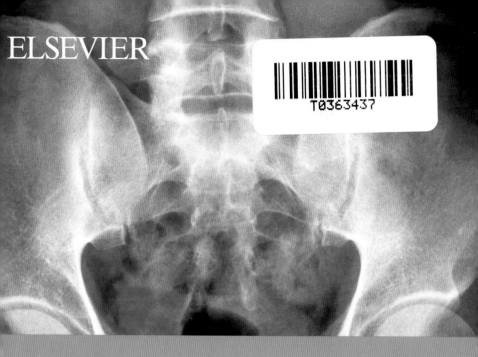

ELSEVIER

T0363437

Help us make our content even better

We are very interested in hearing your feedback about the quality and content of our books. A short survey is all that is required to ensure we continue to deliver the best content in medical publishing.

Elsevier will make a monthly donation to a selected charity on behalf of readers who have completed our survey. A list of eligible charities from which you may choose will be made available during the survey process and each month the charity obtaining the highest number of votes will receive the donation from Elsevier.

Please follow the link to complete the short online survey and help us to help others.

http://www.elsevier.com/booksfeedback

MARSHALL & RUEDY'S

On Call

Principles & Protocols

AUSTRALIAN AND NEW ZEALAND 3RD EDITION

MARSHALL & RUEDY'S

On Call

Principles & Protocols

AUSTRALIAN AND NEW ZEALAND 3RD EDITION

Australian adaptation by
Anthony FT Brown MB ChB, FRCP, FRCS (Ed), FACEM, FRCEM
Professor, Discipline of Anaesthesiology and Critical Care,
School of Medicine MD Program, University of Queensland, Brisbane.
Senior Staff Specialist (Pre-Eminent Status), Department of Emergency
Medicine, Royal Brisbane and Women's Hospital, Brisbane.

Mike Cadogan MA (Oxon), MB ChB, FACEM
Staff Specialist in Emergency Medicine, Department of
Emergency Medicine, Sir Charles Gairdner Hospital, Perth.
Team Physician, Wallabies and the Western Force.

Antonio Celenza MB BS, MClinEd, FACEM, FRCEM
Professor of Emergency Medicine and Medical Education,
Faculty of Medicine, Dentistry and Health Sciences,
University of Western Australia, Perth. Staff Specialist,
Department of Emergency Medicine, Sir Charles Gairdner
Hospital, Perth.

Original edition by
Shane A Marshall MD, FRCPC; Director of Cardiac Care,
Chief of Medicine, King Edward the VIIth Memorial Hospital,
Paget, Bermuda

John Ruedy MDCM, FRCPC, LLD (Hons); Professor (Emeritus)
of Pharmacology, Faculty of Medicine, Dalhousie University,
Halifax, Canada

ELSEVIER

Elsevier Australia. ACN 001 002 357
(a division of Reed International Books Australia Pty Ltd)
Tower 1, 475 Victoria Avenue, Chatswood, NSW 2067

On Call Principles and Protocols, 5th Edition

ISBN: 978-1-4377-2371-7

This adaptation of On Call Principles and Protocols, 5th Edition, by Shane Marshall and John Ruedy, was undertaken by Elsevier Australia and is published by arrangement with Elsevier Inc.

Marshall & Ruedy's On Call Principles & Protocols Australia and New Zealand 3rd edition
Copyright © 2017 Elsevier Australia. Reprinted 2018, 2019, 2021 (thrice), 2022, 2023. 1st edition
© 2007, 2nd edition © 2011 Elsevier Australia
ISBN: 978-0-7295-4262-3
eISBN: 978-0-7295-8625-2

Notice

This publication has been carefully reviewed and checked to ensure that the content is as accurate and current as possible at time of publication. We would recommend, however, that the reader verify any procedures, treatments, drug dosages or legal content described in this book. Neither the author, the contributors, nor the publisher assume any liability for injury and/or damage to persons or property arising from any error in or omission from this publication.

National Library of Australia Cataloguing-in-Publication Data

Title: Marshall & Ruedy's On Call Principles & Protocols
Australian adaptation / by Anthony FT Brown, Mike Cadogan & Antonio Celenza.

Edition: Australian and New Zealand edition. 3rd edition

ISBN: 9780729542623 (paperback)

Notes: Includes index.

Subjects: Emergency medicine—Australia—Handbooks, manuals, etc.
Medical emergencies—Australia—Handbooks, manuals, etc.
Emergency nursing—Australia—Handbooks, manuals, etc.
Communication in emergency medicine—Australia—Handbooks, manuals, etc.

Other creators/contributors:
Brown, Anthony FT, editor.
Cadogan, Mike, editor.
Celenza, Antonio, editor.

Dewey number: 616.0250994

Content Strategist: Larissa Norrie
Content Development Specialist: Lauren Santos
Senior Project Manager: Rosemary McDonald
Edited by: Caroline Hunter, Burrumundi Pty Ltd
Permission/Picture Research by: Sarah Thomas
Design by: Toni Darben, Darben Design
Illustrations by Greg Gaul, Rod McClean and Tor
Ercleve Index by: Innodata
Typeset by: Toppan Best-set Premedia Limited
Printed in China by 1010 International Ltd.

Contents

Foreword

This book is a treasure trove of useful, up-to-date, practical information for newly qualified doctors responding to hospital ward calls. Indeed, such is the scope of its content, many senior doctors in various fields within acute medicine will find it an invaluable resource to have on hand for everyday practice. All three authors are among the finest teachers of emergency medicine in Australasia, with complementary and widely recognised experience in translating knowledge into the clinical performance of students and junior doctors. The book is remarkably well organised, with a clear and easy-to-follow structure that belies the great depth of information provided. It is so relevant to the concerns of junior doctors, and so full of concise clinical wisdom, that it is frankly a joy to read. The book is a source of excitement for those of us who have spent our careers in acute medicine and watched junior staff come and go in the sometimes chaotic and confusing hospital environment, and wished for some more structure and consistency in their teaching.

The authors provide clear guidelines on how to respond to a range of acute emergencies, illuminating the decision-making process in what can be difficult and challenging situations. Few textbooks discuss what might go through one's mind on the way to an emergency; this one does. Similarly, there is often little attention given to what does not need to be done in such emergencies and what is frankly wasting valuable time; this book teaches students and young doctors how to prioritise clinical assessments so that the important issues are addressed in a logical and timely sequence.

The table of contents gives a welcome indication of the importance and priority assigned to highlighting professional, ethical and end-of-life issues before any discussion of managing the critically ill patient. Junior doctors would do well to follow this lead in the development of their careers. The authors have done a great service to acutely ill hospital patients and their attending medical staff by producing this wonderful book. It should make the hospital experience a whole lot better for all concerned! If only a book like this could have been around when I was a junior doctor.

Professor George A Jelinek, MD, DipDHM, FACEM
Professor and Head
Neuroepidemiology Unit
Melbourne School of Population and Global Health
The University of Melbourne, Victoria

Preface to the third edition

Purpose

This new edition provides a structured approach to the initial assessment, resuscitation, differential diagnosis and short-term management of common on-call problems. It is designed to help junior doctors and senior medical students acquire a logical, practical and efficient system, which is essential for problem-based learning and acute management. The entire text has been standardised and updated to include the latest evidence-based guidelines, to optimise both the internal consistency and the external validity.

Clinical problem-solving is a fundamental skill for the doctor on call. Traditionally, the diagnosis and management of a patient's problems are approached with an ordered, structured and sequential system (e.g. history-taking, physical examination and review of available investigations) before formulating the provisional and differential diagnoses and the management plan.

In an emergency, doctors proceed concurrently with resuscitation, history, examination, investigation and definitive treatment. Stabilisation of the airway, breathing, circulation and neurological disability must occur in the first few minutes to avoid death and disability.

This book provides a focused approach to many clinical problems in order to increase efficiency and improve time management.

Structure

Additional reading material, high-quality images, procedural videos and references have been integrated online at http://lifeinthefastlane.com/book/oncall

The book is divided into seven main sections:
A. General principles

An overview of the knowledge and skills that are required to deal with undifferentiated on-call problems.
B. Emergency calls

Life-threatening, time-critical problems involving airway, breathing, circulation, neurological disability and environmental factors (ABCDE). This section outlines a structured approach to managing these emergency situations.

C. Common calls
   These are the calls associated with changes in symptoms or signs that most commonly require review while on call.
D. Interpretation of common investigations
E. Practical procedures
F. Formulary
   A compendium of commonly used medications that are likely to be prescribed by the doctor on call. It is a quick reference for dosages, routes of administration, adverse effects, contraindications and modes of actions.
G. Laboratory values
   A list of the normal reference ranges for all common laboratory investigations.

Within Section C – Common calls, the chapters are further subdivided into:
- Phone call (pertinent questions to ask the ward)
- Corridor thoughts (differential diagnosis)
- Major threat to life (now highlighted in red)
- Bedside (first actions)
- Management (with immediate management also now highlighted in red).

This practical guide to rapid, efficient and effective clinical problem-solving is described in more detail in Chapter 1.

Being a doctor on call

Being 'on call' is an invaluable part of medical training and practice, even if only appreciated in retrospect! It undoubtedly grows the doctor's maturity, competence and confidence by:
- Obtaining experience in rapid, focused patient assessment and emergency treatment
- Honing clinical skills assessing patients with acute pathology
- Encouraging independent thought and actual decision making
- Improving procedural competence
- Providing increased responsibility.

Anthony Brown
Mike Cadogan
Antonio Celenza

About the authors

Anthony FT Brown MB ChB, FRCP, FRCS (Ed), FACEM, FRCEM
Professor, Discipline of Anaesthesiology and Critical Care, School of Medicine MD Program, University of Queensland, Brisbane.
Senior Staff Specialist (Pre-Eminent Status), Department of Emergency Medicine, Royal Brisbane and Women's Hospital, Brisbane.

Professor Tony Brown has written extensively in the medical literature, including a bestselling handbook on emergency medicine now in its seventh edition. He holds a conjoint academic teaching appointment at the University of Queensland School of Medicine, works full-time in clinical emergency medicine and is immediate past Editor-in-Chief of *Emergency Medicine Australasia*. He was awarded the inaugural Teaching Excellence Award 2001 at the Australasian College for Emergency Medicine; the Excellence in Clinical Teaching Award 2001 at the Royal Brisbane Hospital; and the Outstanding Teaching Award 2015 at the Royal Brisbane Clinical School, University of Queensland School of Medicine.

Mike D Cadogan MA (Oxon), MB ChB, FACEM
Staff Specialist in Emergency Medicine, Department of Emergency Medicine, Sir Charles Gairdner Hospital, Perth.
Team Physician, Wallabies and the Western Force.

Mike Cadogan (sandnsurf) has a special interest in medical education, medical informatics and the integration of social media with healthcare. He designs and implements web-based online education programs for undergraduate and postgraduate students. He is the co-founder of LifeInTheFastLane.com, healthengine.com.au and vocortex.com

Antonio Celenza MBBS, MClinEd, FACEM, FRCEM
Professor of Emergency Medicine and Medical Education, Faculty of Medicine, Dentistry and Health Sciences, University of Western Australia, Perth.
Staff Specialist, Department of Emergency Medicine, Sir Charles Gairdner Hospital, Perth.

Professor Tony Celenza is the head of the Discipline of Emergency Medicine and coordinates undergraduate education in emergency medicine at UWA. He also is head of the Faculty Education Centre at UWA and is the Director for the MBBS/MD Program. He has designed and coordinates courses in Critical Illness, Wilderness Emergency Medicine, and Neurological, Cardiovascular and Orthopaedic Emergencies for medical students, emergency trainees and rural general practitioners. He has received numerous awards for Excellence in Teaching, including a Citation for Outstanding Contribution to Student Learning by the Australian Learning and Teaching Council.

Dedication

With heartfelt thanks to my beautiful wife Regina for her encouragement and understanding, and to our inspiring children Edward and Lucy who continue to shine and amaze. [AFTB]

Dedicated to Kat for her love, compassion and unwavering fortitude. [MC]

Thanks to my wife, Helen, and children, Alex, Kate, Anne and Ella, for their continuing support, patience and perseverance for my academic endeavours. To colleagues and students who force me to scrutinise, organise and crystallise my thoughts with every question. [TC]

Acknowledgements

Many thanks in particular to Dr Chris Nickson for his prior review and commentary of the work, and to Dr Tor Ercleve of the University of Western Australia for his expertise in many of the medical illustrations.

In addition, special thanks to Larissa Norrie (Content Strategist, Medicine, Surgery and Integrative Medicine) and Rosemary McDonald (Senior Project Manager, Publishing) at Elsevier Australia, and to our copyeditor, Caroline Hunter. We could not have asked for a more enthusiastic, professional, efficient and effective partnership.

This book would not have been possible without all of your help, and the support of our families. Thank you.

Reviewers

Satyamurthy Anuradha MBBS, FRCS, MPH, PhD, FAFPHM
Senior Medical Officer, Gold Coast Health, Queensland

David A Kandiah MBChB (Hons), MClinEd, MPH, MHL, MBA, PhD, FRACP
University of Western Australia, Western Australia

Kate Lord MBBS
Physician Trainee, The Austin Hospital and The Northern Hospital, Victoria

Kathryn Mayer MBBS
Intern, Hornsby Hospital, New South Wales

Cristina Tedesco Murphy MBBS (Hons)
Junior Medical Officer, Northern Sydney LHD, New South Wales

Paul Nguyen MBBS
Junior Medical Officer, St George Hospital, New South Wales

Chandi Perera MBBS, MPH, GCertHiEd (Medicine), FRACP
Staff Specialist and Director, Rheumatology Unit, Canberra Hospital and Health Services and Network Director of Physician Education for the Canberra Physician Training Network

Erika Strazdins BSc, MD
Student, University of New South Wales, Sydney, New South Wales

Abbreviations

AAA	Abdominal aortic aneurysm	aPTT	Activated partial thromboplastin time
AAD	Acute aortic dissection	ARB	Angiotensin-receptor blocker
Abdo	Abdomen		
ABG	Arterial blood gas	ARDS	Adult respiratory distress syndrome
ACA	Anterior cerebral artery		
		ASD	Atrial septal defect
ACE	Angiotensin-converting enzyme	AST	Aspartate transferase
		ATN	Acute tubular necrosis
ACLS	Advanced cardiac life support	AV	Atrioventricular
		AVM	Arteriovenous malformation
ACS	Acute coronary syndrome	AVPU	Alert, responds to Voice, responds to Pain, Unresponsive
ADH	Antidiuretic hormone		
ADHD	Attention-deficit hyperactivity disorder	AXR	Abdominal X-ray
		BBB	Bundle branch block
AED	Automated external defibrillator	BD	Twice daily
		BGL	Blood glucose level
AF	Atrial fibrillation	BiPAP	Bilevel positive-airway pressure
AFB	Acid-fast bacillus		
AG	Anion gap		
AHD	Advance health directive	BLS	Basic life support
		BP	Blood pressure
AIDS	Acquired immunodeficiency syndrome	BPH	Benign prostatic hypertrophy
		BPPV	Benign paroxysmal positional vertigo
AION	Anterior ischaemic optic neuropathy	BSL	Blood sugar level
AKI	Acute kidney injury	Ca	Calcium
ALOC	Altered level of consciousness	CABG	Coronary artery bypass grafting
ALP	Alkaline phosphatase	CAD	Coronary artery disease
ALS	Advanced life support	cAMP	Cyclic adenosine monophosphate
ALT	Alanine transferase	CAP	Community-acquired pneumonia
AMI	Acute myocardial infarction	CCF	Congestive cardiac failure
AMP	Adenosine monophosphate	CCU	Coronary care unit
ANTT	Aseptic non-touch technique	CDAD	*Clostridium difficile* associated diarrhoea
AP	Anteroposterior	cGMP	Cyclic guanosine monophosphate
APO	Acute pulmonary oedema	CHB	Complete heart block

CHF	Congestive heart failure	DIC	Disseminated intravascular coagulation
CK	Creatine kinase	DKA	Diabetic ketoacidosis
CLL	Chronic lymphocytic leukaemia	DM	Diabetes mellitus
CMV	Cytomegalovirus	DOAC	Direct oral anticoagulant
CNS	Central nervous system	DRS ABCDE	Danger, Response, Send for help, Airway, Breathing, Circulation, Disability, Environment
CO	Cardiac output		
CO_2	Carbon dioxide		
COPD	Chronic obstructive pulmonary disease		
CPAP	Continuous positive airways pressure	DT	Delirium tremens
		DVT	Deep venous (vein) thrombosis
CPR	Cardiopulmonary resuscitation	EACA	Epsilon aminocaproic acid
CrCl	Creatinine clearance		
CRF	Chronic renal failure	ECF	Extracellular fluid
CRP	C reactive protein	ECG	Electrocardiogram
CRT	Capillary refill time	ED	Emergency Department
CSF	Cerebrospinal fluid		
CSM	Carotid sinus massage	EDH	Extradural haemorrhage
CSU	Catheter specimen of urine	EDTA	Edetate disodium
CT	Computed tomography	EEG	Electroencephalo-graphy
CTA	Computed tomography angiogram	eGFR	Estimated glomerular filtration rate
CTPA	Computed tomography pulmonary angiogram	ELFTs	Electrolytes and liver function tests
		ELISA	Enzyme-linked immunosorbent assay
CTR	Cardiothoracic ratio		
CTV	Computed tomography venogram	ENDO	Endocrine
CVA	Cerebrovascular accident (stroke)	ENT	Ear, nose and throat
		EOM	Extraocular muscles
CVC	Central venous cannula	EPA	Enduring power of attorney
CVL	Central venous line	ERCP	Endoscopic retrograde cholangiopancreato-graphy
CVP	Central venous pressure		
CVS	Cardiovascular system	ESR	Erythrocyte sedimentation rate
CXR	Chest X-ray	EST	Exercise stress testing
DBP	Diastolic blood pressure	$ETCO_2$	End-tidal carbon dioxide
DC	Direct current	ETT	Endotracheal tube
DDAVP	1-deamino-8-D-arginine vasopressin (desmopressin acetate)	Ext	Extremities
		FBC	Full blood count
DI	Diabetes insipidus	FDP	Fibrin degradation products

FEV$_1$	Forced expiratory volume in 1 second	HLA	Human leucocyte antigen
FFP	Fresh frozen plasma	HOCM	Hypertrophic
FiO$_2$	Fraction of inspired oxygen		obstructive cardiomyopathy
FVC	Forced vital capacity	HONK	Hyperosmolar,
G&H	Group and hold		non-ketotic
G6PD	Glucose-6-phosphate dehydrogenase	HPC	History of presenting complaint
GABA	Gamma-aminobutyric acid	HR	Heart rate
		HSV	Herpes simplex virus
GBS	Guillain–Barré syndrome	HU	Hounsfield unit
		HUS	Haemolytic–uraemic syndrome
GCS	Glasgow Coma Scale		
GCSE	Generalised convulsive status epilepticus	IBD	Inflammatory bowel disease
GGT	Gamma glutamyl transferase	ICC	Intercostal catheter
		ICF	Intracellular fluid
GHB	Gamma-hydroxy butyrate	ICH	Intracerebral haemorrhage
GI	Gastrointestinal	ICP	Intracranial pressure
GIT	Gastrointestinal tract	ICU	Intensive care unit
GN	Glomerulonephritis	IDC	Indwelling catheter
GORD	Gastro-oesophageal reflux disease	Ig	Immunoglobulin
		IHD	Ischaemic heart disease
GTN	Glyceryl trinitrate	IJV	Internal jugular vein
GU	Genitourinary	IM	Intramuscular
Hb	Haemoglobin	INR	International
hCG	Human chorionic gonadotropin		normalised ratio
		iSBAR	Identify, Situation, Background, Assessment, Recommendation
HCM	Hypertrophic cardiomyopathy		
HDL	High-density lipoprotein	ISI	International Sensitivity Index
HDU	High dependency unit	ITP	Idiopathic thrombocytopenic purpura
HEENT	Head, eyes, ears, nose and throat		
		IV	Intravenous
HELLP	Haemolysis/elevated liver enzymes/low platelets	IVC	Inferior vena cava
		IVH	Intraventricular haemorrhage
HEMS	Helicopter Emergency Medical Service	IVU	Intravenous urogram
HHS	Hyperosmolar, hyperglycaemic state	J	Joule
		JVP	Jugular venous pressure
HITS	Heparin-induced thrombocytopenia syndrome	K	Potassium
		kg	Kilogram
HIV	Human immunodeficiency virus	KUB	Kidneys, ureter, bladder (plain abdominal X-ray)

L	Litre	MRSA	Methicillin-resistant *Staphylococcus aureus*
LAD	Left axis deviation		
LBBB	Left bundle branch block	MRSE	Multidrug-resistant *Staphylococcus epidermidis*
LDH	Lactate dehydrogenase		
LDL	Low-density lipoprotein	MSA	Multiple system atrophy
LFT	Liver function tests	MSOF	Multiple system organ failure
LLL	Left lower lobe		
LLQ	Left lower quadrant	MSS	Musculoskeletal system
LMA	Laryngeal mask airway		
LMN	Lower motor neuron	MSU	Midstream urine
LMW	Low molecular weight	MTP	Metatarsophalangeal
LMWH	Low-molecular-weight heparin	Na	Sodium
		NASH	Non-alcoholic steatohepatitis
LOC	Loss of consciousness		
LP	Lumbar puncture	NBM	Nil by mouth
LRTI	Lower respiratory tract infection	NETS	Neonatal Emergency Transport Service
LUQ	Left upper quadrant		
LV	Left ventricle	Neuro	Neurological system
LVAD	Left ventricular assist device	NFR	Not-for-resuscitation
		NG	Nasogastric
LVF	Left ventricular failure	NGT	Nasogastric tube
LVH	Left ventricular hypertrophy	NIBP	Non-invasive blood pressure
Mane	In the morning	NIH	National Institutes of Health
MAOI	Monoamine oxidase inhibitor		
		NIV	Non-invasive ventilation
MAP	Mean arterial pressure		
MCA	Middle cerebral artery	NMDA	N-methyl-D-aspartic acid
MCH	Mean corpuscular haemoglobin	NMJ	Neuromuscular junction
MCS	Microscopy, culture and sensitivity	NMS	Neuroleptic malignant syndrome
MCV	Mean corpuscular volume	NOAC	New oral anticoagulant
MET	Medical emergency team	NPH	Neutral protamine Hagedorn (insulin)
Mg	Magnesium	NPV	Negative predictive value
MG	Myasthenia gravis		
mL	Millilitre	NSAID	Non-steroidal anti-inflammatory drug
MH	Malignant hyperpyrexia		
MI	Myocardial infarction	NSTEMI	Non-ST-elevation myocardial infarction
MOFS	Multiorgan failure syndrome		
		O_2	Oxygen
MRA	Magnetic resonance angiography	OD	Overdose
		O&G	Obstetrics and gynaecology
MRI	Magnetic resonance imaging	P_2	Pulmonary second sound

PA	Posteroanterior	PUPPP	Pruritic urticarial papules and plaques of pregnancy
PAC	Premature atrial contraction		
$PaCO_2$	Partial pressure of carbon dioxide	PV	Per vaginam
		PVC	Premature ventricular contraction
PAN	Polyarteritis nodosa		
PaO_2	Partial pressure of oxygen	pVT	Pulseless ventricular tachycardia
PCA	Posterior cerebral artery	QID	Quater in die (four times daily)
PCI	Percutaneous coronary intervention	QDS	Four times daily
		RA	Rheumatoid arthritis
PCP	Pneumocystis pneumonia	RAD	Right axis deviation
		RBBB	Right bundle branch block
PCR	Polymerase chain reaction		
		RBC	Red blood cell
PE	Pulmonary embolus	Resp	Respiratory system
PEA	Pulseless electrical activity	RFDS	Royal Flying Doctor Service
PEEP	Positive end-expiratory pressure	RLL	Right lower lobe
		RLQ	Right lower quadrant
PEFR	Peak expiratory flow rate	ROM	Range of movement
		ROSC	Return of spontaneous circulation
PERLA	Pupils equal react to light and accommodation	RR	Respiratory rate
		RSV	Respiratory syncytial virus
PID	Pelvic inflammatory disease	RTA	Renal tubular acidosis
PMR	Polymyalgia rheumatica	RUQ	Right upper quadrant
		RV	Right ventricle (ventricular)
PND	Paroxysmal nocturnal dyspnoea		
		RVH	Right ventricular hypertrophy
PO	Per os (by mouth)		
PPE	Personal protective equipment	S_3	Third heart sound
		SAED	Semi-automated external defibrillator
PPI	Proton pump inhibitor		
PPV	Positive predictive value	SAH	Subarachnoid haemorrhage
PR	Per rectum	SaO_2	Oxygen saturation
PRN	Pro re nata (as needed)	SBE	Subacute bacterial endocarditis
PSI	Pneumonia Severity Index	SBP	Systolic blood pressure
		SC	Subcutaneous
PSVT	Paroxysmal supraventricular tachycardia	SCM	Sternocleidomastoid
		SDH	Subdural haemorrhage
		SG	Specific gravity
Psych	Psychiatric	SI	International system of units
PT	Prothrombin time		
PTH	Parathyroid hormone	SIADH	Syndrome of inappropriate antidiuretic hormone secretion
PUD	Peptic ulcer disease		
PUO	Pyrexia of unknown origin		

SIRS	Systemic inflammatory response syndrome	TPN	Total parenteral nutrition
SJS	Stevens–Johnson syndrome	TPR	Total peripheral resistance
SL	Sublingual	TRALI	Transfusion-related acute lung injury
SLE	Systemic lupus erythematosus	TSH	Thyroid-stimulating hormone
SNRI	Serotonin and noradrenaline reuptake inhibitor	TTP	Thrombotic thrombocytopenic purpura
SOB	Shortness of breath	TURP	Transurethral resection of the prostate
SOL	Space-occupying lesion		
SR	Slow release		
SS	Serotonin syndrome	U&E	Urea and electrolytes
SSRI	Selective serotonin reuptake inhibitor	UA	Unstable angina
		UA	Urinalysis
SSS	Sick sinus syndrome	UFH	Unfractionated heparin
Stat	Statum (immediately)		
STEMI	ST elevation myocardial infarction	UMN	Upper motor neuron
		UO	Urine output
SV	Stroke volume	USS	Ultrasound scan
SVT	Supraventricular tachycardia	UTI	Urinary tract infection
		VBG	Venous blood gas
T_4	Thyroxine	VBI	Vertebrobasilar insufficiency
TACO	Transfusion-associated circulatory overload	VF	Ventricular fibrillation
TB	Tuberculosis	VICC	Venom-induced consumptive coagulopathy
TBW	Total body water		
TDS	Three times daily		
TEN	Toxic epidermal necrolysis	VLDL	Very low-density lipoprotein
TFT	Thyroid function tests	V/Q	Ventilation perfusion
		VRE	Vancomycin-resistant enterococci
TIA	Transient ischaemic attack		
TMJ	Temperomandibular joint	VT	Ventricular tachycardia
		WBC	White blood cell
TNF	Tumour necrosis factor	WCC	White cell count
TOE	Transoesophageal echocardiogram	WPW	Wolff–Parkinson–White
tPA	Tissue plasminogen activator		

SECTION A

General principles

1

Approach to the diagnosis and management of on-call problems

Clinical problem-solving is a fundamental skill for the doctor on call. Traditionally, the doctor approaches diagnosis and management of a patient's problems in an orderly, systematic manner. This includes focused history-taking and physical examination, review of available investigations, formulation of the provisional and differential diagnoses and finally, making a management plan.

History-taking and physical examination may take 20–30 minutes for a patient with a single problem seeing a new doctor for the first time. Or they may take up to 60 minutes for an older patient with multiple complaints.

Clearly, if a patient is found unconscious in the street, the chief complaint is 'coma' and the history of the presenting illness is limited to the information provided by witnesses, the ambulance officers or the contents of the patient's wallet. In this situation, the doctor is trained to proceed with a simultaneous history, examination, investigation and treatment approach, often starting with treatment. How this should be achieved is not always obvious, although the initial steps that must be completed within the first 5–10 minutes to save life are known as the DRS ABCDE approach (Danger, Response, Send for help, Airway, Breathing, Circulation, Disability, Environment).

The trainee doctor first confronts on-call problem-solving in the final years of medical school. At this stage a structured history-taking and physical examination direct the approach to evaluating the patient. When on call, the trainee or junior doctor is faced with a well-defined problem (e.g. fever, chest pain, collapse), yet may feel ill-equipped to begin clinical problem-solving unless the complete history and physical examination are obtained. Anything less induces guilt over a task only partially completed. However, few if any on-call problems should involve more than 30–60 minutes of the doctor's time, because

2

excessive time spent with one patient may deny adequate treatment time to another more seriously ill patient.

Therefore, the approach recommended in this book is based on a structured system that is easily adapted to most situations. It is intended as a practical guide to aid rapid, effective and efficient clinical problem-solving on call. Each clinical chapter is similarly divided into five parts:
1. Phone call
2. Corridor thoughts
3. Major threat to life
4. Bedside
5. Management.

Phone call

Most problems are first communicated by telephone. The on-call doctor must be able to determine the severity of the problem and thus prioritise patients based on this initial telephone information. The phone call section is divided into three parts:
1. **Questions:** pertinent initial questions to help determine the urgency of the problem.
2. **Instructions:** phone orders for the nurse at the bedside to expedite the investigation and management of the patient's immediate problem.
3. **Prioritisation:** assessment of the urgency of the problem to determine which patients need to be seen immediately.

Corridor thoughts

The time spent going to the ward should be used to consider the differential diagnoses and potential life-threats of the problem at hand. This 'travel time' is also useful for organising a plan of action at the bedside.

The differential diagnosis lists presented in this book are not exhaustive—they focus on the most common or most serious causes that should be considered in hospitalised patients.

Major threat to life

Identifying a potential major threat to life follows logically from consideration of the differential diagnoses, and provides a focus for subsequent investigation and management of the patient. It is more useful to appreciate the most likely threats to life and use them to direct questions and the physical examination, than to simply arrive at the bedside with a memorised list of all possible diagnoses. This risk-analysis process ensures that seeking and treating the most serious life-threatening possibility in each clinical scenario is emphasised.

Bedside

The evaluation of the patient at the bedside is divided into the following areas:

* Quick-look test
* Airway and vital signs
* Immediate management
* Selective history and chart review
* Selective physical examination
* Bedside and other investigations.

Thus, the bedside assessment begins with the quick-look test, which is a rapid visual assessment to categorise the patient's condition in terms of severity: well (comfortable), sick (uncomfortable or distressed) or critical (about to die).

Next is an assessment of the airway and vital signs, which are critically important in the evaluation of any potentially sick patient.

The order of the remaining parts is not uniform, due to the nature of the various problems that require assessment when on call. For example, the selective physical examination may either precede or follow the selective history and chart review, and either of these may be superseded by immediate management when the clinical situation dictates.

Occasionally, the physical examination and management sections are further subdivided to focus on urgent, life-threatening problems, leaving the less urgent problems to be reviewed later.

Management

General supportive and specific management include monitoring, stabilisation and therapy, both pharmacological and procedural. Immediate resuscitation with attention to the DRS ABCDE approach is dealt with first. Next, disease-specific management issues are considered.

The principles and protocols offered in this book provide a logical, efficient and safe system for the assessment and management of common on-call problems. The aim is to make an already stressful situation easier to handle, for the benefit of patients and the relief of the doctor involved.

2

Professionalism and teamwork

Interaction with ward staff

Other hospital staff will have certain expectations of the behaviour of the on-call doctor. These include:
* Punctuality, time management and prioritising of workload.
* Being at work when rostered, and calling in sick as soon as it is recognised (never at the last minute).
* Reasonable dress and appearance. Medicine is traditionally considered a conservative profession, and patients and other staff expect the doctor to look 'professional'. Rightly or wrongly, appearance can determine others' perceptions of your competence and affect the development of patient rapport, trust and compliance.
* Answering your pager promptly or delegating to someone who can answer if you are busy.

Consultants (specialists) and registrars (specialist trainees) have managerial, supervisory, training and education roles. They have a wide variety of personalities, expectations and opinions.
* They consider medical students and junior doctors to be part of a team and expect you to ask for their assistance.
* Your interest and motivation for work will be directly reflected back in their attitude to support, supervision and teaching. The more keen and enthusiastic you are, the more supportive they will be.

Nursing staff provide the continuous care for the patient. They know the patient's hopes and fears, personality and prejudices, and are familiar with the patient's family.
* Although many nurses are highly experienced, they will still consider the doctor fully responsible for each patient.
* They are an invaluable source of advice and assistance, and key members of the team. They expect you to act on their concerns.

Teamwork

When dealing with on-call problems, you are part of a team. You may be called upon to lead the team, particularly if more senior help is some time away. Remember that your medical colleagues, nurses, pharmacists, physiotherapists, occupational therapists, social workers, orderlies and clerks on the ward can all aid the assessment and treatment of patients. For example:

- **Clerks** can help find documentation and request forms, obtain investigation results, know how best to order urgent tests, will help page other people or the switchboard, know the commonly used numbers and know how to operate the information technology systems.
- **Orderlies** help move patients on the bed, obtain equipment and restrain patients when indicated.
- **Medical colleagues** can assist in particular tasks or provide an extra pair of hands in complex procedures.
  - It is always useful to 'bounce ideas' to help crystallise thoughts, prevent errors and determine a clear management plan.
  - Having a helper allows for the concurrent or simultaneous performance of tasks (horizontal tasking), rather than having to do them alone in series. You can still maintain a vertical DRS ABCDE prioritisation, but it enables multiple tasks to be completed more rapidly.
- **Nurses** will be able to provide background information, implement therapy and help prepare, assist with or perform certain procedures.
  - They also act as an essential layer of safety, to identify problems and to prevent errors.
  - Experienced senior nurses often have more immediately practical knowledge and skills than some junior doctors, so listen carefully to what they suggest.
  - Importantly, nurses act as a patient comforter during the crisis when the patient is frightened and the doctor too busy to communicate effectively.
- **Pharmacists, physiotherapists, occupational therapists, speech therapists, social workers, aged-care workers and many other allied health specialists** complete the team with their own particular areas of expertise. Use their help.

Teamwork problems

Members of a team (e.g. the Medical Emergency Team or Cardiac Arrest Team) may be strangers who come together only at time-critical and stressful moments. The problems they may face include:

- Unknown personality and experience of each individual
- Unfamiliar environment/equipment/processes
- Need for rapid and/or complex decision making
- Mismatch of an individual's confidence and actual competence
- Lack of leadership, with ill-defined roles and/or no delegation
- Unclear communication (e.g. orders called out, but not directed at anyone)

- Fragmented information and uncertain goals
- Lack of a unified framework of behaviour between different disciplines
- Frequent interruptions
- Reluctance to question those more senior.

Team leadership

The team leader must take control and direct the team members in patient care (see Box 2.1). Effective leadership improves patient outcome, especially in a medical crisis. As a junior doctor, you might start as the team leader until a more senior colleague arrives, so it is important to understand the most important facets of the role. Leadership involves:

- Assembling, introducing and briefing team members
- Setting clear goals and priorities
- Establishing communication paths, obtaining and disseminating information
- Delegating tasks and responsibilities to team members
- Stepping back 'hands off' and maintaining an overview of proceedings
- Giving positive direction and constructive feedback by encouraging members.

In addition, during this phase of care, the team leader must:

- Continuously monitor progress and task completion
- Engage team members in the phases of care
- Balance workload within the team, but call for help if necessary
- Be vigilant for errors and potential pitfalls (situational awareness), and know how to deal with these
- Access educational aids (e.g. guidelines or pathways, textbooks, internet, phone apps).

BOX 2.1 Hints for the team leader in a crisis situation

During a crisis the team leader should ascertain:

- Who is watching the patient.
- Whether the entire team appreciate the:
  - Priorities and plan
  - Working diagnosis
  - Urgency of the task(s)
  - Communication pathways and expectations.
- Whether team members know their roles and responsibilities.
- Whether there are adequate resources, and/or if additional help is needed.
- What the next step will be … and the step after that.

Finally:
- Determine when the job is complete.
- Stand the team down, debrief as soon as possible (make the time) and thank everyone for their participation.

Effective team communication

One of the main difficulties in teamwork is ambiguous or confronting communication. Each team member should:
- Introduce themselves to one another
- Address each other directly, using clear diction and tone, congruent body language and non-judgemental terms
- Define the urgency of the situation and tasks
- Think aloud when the opportunity arises—this crystallises ideas, generates new ones and avoids fixation on any single idea
- Provide relevant information
- Acknowledge/verify information received from one another
- Work for the best interests of the patient.

Making decisions and avoiding errors

Decision making

Students and junior doctors (novices) require more data to make decisions than experienced practitioners (experts).
- Novices have limited pattern-recognition skills (clinical gestalt), have less concept of the course a particular event will take and do not yet have shortcuts or tricks (medical heuristics) for rapid patient assessment and management.
- Experts have seen many different variants of the particular presentation, how it responds to treatment and its expected course.
- Thus, experts make decisions based on a wealth of prior experience, whereas novices have only limited experience and must rely on what they have been taught, which will never fully cover real-life variations and complexity.

When on call, the decision-making process may be simplified to:
- Is the patient in a critical condition and in need of immediate resuscitation?
- Have you called your senior?
- Could the patient have a potentially life-threatening condition that needs early diagnosis or rapid exclusion?
- Are any immediate general supportive or specific interventions required?
- Can the patient receive symptomatic treatment while awaiting further review, perhaps in the morning?

Avoiding errors

An adverse medical event or error causes unintentional harm or injury to a patient as the result of a medical intervention rather than the underlying medical condition. Approximately 10% of patients in hospital suffer an adverse event, 50% of which are preventable and up to 20% of which lead to disability or even death.

An adverse event is always multifactorial, occurring when several events happen in unison (known as the 'Swiss-cheese effect'). Common factors that may culminate in an adverse event include:
• Patient misidentification
• Failure to take an adequate history or physical examination
• Technical and skill-based errors
• Inadequate documentation or communication with other staff
• Failure to perform an indicated test
• Failure to act on the results of a test or known finding
• Inappropriate use of medication, drug interactions or drug side effects, particularly in patients who are older, have renal impairment or are taking multiple medications (especially antibiotic, cardiovascular and anticoagulant drugs)
• Acting outside one's area of expertise.

3Cs protocol

The 3Cs protocol is a useful checklist that can be used to minimise patient harm in any invasive diagnostic or treatment procedure. It ensures that you have the correct patient, the correct site/side and the correct procedure is to be performed. The 3Cs protocol may be used repeatedly, particularly when the patient is handed over, or if more than one procedure is to be performed on the same patient.
• **Correct patient:** check the patient's identity using at least three different pieces of information such as family and first name, date of birth and medical record number.
• **Correct site/side:** check that the correct site or side is clearly marked whenever possible, such as the initials of the person performing the procedure using an indelible pen. Crosscheck this verbally with the patient and with the patient's notes or X-rays (i.e. for an intercostal catheter).
• **Correct procedure:** check that the correct procedure has been chosen and obtain valid, informed consent (i.e. the patient understands what is to be done, why, any complications and the loss if he or she decides not to proceed). Written consent is preferred where possible. A parent/guardian can sign for a child, and a substitute decision maker can sign for an adult with diminished decision capacity.

These are followed by a team 'final check' immediately before performing the procedure itself.

Patient safety and risk management

Every clinician should adopt personal strategies to practise as a good doctor, to improve patient outcomes and to minimise medicolegal risk (see Box 2.2). These strategies include:

- Avoid stereotyping a patient, trivialising complaints or jumping to an easy conclusion.
- Communicate openly with the patient, medical colleagues and nursing staff.
- Never conceal or withhold important information, although it is important to choose a suitable time if the news is bad or unexpected.
- Ask more senior staff for advice when unsure.
- Follow guidelines for good record keeping.
- Notify a senior doctor immediately if an incident occurs that could lead to a complaint or claim, including:
  - An adverse outcome
  - A missed or delayed diagnosis
  - An angry or disgruntled patient
  - Communication breakdown
  - A 'gut feeling' that something is not quite right.
- If an adverse event occurs, always speak honestly with the patient and/or relatives to ameliorate their sense of confusion, anger and disappointment.

Adverse event resolution

Good, caring and open communication decreases the likelihood of the patient lodging or pursuing a complaint. It is best to:

- Talk the problem through with the patient in layperson's language.
- Be truthful and honest, employ 'open disclosure' and do not come across as defensive or evasive.
- Express understanding, regret, concern and empathy. Saying sorry is fine, and is not an admission of guilt.
- Ensure the patient and/or carer are supported after an adverse event.
- Keep the patient informed of ongoing developments and remedial action.

Many patients are concerned that an error may occur again to someone else and want to be sure that preventive action will be taken. This includes education and remediation, system changes, improved resource use and regular audit with feedback.

- In general, when the patient and relatives believe that concern and consideration were shown, they are more likely to accept the event.
- Additionally, the doctor involved in a potential significant adverse event should:
  - Continue liaising with the medical team to ensure proper follow-up.

BOX 2.2 National Patient Safety Education Framework

1. Communicating effectively
   - Involving patients and carers as partners in healthcare, providing information when they need it
   - Communicating risk in an appropriate way
   - Communicating honestly with patients after an adverse event (open disclosure)
   - Obtaining consent and respecting a patient's right to make decisions about their healthcare
   - Being culturally respectful and knowledgeable of different backgrounds and beliefs
2. Identifying, preventing and managing adverse events and near misses
   - Recognising, reporting and managing adverse events and near misses with suitable systems
   - Managing risk, including creating and maintaining safe systems of care
   - Understanding healthcare adverse events and near misses
   - Managing complaints with appropriate and timely responses
3. Using evidence and information
   - Employing best available evidence-based practice, tools and guidelines
   - Using information technology to enhance safety
4. Working safely
   - Showing leadership, being a team player
   - Understanding how workers can make mistakes
   - Understanding complex organisations
   - Providing continuity of care
   - Establishing a framework to manage fatigue and stress
5. Being ethical
   - Maintaining fitness to work or practice
   - Ensuring professionalism and ethical conduct
6. Continuing learning
   - Being a workplace learner
   - Being a workplace teacher
7. Specific issues
   - Preventing wrong patient, wrong procedure, wrong site
   - Dispensing and administering medications safely

Adapted from Australian Council for Safety and Quality in Health Care. National Patient Safety Education Framework. Canberra: Commonwealth of Australia, 2005.

- Contact the medical defence organisation (MDO) and the hospital's legal department as early as possible (usually the same day or the next day).
- Document events meticulously, but never backdate, alter or delete a medical record.

3

Documentation and communication

An important aspect of the management of on-call problems is your documentation and communication of events. These are essential for the continuity of effective care of the patient.

The medical chart is a medicolegal document, and must be as accurate and complete as possible. Documentation is required for every clinical evaluation of the patient, whether comprehensive or brief. If the problem was straightforward, a short note is sufficient. However, if the problem was complicated, the clinical note must be thorough but concise.

On-call problems do not require a complete history and physical examination, as these were done when the patient was first admitted. Instead, your on-call history, physical examination and chart documentation should be focused and directed (i.e. problem oriented), which should include relevant negative findings.

Documentation in the patient's chart

Begin by recording the date, time and who you are. For example:

1 June 2016: 02:00 hours. 'Resident on-call note.'

State who called you and at what time you were called. For example:

Called by nursing staff at 01:30 hours to see a patient who 'fell out of bed'.

If your assessment was delayed by more urgent problems, say so. A brief summary of the patient's admission diagnosis and major medical problems should follow. For example:

74-year-old female.
Admitted 10 days ago with joint pain and poor mobility.
Medical history: chronic renal failure, type 2 diabetes mellitus, rheumatoid arthritis.

Next, describe the history of the presenting complaint (HPC)—that is, the 'fall out of bed'—from the viewpoint of both the patient and any witnesses. This HPC is no different from the HPC you would document in an admission history. For example:

> *HPC: Unwitnessed fall. Patient states was going to the bathroom, when tripped on bathrobe. Fell to the floor, landing on left side. Denies prior palpitations, chest pain, light-headedness, nausea or hip pain. No pain afterwards and no difficulty walking unaided. Nurse found the patient lying on the floor. Vital signs were normal.*

If your chart review has other relevant findings, include these in your HPC. For example:

> *Note has had three previous 'falls out of bed' on this admission. Patient has no recollection of these.*

Documentation of your examination findings should be selective. Thus, a call regarding a fall out of bed requires you to examine the vital signs, as well as components of the musculoskeletal, head and neck, cardiovascular and neurological systems. It is not necessary to examine the respiratory system or the abdomen unless there was direct injury, or there is a separate second problem (e.g. you arrive at the bedside and find the patient breathless).

It is useful to underline the abnormal physical findings both for yourself (it aids your summary) and for the staff who will be reviewing the patient in the morning.

Vitals	HR: <u>104/min</u>
	BP: 140/85
	RR: <u>36/min</u>
	O$_2$ sats: 99%
	Temp: 36.9°C PO
HEENT	No tongue or cheek lacerations
	No scalp or face lacerations or haematomas
	No haemotympanum
CVS	Pulse rhythm regular; JVP 2 cm > sternal angle
MSS	Spine and ribs normal
	Full, painless ROM of all 4 limbs
	<u>7 × 9 cm bruise left thigh</u>
Neuro	Alert; oriented to time, place and person
	Cranial nerves—PERLA, EOM full. Otherwise not assessed
	Tone/power/reflexes/sensory—all normal

Then note relevant laboratory, electrocardiographic or X-ray findings. Again, it is useful to underline abnormal results. For example:

Glucose	*6.1 mmol/L*
Sodium	*141 mmol/L*
Potassium	*3.9 mmol/L*
Calcium	*Not available*
Urea	*12 mmol/L*
Creatinine	*180 mmol/L*

Your conclusions regarding the diagnostic problem for which you were called must now be clearly stated. It is not enough to simply write '*Patient fell out of bed*'. The nurse could have written that without consulting you! You need to synthesise the information gathered and formulate a problem list.

Your provisional or 'working' diagnosis should be followed by potential differential diagnoses, listing the most likely alternative explanations in order, then any complications. For example:

1. *Unwitnessed fall on way to bathroom.*
   Presumed mechanical fall (?diuretic-induced nocturia, ?contribution of sedation).
2. *Large bruise to left thigh, but no obvious bony injury. No other findings.*

Then clearly state the management, outlining the measures taken during the night, and the investigations or treatment arranged or recommended for the morning. For example:

- *Simple analgesia*
- *Ice pack to thigh haematoma*
- *Review mobility by inpatient team mane.*

Avoid writing '*Plan—see medication orders*', as it is not always obvious to staff handling the patient's care the next morning why certain measures were taken.

If you informed another resident, registrar or consultant about the problem, document at what time and with whom you spoke and state the recommendations given. For example:

Discussed with Medical Registrar at 02:30 hours.
Suggests: team to reassess mobility in the morning, and role of diuretics and sedation.

Record whether any of the patient's family members were informed of the problem and what they were told.

Finally, sign the clinical note and clearly *print* your name and designation (e.g. medical ward call resident; surgical intern) so staff know who to contact if there are any questions about the overnight management of the patient.

Communication of the patient's problem

When you call to inform a colleague what has happened, make sure you use a consistent approach to frame your conversation, particularly when the situation is critical.

Use a standardised format to provide concise information with the right level of detail, to avoid unnecessary repetition or confusion, and to facilitate a positive, proactive interaction.

One such communication tool is 'iSBAR' (identify, Situation, Background, Assessment, Recommendation).

iSBAR

Identify state who you are, where you are calling from and the name of the patient.

Situation describe your concern and the reason you are calling.

Background state a brief history of why the patient was admitted, any relevant past medical history, current treatment and important investigation results.

Assessment give your assessment of the patient's condition including vital signs, whether stable or deteriorating, your clinical impression and immediate concerns.

Recommendation state exactly what you would like to happen, making clear suggestions and clarifying your expectations.

Thus for the patient who fell out of bed, the call to your registrar might go like this:

Hello Mike, sorry to call you so late, Tony here. I just wanted to let you know I am on Ward X seeing a 74-year-old lady Mrs Y. She had an unwitnessed fall on her way to the bathroom with no prodromal symptoms. Although she only has a bruise on her left thigh, I just wanted to check I had not forgotten anything.

Mrs Y was admitted 10 days ago with poor mobility on a background of known rheumatoid arthritis, chronic renal failure and type 2 diabetes mellitus. I note she has had three previous falls this admission, and is on diuretics and sleeping tablets. Her last urea was 12 and creatinine 180.

Her vital signs are OK with a slight tachycardia at 104, but normal BP for her at 140/85. Her resp rate is 36, but she is upset at all the fuss, and her sats are normal on room air. Otherwise, I really could not find anything abnormal examining her, apart from a 7×9 cm bruise on her thigh, with no underlying bony injury as she can still walk unaided. I think this was most likely a mechanical fall, maybe related to her tablets, and I have given her some paracetamol.

I have asked the medical team to reassess her mobility in the morning. Should I come back later to see her myself before that, only I still have another five calls to complete?

No Tony, I think you have done enough, it all sounds fine. I suggest you make an additional note for the day team to ask them to review her medications, to see if they are causing her to fall. Thanks for calling.

4

Ethical and legal considerations

Consent and competence

Consent

An individual has a right to not be touched, which derives from the ethical principle of 'autonomy', whereby each person is presumed to know what is best for him or her. This contrasts with 'paternalism', which assumes that a healthcare worker knows and does what is best for the patient, irrespective of the patient's wishes.

Assault and battery are entities specifically recognised in both civil (tort) and criminal law. The current legal principles are that 'assault' is an act that causes another person to feel apprehension of an imminent, harmful or offensive contact. 'Battery' is intentional physical contact with a person without his or her consent that results in bodily harm or is offensive to a reasonable sense of dignity, regardless of whether this contact is beneficial. An 'assault and battery' is the combination of a threat with physical violence.

Obtaining consent

Consent is therefore required for every occasion of bodily contact to prevent the assumption of battery. Consent may be implied (by submission, e.g. offering an arm for a blood test) or expressed (by formal verbal or written permission).

The features required to obtain valid consent are:
- Consent must be well-informed. An adequate explanation of the risks and benefits needs to be given *and* understood by the patient.
- The patient is both mentally and legally competent (see later).
- Consent needs to be specific (i.e. to cover what is actually being done).
- Consent must be given freely without coercion.
  Based on these principles, the patient is then asked to sign a consent form, which may be procedure-specific with a list of particular risks and

their individual likelihood, plus an accompanying information sheet, where these are available.

Under common law, a doctor may proceed without consent in an emergency, presuming that 'a reasonable person' would want to be treated (e.g. an emergency craniotomy for a person in a coma, secondary to an extradural haematoma). If in doubt, *always* seek a second senior opinion.

Understanding consent

Clearly, the patient must understand the implications and nature of the treatment proposed, or of not accepting the treatment, when obtaining consent. The doctor has a duty to inform of material risks inherent in the proposed treatment and to give sufficient information for the patient to understand these risks and benefits.

The difficulty is judging the depth to which this explanation should be given, as the number of potential risks may be large for complex interventions. The degree of explanation depends on whether the particular individual patient is likely to attach significance to the risk in his or her own case, and will vary from patient to patient on direct questioning.

The questions that need to be considered are:
- **Would a reasonable person attach significance to that particular risk?** This gives an idea of what should be the minimum information given to all patients.
- **Would this particular patient attach significance to the particular risk?** This would be additional information given to a particular patient depending on specific concerns.

Refusal of treatment

Competent, informed patients have a right to refuse to stay in hospital or to refuse a recommended treatment plan (e.g. a Jehovah's Witness will refuse a blood transfusion or blood products). Patients may be permitted to discharge themselves against advice, provided they fully understand the consequences of their actions.

Meticulous notes must be made of exactly what was said to the patient and their response, demonstrating that the patient fully understood the issues. The patient can sign an appropriate form, accepting responsibility for his or her own actions. However, documenting carefully in the medical notes exactly what was said to the patient and what the patient understood is of *far greater value* than a mere signature on a 'Left against medical advice' form.

Negligence

Negligence occurs by an act or omission of a healthcare provider when that care deviates from accepted standards of practice in the medical community and causes harm. The four elements required for a successful malpractice claim are a duty of care, a breach of that duty by substandard care, that the breach was the proximate cause of injury, and damages are sought.

The levels of evidence required for a successful determination differ. In civil negligence (tort law), evidence must prove 'on the balance of probabilities' (i.e. 51%). However, in the rare circumstance of criminal negligence, a much higher level of proof is required (i.e. 'beyond all reasonable doubt').

Informed consent is thus one way to deter civil negligence. Even if the patient allows contact, but the doctor does not obtain valid consent for a proposed intervention, the patient may be able to sue for damages if a poor outcome results.

However, valid consent would still not prevent legal action for criminal negligence when extreme damage such as death resulted from recklessly unacceptable actions on the part of the doctor (i.e. from intoxication by drugs or alcohol).

Competence and capacity
Legal competence
A child of or over 16 years of age may give consent for medical treatment.

In certain circumstances, a patient under the age of 16 years can consent to medical treatment without the knowledge or required acceptance of a parent or guardian. These include:

- Under common law principles or as set out in local legislation, provided the patient is deemed competent
- Dependent on the patient's maturity, marital status, economic independence and ability to understand the benefits and risks of what is proposed
- An emancipated minor (i.e. a child who is married or living independently) who is usually legally able to provide consent.

For major or complex treatment, it is appropriate to seek consent from a parent or guardian on the assumption that the younger patient will not fully comprehend the circumstances and cannot therefore give truly informed consent. Always try to persuade a child to notify the parent.

Mental competence
Mental competence requires that a patient understands what is proposed, the options involved, the treatment and the risks of treatment or lack of it, and the possible outcomes.

- Competence can vary over time.
- Competence is specific and/or can vary with specific tasks. More complicated tasks require a better understanding (e.g. a young child may be able to consent to removal of a splinter, but not to undergoing surgery).

BOX 4.1 Assessing capacity to consent

Understanding

The patient must understand and retain (i.e. be able to relate back) information on the treatment proposed, its benefits, risks and consequences.

- What do you understand about what I have told you about your treatment?
- What are the risks and benefits of treatment, and the consequences of no treatment?

Belief

The patient must believe this information.

- What do you think is wrong with your health?
- Do you believe you need treatment?
- What do you believe the treatment will do for you?
- What do you believe will happen if you do not receive the treatment?

Reasoning

The patient must be able to evaluate the information to reach a reasonable decision.

- How did you reach the decision to have/not have (refuse) treatment?
- What things were important to you in reaching the decision?

Choice

- What have you decided?

- Competence to consent, or 'capacity', incorporates the elements of understanding, belief, reasoning and choice (see Box 4.1). A mental illness does not necessarily imply a lack of capacity to consent, if these elements can still be satisfied. Thus, a person with a stable, chronic psychosis, such as treated schizophrenia, is perfectly able to consent to an appendicectomy.

  In the event that the patient is not capable of giving consent, substituted consent may be provided by the following:
- Parent or guardian, in the case of a child
- Guardian, in the case of a patient with chronic mental incapacity
- Appropriate surrogates as provided for in the *Guardianship and Administration Act* or equivalent in each legal jurisdiction. These may include the next of kin, other relatives, carers or those with an enduring power of attorney. A court order may be required.

Duty of care

Once a therapeutic relationship has been established between patient and doctor, that doctor has a duty of care to that patient. If the patient is not competent to accept (or refuse) medical care, and there is no substituted consent available, the doctor has a duty of care to ensure the patient's safety.

- Under common law, an incompetent patient may receive treatment, because there is the overriding principle of best care by the treating doctor.

- Duty of care may involve patient restraint in some cases to facilitate assessment or treatment despite the patient's protestations. In such cases, only what is absolutely necessary for emergency treatment should be forced on the patient.
- Non-emergency issues can be addressed when either the patient recovers from a temporary incompetence or legal permission to proceed is granted.

Patients with conditions that preclude comprehension of the nature and implications of the treatment proposed may be given emergency treatment without consent, to save life or to prevent serious damage to health. Similarly, patients suffering from mental illness may be involuntarily detained against their will under the relevant *Mental Health Act* if they are a danger to themselves or others.

The doctor's duty of care also implies acceptable standards of care. Both incompetent and competent patients deserve acceptable treatment. To do otherwise may lead to legal action for negligence, irrespective of the lack of informed consent.

Patient confidentiality

There are some instances when the doctor–patient relationship may be breached. Each state or territory will have different legal requirements, but in broad terms, these are:

- When the patient consents in writing to allow personal details to be revealed to a third party.
- If there are other health professionals who have a legitimate therapeutic interest in the care of the patient (this does not necessarily include medical students). That is, another doctor may read the case notes.
- If there is overriding public interest. This is not well-defined, but if the patient was about to commit, or has committed, a serious crime, including murder, battery, rape, child abuse or an act of terrorism, or was the victim of a serious crime, then an appropriate authority such as the police could be informed to reduce likely associated risks.
- Mandatory reporting of certain conditions may be present in certain jurisdictions, such as deaths of unknown cause, some infectious diseases, and domestic or child abuse.

Remember, this duty of confidentiality includes patients under the age of 18 years who do not want their parents notified. A breach of this duty may lead to civil action for damages.

5

Death, dying and breaking bad news

End-of-life orders

Advance health directive and enduring power of attorney

- An **advance health directive (AHD)** or 'living will' is a legal document made in writing by a competent person aged over 18 years expressing an intention to refuse medical treatment for a specified condition or conditions in the future, at a time when he or she may no longer be competent to make that treatment decision.
- An **enduring power of attorney (EPA)** is a legal authorisation for another person to make decisions, including on health and financial issues, when the patient has become incapacitated.

A legally valid AHD for a specific condition should be respected. Treatment against a patient's wishes, as expressed in the AHD, compromises patient autonomy and may constitute battery.

If you are uncertain about the legality of an AHD, provide treatment according to the patient's best interests, while seeking senior assistance and legal advice. Always obtain a *written* copy or certified photocopy of the AHD for verification purposes.

The AHD may apply to a certain condition such as cancer, but does not preclude treatment from an unexpected cause such as a motor vehicle accident.

Not-for-resuscitation order

Advanced life support may reverse death in a small proportion of patients who have suffered a cardiac arrest ('failed sudden cardiac death'). Survival rates for inhospital CPR vary according to ward area and patient mix. Although up to 15–20% survive to leave hospital, only just over half retain good neurological function.

Some hospitalised patients clearly have multiple irreversible medical problems and/or a terminal illness, which limits their quality of life. In many of these patients, CPR is without value or virtue—'futile'—and thus inappropriate. CPR may diminish patient dignity during the dying process and alienate families.

A not-for-resuscitation (NFR) order is an advance directive that indicates beforehand the patient's wishes to refuse lifesaving medical procedures if the situation arises. It authorises an omission to act, which is different from an act causing death, as is the case with euthanasia. It may also be known by alternative terms such as 'not for CPR', 'do not resuscitate' (DNR), or 'do not attempt resuscitation' (DNAR). All orders encompass dying with dignity through empowering the transition to a 'good death'.

The order may be in the form of a 'living will', setting out the patient's wishes, and prescribed in the relevant legislation (e.g. an AHD).

Discussing an NFR order

The NFR order must have been discussed with the patient when competent and with the relatives. This discussion should include:

1. An understanding of the patient's wishes, and opinion on current and likely future quality of life.
2. The expected outcome with or without CPR, including discussion of the likely futility of CPR.
3. The possible harms of CPR, including performance of invasive procedures and potential injury, loss of dignity, loss of privacy and contact with the family during and after the resuscitation.
4. Emphasis that other active or supportive management such as pain relief or fluids is not affected by an NFR order.

The NFR decision must be clearly documented in the medical notes, ideally in a place that is easily found, such as in an Acute Resuscitation Plan (ARP) at the front of the patient's notes.

- The NFR decision must also be discussed with relatives if the patient is incompetent, and a clear, reasoned decision not to resuscitate made in agreement with the family, medical and nursing staff. Once again, the NFR order should be clearly written in the medical notes.
- Nursing staff must be made aware of an NFR order at each shift change.

Dying patients

Patients are frequently admitted to hospital to die.

- This is a challenging situation for hospital staff, for whom the usual aim of treatment is to cure, rather than to focus on the holistic care of dying patients and their relatives.
- Careful planning, comprising symptom control and emotional and spiritual support, is important to ensure that the patient has a comfortable, calm and dignified death.

Pain

Pain is the symptom that causes the most fear and suffering in the dying patient. Providing explanation and support, and gaining trust help raise the pain threshold as an adjunct to prescribing analgesic medication. Treatment depends on the cause and nature of the pain:

- Somatic pain from superficial structures is usually well localised. Commence regular paracetamol or NSAIDs and add an opiate analgesic when required.
- Visceral pain from deeper structures is usually poorly localised. Opioids are frequently necessary, but some pain may improve with steroids such as dexamethasone or prednisolone.
- Neurogenic pain from damage, pressure or stretching of a peripheral nerve is difficult to control. Multiple agents such as opioids, ketamine, antidepressants, anticonvulsants or nerve blocks are necessary.

Dyspnoea and cough

Any underlying cause should be addressed (see Chapter 15). When death is near, symptomatic treatment and a calm, reassuring manner are required. Options include:

- Position the patient to provide maximum comfort, usually sitting up.
- Provide oxygen if hypoxic, or cool air from a fan.
- Prescribe morphine 5–10 mg or lignocaine 50–100 mg via a nebuliser for persistent cough.
- Prescribe a benzodiazepine to relieve anxiety from the worsening dyspnoea (see below).
- Give dexamethasone 4 mg PO or IV to treat dyspnoea associated with lymphangitis carcinomatosis.

'Death rattle'

Gurgling respirations from a dying person unable to clear oropharyngeal secretions is distressing, particularly for the family.

- Repeated suctioning (often through a nasopharyngeal airway) is unpleasant and traumatic.
- Reassure the family, position the patient on their side and administer an anticholinergic agent such as glycopyrrolate 200–400 micrograms SC, or atropine 600 micrograms SC, to reduce the secretions.

Anorexia and nausea

Anorexia and nausea are common symptoms in the dying patient. Causes include opioid analgesia, hypercalcaemia, abdominal malignancy, raised intracranial pressure or hepatic congestion. Treatment options include:

- Metoclopramide 10 mg PO or IV or IM; side effects include dystonia

- Ondansetron 4–8 mg SL or IV
- Domperidone 10–20 mg PO
- Prochlorperazine 5–10 mg PO or 12.5 mg IM or slowly IV; side effects include akathisia (an intolerable sense of restlessness)
- Haloperidol 1 mg PO or IM or IV
- Droperidol 0.5 mg PO or IM or IV
- Lorazepam 1 mg PO or SL
- Dexamethasone 4 mg PO or IM or IV for nausea, regardless of cause; it also acts as an appetite stimulant.

Dry mouth and dehydration

Dry mouth is common and often caused by medication side effects. Try administering frequent mouthwashes, offer sips of water or give ice chips to suck.

- Thirst diminishes in the terminal phase of dying, but dehydration is usually not perceived by the patient.
- However, if fluids are required in a patient who cannot swallow, a subcutaneous infusion is preferable to nasogastric or IV fluids.

Terminal agitation

Agitation may be caused by medication side effects (especially the dysphoric effect of opioids or anticholinergics), intractable pain, a full bladder or loaded rectum, or anxiety and fear. If attempts at reversing the causes are unsuccessful, other options include:

- Lorazepam 1 mg PO or SL
- Midazolam 10–20 mg/24 h or clonazepam 0.5–2 mg/24 h as a continuous subcutaneous infusion.

Pronouncing death

While on call you will be required to pronounce death in a newly deceased patient.

- Be familiar with the medical and legal criteria accepted for the determination of death in the state or territory in which you work.
- A person is dead when irreversible cessation of all brain function has occurred. This can be determined by the prolonged absence of spontaneous circulatory and respiratory functions. A slightly more detailed assessment is recommended, which takes only a few minutes to complete (see next page).
- Although other emergencies take precedence over pronouncing a patient dead, try not to postpone this task for too long, as the time of death is legally the time at which you see and then pronounce the patient dead. It also allows nursing staff to begin

organising the numerous notifications and procedures required once death has been certified.

Expected death

The nurse will page you and inform you of the death of the patient, requesting that you come to the ward and pronounce the patient dead.

- Review the medical notes to obtain the background to this event.
- Identify the patient by the hospital identification tag worn on the wrist or leg.
- Ascertain that the patient does not rouse to verbal or tactile stimuli.
- Look and listen for absent spontaneous respirations.
- Listen for absent heart sounds and feel for an absent carotid pulse.
- Look for absent pupillary reactions to light. (*Note*: fixed dilated pupils are not necessarily synonymous with death and may occur with eye drops, anticholinergic agents, hypoxia etc.)
- Record the time at which your assessment was completed.
- Document your findings on the chart. A typical chart entry may read as follows:

> *Called to pronounce Mr X deceased. Patient unresponsive to verbal or tactile stimuli. No heart sounds heard, no pulse felt. No spontaneous respirations observed and no air entry heard. Pupils fixed and dilated. Patient pronounced dead at 20:30 hours, 1 June 2016.*

This entry is then signed, and your name and designation printed alongside.

When the death is expected, the relatives will usually have been notified to come to hospital. Check the chart to find the contact details for the next of kin and whether there was documentation regarding the need for urgent contact.

- Notify the next of kin as soon as possible, unless it is documented to wait until the morning.
- It is best to call the family in to the hospital to break bad news, but if the death was expected to occur, a phone call may be reasonable.
- If possible, a doctor familiar with the patient, or a senior nurse who knows the family well, should notify the next of kin, as the family will appreciate hearing the news from a familiar voice.

Informing the family

If you are appointed to break the news of death to the family over the phone:

- Spend a few minutes familiarising yourself with the patient's medical history and cause of death.

- Speak to the nursing staff who are familiar with the family, in case there are difficult family situations or other potential problems.
- When calling, identify yourself and ask for the immediate next of kin. Try to establish in advance who this is (i.e. husband/wife/ daughter).
- Deliver the message clearly; for example: *'I am sorry to inform you that your husband died at 8:30 this evening.'*
- You may find that in many instances the news is not unexpected. It is, however, comforting to know that a relative has died peacefully. Continue by stating: *'As you know, your husband was suffering from a terminal illness. Although I was not with your husband at the time of his death, the nurses looking after him assure me that he was comfortable and that he passed away peacefully.'*
- Ask the next of kin if they wish to come to the hospital to see their loved one for one last time and encourage them to do so. Inform the nurse of this decision.
- Questions pertaining to funeral arrangements and the patient's personal belongings are best referred to the nurse in charge, or to the social worker to be sorted out in the morning.
- Requests for an autopsy or tissue donation are ideally introduced during face-to-face contact and should await the arrival of the relatives. This could also be deferred to the patient's usual medical team in the morning.
- Ensure that there is explicit communication of the death to this team and to the patient's general practitioner (GP) as soon as possible.
- Many hospitals have a bereavement program that is of great assistance to relatives during the grieving process.

Breaking bad news

Breaking bad news to relatives concerning sudden unexpected death, or sudden onset of critical illness or injury, is an important skill in a difficult and challenging situation. Doctors may naturally have fears about showing their own feelings about death or even of being blamed for a patient's death.

If the breaking of bad news is poorly handled, the result may be:
- Prolonged and pathological grieving
- Poor image of the doctor and hospital in the eyes of the relative(s)
- Unnecessary complaints
- Increased stress for medical and nursing staff.

Initial contact by phone
- Identify yourself and the person to whom you are talking.
- Do not inform of the death over the phone (unless unavoidable, e.g. the relatives live more than an hour away, or overseas).

- Advise the person to come directly to the hospital, preferably with a friend or relative driving.
- Arrange for relatives to be met on arrival and directed to a private relative's room.

A patient still being resuscitated

- Speak to the relatives as soon as possible and keep them regularly updated, which also gives an opportunity to discuss the realistic expected outcome with the relatives.
- Arrange for a nurse, social worker or pastoral care worker to be with the family while they wait.
- Make sure you ask whether one or more of the relatives wish to witness the resuscitation.
- Make certain that any witness is accompanied at all times by a staff member, who will explain what is happening and what to expect.

The patient who has died suddenly

The senior doctor in charge of the resuscitation should inform the relatives, accompanied by a nurse who has had some time with the family, and ideally by a junior doctor as an observer to learn this important skill. Turn off your pager or phone.

- Introduce yourselves briefly, ascertain who is in the room and their relationship to the patient, and sit down by the next of kin.
- Ask the relatives what they know about the events leading up to death and/or give a brief account of events in hospital. This establishes rapport and sets the scene before telling the bad news.
- Provide accurate information in simple language, pacing the information to the needs of the relatives.
- Sometimes it is more appropriate to tell them immediately that the patient has died, especially if they are expecting this.
- Be precise, use the words 'dead' or 'died' and avoid all euphemisms such as 'gone to a better place'.
- Touching the relative's shoulder may be comforting and shows concern and empathy. Allow a period of silence, avoiding platitudes or false sympathy, but encourage and answer any questions.
- Understand that the relative's reaction may vary from numbed silence, disbelief or acute distress, to anger, denial and guilt. There will be wide cultural and individual variations in this response.
- Answer questions if asked, but silence is appropriate while the initial reaction settles.

- Encourage the relatives, when they are ready, to see and touch the body, and to say goodbye to their loved one.

Following the breaking of bad news

- Inform the relatives of the formal processes such as where the body will go, collecting belongings, issuing of a death certificate or the need for an autopsy.
- Ask whether the relatives wish the hospital chaplain or bereavement counsellor to be contacted.
- Give the relatives a pamphlet with contact numbers and information to aid with the bereavement process. This may take the form of a sympathy card, a follow-up call from the social worker or the offer of an interview with the usual medical team to answer any questions.
- Ensure the appropriate paperwork and communications are completed, including documenting in the medical notes, the death certificate, telephoning or emailing the GP, and reporting to the coronial office if necessary.

Common pitfalls when breaking bad news

This is one of the most stressful life events for the relatives and will be recalled in minute detail for many years. Small points are noticed, may be misinterpreted and are rarely forgotten.

It is therefore important to make this last interaction as professional and empathic as possible:

- Do not break bad news while dishevelled or covered in blood. Change your clothes or cover up.
- Do not forget or mistake the patient's name. A wrong name is devastating, confusing and absolutely avoidable.
- Ensure that you have the correct relatives and that you directly address the next of kin.
- Make sure you use the words 'dead', 'died' or 'dying', and avoid ambiguous phrases such as 'has left us' or 'gone' or 'passed on'.
- Avoid saying *'I know how you feel'* when clearly you do not. Instead you could say *'I can only imagine how it must feel'*.
- Also try not say *'I am sorry'*, which may be misinterpreted as you having made a mistake; phrase this better as *'I am sorry for your loss'*.
- Do not try to control the acute grief reaction. Allow silence, and spend as much time as is needed.
- Tears are an appropriate reaction and are perfectly acceptable from medical or nursing staff.

- Avoid giving a sedative drug if requested by other relatives for the next of kin. This only postpones acceptance of what has happened.

After speaking to the relatives, remember to debrief with the medical and nursing staff involved in the resuscitation at a suitable time, even if only informally. Make sure to thank everyone for their efforts and special contributions, such as the nurse who lays out the body.

6

Preparation of patients for transfer

The interhospital transfer of a patient to a hospital providing more definitive care, usually from a non-tertiary to a tertiary institution, is a frequent occurrence in many countries, whether for medical, geographical or financial reasons. Similar principles of safe mobile care apply to critically ill patients who need to be transferred within a hospital from one department to another (e.g. from a ward to radiology for imaging).

The decision to transfer a patient may have been made during the day by the treating team, but by the time referral phone calls are made, a bed is booked and transport resources are organised, movement of the patient may only be possible after working hours. The responsibility of ensuring that the patient is prepared and ready for this transfer then falls to the on-call doctor.

The transfer of a patient from one hospital to another involves high risk. Equipment can fail, lines can become dislodged or the patient may deteriorate in an environment in which even simple interventions are difficult to perform. However, with careful planning and preparation, patients may be moved safely even if intubated, ventilated and on multiple infusions (a doctor trained in critical care would then be responsible for the transfer).

Successful patient transfer requires meticulous planning and preparation, medical stabilisation, good communication and appropriate levels of crew selection. Any procedure that might be required should always be done prior to the patient being moved, as many if not most are technically challenging or near impossible once in transit.

Referring doctor's responsibilities

Responsibility for the preparation of the patient for transfer lies principally with the referring doctor or, in the case of an after-hours transfer, the on-call doctor. Duties of this *referring* doctor include:
- **Communication and facilitation:**
  - Notify the transport retrieval organisation as early as possible, so that an appropriate crew can be assembled.

- Initiate and maintain clear and accurate communication between the receiving hospital and the transport retrieval organisation, ideally using a single, centralised retrieval service telephone number.
- Do not delay a request to the transport retrieval organisation while awaiting results when it is apparent that management of the patient is beyond the capability of your referring hospital. Refer on as soon as this is recognised.
- Contact the receiving hospital early to obtain medical advice regarding specific treatment and to ensure that a bed is reserved.
- Notify any change in the patient's condition to both the transport retrieval organisation and the receiving hospital. Most transport retrieval organisations have limited resources and operate on a priority system. Deterioration in the patient's condition may lead to an earlier retrieval and/or deployment of a more experienced team. Similarly, notification of an improvement in the patient's condition may allow the retrieval team to respond to another more urgent patient.
- **Preparation and stabilisation** of the patient at the referring hospital, prior to transfer:
  - Review the patient's airway, breathing and circulation status. Have a low threshold for organising procedures such as endotracheal intubation or chest drain insertion if there is any concern that the patient's condition may deteriorate en route. With your senior, call anaesthetics or ICU as necessary to help in the preparation.
  - Ensure that a minimum of two IV lines are sited in all but the most stable of patients, and that the lines are patent and well secured.
  - Initiate interim treatment according to the resources available. Treatments such as oxygen, antiemetics, analgesics, antibiotics and anticonvulsants should be given as indicated, spinal immobilisation instituted, fractures splinted, wounds dressed and tetanus prophylaxis given when indicated.
  - If the patient has an intercostal catheter in situ, attach it to a Heimlich flutter valve or transport bag with valve. Underwater drainage systems are not suitable for aeromedical transport.
  - Remember that transfer is not an alternative to timely diagnosis and treatment. Any procedures that are required for the immediate management of the patient must be performed prior to moving the patient to ensure safe transfer.
- **Documentation and administration:**
  - Ensure that the patient is accompanied by X-rays, pathology test results and personal effects.

- Prepare explicit documentation of the initial condition and treatment to date, with a personalised referral letter, to go with the patient.
- Ensure that packaging is appropriate for the transport service, with advice from the transport doctor. Aviation requirements for the safe transport of blood products, for instance, are different to road transport requirements.
- Keep relatives informed at all times, as they may wish to depart early to meet the patient on arrival at the receiving hospital.

Transfer doctor's responsibilities

The interhospital transfer of patients is usually undertaken by a dedicated transport organisation such as the local ambulance servie, a Helicopter Emergency Medical Service (HEMS), Neonatal Emergency Transport Service (NETS) or the Royal Flying Doctor Service (RFDS) in rural Australia.

However, in some circumstances a medical officer from the referring hospital may be required to escort the patient. The fundamental tenet of all medical transfer is that the level of medical care should be either maintained or increased during the transfer phase. Therefore, the transferring doctor must be skilled enough for the job.

Responsibilities of the *transfer* organisation doctor include:
- Assessing the requirement for transfer and determining the degree of urgency:
  - Use a simple three-tiered priority system (1 = life- threatening, 2 = immediate, 3 = all others) based on the patient's clinical condition and the resources available at the referring institution.
- Ensuring that the level of escort is appropriate for the patient's condition. A paramedic or registered nurse may be able to escort a stable patient between hospitals. However, critically ill patients need a doctor with advanced airway and procedural skills as part of the team.
- Giving appropriate advice regarding pre-transfer stabilisation.
- Confirming that the destination is appropriate for the patient.
- Selecting the mode of transport:
  - Fixed-wing aircraft, helicopters and road vehicles all have advantages and disadvantages in terms of range, speed, patient accessibility and requirements for secondary transfer (e.g. an ambulance from an airport to the hospital).
- Checking that there are adequate supplies of medications (including oxygen), fluids, monitoring and other equipment for the duration of the journey, with extra available to cover unanticipated delays:
  - Portability, ability to recharge en route and battery life of all the medical equipment (including a defibrillator) are taken into consideration in the planning and preparation stage.

- Ensuring that the patient is appropriately prepared and stabilised. Prior to departure, perform any essential procedures that have not been done by the referring institution.
- Monitoring and documenting the pre-transfer and intra-transfer condition of the patient.
- Personally handing over the patient to the receiving institution doctor.
  - At all times, safety is the overriding concern in medical transfers, for both the crew and the patient.

Aviation medicine

Some knowledge of aviation medicine will help both an on-call referring doctor and a receiving doctor on call to understand the special requirements and complications associated with travel at altitude.

Dysbarism

Atmospheric pressure decreases with increasing altitude. As pressure falls, gas expands according to Boyle's law. Gas trapped in a cavity will expand at altitude and contract on descent. At the pressurised cabin altitude of around 7000 ft/2100 m (used on many commercial flights and by most fixed-wing aeromedical teams), trapped gas will expand by approximately 25%.

Pathological conditions that are aggravated by flying at altitude include:

- Decompression illness with gas embolism (e.g. after scuba diving)
- Pneumothorax (especially with positive pressure ventilation)
- Intraocular air (posttraumatic or postoperative)
- Aerocele (air inside the cranium)
- Bowel obstruction/postoperative bowel repair
- Middle ear or sinus infection or fracture.

Consider flying at lower altitudes ('sea-level cabin' in a pressurised aircraft) for patients with these conditions, in particular decompression illness. Pressure considerations must be weighed up against increased turbulence, fuel requirements and decreased range when flying at these lower altitudes. Equipment affected by Boyle's law includes:

- Air in the cuff of the endotracheal tube, so use sterile water/saline instead, *or* remove air from the cuff during ascent and instil air during descent (this is the less safe option)
- Air splints
- Drip chambers in IV lines
- Ventilator settings
- Gas-stream sampling devices such as end-tidal CO_2
- Sealed specimen jars (no glass is allowed on flights).

Altitude hypoxia

As barometric pressure falls, the partial pressure of oxygen falls. In healthy people this does not cause a problem up to pressurised cabin altitudes (<8200 ft/2500 m), because of the flat shape of the haemoglobin dissociation curve. However, supplemental oxygen will be required for relative hypoxia in patients with impaired cardiorespiratory reserve (e.g. pneumonia, ischaemic heart disease, anaemia).

Patients already needing high-flow oxygen on the ground will *always* need to be intubated for transfer, as they will not tolerate further desaturation, despite some medical retrieval aircraft being pressurised to sea level.

General risks

Turbulence, vibration, noise, thermal stress, vestibular disturbances, acceleration/deceleration forces, suboptimal lighting and cramped conditions limiting patient access all combine to make transfer by air potentially hazardous to both the patient and the attending staff.

As there is always the risk of a crash, only essential transfers should go by air and only a critical transfer should travel during the night.

Emergency calls

7

The critically ill patient

Serious complications can occur in hospital patients, as they may have been admitted with a critical illness or their condition may deteriorate while in hospital. Major complications include severe hypoxia, shock and multiorgan failure syndrome, ICU admission or cardiac arrest.

Once a patient goes into cardiac arrest, the outcome is generally dismal unless the patient has a monitored VF arrest. Outside of critical care areas such as CCU, ICU or emergency, survival is less than 5% for VF and effectively less than 1% for asystole.

The DRS ABCDE approach addresses potential life threats in a systematic fashion, and is summarised below and discussed in detail in subsequent chapters.

Medical Emergency Team

The Medical Emergency Team (MET) is an example of a rapid-response team that is activated to review an acutely unwell patient in a hospital ward to prevent further deterioration, before the onset of more severe complications and cardiac arrest. Most hospitals have a MET or a similar strategy. A number of principles underlie the rationale for METs:

- **There is time for intervention:** clinical and physiological deterioration are often relatively slow.
- **There are warning signs:** deterioration is preceded by changes in vital signs, which are easy to measure inexpensively and non-invasively.
- **Early intervention improves outcome:** e.g. oxygen and non-invasive ventilation for respiratory failure, fluid therapy for hypovolaemia or adrenaline for anaphylaxis, rather than trying to reverse cardiac arrest once it occurs, which is usually unsuccessful.
- **Expertise exists and can be deployed:** it may not be immediately available on a general ward.

MET activation

The MET can be activated by any member of staff who is worried about the patient's condition.

- You are expected to recognise the critically ill patient and know when to call for help and/or activate the MET response, so you need to become familiar with peri-arrest life threats, such as failure of the airway, respiratory, circulatory, neurological or metabolic functions of the patient.
- This is explored further in subsequent chapters.

Activation criteria

MET activation criteria are usually predefined and relate to measureable deterioration in the ABCDEs (see Table 7.1).
- Following assessment of the critically ill patient, an emergency response is initiated and supportive treatment is commenced (see Figure 7.1).
- Activating an emergency response depends on the location and situation of the patient. There are emergency call buttons in most rooms in hospital wards. Ringing the bedside nurse call bell three times is also commonly regarded as a call for help.
- If in doubt, put out a call. Do not feel you are going to waste other people's time—the patient's life is at stake, and can be saved by prompt action.

Table 7.1 Medical Emergency Team (MET) activation criteria (*may differ according to hospital policy*)

Acute change in	
Airway	Threatened airway
Breathing	Acute respiratory distress
	RR <8 breaths/min
	RR >36 breaths/min
	Oxygen saturation <90%
Circulation	HR <40 beats/min
	HR >140 beats/min
	Systolic BP <90 mmHg
	Unexplained fall in urine output to <100 mL over 4 h
Neurology	Sudden decrease in level of consciousness (fall in GCS score >2 points)
	Prolonged or repeated seizures
Other	Any concern that does not fit the above criteria

Initial assessment and management of the critically ill patient

DRS ABCDE approach (see also Figure 7.2)
Dangers

Ensure that the patient and staff are safe to continue further assessment and resuscitation.
- Check for dangers such as a live electrical wire, smoke, fluids on the floor constituting a slip hazard, or discarded needles.
- Ensure staff wear gloves to minimise exposure to body fluids.

SECTION B – Emergency calls

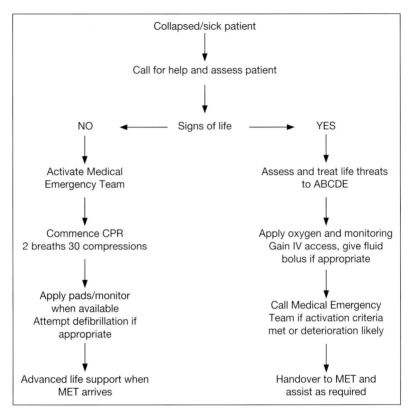

Figure 7.1 Approach to the critically ill patient in hospital.

Response and Send for help

Assess responsiveness: call the patient's name and observe the response to a stimulus such as gently shaking by the shoulders.

- Commence CPR in an unresponsive patient with no signs of life. Call the MET.
- Unresponsiveness suggests CNS failure, severe hypoxia or hypotension, the potential for airway obstruction, and lack of airway protection with the risk of aspiration.
- An unresponsive patient needs emergency care, irrespective of the cause. Call a MET response.
- Normal mental status and speech suggest adequacy of airway, breathing and circulation. The responsive patient undergoes a primary survey of ABCDE, more measured assessment of vital functions and elucidation of underlying cause(s).

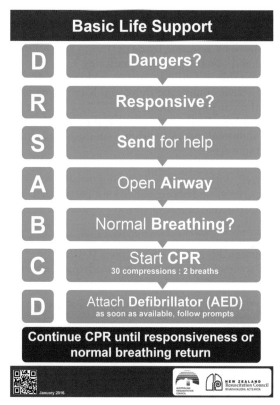

Figure 7.2 Basic Life Support algorithm for adults. Reproduced with permission from the Australian Resuscitation Council and New Zealand Resuscitation Council; January 2016.

Airway

Assess for airway patency, obstruction and protective reflexes.
- Open and clear the airway and prevent aspiration.
- Use airway positioning, suction, airway adjuncts (oropharyngeal Guedel, nasopharyngeal or laryngeal mask airway). Endotracheal intubation is to be done by experienced staff *only*.
- Treat the underlying cause.

Breathing

Assess for work and efficacy of breathing, including pulse oximetry.
- Give oxygen and provide assisted ventilation if ventilatory failure is present.
- Treat the underlying cause.

Circulation

Recheck vital signs.
* Look for shock by assessing tissue perfusion and volume status.
* Place ECG and non-invasive BP monitoring.
* Look for unstable arrhythmias or any evidence of ACS.
* Obtain IV access: commence fluids and haemodynamic support if evidence of circulatory failure.
    * Give 20 mL/kg IV fluid rapidly if hypovolaemic shock.
* Optimise abnormal cardiac rhythm with cardioversion, pacing or antiarrhythmic agent.
* Commence inotropes if no improvement, once hypovolaemia has been reversed, with invasive monitoring usually in ICU.
* Treat time-critical underlying conditions, particularly anaphylactic, septic or obstructive causes of shock.

Disability

Assess for depressed level of consciousness (GCS).
* A GCS score of 8 or less indicates inadequate airway protection. See Table 7.2.

Table 7.2 **Glasgow Coma Scale**	
Response	**Score**
Eye opening	
Spontaneously	4
To verbal command	3
To pain	2
No response	1
Best motor response	
Obeys commands	6
Localises to pain	5
Withdraws to pain	4
Abnormal flexion	3
Abnormal extension	2
No response	1
Best verbal response	
Orientated	5
Disorientated	4
Inappropriate words	3
Incomprehensible sounds	2
No response	1
Normal score is 15 A confused patient will score 14 Score of 8 or less indicates coma	
Glasgow Coma Scale © Sir Graham Teasdale, http://glasgowcomascale.org	

- An altered mental status may be due to cerebral hypoxia or hypoperfusion.
- Optimising ABC is the best initial management for altered mental status.
- Note pupil size and lateralising signs.
- Seek and treat the cause of depressed consciousness.

Environment, exposure and examination

- Measure and normalise body temperature.
- Measure and normalise blood glucose.
- Consider antidote such as naloxone, electrolyte replacement and other specific therapy as indicated.
- Perform a full top-to-toe examination (secondary survey).
- Obtain a history from any source (patient, medical staff, relative, allied health worker, old notes).
- Decide on a working diagnosis and definitive management plan.
- Document carefully.

8

Cardiac arrest

Cardiopulmonary resuscitation (CPR) is aimed at treating sudden cardiac arrest from reversible causes, particularly malignant arrhythmias, *not* for prolonging life in a patient who is dying from an irreversible acute or chronic/terminal illness.

CPR is probably futile in acute illnesses when a patient has deteriorated *despite* maximal medical management, or among those dying from a terminal condition. These patients need all the medical effort directed beforehand to prevent cardiac arrest from occurring in the first place, or to have a clear decision documented that they are not for resuscitation.

You may be part of the Cardiac Arrest Team or Medical Emergency Team (MET), either as the on-call doctor or as part of an attachment in anaesthesia, intensive care or emergency medicine. Cardiac arrest calls are stressful experiences for junior doctors and require a rapid and organised approach. As there is no time to look up information, CPR algorithms outline the initial management of sudden cardiac arrest with a nationally or internationally agreed consensus approach.

Cardiac arrest management

The best outcome for cardiac arrest occurs if the victim is witnessed to collapse, and quality basic life support with expired air or mask resuscitation and external cardiac compression is commenced immediately and continued with minimal interruption. Compression-only CPR can be used if the rescuer is unwilling or unable to perform mouth-to-mouth rescue breathing.

Chain of survival
The 'chain of survival' refers to the four links that, acting together, improve the victim's chance of survival in cardiac arrest:
1. Early recognition and activation of the emergency response
   e.g. hospital MET (or calling an ambulance) to transport a
   defibrillator to the victim.
2. Early basic life support (until a defibrillator arrives).
3. Early defibrillation.
4. Post-resuscitation care.

Verify cardiac arrest

- Look for signs of life.
- A patient who is unresponsive and has no effective respiration is assumed to be in cardiac arrest.
- Checking for a pulse such as the carotid may be difficult or inaccurate.
- *Note:* intermittent gasping respirations or agonal breaths are not a sign of life; assume that the patient is in cardiac arrest.

Activate the emergency response

Once cardiac arrest has been diagnosed, call for help to bring other staff quickly, and commence resuscitation. If no one is around, leave the patient briefly while you activate the emergency response yourself.

Basic life support

Basic life support (BLS) is a temporising measure that provides, at best, around 20–30% of normal cardiac output and oxygenation. It may prolong survival for short periods until defibrillation is available, or until reversible causes are diagnosed and/or treated.

- Place the patient in the supine position.
- Open the airway by head tilt and chin lift or jaw thrust, and look again for signs of life (generally regarded as adequate respiratory efforts).
- If no signs of life, commence external cardiac compressions by giving 30 external chest compressions at the rate of 100–120/min.
  - Place the heel of one hand in the centre of the patient's chest. Place the heel of the other hand on top, interlocking the fingers.
  - Keep the arms straight and apply vertical compression force. Depress the sternum approximately one-third of the anteroposterior diameter of the chest.
  - Do not apply pressure over the upper abdomen, lower end of the sternum or the ribs, and take equal time with compression and release.
- After 30 compressions, give two ventilations by either mouth-to-mouth or preferably via a self-inflating bag and mask device such as the Laerdal or Ambu bag. This may be helped by the insertion of an oropharyngeal Guedal airway (see Chapter 10).
- Continue the 30 compressions to two ventilations (30:2) ratio, only pausing compressions while ventilating the patient.
- Attach a defibrillator as soon as possible.

Maximally effective CPR

- External cardiac compressions
  - Avoid interruptions (even for checking a pulse), although a brief pause is required for ventilations.

SECTION B – Emergency calls

- Change operators frequently, at least every 2 minutes, as fatigue decreases the efficacy of cardiac compressions.
- Adequacy of oxygenation and ventilation
  - Ensure adequate chest rise.
  - Use supplemental oxygen.
  - Avoid hypo- or hyperventilation (too slow or too fast).
- Minimise time to first defibrillation to increase the likelihood of success.

Advanced life support

Advanced life support (ALS) is the addition of invasive techniques such as defibrillation, advanced airway management and IV drugs.
- Attach a monitor/defibrillator while BLS is ongoing.
- Determine the cardiac rhythm—see Figure 8.1:
  - Shockable: ventricular fibrillation (VF) or pulseless ventricular tachycardia (pVT)
  - Non-shockable: asystole or pulseless electrical activity (PEA).
- Search for and correct reversible causes (the 4 Hs and 4 Ts, see below).

Shockable rhythms: ventricular fibrillation or pulseless ventricular tachycardia

Defibrillation is the only proven successful treatment for VF and pVT. Its efficacy decreases with time. Do not delay defibrillation for *any* other procedure such as IV access or endotracheal intubation, as every 1-minute delay decreases survival by 7–10%.
- **Attaching a defibrillator**
  - Place one self-adhesive defibrillation pad or conventional paddle to the right of the sternum below the clavicle and the other adhesive pad or paddle in the mid-axillary line at the 5th or 6th intercostal space.
  - Do not defibrillate over ECG electrodes or leads, GTN patch, internal devices such as a pacemaker, or jewellery.
  - If there is inadequate pad/paddle contact because of excessive hair, it should be immediately shaved off.
- Listen to the prompts if using an automated or semi-automated external defibrillator (AED/SAED). Check the monitor to confirm shockable rhythm if using a manual defibrillator.
- **Defibrillate** (administering shocks using a manual defibrillator):
  - CPR should continue during charging of the defibrillator (State loudly: '*CPR continue*') to minimise CPR interruptions.
  - Ensure that no one else is in contact with the bed, IV fluid or the patient, and that flowing oxygen is moved from the patient before charging the defibrillator (State loudly: '*Everyone else away, oxygen away*').

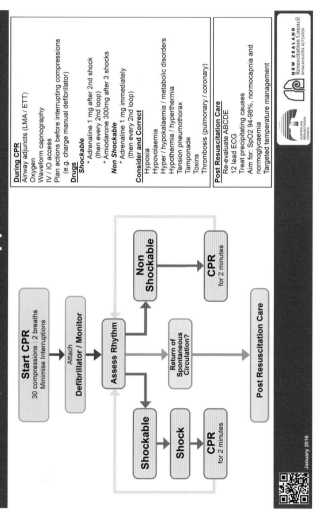

Figure 8.1 Advanced Life Support algorithm for adults. Reproduced with permission from the Australian Resuscitation Council and New Zealand Resuscitation Council; January 2016.

- Charge the defibrillator to 200 J biphasic (State loudly: *'Charging defibrillator'*).
- Once the defibrillator is charged, state loudly: *'Stop CPR and move away.'*
- Once you have ensured it is safe, and confirmed that it is still a shockable rhythm on the monitor, deliver the shock (State loudly: *'Delivering shock'*).
- Recommence CPR immediately after shock delivery (State loudly: *'Recommence CPR'*) without checking the rhythm or pulse. Try to minimise any interruption to CPR to less than 5 seconds.
- **Reassess the patient and monitor rhythm** after one cycle (five sets of 30 compressions : 2 breaths over approximately 2 minutes).
- Repeat a single shock if there is persistent VF or pVT.
- Obtain IV access and administer adrenaline 1 mg IV after the second shock.
- Continue the **reassess–defibrillate–CPR** cycle.
- Give amiodarone 300 mg IV diluted in 5% dextrose up to 20 mL after the third shock.
- Repeat adrenaline 1 mg IV after the fourth shock and every two cycles thereafter (approximately 4 minutes).
- An additional dose of amiodarone 150 mg IV can be considered.
- Reassess the patient and rhythm every 2 minutes.
- If at the 2-minute reassessment organised electrical activity is present, dump the charge of the defibrillator and feel for a pulse:
  - If no pulse, continue CPR but switch to the non-shockable algorithm.
  - If a pulse is present, commence post-resuscitation care.

Non-shockable rhythms: asystole or pulseless electrical activity

These rhythms do not respond to defibrillatory shocks. Check that the leads are connected, the monitor gain is turned up and/or try a different lead.
- Continue CPR at the 30:2 compression–ventilation ratio.
- Obtain IV access and administer adrenaline 1 mg immediately.
- Reassess the patient and rhythm every cycle (five sets of 30 compressions : 2 breaths over approximately 2 minutes).
- Give further adrenaline 1 mg IV every two cycles (approximately every 4 minutes).
- Reassess the patient and rhythm every 2 minutes:
  - If VF/pVT is present, switch to the shockable rhythm algorithm.
  - If a pulse is present, commence post-resuscitation care.

In every case of cardiac arrest

- Search for and correct reversible causes: the 4 Hs and 4 Ts (see below).

- If trained to do so, insert a supraglottic airway such as an LMA, or place an ETT when practical, then confirm placement with capnography. Ventilate 10 times per minute once a definitive airway is in place without pausing for compressions, while monitoring using continuous waveform capnography, if available.
- Give at least 20 mL of normal saline to flush any drugs administered and elevate the limb for 10–20 seconds to facilitate drug delivery to the central circulation.
- Establish a second IV line unless the cardiac resuscitation is rapidly successful.
- Try the use of a CPR prompt or feedback device to improve the quality of CPR.
- Consider extracorporeal CPR in selected patients in specialised centres.

Reversible causes

Always look out for the following potentially reversible conditions that may precipitate cardiorespiratory arrest or decrease the chances of successful resuscitation, known as the 4 Hs and 4 Ts.

Perform bedside cardiac ultrasound during resuscitation if the skill is available. It must not interfere with CPR, but does help find potentially reversible causes.

4 Hs

- **Hypoxaemia**
  - Deliver high-flow 100% oxygen and ensure ventilations create a visible rise and fall of both sides of the chest.
- **Hypovolaemia**
  - Severe blood loss following surgery or internal haemorrhage, and volume loss in anaphylaxis or sepsis may cause cardiac arrest. Search for and control any potential source of bleeding.
  - Give fluid/blood replacement rapidly if hypovolaemia is likely and alert the relevant surgeon and theatre.
- **Hyper-/hypokalaemia, hypocalcaemia, acidaemia and other metabolic disorders**
  - Rapidly check the potassium, glucose and calcium levels, as suggested by the medical history (e.g. in DKA or renal failure).
  - Give 10–20 mL of 10% calcium chloride solution IV immediately for hyperkalaemia, such as in a renal patient who has a cardiac arrest.
  - Consider 50 mL of 8.4% $NaHCO_3^-$ if the patient is severely acidaemic (pH < 6.8) and is undergoing prolonged resuscitation or post-resuscitation care; or if there is hyperkalaemia.
- **Hypothermia**
  - Check the core temperature with a low-reading thermometer, particularly in any immersion or exposure incident. Moderate

(29–32°C) or severe (<29°C) hypothermia requires active core rewarming with warmed pleural or peritoneal lavage, or cardiopulmonary bypass.

4 Ts

- **Tension pneumothorax**
  - Usually follows a traumatic rather than a spontaneous pneumothorax, particularly when the patient has positive-pressure ventilation. Immediately insert a needle into the chest to decompress if there are asymmetrical chest movements and ventilation requires high pressures.
- **Tamponade**
  - Cardiac tamponade is usually traumatic, but may occur following cardiothoracic surgery, myocardial infarction, dissecting aortic aneurysm, pericarditis or in an oncology, rheumatology or renal patient as a complication of the disease.
  - Perform pericardiocentesis if the patient is in cardiac arrest or peri-arrest from a medical cause. Thoracotomy is indicated following trauma—unlikely on a ward call.
- **Toxins/poisons/drugs**
  - Many substances cause cardiac arrest following accidental or deliberate ingestion (e.g. tricyclic antidepressants, calcium-channel blockers, digoxin or beta-blockers).
  - Consider these based on the history and treat supportively or with antidotes where available.
- **Thrombosis (PE or ACS)**
  - Perform vigorous external chest compressions to attempt to break up a massive PE when this is likely, and give a fluid load bolus of 20 mL/kg.
  - If high clinical suspicion of a massive PE (or ACS) causing cardiac arrest, a fibrinolytic agent can be given.

Indications for other drugs

- **Calcium:** give 10 mL of 10% calcium chloride or 20 mL of 10% calcium gluconate IV for hyperkalaemia, hypocalcaemia or calcium-channel blocker overdose and repeat as necessary.
- **Lignocaine:** initial bolus of 1 mg/kg IV for VF or pVT, when amiodarone is not available, followed by 0.5 mg/kg if necessary. Omit if amiodarone has been given.
- **Magnesium:** give 2.5 g (10 mmol or 5 mL) of 49.3% magnesium sulfate IV in suspected hypomagnesaemia such as in patients with torsades de pointes, on potassium-losing diuretics or with digoxin toxicity.
- **Sodium bicarbonate:** give 50 mmol of 8.4% (50 mL) IV boluses for hyperkalaemia, tricyclic antidepressant or other sodium-channel blocker overdose or severe metabolic acidosis.

Post-resuscitation care

- **Continue respiratory support**
  - Give supplemental oxygen, even if the patient has rapidly returned to consciousness.
  - Avoid both hypoxia and hyperoxia, and maintain normocarbia in ventilated patients. Monitor ABG and titrate inspired oxygen to achieve oxygen saturations of 94–98%.
  - Ensure the ETT is correctly positioned and secure, and organise an immediate CXR.
  - Place a nasogastric tube to decompress the stomach if the patient is still comatose and/or intubated. Confirm placement with the CXR.
- **Maintain cerebral perfusion**
  - Maintain SBP at greater than 100 mmHg.
  - This may require intermittent boluses of adrenaline 50–100 micrograms IV or an adrenaline infusion under close supervision.
  - Ensure there is adequate intravascular volume by looking again for sources of hypovolaemia, checking the JVP or arranging for the insertion of a CVL.
  - Treat and prevent cardiac arrhythmias, which may include an infusion of an antiarrhythmic.
- **Repeat investigations** including a 12-lead ECG, blood glucose, ABG or VBG and electrolytes. Ensure all tubes and lines are in the correct position and functioning.
- **Avoid hypo-/hyperglycaemia or acidosis and control seizures**, as all of these worsen neurological outcome.
- **Commence targeted temperature management** which may improve survival and neurological outcome. Maintain a chosen temperature between 32°C and 36°C according to local policy.
- **Seek and treat the underlying cause** of the cardiac arrest, and/or any complications of the resuscitation itself, such as a pneumothorax from a broken rib or pulmonary aspiration.
- **Consider immediate coronary angiography** and PCI, particularly in a patient with collapse following chest pain, or with ST elevation on ECG.
- **Transfer the patient to an intensive care area**, cardiac catheter lab or coronary care unit.

Acute airway failure

A patent, functioning airway is necessary to provide oxygen, allow ventilation and avoid aspiration.

- Airway assessment is traditionally the first component of assessing a critically ill patient, as complete obstruction causes hypoxia and death within minutes.
- The partially obstructed airway is also a serious problem, as it may interfere with ventilation or progress to total obstruction.

Causes of acute airway failure

- **Depressed level of consciousness**
  - Loss of airway muscle tone can lead to partial or complete obstruction.
  - Loss of protective airway reflexes increases the risk of airway obstruction and aspiration of stomach contents.
- **Mechanical obstruction**
  - Foreign material (food bolus, vomit, blood, dentures)
  - Laryngospasm (multiple causes, including aspiration)
  - Angio-oedema, alone or as part of anaphylaxis
  - Infection (para- or retropharyngeal abscess, croup, epiglottitis)
  - Tumour, either within or compressing the airway
  - Burns, either inhalational or secondary to caustic ingestion
  - Trauma (fractured mandible, neck haematoma, thyroid cartilage fracture)

Assessment of acute airway failure

- Assess airway function (airway patency, potential for obstruction and protection against aspiration).
- Call your senior immediately.
- Search for and treat the underlying cause of the acute deterioration.

Airway function

- The airway is patent if the patient can talk normally and is conscious and alert.

Look for signs of partial airway obstruction
- Hoarse voice, inability to speak or cough
- Stridor, snoring or gurgling secretions
- Soft-tissue retraction—tracheal tug, rib or abdominal recession
  - Loss, or an uncoordinated rise and fall, of the chest and/or abdomen
- Altered level of consciousness or mental status
  - Agitation (hypoxia)
  - GCS < 9 is a better predictor of inadequate airway function with the risk of aspiration than a reduced or absent gag reflex alone
- Cyanosis and a low pulse oximeter reading are late signs; normal pulse oximetry gives no information regarding the degree of airway obstruction or the adequacy of ventilation

Look for compensatory features of partial airway obstruction
- Sitting up and leaning forwards (tripod position)
- Reluctance to speak or cough
- Increased work of breathing with nasal flaring, accessory muscle use, pursed lips

Look for potentially reversible causes of airway obstruction
- Inspect the upper airway for foreign material—may require laryngoscopy to visualise.
- Inspect for erythema or urticaria with lip, tongue or palatal swelling, listen for bronchospasm and examine for circulatory features that suggest anaphylaxis.
- Inspect for localised trauma, burns, infection or tumour.
  - Palpate the anterior neck, including the thyroid cartilage, for pain, inflammation, crepitus, swelling or masses.
- Investigate any cause of depressed consciousness.
  - Especially a rapidly reversible cause such as hypoglycaemia or opioid intoxication.
  - Ensure the patient is not hypoxic or hypotensive.
- Inspect for evidence of head and/or neck trauma, focal neurological features, meningism or seizure activity.

Complete airway obstruction leads to:
- No stridor, airway sounds or breath sounds on lung auscultation.
- Inability to ventilate the patient with a bag-mask.
- Rapid development of cyanosis and unconsciousness.

A MET call should ideally have been made before this occurs, in any patient with even partial airway obstruction.

Management of acute airway failure

Management is carried out simultaneously with assessment of the patient. The underlying cause of the airway compromise should be addressed while optimising airway patency, oxygenation and ventilation and protecting against aspiration.

SECTION B – Emergency calls

General measures

- Administer high-flow oxygen and reverse the cause of depressed consciousness if possible (e.g. check for, and treat, hypoglycaemia or opioid intoxication).
- Apply non-invasive monitoring, including ECG, pulse oximeter and BP.
- Obtain reliable IV access.
- Call your senior for help and summon staff experienced in airway management.
- Reposition the patient to optimise the airway if in coma (see Figure 9.1):

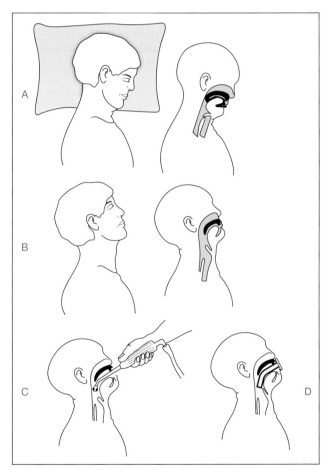

Figure 9.1 Airway management requires correct positioning of the head and neck, correct suctioning and correct insertion of an oral airway. **A** Neck extension and/or head flexion close the airway. **B** Head extension with neck flexion in the sniffing position opens the airway. **C** Suctioning. **D** Placement of the airway.

- Flex the neck at the cervicothoracic junction and extend the head at the cervico-occipital junction ('sniffing the morning air' position), providing there is no trauma to the neck. This usually requires placement of a pillow or support behind the head.
- **Head tilt**–tilt the head gently back with pressure on the forehead.
- **Jaw thrust**–this is most effective when applied together with head tilt. Use jaw thrust alone if there is *any* possibility of spine injury, as this technique avoids excessive movement of the spine.
  - Place the fingers behind the angle of the mandible and push the jaw forwards to lift the soft tissues away from the pharynx to relieve obstruction.
- **Chin lift**–usually best reserved for single operators at the side of the patient for expired air resuscitation, when combining with external cardiac compressions (as in BLS for cardiac arrest).
- **Recovery position**–the left lateral position is used to keep the airway open and assists in drainage of secretions in certain situations (see Figure 9.2).
- Clear foreign material:
  - Manually remove any intra-oral foreign body (e.g. broken or loose-fitting dentures).
  - Suction secretions and smaller foreign material using a large-bore rigid (Yankauer) sucker. Use a laryngoscope and Magill forceps if material is still lodged in the upper airway.

The above measures should be sufficient to keep the airway open. If not, supplement these basic manoeuvres with the use of airway adjuncts.

Airway adjuncts

- **Oropharyngeal (Guedel) airway:** a curved semirigid plastic tube placed in the mouth and designed to lift the tongue away from the pharynx and palate, plus is a bite guard and allows suctioning.
  - The size is approximately the distance from the angle of the jaw to the centre of the lips.
  - Insert upside down, then rotate 180 degrees until the flange rests against the lips.
    - *Note:* if inserted incorrectly, it can worsen airway obstruction by pushing the tongue further back.
  - It is not tolerated or indicated in a semiconscious patient, who will gag or develop laryngospasm. Remove if this is happening.
  - After insertion, head tilt, jaw thrust or chin lift may still be needed to maintain airway patency. Suction secretions through the lumen of the Guedel airway as necessary, using a flexible suction catheter.

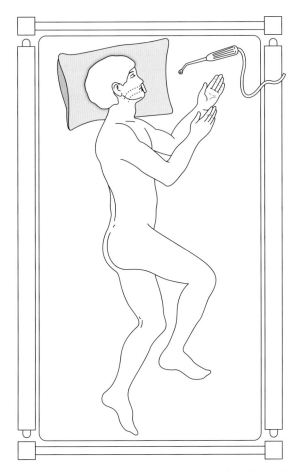

Figure 9.2 Positioning of the patient to prevent aspiration of gastric contents.

- **Nasopharyngeal airway:** a soft plastic tube inserted through the nostril and down the nose to sit in the pharynx, separating the palate and tongue from the posterior pharyngeal wall.
  - Size from the tip of the nose to the tragus of the ear: a size 6 or 7 is suitable for adults.
  - If time allows, spray the nasal cavity with vasoconstrictor/ anaesthetic spray to prevent bleeding and decrease discomfort.
  - Insert a safety pin in the flange in some models to prevent the device disappearing into the nose.

- Lubricate the airway thoroughly and insert horizontally through the nares at right angles to the face, and direct the tube along the floor of the nasal cavity. Push in until the flange rests at the nares.
  - *Note:* this device is better tolerated in a semiconscious patient and may be used in patients with clenched jaws or trismus (e.g. during or following a seizure).
  - Nasopharyngeal airways must be used with extreme caution in a patient with facial injuries, as it is possible to insert upwards in the wrong direction and pierce the anterior cranial fossa of the brain.
- Pass a suction catheter through the airway to help clear secretions.
- **Laryngeal mask airway (LMA):** a plastic tube similar to an endotracheal tube (ETT), but with an elliptical inflatable cuff designed to fit around and above the laryngeal opening (not through it, as with the ETT).
  - It is much simpler to insert after minimal training, provides an open airway and allows positive-pressure ventilation, with some degree of protection against aspiration.
  - It requires little neck movement for insertion, so is suitable for a patient with potential spinal injury.
  - It is not tolerated unless the patient is unconscious.
  - Most LMAs have a patient weight range printed on them, assisting the choice of the correct size (e.g. size 4 suits 50–70 kg).
  - The outer lip of the cuff must be lubricated, then the LMA is inserted through the mouth and pushed backwards against the palate with a confident thrust until resistance is felt from the pharynx.
  - The cuff is inflated and ventilation commenced.

After each of these techniques, reassess the airway to ensure adequacy of treatment or to identify any deterioration.

- **Endotracheal tube intubation** for definitive airway management.
  - To obtain, maintain or protect an airway when temporising measures fail.
  - To provide mechanical ventilation in respiratory failure.
  - Semi-electively used in certain progressive clinical emergencies with a high risk of airway compromise, such as burns or local infection.
  - *Never* attempt until you have been fully trained.

Specific causes of airway compromise

Use the above methods of airway opening in the following situations until or as the cause is being addressed, particularly if progressive airway obstruction is possible.

Local trauma
- Stabilise fractures, re-position, stop bleeding by local pressure or pack. Call a surgeon.

Local infection
- Call ENT and commence antibiotics, drain any abscesses, such as in Ludwig angina, and consider IV steroids to decrease oedema.

Local tumour
- Consider steroids to decrease oedema and arrange urgent ENT assessment.

Angio-oedema
- This is oedema involving the deep tissues of the face, eyelids, lips, tongue and occasionally the larynx. It is often related to ACE inhibitor use (pruritus is absent), or can occur as part of generalised anaphylaxis, usually with pruritus.
- Rarely, it is due to hereditary angio-oedema, an autosomal dominant hereditary condition caused by C1 esterase inhibitor deficiency that also does not include pruritus.
- Angio-oedema may respond poorly to adrenaline (see *Anaphylaxis* below), particularly hereditary angio-oedema, which needs urgent C1 esterase inhibitor IV, or the bradykinin B2-receptor antagonist icatibant 30 mg in 3 mL SC.

Anaphylaxis
Allergic anaphylaxis is an IgE-mediated multisystem reaction that may rapidly follow drug ingestion or injection, Hymenoptera stings (bees, wasps, ants) or ingestion of food such as nuts, fruit or seafood.

Non-allergic anaphylaxis (old term 'anaphylactoid') can follow radio-contrast media, N-acetylcysteine, aspirin or NSAID exposure and is non-IgE mediated—i.e. not an immune response.
- **Clinical systemic manifestations:**
  - **Airway**
    - Laryngeal oedema with hoarseness, stridor and potential for obstruction.
  - **Respiratory**
    - Bronchospasm with rapid onset
    - Cough, excessive secretions, rhinitis and conjunctivitis.
  - **Circulatory**
    - Tachycardia (very occasionally bradycardia)
    - Vasodilation and capillary leakage causing sudden hypotension and distributive shock; can occur rapidly enough to cause syncope.
- **Other features:**
  - Erythema, pruritis, local or widespread urticaria, angio-oedema. Useful as cutaneous markers of generalised allergic reaction.

Not anaphylaxis unless associated with the systemic manifestations above.

• Abdominal cramps or pain, vomiting, diarrhoea.

Generalised allergic reaction

Skin manifestations ± mild angio-oedema only.

• Remove allergen if possible.
• Give oral antihistamine (e.g. cetirizine 10 mg).
• Give prednisolone 50 mg and ranitidine 150 mg PO if urticaria present for many hours or days.
• If no response, or rapidly progressive symptoms with systemic features developing, treat as anaphylaxis.

Anaphylaxis

Systemic features such as upper airway swelling, bronchospasm and/or shock.

• Give high-dose oxygen via a mask, aiming for an oxygen saturation > 94%.
• Give 0.01 mg/kg adrenaline up to 0.3–0.5 mg (0.3–0.5 mL of 1 : 1000 solution) IM into the upper lateral thigh.
• Attach patient to pulse oximetry and ECG monitoring, obtain large IV access.
• If no response, treat as critical anaphylaxis.

Critical anaphylaxis

Impending airway obstruction, hypoxia or hypotension with immediate threat to life.

• Ensure two large-bore IV lines.
• Repeat the dose of adrenaline 0.01 mg/kg IM up to 0.3–0.5 mg every 3–5 minutes.
• Alternatively, place adrenaline 1 mg (1 mL of 1 : 1000) in 100 mL of normal saline and administer IV at 60–120 mL/h (10–20 microgram/min) titrated to response.
  • Must be on an ECG monitor. Give faster in cardiopulmonary collapse/arrest.
• **Hypotension**
  • Lay the patient supine and elevate the legs. Give adrenaline as above.
  • Give a normal saline bolus 20 mL/kg IV under pressure, repeat twice more as necessary.
  • Give glucagon 1 mg IV repeated every 5 minutes in patients on a beta-blocker who are resistant to the above treatment.
  • Give atropine 0.6 mg IV boluses if bradycardia unresponsive to adrenaline.
• **Cardiac arrest**
  • Give usual adrenaline 1 mg IV dose and repeat according to response. Large doses of adrenaline 3–5 mg IV or more have been used successfully.
  • Deliver rapid boluses up to 60 mL/kg of normal saline.

Adjunctive agents for specific indications:
- Laryngeal oedema
  - Give 1:1000 adrenaline 5 mg (5 mL) nebulised with oxygen.
  - Call the anaesthetist. Prepare for surgical airway.
- Wheeze and/or a history of asthma
  - Give hydrocortisone 200 mg IV or prednisone 50 mg PO.
  - Give nebulised salbutamol 5 mg and repeat up to continuously as necessary.
- H1 and or H2 antihistamines
  - Cetirizine 10 mg PO or fexofenadine 180 mg PO, plus ranitidine 150 mg PO are of no value during anaphylaxis. They may be given for a generalised cutaneous reaction alone, or as discharge medication following full recovery from the anaphylaxis.

Observation
- Observe patient closely for at least 4–6 hours after the resolution of all clinical features, as late deterioration may occur in up to 5% (known as biphasic anaphylaxis). If symptoms continue or recur, admit to ICU.
- Ensure an alert is placed in the patient's record and on the medication chart if allergy was caused by medication. Also document carefully the severity of the reaction, with exact description of what occurred when.
- Organise referral of all significant or recurrent attacks to an allergist, and arrange an EpiPen or Anapen prescription.
- Discuss an Anaphylaxis Management Plan with the patient prior to discharge.

Choking

A patient may choke on food or foreign material to cause a partial or complete airway obstruction.
- Allow the patient to clear the obstruction by coughing, which will usually be more effective than chest compression. Be prepared to assist if the patient has a weak cough or depressed consciousness.
- Give five firm blows to the back if the patient cannot breathe or cough. If this is unsuccessful, give five chest compressions, similar to CPR compressions, but performed more slowly with a more prolonged compression time.
- Continue this cycle until the obstruction is cleared or the patient becomes unconscious.
- If the patient becomes unconscious, commence CPR, suction the airway and, under direct visualisation at laryngoscopy, remove the foreign material with Magill forceps.
- Only use a finger sweep to clear an airway if solid material is visible and no equipment is to hand.

10

Acute respiratory failure

Acute respiratory failure causes hypoxia and/or impaired ventilation with hypercapnoea, leading to severe hypoxaemia and rapid deterioration in the patient's status.

The patient's own physiological mechanisms may compensate and prevent respiratory failure, depending on the severity of the insult and the patient's ability to increase the work and efficacy of breathing.

If compensation is insufficient, inadequate gas transfer and ventilation will lead to hypoxaemia and hypercarbia.

There are two main types of respiratory failure:
- **Type 1:** hypoxaemia with normal (or low) $PaCO_2$
  - Primarily a failure of oxygenation.
  - Usually responds to oxygen therapy.
- **Type 2:** hypoxaemia with an increased $PaCO_2$
  - Failure of ventilation as well as oxygenation.
  - Requires ventilatory assistance, as well as supplemental oxygen.

Confirm the diagnosis of acute respiratory failure by ABG determination. PO_2 <60 mmHg or PCO_2 >50 mmHg while breathing room air indicates respiratory failure. An associated pH <7.30 is also suggestive.

Causes of acute respiratory failure

See Chapter 9 and Chapter 15.
- **Airway obstruction** (any cause)
- **Pulmonary:**
  - Bronchospasm with wheeze (asthma, COPD, anaphylaxis)
  - Pneumonia, aspiration, pneumonitis, ARDS
  - Pneumothorax
  - Massive pleural effusion
  - Interstitial lung disease (sarcoid, autoimmune diseases, occupational, drugs, hypersensitivity, idiopathic)
  - Pulmonary hypertension

- **Cardiovascular:**
  - Acute pulmonary oedema (cardiogenic, occasionally non-cardiogenic)
  - PE
- **Neuromuscular:**
  - Depressed level of consciousness
  - Muscular weakness (Guillain–Barré syndrome, myasthenia gravis, muscular dystrophy)
  - Drug intoxication (opioid, sedative)
  - Poisoning (carbon monoxide, opioid)

Assessment of acute respiratory failure

Assess the work of breathing (degree of respiratory distress) and its efficacy at providing oxygenation, ventilation (exhaling CO_2), speech and cough. After this, determine the cause of the acute deterioration.

Work of breathing

Increased work of breathing is a physiological mechanism to compensate for an acute insult causing impaired respiratory function. Hypoxia and hypercarbia both stimulate the brain to increase the respiratory rate and respiratory effort. However, patients with acute respiratory failure secondary to a depressed conscious level (e.g. drug toxicity) may be unable to increase the work of breathing, as the physiological compensatory mechanisms are non-functional.

Signs associated with increased work of breathing (respiratory distress) include:
- Increased respiratory rate
- Use of accessory muscles
- Soft-tissue recession—tracheal tug, rib or abdominal recession
- Increased pulse rate
- Increased sweating or clammy skin
- Anxiety or agitation
- Exhaustion, confusion.

Effectiveness of respiratory function

Oxygenation is the most critical respiratory function. Assessing this is a priority, followed by adequacy of ventilation and removal of CO_2. Look for the following:
- **Hypoxia**
  - Cyanosis, low pulse oximetry (oxygen saturation <88%)
  - Cardiac ischaemia or arrhythmias from cardiac muscle hypoxia

- Anxiety, agitation or (later) depressed consciousness from cerebral hypoxia
- Acidosis from tissue hypoxia, usually a lactic acidosis
- Increased A–a gradient on ABG—if adequate oxygen saturation can be achieved only with high-flow oxygen, lung gas exchange must be significantly impaired
- **Hypoventilation**
  - Vasodilation
  - Headache, drowsiness and lethargy
  - Asterixis (tremor of fingers and hands, which is also seen in liver and renal failure)
  - Acidosis—respiratory acidosis from inadequate removal of CO_2; raised bicarbonate if chronically compensated
- **Mechanical compromise**
  - Inability to speak in sentences or to cough properly
  - Accumulation of secretions.

Respiratory decompensation

A severe or prolonged respiratory insult, with exhaustion or a reduction in the patient's physiological reserves, may lead to decompensation. Decompensation is associated with a decrease in both the work and the effectiveness of breathing.

   Signs of decompensation:
- Gasping respirations
- Decreased respiratory effort, even a silent chest
- Tachycardia followed by bradycardia (a preterminal sign) from worsening hypoxia
- Sweating, lethargy, apathy, drowsiness and coma
- Respiratory arrest followed by cardiac arrest.

   Call senior staff and a MET immediately to help with a patient who has any features of decompensation.

Diagnosing the cause

Look for these common conditions, which can rapidly progress to severe respiratory failure:
- Pneumonia
- Exacerbation of COPD
- Acute pulmonary oedema
- Asthma (a rising $PaCO_2$ is a late sign indicating imminent respiratory arrest)
- Pulmonary embolism
- Pneumothorax.

   Specific diagnostic features of these conditions are described in Chapter 15. Pulse oximetry, cardiac monitoring, ECG, ABG and a CXR are important in a patient with respiratory failure.

Management of acute respiratory failure

Management is carried out simultaneously with assessment of the patient. The underlying cause of the respiratory failure must be specifically addressed while optimising oxygenation and ventilation.

Oxygenation

- Use supplemental oxygen in all hypoxic patients (see Table 10.1), with high-flow oxygen at 15 L/min through a mask with a reservoir.
- The only exception is patients who chronically retain CO_2 (e.g. COPD) and who require a titrated, low-dose oxygen delivery system (Venturi mask).
- Table 10.1 is a guide only. Inspired oxygen concentration depends on the concentration delivered, the flow rate and positioning and the fit of the device on the face, balanced against the patient's ventilation (respiratory rate and tidal volume).
- Thus, a patient who is hypoventilating may receive a higher effective inspired oxygen concentration, whereas a hyperventilating patient will receive the opposite.
- The initial concentration of O_2 ordered depends on your judgement of how sick the patient is. An accurate enough assessment of oxygenation is made by pulse oximetry, although this provides no information about ventilation or pH.
- Blood gases are therefore necessary to determine the adequacy of ventilation. If adequate pulse oximetry is available, this blood gas can be a venous or arterial sample, as the minor differences between these should not influence immediate management decisions.

Titrated oxygen therapy

Some patients with COPD chronically hypoventilate and retain CO_2. Giving uncontrolled oxygen therapy to these patients may increase their $PaCO_2$. This will depress consciousness and further depress ventilation, with a vicious cycle leading to respiratory acidosis and worsening hypoxia. The excessive rise in $PaCO_2$ is caused by:

- Changes in pulmonary vasoconstriction, dead space and shunting i.e. V/Q mismatch
- Haldane effect (haemoglobin molecules release CO_2 in the presence of oxygen)
- Blunting of the hypoxic drive. These patients are dependent on mild hypoxia to stimulate the respiratory centre.

Check for any previous blood gas results. A patient with a recent low or normal $PaCO_2$ (and/or normal bicarbonate) is not a chronic CO_2

Table 10.1 **Oxygen delivery systems**

Delivery system	Oxygen flow (L/min)	Delivered oxygen concentration	Use
Nasal prongs	1	24%	Chronic administration in certain patients
	2	28%	Mouth breathing will decrease FiO_2
	3	32%	*Note:* higher flow rates are irritating to the nasal passages and do not significantly increase the FiO_2
	4	36%	
Simple mask	4	40%	General use
	6	45%	
	8	50%	
	10	55%	
	12	60%	
	14	65%	
Mask with reservoir ('non-rebreathing')	8	60%	High-concentration oxygen administration
	10	70%	
	15	80%	
Venturi mask	Flow varies according to setting on mask	24%	Titrated oxygen delivery, for CO_2 retainers in particular
		28%	
		35%	
		40%	
		(50%)	
		(60%)	

Least commonly-used Venturi mask sizes are in brackets.

retainer and does not require titrated oxygen therapy. If unsure, or there is documented chronic CO_2 retention, titrate oxygen therapy initially.

- Begin empirical O_2 treatment under pulse oximetry monitoring.
- Increase (or decrease) oxygen delivery until O_2 saturation is 88–92%. This is done by using differing oxygen mixers on a Venturi mask or by changing the oxygen flow rate through a simple mask if unavailable.
- Recheck the blood gases and watch for a change in PCO_2:
  - Continue with current therapy if CO_2 is normalising.
  - Decrease oxygen delivery if CO_2 is increasing, but maintain O_2 saturation 88–92% and recheck blood gases.
- If CO_2 is increasing, and you are unable to maintain oxygen saturation >88%, the patient may require assisted ventilation such

as non-invasive, bilevel (BiPAP) ventilation (see below). Get help urgently.

Controlled oxygen therapy is *not* given to a patient with acute CO_2 retention from acute pulmonary oedema, pneumonia, PE or asthma, as the PCO_2 is acutely raised by the impaired respiratory pathology, with no risk from blunting of any hypoxic drive. These patients require high-flow oxygen as a priority.

Ventilation

Ensure that the patient has not received opioids or other respiratory depressant drugs in the past 24 hours. Pupillary constriction may provide a clue that an opioid is responsible.

- Give naloxone 0.2 mg up to 2 mg IV, SC or IM every 5 minutes repeated until alert, but be careful not to precipitate an acute withdrawal reaction in the opiate-dependent patient. Start at 100 micrograms IV in those patients.
  Assisted manual ventilation:
- Bag-valve-mask assisted manual ventilation may be required in the patient with a depressed level of consciousness until definitive ventilation is provided.
- Consider non-invasive ventilation (NIV), such as continuous positive airway pressure (CPAP) ventilation or bilevel positive airway pressure (BiPAP) ventilation, if there is a rising PCO_2 or inadequate oxygenation despite maximal oxygen therapy.
  - NIV machines provide positive-pressure assistance through a closed gas circuit and tight-fitting mask. The patient derives benefit because:
    - Higher inspired oxygen, up to 100%, may be delivered, as it is a closed circuit
    - Less effort is required to ventilate the lungs, which helps a tiring patient
    - Reduced ventilation–perfusion mismatch, decreased airway collapse and decreased pulmonary congestion by reducing cardiac preload.

If there is no improvement, contact ICU and make arrangements for possible ETT intubation by an anaesthetist. Acute respiratory acidosis with a pH <7.2 usually requires mechanical ventilation until the precipitating cause of the respiratory deterioration can be reversed.

11

Acute circulatory failure

'Shock' is defined as acute circulatory failure leading to inadequate end-organ tissue perfusion with oxygen and nutrients. It is a clinical diagnosis, with a high mortality that depends on the underlying cause, its duration and response to treatment. See also Chapter 18.

It progresses from initial insult to compensated (reversible), decompensated (progressive) then finally refractory (irreversible) shock. A patient may present in any stage, but the aim is to identify abnormal tissue perfusion early, ideally before the SBP drops, treat aggressively and avoid the irreversible phase.

Compensatory mechanisms:
- Following the acute insult, physiological mechanisms initially compensate to combat the circulatory failure, including hyperventilation as a result of acidosis, sympathetic mediated tachycardia and vasoconstriction, and diversion of blood from the GI and renal tracts to the brain, heart and lungs.
- Success depends on the severity and duration of the insult, and the individual's physiological capacity to maintain cardiac output (CO).

Decompensated shock:
- When this compensation fails, inadequate tissue perfusion results in increasing anaerobic glycolysis and metabolic acidosis, cytokine-mediated cellular injury with fluid and protein leakage, and deteriorating CO from vascular dilation and myocardial depression.
- Eventually irreversible shock ensues, when vital organs fail and cell death is occurring.
- Severe and progressive shock states cause multiorgan failure syndrome (MOFS) or end in cardiac arrest with pulseless electrical activity. Once shock deteriorates to this degree, it is difficult or impossible to reverse.

Causes of acute circulatory failure

Pathophysiology
- Shock is directly related to the physiological determinants of BP, CO and total peripheral resistance (TPR).
- Tissue perfusion pressure relates to MAP, which depends on CO and TPR.

- In turn, the cardiac output CO = HR × SV.
- Stroke volume (SV) depends on the venous return or preload (a function of intravascular volume and free flow to the heart), cardiac function (rhythm, myocardial contractility and efficient cardiac valves) and afterload (aortic and pulmonary pressure).
- Thus, BP relates directly to the combination of cardiac function, TPR and venous return.

Classification

Shock can thus be classified using four broad categories: hypovolaemic shock ('insufficient circulatory volume'); cardiogenic shock ('pump failure'); distributive shock ('circulation unable to be filled'); and obstructive shock ('obstruction to circulation'); see Figure 11.1. Often, more than one mechanism is present.

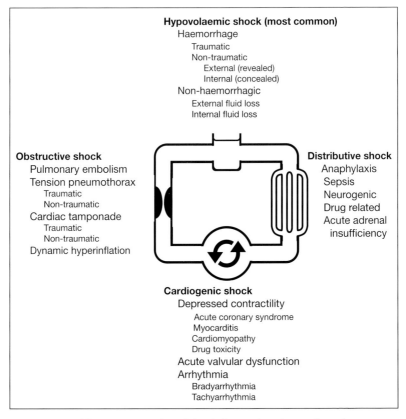

Figure 11.1 The four categories of shock (hypovolaemic, cardiogenic, distributive, obstructive). Copyright Tor Ercleve.

Note: the causes of shock have some similarities to the 4 Hs and 4 Ts of the potentially reversible causes of cardiac arrest (see Chapter 8).

Hypovolaemic shock (most common type)

• Haemorrhagic:
  • Traumatic
    – **External** (revealed): arterial laceration; limb amputation; compound fracture; scalping injury
    – **Internal** (concealed): haemothorax; haemoperitoneum (liver, spleen, mesentery); retroperitoneal haemorrhage (pelvis, aorta, renal); closed fracture
  • Non-traumatic
    – **External** (revealed): epistaxis; haemoptysis (bronchiectasis, cystic fibrosis, neoplasm, sarcoidosis, tuberculosis, other infections); GI bleed (haematemesis, PR bleeding); PV bleed (non-pregnant, pregnant or postpartum); haematuria (bladder neoplasm, prostatic hypertrophy, AV malformation)
    – **Internal** (concealed): haemothorax; haemoperitoneum (ruptured AAA, ruptured ectopic pregnancy, bleeding diathesis including anticoagulation, hepatic tumour or secondary, iatrogenic); retroperitoneal haemorrhage (ruptured AAA, bleeding diathesis including anticoagulation, renal, adrenal, spontaneous)
• Non-haemorrhagic:
  • **External** (e.g. GI losses from diarrhoea and vomiting, burns, severe skin disease, hyperthermia, high-output fistulae)
  • **Internal** (e.g. bowel obstruction, pancreatitis, other capillary leak syndromes)

Cardiogenic shock

• **Depressed contractility:**
  • Acute coronary syndrome (the most common cause), myocarditis, myocardial contusion, vasculitis, end-stage cardiomyopathy, drug overdose such as calcium antagonist or beta-blocker, severe acidaemia
• **Acute valvular dysfunction:**
  • Papillary muscle rupture, chordae tendineae rupture (e.g. ischaemia, trauma)
  • Acute valve leak (infective endocarditis)
  • Severe aortic stenosis (increased afterload), mitral stenosis
• **Arrhythmia:**
  • Tachycardia (ventricular, atrial fibrillation, SVT)
  • Bradycardia (heart block, sinus)

Distributive shock

- **Anaphylaxis:**
  - Vasodilation with increased capillary permeability
- **Sepsis:**
  - Vasodilation with increased capillary permeability, and cardiogenic dysfunction from myocardial depression
- **Neurogenic:**
  - Loss of sympathetic tone from high spinal cord trauma or epidural anaesthesia
    - *Note*: spinal shock refers to temporary recoverable spinal cord neurological dysfunction
- **Drug-related:**
  - Vasodilator antihypertensive agents, nitrates, strong analgesics, excessive sedation
- **Acute adrenal insufficiency:**
  - Discontinuing long-term steroids, inadequate steroid therapy, Addison's disease

Obstructive shock

- **Pulmonary embolism:**
  - Thrombotic, air, amniotic fluid, fat
- **Tension pneumothorax:**
  - Traumatic (penetrating or blunt)
  - Non-traumatic (e.g. severe asthma, COPD, mechanical ventilation, iatrogenic)
- **Cardiac tamponade:**
  - Traumatic (penetrating or blunt)
  - Non-traumatic (pericarditis, aortic dissection, uraemia, malignancy, post-surgery, postinfarction)
- **Dynamic hyperinflation:**
  - Excessive ventilation with severe bronchospasm (asthma, COPD)

Assessment of acute circulatory failure

Specific details on the assessment and treatment of shock are described in Chapter 18.

- Initially, assess shock severity according to the vital signs and degree of inadequate tissue perfusion.
- Start to identify the possible cause as described above by assessing volume status and JVP, and examining the ECG.
  - A low/non-visible JVP is seen in hypovolaemic and distributive shock.
  - A raised JVP is seen in cardiogenic and obstructive shock.

- A normal ECG makes cardiogenic shock highly unlikely, although ECG changes may be the cause or the effect of the shock state.

Assessing the severity of shock

Shock severity correlates with the degree of physiological compensation, which includes a complex activation of the sympathoadrenal autonomic nervous system to maintain BP.

With increasing severity of shock, the HR and RR increase, and there is progressive vasoconstriction to direct the remaining CO to the vital organs.

Minor insult (early)

The body's response to a minor insult is venoconstriction and increasing the heart and respiratory rates. The patient may be largely asymptomatic and only have abnormal vital signs on standing (orthostatic change).

- Always check a postural HR and BP:
  - Repeat the HR and BP after the patient sits or stands for *at least* 2 minutes (specifically ask the nurse to wait this long).
  - If the patient is unable to stand alone, ask for assistance or have the patient sit up with legs over the side of the bed.
  - An increase in HR >20 beats/min, a fall in SBP >20 mmHg or any fall in DBP indicates postural hypotension. This signifies intravascular volume depletion in the context of volume loss (hypovolaemia) or volume redistribution (early distributive shock).

Compensated shock

Initial vasoconstriction of skin and muscles leads to pallor, clamminess, cool mottled peripheries, agitation then lethargy.

- Assess the capillary refill time (CRT) by pressing on a nailbed (held at the level of the heart) for 5 seconds. Measure the time taken to refill the blanched area with blood. Over 2 seconds is regarded as prolonged and indicates hypoperfused or cool peripheries.
- As shock progresses, renal and splanchnic perfusion decrease, leading to reduced urine output and diminished gut motility. Measurement of urinary output is vital.

Decompensated shock

In severe shock, compensatory mechanisms are insufficient to maintain perfusing pressure to the heart and brain, leading to altered mental status, severe hypotension with cardiac ischaemia, anuria and gut ischaemia.

The absolute value of the SBP associated with poor perfusion varies greatly (see Chapter 18), but a SBP <90 mmHg is usually insufficient to maintain adequate vital organ perfusion.

Haemorrhagic shock

A simple classification of the severity of haemorrhagic shock in terms of the physiological and clinical manifestations as well as initial response to treatment is shown in Table 11.1. Treatment is best guided by the response to initial therapy (10–20 mL/kg of crystalloid followed early by blood), rather than simply the physiological and clinical features alone.

Assessment of volume status

In shock, accurate volume status assessment is essential to determine the cause (reduced preload signs occur in hypovolaemic and distributive shock) and to monitor treatment effects.

Normal fluid distribution within body compartments:
- The human body is composed mostly of water, with the total body water (TBW) of 42 L representing 60% of the weight of a 70 kg adult male (see Figure 11.2). This percentage is higher in infants and lower in adult women and the elderly.
- Two-thirds of this fluid (28 L) is intracellular (ICF) and one-third (14 L) is extracellular (ECF).
- Two-thirds (9 L) of the ECF is interstitial fluid, which bathes the cells and tissues, and one-third (5 L) is intravascular fluid, which comprises the blood and lymphatic system.
- Clinically, it is the ECF compartment consisting of intravascular and interstitial fluid that is assessed when determining the volume status of a patient.

Skin and mucous membranes:
- Volume status can be assessed by examining the oral mucous membranes.
- An adequately hydrated patient has moist mucous membranes and a small pool of saliva at the undersurface of the tongue in the area of the frenulum.
- Lack of axillary sweating or tears may suggest a fluid deficit.
- Check tissue turgor by raising a fold of skin from the anterior chest area over the sternal angle.
  - The skin should return promptly to its usual position in a normovolaemic patient.
  - A sluggish return suggests fluid deficit from dehydration.
- Intravascular volume:
  - This can be assessed by measuring CRT, HR, SBP, pulse pressure (widened in distributive shock, narrowed in hypovolaemic shock due to vasoconstriction), JVP (low in

Table 11.1 Classification of haemorrhagic shock

	Mild	Moderate	Severe
Percentage of circulating blood volume loss (normal 70 mL/kg or 5 L in average adult male)	<20% (<1 L)	20–40% (1–2 L)	>40% (>2 L)
Tissue perfusion	Non-essential tissue vasoconstriction (skin, muscles) Slight reduction urine output	Vasoconstriction of most vascular beds (decreased urine output, poor splanchnic perfusion) Trying to maintain vital organ perfusion	Critically inadequate vital organ perfusion
Vital signs	HR usually <100 beats/min Narrowed pulse pressure, but SBP maintained Postural changes in vital signs No significant tachypnoea	HR rises (>100 beats/min) SBP begins to fall Tachypnoea Oliguria Agitation and restlessness	HR >120 beats/min RR >30/min SBP <90 mmHg Anuria Coma (>50%/2.5 L loss)
Compensation	Fully compensated in most patients by veno- and vasoconstriction, and mild tachycardia	Patient will begin to decompensate in this range Occurs earlier in those with pre-existing altered/damaged physiology	Decompensated shock
Response to initial fluid resuscitation	Rapid response	Transient response (suggests ongoing loss or inadequate resuscitation) Needs blood or surgery	No response

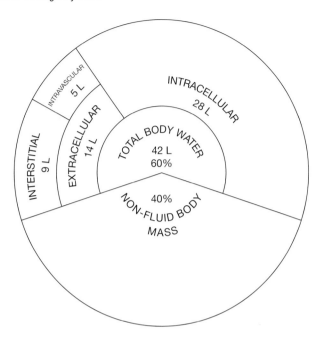

Figure 11.2 Fluid compartments totalling 42 L with their proportions in a 70-kg male

hypovolaemic or distributive shock; distended in cardiogenic or obstructive shock). See Box 11.1 and Figure 11.3.
  — *Note*: Kussmaul's sign is an unexpected rise in JVP on inspiration seen in obstructive shock (classically cardiac tamponade) and right ventricular failure. The JVP usually falls on inspiration.
- Volume overload:
  • Excessive volume causes a raised JVP, peripheral oedema with taut, non-compliant skin, pre-sacral or ankle oedema and an enlarged, tender liver with a positive hepatojugular reflux (pressing on the liver persistently elevates the JVP).
  • An S_3 gallop, lung crackles and pleural effusions are signs of pulmonary oedema from volume overload or cardiogenic shock.

Management of acute circulatory failure

- Management is carried out simultaneously with assessment of the patient.
- Treat the patient initially with oxygen and rapid IV fluid replacement (provided there is no evidence of cardiac failure).
- Call early for a senior doctor to help.

BOX 11.1 Assessment of jugular venous pressure

- The JVP can be assessed with the patient at any inclination from zero to 90 degrees. By tradition, begin looking for the JVP pulsation with the patient at a 45-degree inclination. Either the internal or the external jugular veins can be used.

- If unable to visualise the neck veins at 45 degrees, this signifies that the JVP is either low (in which case, lower the head of the bed) or high (in which case, sit the patient upright to see the top of the column of blood in the jugular vein).

- Once the jugular vein pulsation is identified, measure the perpendicular distance above the sternal angle to the top of the column of blood.

- This distance represents the patient's JVP in centimetres of water above the sternal angle. It represents a composite of the volume of venous return to the heart, the central venous pressure and the efficiency of right atrial and right ventricular emptying.

- A JVP of 2–3 cm above the sternal angle is normal in adult patients.

- A significantly volume-depleted patient has invisible, flat or empty neck veins, which may fill only when the patient is placed in the head-down, Trendelenburg position.

- Pressing on the abdomen induces the hepatojugular reflux, which increases the level of the JVP. This helps determine the level of the JVP if it is difficult to visualise, or temporarily raises a low JVP so that it becomes visible in the neck.

- A volume-overloaded patient has an elevated JVP > 3 cm above the sternal angle.

- A high JVP may only be visualised as a pulsating earlobe at 45 degrees, but the top should become visible when the patient sits fully upright.

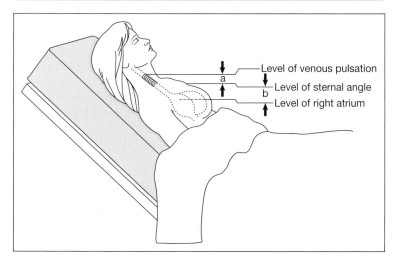

Figure 11.3 Measurement of jugular venous pressure. **a,** The perpendicular distance from the sternal angle to the top of the column of blood. **b,** The distance from the centre of the right atrium to the sternal angle, commonly accepted as measuring 5 cm, regardless of inclination.

- The underlying cause of the shock needs to be specifically sought and addressed, while optimising the cardiorespiratory function to prevent ongoing tissue damage from hypoperfusion and the development of irreversible end-organ damage.

Overview of shock management

- Ensure accurate haemodynamic monitoring:
  - Pulse oximetry, ECG, BP, urine output, invasive arterial and venous monitoring (ICU).
- Optimise oxygenation and ventilation:
  - High-flow oxygen and assisted ventilation (bag-valve-mask) if necessary.
- Optimise heart rate and rhythm:
  - Cardioversion of a cardiac tachyarrhythmia if causing hypotension.
  - Atropine, adrenaline and pacing if bradycardia causing hypotension.
- Optimise preload and haemoglobin:
  - Give 10–20 mL/kg normal saline rapidly IV and repeat until JVP is 3–5 cm above sternal angle.
    - *Note:* do not give fluids if JVP is already raised and the patient is in pulmonary oedema.
  - Give blood early for ongoing haemorrhage, and arrange urgent surgery according to the cause (ruptured spleen, AAA, ectopic etc). Aim for Hb >90–100 g/L.
- Optimise afterload:
  - Give a vasopressor if vasodilated from anaphylaxis or sepsis (e.g. adrenaline or noradrenaline infusion, respectively).
    - *Note:* do *not* use a vasopressor in hypovolaemia, particularly haemorrhagic shock. Address the underlying cause with blood or surgery.
- Optimise cardiac function:
  - Inotropic support (e.g. low-dose adrenaline, dobutamine or dopamine infusion) if still shocked despite above measures.
- Treat sepsis:
  - Give broad-spectrum antibiotics early if septic shock is suspected.

General principles when choosing intravenous fluids

The goal of fluid replacement therapy is to replenish the intravascular space to maintain cardiac preload. This ensures adequate end-organ perfusion and oxygenation, and decreases the risk of ischaemia or tissue infarction.

- Volume status abnormalities should be corrected at a rate similar to that at which they developed.

- Thus, in significant dehydration, it is safest to correct half the deficit, then re-evaluate. See Box 11.2 for an overview of fluid replacement in severe dehydration.
- There is no substitute for frequent, repeated examination of the patient at the bedside when effecting change in volume status.
- There are many replacement fluids to choose from (see Table 11.2). The correct choice is determined by:
  - Cause(s) of the fluid deficit
  - Aim(s) of the fluid replacement
  - Required rate and volume
  - Personal preference.

BOX 11.2　Fluid replacement in severe dehydration

1. Resuscitate the intravascular volume with 20 mL/kg boluses of crystalloid until perfusion is normalised. If more than 60 mL/kg is required, check Hb to determine need for blood transfusion. Normal saline is the first-line resuscitation agent.

2. Calculate fluid losses (generally at least 10% body weight if the patient with dehydration is hypotensive). Thus a 70-kg patient will be depleted of at least 7 L of body fluid.

3. Subtract from this deficit the amount of fluid already given for resuscitation. If 2 L of fluid was required for resuscitation, a further 5 L needs to be replenished.

4. Replace this fluid over the next 24 hours, together with maintenance fluid and ongoing losses, approx 110 mL/h. For example:
   - 5 L of lost fluid remaining
   - Maintenance for a 70-kg person approx 2.5 L/day
   - Assume no abnormal ongoing losses
   - Total to be replaced over next 24 hours is thus 7.5 L.

5. Replace half of this in the first 8 hours, the remainder in the next 16 hours. Therefore:
   - 3.75 L over 8 hours (i.e. ≈ 450 mL/h)
   - 3.75 L over next 16 hours (i.e. ≈ 230 mL/h).

6. Monitor the adequacy of replacement by:
   - Perfusion and vital signs
   - Urine output
   - Electrolyte changes.

7. Speed of fluid replacement will depend on:
   - Rapidity of progression of the dehydration. Generally, the faster it has occurred, the faster it can be corrected.
   - Severity of haemodynamic compromise. The more severe the insult, the faster it should be corrected.
   - Comorbidities that restrict aggressive fluid infusions. Patients with cardiac, renal or hepatic impairment may need to have their dehydration corrected slowly over 48 hours, to avoid large fluid and electrolyte shifts, acute pulmonary oedema and/or CCF.

Table 11.2 Composition of commonly used intravenous fluids

	Na (mmol/L)	Cl (mmol/L)	K (mmol/L)	Ca (mmol/L)	Mg (mmol/L)	Other constituents	Osmolarity mOsm/L (osmolality mOsm/kg)	pH
Crystalloids								
Compound sodium lactate (Hartmann's solution)	131	111	5	2	—	29 mmol/L lactate	280 (254)	5.0–7.0
Modified Hartmann's	131	135	29.5	2	—	29 mmol/L lactate	329 (304)	
Ringer's lactate	130	109	4	3	—	28 mmol/L lactate	272	
0.9% sodium chloride (normal saline)	154	154	—	—	—	—	308 (300)	6.0–7.5
0.45% sodium chloride (half normal saline)	77	77	—	—	—	—	154 (150)	4.0–7.0
5% dextrose	—	—	—	—	—	50 g/L dextrose	278 (252)	3.5–6.5
10% dextrose	—	—	—	—	—	100 g/L dextrose	556 (505)	3.5–6.5
50% dextrose	—	—	—	—	—	500 g/L dextrose	2778 (2525)	3.5–6.5

Table 11.2 Composition of commonly used intravenous fluids—cont'd

	Na (mmol/L)	Cl (mmol/L)	K (mmol/L)	Ca (mmol/L)	Mg (mmol/L)	Other constituents	Osmolarity mOsm/L (osmolality mOsm/kg)	pH
3.3% dextrose, 0.3% sodium chloride ('3 and a 1/3')	51	51	—	—	—	33 g/L dextrose	286 (284)	3.5–6.5
4% dextrose, 0.18% sodium chloride ('4 and a 1/5')	30	30	—	—	—	40 g/L dextrose	284 (282)	3.5–6.5
8.4% sodium bicarbonate	1000	—	—	—	—	1000 mmol/L HCO_3^-	—	—
Plasma-Lyte 148	140	98	5	—	1.5	27 mmol/L acetate; 23 mmol/L gluconate	294 (294)	6.5–8.0
Plasma-Lyte 148-replacement and glucose 5%	140	98	5	—	1.5	27 mmol/L acetate; 23 mmol/L gluconate; 50 g/L dextrose	547 (573)	4.0–6.0
Plasma-Lyte 56-maintenance and 5% glucose	40	40	13	—	1.5	16 mmol/L acetate; 50 g/L dextrose	363 (401)	

Continued

SECTION B – Emergency calls

SECTION B – Emergency calls

Table 11.2 Composition of commonly used intravenous fluids—cont'd

	Na (mmol/L)	Cl (mmol/L)	K (mmol/L)	Ca (mmol/L)	Mg (mmol/L)	Other constituents	Osmolarity mOsm/L (osmolality mOsm/kg)	pH
Colloids								
Albumin 4%	140	128	<2	—	—	40 g/L albumin; 6.4 mmol/L octanoate	260	6.7–7.3
Gelofusine	154	120	—	—	—	40 g/L succinylated gelatin	274	7.4±0.3
Dextran 40 in 0.9% saline	150	150	—	—	—	Dextran 40 g/L	(325)	6.0
Dextran 40 in 5% dextrose	—	—	—	—	—	Dextran 40 g/L; dextrose 50 g/L	(349)	5.0
Dextran 70 in 0.9% saline	150	150	—	—	—	Dextran 70 g/L	(306)	6.0
Dextran 70 in 5% dextrose	—	—	—	—	—	Dextran 70 g/L; dextrose 50 g/L	(325)	4.5

Note: Some texts will refer to osmolarity and some to osmolality when discussing composition of electrolyte solutions. We have given both where available.

- The replacement fluid should be isotonic, with roughly the same solute concentration as blood to minimise fluid shifts.
- The time over which the fluid is replaced is variable and depends on both the rapidity and the severity of the deficit, the type of fluid lost and the ability of the patient to tolerate large volumes of fluid.
- Frequent re-evaluation of the patient's response to fluid administration ensures a balance between adequate rehydration and the risk of overhydration.

Three plasma solutes—sodium, albumin (or other colloids) and glucose—must be considered to correctly diagnose and treat disorders of fluid balance. Sodium is limited primarily to the extracellular space, whereas colloids remain longer in the intravascular space. However, glucose distributes widely throughout both the intracellular and the extracellular spaces and so is of no value in acute volume resuscitation.

Crystalloid is the most widely used fluid replacement. It is readily available, inexpensive and suitable as a primary replacement fluid, volume expander and maintenance fluid.

- **Normal saline** has an osmolality of 300 mOsm/kg and, although slightly hypertonic, is not sufficiently different from blood tonicity to cause cell shrinkage.
  - It stays predominantly in the extracellular space and is therefore useful as an intravascular volume expander.
  - The half-life of normal saline in the intravascular space is around 1–3 hours.
  - As normal saline is more readily available and inexpensive, it is the treatment of choice for the initial resuscitation of a volume-depleted patient.

Colloids stay in the intravascular space for many hours as they are larger molecules that do not readily traverse the endothelial pores of the blood vessels.

- The half-life of albumin within the intravascular space is 17–20 hours.
- Colloids can be used in place of normal saline, although they are more expensive, and may cause an allergic reaction.

5% dextrose consists of 50 g of dextrose dissolved in 1 L of water.

- It is iso-osmolar, and equilibrates rapidly among the intravascular, interstitial and intracellular spaces, with water following quickly by osmosis.
- Infusion of 5% dextrose does *not* support the intravascular volume, as the glucose and water re-distribute rapidly throughout the interstitial and extravascular spaces, leaving the intravascular compartment. It therefore has no role in fluid resuscitation for shock.

12

Disability: acute neurological failure

Coma implies unresponsiveness with significant depression of the level of consciousness. It is potentially life-threatening due to its immediate effects on airway, breathing and circulation, irrespective of the underlying cause(s).

A patient is regarded as comatose if requiring a painful stimulus to rouse or if the Glasgow Coma Scale (GCS) score is 8 or less (see Table 7.2 in Chapter 7). Urgent active assessment and support of the airway, respiration and circulatory functions are essential, if a rapidly reversible cause is not found and treated (such as hypoglycaemia or opioid toxicity).

Immediate risks from coma:
- **Airway**
  - Decrease in the tone of the palatal, tongue and pharyngeal muscles, with resultant airway obstruction.
  - Depressed protective airway reflexes with the risk of pulmonary aspiration of oral secretions or gastric contents.
- **Breathing**
  - Depression of the brainstem respiratory centres, resulting in hypoventilation. When severe, the rise in accumulating CO_2 leads to respiratory acidosis and worsening hypoxia.
- **Circulation**
  - Cardiovascular depression with resultant hypoperfusion of tissues.

Causes of acute neurological failure

See Chapter 20 for a full discussion of the aetiology and management of an altered mental status. Important causes that should be considered rapidly at the bedside include:
- Hypoglycaemia
- Opioid/sedative toxicity
- Hypoxia/respiratory failure
- Hypoperfusion
- Stroke such as intracerebral bleed or subarachnoid haemorrhage

- CNS infection such as meningitis
- CNS trauma such as an epidural or subdural haematoma
- Post-ictal state (search for the underlying cause of the seizure)
- Hyperthermia, including sepsis
- Hepatic, renal or endocrine failure.

Assessment of acute neurological failure

Airway, breathing, circulation
The initial assessment and management of ABC are of paramount importance. After oxygenation and perfusion are stabilised, rapid assessment of depressed consciousness involves the following.

Disability
Verify the degree of depression of the level of consciousness:
- Objective assessment is made using the GCS score.
- A more rapid, but less meaningful, alternative is to use the AVPU scale:
  - Alert, responds to Voice, responds to Pain, Unresponsive.
- Use a noxious stimulus to confirm unresponsiveness if the patient fails to respond to verbal stimuli:
  - Sternal rub
  - Supraorbital nerve pressure
  - Earlobe pressure
  - Corneal reflex using a wisp of cotton or tissue.

Environment, exposure and extended examination
Assess rapidly for a cause:
- Temperature
- Fingerprick glucose
- Focused neurological examination:
  - Pupillary constriction suggests opioid toxicity or brainstem pathology.
  - Neck stiffness suggests meningitis or SAH.
  - Subtle facial or ocular twitching suggests ongoing seizure activity.
  - Evidence of head or spine trauma—palpate the skull and neck, and look in the ears for haemotympanum (basal skull fracture).
  - Lateralising signs including on fundoscopy, indicating a possible stroke or intracranial space occupying lesion.

Management of acute neurological failure

Management is carried out simultaneously with assessment of the patient. The underlying specific cause(s) of depressed consciousness must be diagnosed and addressed. Make certain you have called your senior.

Early coma management aims to stabilise the airway, breathing and circulation, which may treat the cause and will also help prevent secondary brain injury from hypoxia, hypoperfusion, seizures and hyperthermia.

Immediate management includes:
- Supplemental oxygen with pulse oximetry monitoring.
- Spinal immobilisation (if possibility of trauma).
- Non-invasive ECG and BP monitoring.
- Reliable IV access.
- Giving 50 mL of 50% glucose IV (if fingerprick glucose <2.5 mmol/L).
  - Administer thiamine 250 mg IV prior to this if the patient is alcoholic or appears malnourished, to avoid precipitating Wernicke's encephalopathy.
- Titrating 200-microgram boluses of naloxone IV every 5 minutes (if evidence of opioid toxicity).
- Rapid IV fluid resuscitation (if hypotensive or shocked).
- Antibiotics (if fever and/or neck stiffness—see Chapter 22).
- Commencing cooling or warming (if temperature abnormal).
- Ordering an urgent CT scan in an unresponsive patient with any evidence of head trauma, lateralising neurological signs suggestive of an intracranial pathological feature or undiagnosed coma (discuss with your senior).

13

Environment, exposure and examination

Once the primary survey has been performed in the critically ill patient, and airway, breathing, circulation and disability have been stabilised, re-evaluate the patient using a systematic approach. The physical and physiological environment of the patient must be assessed with the patient fully undressed to complete a full physical examination (secondary survey), together with bedside investigations.

If the patient's condition deteriorates, or undergoes a major therapeutic intervention or procedure, repeat the primary survey again to re-assess the ABCDE. Keep doing this until the patient's condition has stabilised.

Environment

The patient's environment includes the physical (temperature) and physiological (blood glucose, electrolytes, toxins etc), as well as ongoing documentation of all the findings.
- Measure the temperature accurately. In critically ill patients, invasive temperature monitoring using rectal, bladder or oesophageal probes is used in ICU.
- Assess the patient for potential drug toxicity and clinical toxidromes (symptoms and signs characteristic of a certain poisoning).

Assessment of the physiological environment also requires the use of investigations. **Bedside tests** to perform early in all critically ill patients include:
- Pulse oximetry
- Fingerprick glucose
- VBG or ABG
- Spirometry if available
- Urinalysis and monitoring of urine output
- Electrocardiogram (ECG)
- Chest X-ray (CXR).

Laboratory tests include:
• Full blood count (FBC)
• Electrolytes
• Liver function tests (LFTs) (coagulation profile is rarely indicated or helpful)
• Blood cultures (sepsis suspected)
• Blood levels (of a measurable drug thought to be causal).
  Other investigations may include:
• Computed tomography (CT) head scan or lumbar puncture (LP), which will depend on the likely causes to be ruled out.

Exposure and examination

The patient must be completely undressed for a proper physical examination:
• Head and neck—including ears, nose, teeth, oral cavity
• Chest
• Abdomen
• Perineum—including rectal and vaginal examinations as appropriate
• Back—may require a 'log roll' in trauma cases to keep the patient's spinal column straight and protected
• Limbs—including peripheral circulation, skin, muscles, bones, joints
• CNS—including eyes and cranial nerves, limbs and higher cerebral functions.

During this time, a full history should be obtained from the patient or by using as many collateral sources of information as possible, including the nursing staff, other patients, relatives or friends, paramedics (if just arrived on the ward), medical records, laboratory and imaging reports. Sometimes it is justified to contact medical staff who have recently seen the patient (particularly those already on call).

Once this has been done, there is usually sufficient information to develop a working diagnosis and commence specific management. Make certain you have contacted your senior early.

14

Hospital-based emergency response codes

The emergency codes are hospital-based responses to critical internal or external events. Each is colour-coded according to the Australian Standards Association (AS 4083-2010).

The most commonly encountered are Code Blue (medical emergency) and Code Black (personal threat). The codes are usually activated by calling the switchboard emergency number. Switchboard will then continue the cascade of calls to the appropriate personnel for that code.

You may be the person to call a code or be allocated a role within the response. As these are uncommon events, most hospital wards or departments have a folder of all the actions needed for each code.

Look at this as soon as you commence working in a new ward area and refer to it when required. Take advice from senior staff.

Emergencies can be divided into four distinct phases:

1. **Prevention**—identification of potential hazards and minimising their impact. This means using the Medical Emergency Team (MET) activation criteria in a medical emergency, rather than leaving it until full cardiac arrest ensues.
2. **Preparation**—the response must be functional even when minimal personnel are present, using the resources that are on site, as an event can occur at any time. This often means the on-call doctor plays a significant role.
3. **Response**—emergency procedure manuals are available in all ward and department areas, with action cards that detail individual roles. These events are uncommon and the details are hard to memorise, so make use of the cards.
4. **Recovery**—return to normal conditions once the crisis is over. Includes debriefing and a review to improve the system for the next episode.

Code Blue (medical emergency)

Code Blue is usually called to prevent critical deterioration in a patient's condition to *avert* the risk of cardiac arrest. However, some hospitals only call this in *response* to cardiac arrest.

* You may be the one to call a medical emergency if a patient you are treating deteriorates or you may be a part of the response team that is called to a ward, usually by the nursing staff.
* You should be familiar with the requirements for activation, as well as your initial role and response when you arrive at a Code Blue as part of the MET or a Cardiac Arrest Team (see Chapter 7).

Code Black (personal threat)

It is exceedingly uncommon to be involved in an armed confrontation or 'hold-up' in hospital. Your role is not to subdue the aggressor—do what you are told!

* Ensure a Code Black has been activated and keep yourself, other staff and patients out of danger. This may require alerting other staff to call the Switchboard, using hidden distress alarms or calling Switchboard yourself if it is safe to do so.
* Much more common is a patient (or relative) who exhibits offensive, agitated or aggressive behaviour because of medical or psychiatric illness, drug intoxication, personality disorder or frustration.
  * A Code Black should be activated while staying out of danger. In certain circumstances, attempting to calm the aggressor may be appropriate, depending on the potential danger, the person's level of arousal and the precipitating event.
* Never tackle a patient alone, however small or frail-looking. You will get hurt or cause harm. Await the arrival of security staff.

Code Red (fire/smoke)

You are usually not required to attend this Code, but you may be the person activating it. If you discover a fire, the following should be done (RACE):

* **Remove** anyone from immediate danger.
* **Activate** the Code Red by calling Switchboard.
* **Contain** the fire by closing doors and windows.
* **Extinguish** the fire (if smaller than a wastepaper basket and safe to do so).

Following these actions, you should remain out of danger and take instructions from the emergency service personnel.

Code Purple (bomb threat)

You might be the person who receives the telephone threat. You need to alert staff to activate a Code Purple via Switchboard, while asking pertinent questions of the caller regarding the bomb (e.g. time of detonation, location, appearance, type of bomb, detonating mechanism).

After the caller has hung up, *do not* hang up the phone—wait for the arrival of the emergency response team.

Code Yellow (internal emergency)

A Code Yellow is called in response to an infrastructure failure such as electricity, gases, water or drainage. It will usually require engineering and security staff, rather than being a medical problem.

You should take directions from the emergency response team.

Code Orange (evacuation)

A Code Orange may follow a Code Red, Purple or Yellow. You should be under the direction of the emergency response team when helping evacuate the hospital. In general, this means assisting staff to move patients:

- Away from immediate danger
- Laterally on the same level
- Vertically down stairwells (e.g. through a set of fire doors)
- Out of the building to an external evacuation point.

You should take instructions from senior staff during these episodes.

Code Brown (external emergency)

Each hospital will have its own plan for coping with large numbers of patients from a mass casualty incident, known as a Major Disaster Plan, that is centred around the Emergency Department.

It is likely you will form part of this plan, and your roles and responsibilities are summarised on action cards.

Make certain that Switchboard has a reliable contact telephone number for the purpose of an emergency call-out. In addition, make sure you know where the Major Disaster Plan information is located and understand your role within that plan.

SECTION B – Emergency calls

Common calls

15

Shortness of breath, cough and haemoptysis

Calls to a patient with respiratory difficulty are common. The most important causes of SOB in hospitalised patients are upper airway obstruction, acute pulmonary oedema, PE, pneumonia and broncho-spasm from severe asthma or COPD, particularly with sudden pneumothorax.

Phone call

Questions

1. **Is the patient cyanosed?** Central cyanosis indicates significant hypoxia and necessitates immediate patient review.
2. **How long has the patient had SOB?** Sudden onset of SOB suggests PE or a pneumothorax and also requires immediate review.
3. **What are the vital signs?**
4. **Are there any associated symptoms?** Additional symptoms of chest pain, cough, fever, stridor, wheeze and facial oedema help define the cause.
5. **Does the patient have a history of heart failure or acute pulmonary oedema, or of asthma or bronchitis (COPD)?** Patients who retain carbon dioxide (CO_2) ('blue bloater') depend on a hypoxic respiratory drive and must be given controlled oxygen at no more than 28% initially.
6. **What was the reason for admission?**
7. **Does the patient have massive haemoptysis?** Significant bleeding requires immediate assessment.

Instructions

- Ask for measurement of the oxygen saturation by non-invasive pulse oximetry.
- Give oxygen by mask to maintain saturation >95%.
  - Request as high a concentration of O_2 in the short term, unless the patient has significant COPD, in which case specify 28% O_2 by Venturi mask and reassess at the bedside.

- Ask the nurse to bring the resuscitation trolley to the bedside, attach an ECG monitor to the patient and gain IV access.
- Request nebulised salbutamol 5 mg (1 mL) diluted with 3 mL of normal saline if the patient has asthma or wheeze.
- Request GTN SL (0.4 mg by spray or 0.6 mg tablet) if the patient is hypertensive, has chest pain or a history of heart failure. Repeat in 5–10 minutes provided the SBP remains >100 mmHg.
- Request an urgent CXR if the patient is tachypnoeic, tachycardic, hypoxic or confused.

Prioritisation

See the patient with upper airway compromise, SOB or massive hae-moptysis immediately. Patients with cough or blood-streaked sputum but without respiratory distress may be seen less urgently.

Corridor thoughts

What causes shortness of breath? (* = major threat to life)
- **Pulmonary causes:**
  - Pneumonia*
  - Bronchospasm with wheeze (asthma*, COPD*, anaphylaxis*)
  - Pneumothorax
  - Massive pleural effusion
  - Aspiration of gastric contents or other foreign material
  - Collapse or atelectasis, especially postoperatively
  - Interstitial lung disease (sarcoid, autoimmune diseases, occupational, drugs, hypersensitivity, idiopathic)
  - Pulmonary hypertension
- **Cardiovascular causes:**
  - Acute pulmonary oedema*
  - PE*
  - Cardiac tamponade* (shock usually dominates—see Chapter 11)
- **Miscellaneous causes:**
  - Upper airway obstruction* (with stridor)
  - Metabolic acidosis* (DKA, sepsis)
  - Neuromuscular weakness* (Guillain–Barré syndrome, myasthenia gravis, muscular dystrophy)
  - Anaemia
  - Hyperthyroidism
  - Poisoning* (aspirin, carbon monoxide)
  - Massive ascites
  - Pregnancy (physiological tachypnoea)
  - Anxiety (diagnosis of exclusion *only*)

What causes cough? (* = major threat to life)
- Any of the cardiopulmonary causes above
- Upper airway stimuli:
  - Viral illness or postviral syndromes
  - Sinusitis
  - Gastro-oesophageal reflux
  - Inhalational injury*
  - Allergy*
  - Malignancy*
  - ACE inhibitors (plus angio-oedema*)
  - Anxiety, tics

What causes haemoptysis? (* = major threat to life)
- Chest infection, including pneumonia*, COPD* and TB*
- Lung cancer*
- Benign tumours or arteriovenous malformations
- PE* (pulmonary infarction)
- Bronchiectasis
- Acute pulmonary oedema* (blood-stained frothy sputum)
- Pulmonary vasculitis* (Goodpasture, Wegener)
- Pulmonary hypertension, including mitral stenosis
- Upper airway origin*
- Foreign body* (especially children)

Major threat to life

- **Hypoxia with inadequate tissue oxygenation**
- **Upper airway failure** (see Chapter 9)
- **Acute respiratory failure** (see Chapter 10)
- **Tension pneumothorax** results from increased intrathoracic pressure that decreases venous return to the heart with compression of the ipsilateral lung, causing hypotension and hypoxia with extreme respiratory distress
- **Massive haemoptysis**
  - Haemoptysis of 100–200 mL can cause complete airway flooding and asphyxiation

Bedside

Quick-look test
Does the patient look well (comfortable), sick (uncomfortable or distressed) or critical (about to die)?
Hypoxia causes cyanosis, agitation and altered mental status with confusion. Life-threatening CO_2 retention causes tachypnoea, lethargy and depressed consciousness, but note that hypoventilation of itself is a

cause of CO_2 retention. A patient who is volume-overloaded looks puffy, anxious and restless and sits upright.

Airway and vital signs

Is the patient ventilating adequately?
This requires both a patent airway **and** effective breathing effort.
- Is the airway patent? (see Chapter 9)
  - Suspect upper airway obstruction if the patient is making breathing efforts (tachypnoea, agitation, increased work of breathing), but has noisy breathing (stridor) and impaired air entry.
- Upper airway obstruction may be caused by:
  - Pharyngeal soft-tissue obstruction from loss of airway tone in coma
  - Infection such as croup or epiglottitis (now rare with Hib vaccine)
  - Angio-oedema from anaphylaxis or medications (ACE inhibitors)
  - Food bolus or other foreign material in the posterior pharynx, larynx or trachea
  - Burns secondary to inhalational injury or caustic ingestion
  - Tumour
  - Laryngospasm due to aspiration.

What is the respiratory rate and pattern?
- Is the patient making adequate breathing efforts (see Chapter 10)?
- RR <10 breaths/min suggests central depression of ventilation, usually due to an intracerebral event, drug toxicity (e.g. opioid) or profound hypercarbia with CNS depression.
- RR >20 breaths/min suggests increased work of breathing secondary to hypoxia, acidosis, reflex stimulation or pain. Anxiety is a diagnosis of exclusion *only*.
- Look out for thoraco-abdominal dissociation, which inhibits adequate gas exchange. The chest cage and abdominal wall normally move in the same direction; if they are not synchronised (see-saw movements), suspect acute respiratory failure.
- Look for unequal chest expansion associated with hyperresonance and hyperinflation with tracheal deviation to the opposite side (tension pneumothorax).

What is the heart rate?
- Sinus tachycardia accompanies hypoxia. Vascular beds supplying hypoxic tissue dilate, and a compensatory sinus tachycardia occurs in an effort to increase cardiac output and thereby improve oxygen delivery.
  - Bradycardia from hypoxia is a preterminal event.
- Tachycardia is also associated with fever (pneumonia), PE, shock, ACS, CCF, arrhythmias and beta-agonist therapy (asthma/COPD).

What is the blood pressure?
- Hypotension may indicate tension pneumothorax, cardiac tamponade, massive PE, septic shock, cardiogenic shock or occult haemorrhage.
- Hypertension may be associated with acute respiratory distress, in particular acute pulmonary oedema.

What is the JVP?
- A raised JVP suggests a massive PE, cardiogenic shock, tension pneumothorax or cardiac tamponade.

What is the temperature?
- An elevated temperature suggests infection (pneumonia, bronchitis or bronchiectasis). A low-grade fever also occurs with a PE, particularly in those aged under 35 years.

Selective physical examination

Vitals	Repeat now
Mental	Check the level of consciousness—is the patient alert, confused, drowsy or unresponsive?
	Agitation, confusion (hypoxia), depressed conscious level (CO_2 retention)
HEENT	Check for central cyanosis (blue-tinged tongue and mucous membranes).
	Cyanosis does not occur until there is severe Hb desaturation of at least 50 g/L (5 g/dL), so may not occur at all in an anaemic patient.
	If hypoxia is suspected, confirm by pulse oximetry (an ABG measurement is not immediately necessary).
	Remember: cyanosis is ominous if it is present, but its absence does not mean that the PO_2 is adequate.
Resp	Check for wheeze, crackles, consolidation (bronchial breathing), pneumothorax or pleural effusion (absent).

Management

Immediate management of the hypoxic patient
- **If the patient is not breathing or is making inadequate breathing efforts**, perform a head tilt–chin lift or a jaw thrust to open the airway and begin ventilation with a bag-mask device connected to high-dose oxygen.
  - Call your senior and intensive care or anaesthetics immediately.
- **Ensure the airway is clear of foreign material using suction.** Insert an oropharyngeal airway if tolerated by the patient.
  - Endotracheal intubation will need to be performed only by an experienced airway doctor.

- Do not interfere if the patient is coughing and able to clear the airway. Treat as per choking (Chapter 9) if the coughing becomes ineffective or the patient loses consciousness.
- **If the patient is making adequate respiratory efforts:**
  - **Deliver enough oxygen:**
    - Give 4–15 L/min oxygen by mask to keep oxygen saturation >95%.
    - Titrating oxygen therapy occurs once the patient is stabilised and further information is gained regarding the possibility of chronic ventilatory failure (hypoxic drive).
  - **Evaluate adequacy of oxygen delivery:**
    - Attach pulse oximetry—this estimates the arterial Hb saturation (SaO_2), which is closely linked to the PaO_2. SaO_2 saturation <88% indicates a PaO_2 <60 mmHg (8 kPa).
- Obtain IV access, take blood for FBC, U&E, request a portable CXR and perform an ECG.
- Obtain a VBG, or ABG—will help determine respiratory acidosis and assist in accurately titrating the supplied oxygen to achieve PaO_2 >60 mmHg or SaO_2 >88%.
- Provide urgent intervention for life-threatening causes:
  - When tension pneumothorax is suspected, immediate needle decompression of the chest is necessary if the patient is in extreme respiratory distress or hypotense. Insert a wide-bore cannula into the second intercostal space in the mid-clavicular line.
  - Give nebulised salbutamol 5 mg diluted in 3 mL of normal saline for wheeze.
  - Give GTN 0.6 mg SL and repeat twice further, provided SBP is >100 mmHg, if chest has crackles and acute pulmonary oedema suspected.

Selective history and chart review

Further refine your differential diagnosis following immediate management and stabilisation to determine why the patient is short of breath or hypoxic.

Was the onset of SOB gradual or sudden?
- Sudden onset occurs in pneumothorax, PE and inhaled foreign body. Rapid progression over a few minutes occurs with acute LVF. Gradual onset occurs in pneumonia.
- Ask about a history of increased SOB when lying flat (orthopnoea) and night waking with acute respiratory distress (PND); both are associated with LV failure.

Does the patient have chest pain, and what is its nature?
- Central, heavy chest pain radiating to the neck, jaw or arms suggests the possibility of ACS and LVF.
- Pleuritic chest pain with associated SOB may indicate pneumonia, PE or pneumothorax.
  - PE is characterised by sudden SOB with non-radiating chest pain, which can be a central, constant ache or lateral pleuritic pain.

Is there a cough, and is it productive of sputum?
- Coloured sputum (green, yellow, brown or blood-streaked) suggests an infective source.
- Blood-stained frothy sputum is usually associated with acute LVF.
- Mucoid sputum, produced on a regular basis, is most commonly associated with chronic bronchitis.
- Dry, persistent cough may be caused by an ACE inhibitor, asthma, sinusitis, postviral syndrome or gastro-oesophageal reflux.

Has there been any haemoptysis? What was its estimated volume?
- Enquire about a history of malignancy, TB, pulmonary vasculitis or pulmonary hypertension.
- A history of chest pain, SOB and haemoptysis is characteristic of PE. However, the majority of PEs do not cause pulmonary infarction and therefore haemoptysis is rare.

Is there any audible wheeze?
- This is usually a sign of reversible airway obstruction in patients with a known history of asthma or COPD.
- Bronchospasm can also occur in LVF, PE, inhalational injury or anaphylaxis (look for cutaneous signs of urticaria or erythema).

Is there fever or chills?
- Fever and chills suggest a respiratory infection. Check the temperature chart since admission.
- PE and postoperative atelectasis are also associated with low-grade fever.

Has the patient had recent surgery?
- All postoperative patients are at risk of atelectasis with collapse-consolidation and/or a PE.
- Thoracic surgery increases the possibility of pneumothorax, haemothorax and cardiac tamponade as postoperative complications.
- Breathing is often painful after abdominal surgery. Splinting with poor lung expansion is the rule, which increases the likelihood of postoperative atelectasis and pneumonia.
- Abdominal distension secondary to ileus or bowel obstruction also leads to reduced lung ventilation and dyspnoea.

Has a central line been placed recently?
- CVL placement may be associated with iatrogenic pneumothorax (common) or cardiac tamponade (rare).

SECTION C – Common calls

Confirm any past medical history or presenting problem that may be the cause of the symptoms. For example:

- Asthma or COPD
- Heart failure, hypertension or cardiac disorder (acute LVF)
- Thromboembolic disease or risk factors predisposing to PE (see Table 15.1)
- Chronic lung disease such as bronchiectasis, recent episodes of unconsciousness with possible aspiration, or immunosuppression predisposing to chest infection
- Recent CVL placement causing pneumothorax
- TB, cancer or bronchiectasis causing massive haemoptysis.

Check the observation chart

- Check previous vital signs to determine whether this is an acute change or a gradual deterioration.
- Review the fluid balance. Progressive weight gain or persistent positive fluid balance may be associated with fluid overload and acute LVF.

Table 15.1 Risk factors for venous thromboembolism

Acute provoking factors

Hospitalisation (i.e. reduced mobility)

Surgery—particularly abdominal, pelvic or leg

Trauma or fracture of lower limbs or pelvis

Immobilisation (including plaster cast)

Long-haul travel (>5000 km)

Recently commenced oestrogen therapy (e.g. within previous 2 weeks)

Intravascular device (e.g. venous catheter)

Chronic predisposing factors

Inherited	Acquired	Inherited or acquired
Natural anticoagulant deficiency such as protein C, protein S, antithrombin III deficiency	Increasing age	High plasma homocysteine
	Obesity	High plasma coagulation factor VIII, IX or XI
	Cancer (chemotherapy)	
	Leg paralysis	
Factor V Leiden	Oestrogen therapy	Antiphospholipid syndrome (anticardiolipin antibodies and lupus anticoagulant)
Prothrombin G20210A mutation	Pregnancy or puerperium	
	Major medical illness*	
	Previous venous thromboembolism (DVT/PE)	

*Chronic cardiorespiratory disease, inflammatory bowel disease, nephritic syndrome, myeloproliferative disorders.

Ho WK, Hankey GJ et al. Venous thromboembolism: diagnosis and management of deep venous thrombosis. *Med J Aust* 2005; 182(9): 476–481. © Copyright 2005 The Medical Journal of Australia—adapted and reproduced with permission.

Check the medication list

- Look for newly introduced drugs. Beta-blockers and NSAIDs may precipitate bronchospasm or worsen CCF.
- Have any medications recently been stopped? Some medications may be ceased prior to surgery and not recommenced (e.g. diuretics, steroids or preventive inhalers).
- Recent administration of IV antibiotics or radiographic contrast may precipitate anaphylaxis. Check for other known drug allergy.
- ACE inhibitors may cause chronic cough.
- *Note:* make certain postoperative, immobile or obese patients have been prescribed prophylactic anticoagulants to reduce their risk of DVT and PE.

Selective physical examination

Vital signs	Repeat now
HEENT	Oral or facial oedema (angio-oedema, anaphylaxis)
CVS	Distended neck veins (massive PE or cardiogenic failure, tension pneumothorax, cardiac tamponade)
	Peripherally shut down with clammy skin (cardiogenic, obstructive or hypovolaemic shock)
	Arrhythmia (LVF, PE)
	S_3 gallop (most specific finding for LV failure)
	Loud P_2 (COPD/pulmonary hypertension)
	Systolic murmur (LVF)
	Wheeze (asthma, COPD, LVF, foreign body aspiration when localised)
Resp	Stridor, hoarse voice, inability to speak (upper airway obstruction, anaphylaxis)
	Limited inspiration and splinted chest wall secondary to pleuritic chest pain (pneumothorax, pneumonia, PE)
	Basal crackles (LVF)
	Hyperexpanded, hyperresonant hemithorax (pneumothorax)
	Subcutaneous emphysema (pneumothorax)
	Pleural friction rub (pneumonia, pleurisy or PE with infarction)
	Pleural effusion (LVF, malignancy, PE, pneumonia)
	Pulmonary consolidation (pneumonia, PE with infarction)
GIT	Distension and ascites with tender hepatomegaly (RV failure or CCF)
Other	Peripheral oedema with accentuated skin creases on posterior thorax and taut, noncompliant skin (RV failure or CCF)
	Tender swollen thigh (DVT with PE)

SECTION C – Common calls

Investigations
Chest X-ray
- Review the CXR (see Box 15.1) as it provides a wealth of diagnostic information.
- CXR is *not* required in exacerbations of asthma that respond promptly to treatment.

Electrocardiogram
- Review the ECG for evidence of cardiac disease (such as LVH, ischaemia, arrhythmia) or indirect evidence of PE.
- The most common finding in PE is a sinus tachycardia. Significant PE may cause right axis deviation and right BBB. The S1 QIII TIII pattern is neither specific nor sensitive for PE.

Bedside
- **Peak expiratory flow rate** (PEFR) or spirometry is useful to quantify bronchospasm. Improvement after bronchodilator therapy suggests 'reversible' bronchospasm.

BOX 15.1   Clinical features on chest X-ray

Pneumonia
- Infiltrates (unilateral, bilateral, lobar, patchy)
- Parapneumonic effusion

COPD/asthma (CXR *not* routine in asthma)
- Hyperinflation of the lungs with flattened diaphragms
- Increased anteroposterior diameter
- Occasional infiltrates
- Occasionally pneumomediastinum

Left ventricular failure (see Figure 15.1)
- Cardiomegaly
- Bilateral interstitial or alveolar opacities, with perihilar congestion ('batwing' configuration)
- Upper lobe distribution of pulmonary vascular markings
- Pleural effusion
- Interstitial oedema (septal lines)
- Kerley B lines (1–2 cm horizontal, peripheral engorged subpleural lymphatics)

Pulmonary embolus
- CXR is frequently normal in patients with PE
- Plate or linear atelectasis
- Unilateral pleural-based wedge-shaped pulmonary infiltrate
- Unilateral pleural effusion (blunted costophrenic angle)
- Raised hemidiaphragm
- Dilated pulmonary artery (massive PE)
- Areas of oligaemia (massive PE)

- **Venous or arterial blood gases**—rapid assessment of pH, $PaCO_2$, PaO_2 and HCO_3^-. Previous VBG or ABG analysis is helpful to compare chronic ventilatory failure and CO_2 retention in patients with COPD. Look for a high bicarbonate level (chronic metabolic compensation).

Laboratory
- Take blood for FBC, U&E, cardiac enzymes and LFTs.
- Anaemia may be associated with dyspnoea, and may mask significant cyanosis.
- U&E and LFTs reflect renal function and hepatic congestion.
- Cardiac markers—only request if suspicious of ACS as precipitating event, or worsened CCF.

Specific management
Acute left ventricular failure (acute pulmonary oedema)
Acute LVF is a common emergency call in the middle of the night. The presentation develops over minutes with severe breathlessness, coughing frothy pink (bloodstained) sputum, orthopnoea and PND.
- The patient is distressed, unable to lie flat and usually peripherally shut down and clammy. Examination classically reveals tachypnoea, tachycardia, hypertension with widespread basal crackles, and possibly expiratory wheeze ('cardiac asthma').
- Fluid overload is not always causally associated with acute LVF, being more a feature of CCF (a different clinical syndrome).
- Cardiogenic shock is severe LVF associated with hypotension.
- The CXR is characteristic in acute LVF (see Figure 15.1), or may show a precipitating cause such as pneumonia or provide an alternative diagnosis.

Medical management
- Sit the patient upright and give high-flow oxygen via a reservoir mask aiming for oxygen saturation >95%.
- Decrease preload by giving GTN or starting non-invasive ventilation (CPAP).
  - GTN is the drug of choice as most patients are acutely hypertensive.
  - Give GTN 0.3–0.6 mg SL. Repeat after 5 minutes if SBP remains >100 mmHg. Remove the tablet if excessive hypotension occurs.
  - Commence a GTN infusion IV as per hospital guidelines once the patient is fully monitored. Infuse initially at 1 mL/h, maintaining SBP >100 mmHg. Quickly increase by doubling the infusion rate every 5 minutes to 20 mL/h or more, titrated to SBP.
- In patients with evidence of systemic fluid overload, give frusemide 40 mg IV, or twice the usual daily dose IV (if already on frusemide).

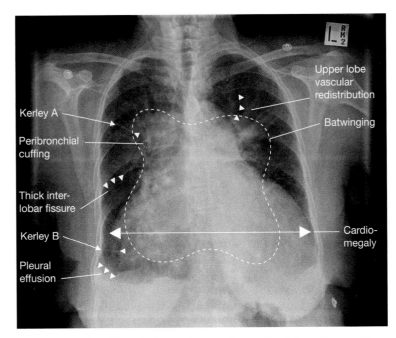

Figure 15.1 Chest X-ray features of congestive cardiac failure. Copyright Tor Ercleve.

- Commence mask CPAP ventilation if the patient does not respond quickly to the above measures, remains distressed or is persistently hypoxic despite maximal oxygen delivery:
  - Use a dedicated, high-flow oxygen circuit and a tight-fitting mask with initial PEEP resistance of 5–10 cm H_2O.
  - A trained nurse *must* remain in attendance at all times, as some patients will not tolerate the mask.
  - Hypotension may occur due to decreased venous return. Decrease the PEEP resistance to <5 cm H_2O or change back to a reservoir mask.
  - Once the patient improves, wean the inspired oxygen concentration and PEEP until the patient is comfortable with a normal oxygen mask.
- If the patient is hypotensive with poor peripheral perfusion, make sure you have called your senior and intensive care and treat as for cardiogenic shock. Endotracheal intubation is usual (see Chapter 19).

Determine the precipitating cause for the acute episode
Acute LVF is a serious condition. Once stabilised, determine the reason(s) for the acute episode. Six major aetiologies exist:
- Ischaemic heart disease
- Hypertension

- Valvular disease (mitral incompetence, aortic stenosis)
- Cardiomyopathy (dilated, restrictive, hypertrophic)
- Pericardial disease
- Congenital heart disease.
  The most common precipitating factors include:
- ACS
- Arrhythmia
- Fever, infection
- PE
- Increased sodium or fluid load (parenteral, medicinal, dietary)
- Cardiac depressant drug (e.g. beta-blockers, calcium-channel blockers)
- Sodium-retaining agents (e.g. NSAIDs)
- Renal disease
- Anaemia
- Non-compliance with diet or medication (e.g. dialysis patient).

Pulmonary embolism

The best way to avoid missing this critical diagnosis is to consider it in every patient with SOB.

A small PE causes sudden dyspnoea, pleuritic pain and possibly haemoptysis, with few physical signs. Look for a low-grade pyrexia (>38°C), tachypnoea (>20/min), tachycardia and a pleural rub.

A major PE causes dyspnoea, chest pain and light-headedness or collapse, followed by recovery. Look for cyanosis, tachycardia, hypotension, a parasternal heave, raised JVP and a loud delayed pulmonary second sound.

- Perform an ECG to exclude other diagnoses such as ACS or pericarditis.
  - The ECG is abnormal in approximately 85% of PE cases, but usually with non-specific changes. It may show a tachycardia alone or possibly right-axis deviation, right heart strain, right BBB or AF.
- Request a CXR mainly to exclude other diagnoses such as pneumonia or pneumothorax.
  - Positive findings on CXR generally depend on the presence of a pulmonary infarction (see Box 15.1). An entirely normal CXR in the setting of severe shortness of breath and hypoxia is highly suggestive of a PE.
- Consider performing ABGs. Do *not* perform routinely unless pulse oximetry is unreliable or demonstrates unexplained hypoxia on room air. Characteristic findings include acute respiratory alkalosis, or hypoxia and a raised A–a gradient.
- Calculate the clinical pre-test probability of PE (see Table 15.2) *before* requesting any diagnostic imaging.

Table 15.2 **Estimation of the clinical pre-test probability for suspected pulmonary embolus**

Clinical feature	Score
Clinical signs and symptoms of DVT (minimum of leg swelling and pain with palpation of the deep veins)	3
Alternative diagnosis less likely than PE	3
Heart rate >100 beats/min	1.5
Immobilisation or surgery in previous 4 weeks	1.5
Previous DVT or PE	1.5
Haemoptysis	1
Cancer	1

Pre-test probability	Score	Probability of PE
Low	<2	3.6%
Moderate	2–6	20.5%
High	>6	66.7%

Modified from Wells PS, Anderson DR, Rodger M et al. Excluding pulmonary embolism at the bedside without diagnostic imaging: Management of patients with suspected pulmonary embolism presenting to the emergency department by using a simple clinical model and d-dimer. *Ann Intern Med* 2001; 135:98–107.

- D-dimer is used to exclude PE in patients with a low probability of PE, if normal. However, according to the test's sensitivity, an ELISA D-dimer, when normal, may also be used to exclude PE in intermediate probability patients.
  - Only send a D-dimer test in a patient ≥50 years with a low pre-test probability, or in any patient under 50 with a low pre-test probability but who fails to fulfil one or more PERC criteria (see Table 15.3).
  - If all PERC criteria are fulfilled, the patient does not have a PE and does *not* need a D-dimer test sent.
  - Check with your laboratory which D-dimer test is used and the test's reference ranges. A negative D-dimer test then rules out a PE.
- Arrange a CTPA or V/Q lung scan in all patients with a high or intermediate pre-test probability, or in those with a positive D-dimer. Choice depends on local guidelines and test availability.
- **CTPA**
  - This test is more useful if the CXR is abnormal, which makes the V/Q scan difficult to interpret.
  - CTPA has over 95% sensitivity for segmental or larger PEs and about 75% for subsegmental.
  - Arrange sequential testing with **V/Q scan** plus or minus a lower limb Doppler ultrasound or CT venogram, to finally make (or usually exclude) the diagnosis when doubt remains.

Table 15.3 **Pulmonary embolism rule-out criteria (PERC) rule in the low pre-test probability patient**

Age <50 years
Pulse <100 beats/min
Pulse oximetry >94%
No unilateral leg swelling
No haemoptysis
No recent trauma or surgery
No prior pulmonary embolism or deep vein thrombosis
No oral hormone use

If all eight factors are fulfilled (i.e. top three are positive and bottom five are negative), no further testing is required, so do *not* send a D-dimer.
Modified from Kline JA, Mitchell AM, Kabrhel C et al. Clinical criteria to prevent unnecessary diagnostic testing in ED patients with suspected pulmonary embolism. *J Thromb Haemost* 2004; 2: 1247–55.

- **V/Q scan**
  - V/Q scan is preferred if the patient is allergic to contrast dye, has renal failure, when the CXR is normal, particularly in the younger female, or if CTPA is unavailable.
  - A normal V/Q scan rules out clinically important PE in patients with low-to-moderate clinical pre-test probability, and a high-probability scan gives a likelihood of PE up to 90%.
  - However, a low-probability scan still has a PE likelihood of approximately 15%, and an intermediate-probability scan still has a likelihood of 30%.
  - As overall more than 50% of results are low or intermediate probability, the V/Q scan must then be followed by further testing (lower-limb Doppler or CTPA/CTV).
- **Echocardiography**—if the patient is too unstable to undergo a CTPA or V/Q scan, a bedside echocardiogram gives diagnostic information by demonstrating RV dilation with small but actively contracting left-sided chambers, pulmonary hypertension or visible pulmonary artery clot. Echo will also help exclude other diagnoses such as cardiac tamponade.

Management
- Give high-dose oxygen via mask, aiming for oxygen saturation >95%.
- Give IV normal saline to support BP if necessary. Avoid excessive fluid, which can worsen RV dilation and cause septal shift, thereby worsening LV function.
- Relieve pain with titrated morphine 2.5 mg IV boluses.

Anticoagulation therapy
- Commence anticoagulation therapy once the diagnosis is confirmed or when there is an intermediate or high pre-test

probability of PE, but a delay to testing, in the absence of contraindications.

- Give low-molecular-weight heparin (LMWH) such as enoxaparin 1 mg/kg SC BD. Patients receiving LMWH do not require aPTT monitoring.
- Alternatively, particularly with haemodynamic compromise, give unfractionated heparin (UFH) (80 U/kg IV bolus) followed by a maintenance infusion of 18 U/kg/h titrated to aPTT (1.5–2.5-fold the control value).

- Patients with contraindications to anticoagulation require definite confirmation of PE prior to decisions on anticoagulation.
- Consult the cardiothoracic team for consideration of transvenous vena caval filter, particularly if a PE has occurred in a patient already taking warfarin.
- Commence the first dose of warfarin 5 mg PO on the first day of heparin therapy and titrate the subsequent daily doses to achieve an INR of 2.5–3.5.
  - *Note*: heparin must be continued until therapeutic warfarinisation is achieved (usually by 3–5 days).
- Instead, a new oral anticoagulant (NOAC) such as rivaroxaban 15 mg PO 12-hourly, or apixaban 10 mg PO 12-hourly may be started in place of the heparin and warfarin.
  - NOACs do not require INR testing, have fewer drug interactions than warfarin and the two above can be used alone without an initial heparin transition period. However, dabigatran 150 mg PO 12-hourly requires at least 5 days of parenteral anticoagulant to be given first.
  - Dosing modifications according to renal function (CrCl) are essential.

Fibrinolytic therapy

- Consider fibrinolytic therapy when the probability of PE is high (and preferably confirmed) and the patient is hypotensive despite fluid resuscitation, has evidence of acute RV failure and/or is peri-arrest.
- Call for immediate senior help and contact intensive care.
- Give tissue plasminogen activator (tPA) 10 mg IV over 1–2 min, then 90 mg IV over 2 hours together with heparinisation. Streptokinase and urokinase have also been used.
- Stat fibrinolytic doses can be given in cases of cardiac arrest considered related to a massive PE.
- Operative embolectomy is another heroic option in massive PE with shock.

Pneumonia

Community-acquired pneumonia (CAP) is a frequent cause for hospital admission and nosocomial pneumonia is a common complication in hospital, particularly in the ICU.

- Risk factors for CAP include: age over 50 years; smoking; chronic respiratory disease; cardiac, renal, cerebrovascular or hepatic disease; diabetes; alcoholism; malignancy; nursing home resident; and immunosuppression.
- **Common organisms:**
  - *Streptococcus pneumoniae* (>50%); *Haemophilus influenzae* (especially in COPD), 'atypical' organisms such as *Legionella* spp., *Mycoplasma* and *Chlamydia*, and viruses, including influenza and chickenpox.
  - Less common are *Staphylococcus aureus* (following a viral infection, or MRSA-related) and Gram-negative organisms (alcoholism).
  - In tropical areas, consider *Acinetobacter baumanii* and melioidosis caused by *Burkholderia pseudomallei*, especially among patients with diabetes, alcohol abuse, chronic lung disease and chronic renal failure. *Pneumocystis jiroveci* infects patients with HIV/AIDS and other severe immunosuppression.
- **Clinical features:**
  - Dyspnoea, fever, productive cough, pleuritic chest pain and haemoptysis. However, patients may present less classically with referred upper abdominal pain, diarrhoea, an acute confusional state, particularly in the elderly, and septicaemia with shock.
  - Protracted fever, night sweats, haemoptysis, weight loss and recent travel or past exposure are vital historical clues when to suspect TB.
- Examine for respiratory signs of lobar infection, such as a dull percussion note and bronchial breathing, although usually there are only localised moist crepitations with diminished breath sounds.
- **Investigations:**
  - Send blood samples including FBC, BSL, U&E, LFTs and blood cultures if severe or in nosocomial pneumonia.
  - Send a sample of sputum for microscopy and culture in suspected staphylococcal pneumonia or suspected TB (request Ziehl–Neelsen staining for TB).
  - Perform a CXR to confirm the diagnosis and exclude other pathological features such as COPD, malignancy, atelectasis, pulmonary oedema, hypersensitivity pneumonitis or a PE.
    - Findings vary from reticular shadowing through to patchy diffuse infiltrates to lobar consolidation. Pleural effusions and multilobar infiltrates are associated with increased mortality.
  - Antigen testing and serology: *Legionella* urinary antigen; pneumococcal urinary antigen; nose and throat swabs for respiratory viruses including influenza PCR; acute and convalescent serology for viruses, *Chlamydia*, *Legionella* and *Mycoplasma*, especially in younger adults or clustered disease outbreaks.

SECTION C – Common calls

Management

- Give the patient high-dose oxygen, aiming for oxygen saturation >95%.
- Obtain IV access in patients with moderate or severe pneumonia, and give normal saline IV. Many of these patients are dehydrated or have hypovolaemia from sepsis.
- Determine the severity of CAP using a validated scoring system such as the SMART-COP score (see Table 15.4), with a score of 5 or greater indicating severe disease requiring hospital admission, empirical IV antibiotics and referral to intensive care.
- Alternative severity scoring systems include the CURB-65 score (see Table 15.5) or the Pneumonia Severity Index (PSI).
- Other general markers of severity include:
  - Chronic disease and immunosuppression
  - FiO_2 0.35 to maintain SaO_2 >90%
  - Multilobar CXR changes
  - WCC $<4 \times 10^9$/L or $>30 \times 10^9$/L

Table 15.4	**SMART-COP score, once CAP confirmed on CXR**		
S	Systolic BP <90 mmHg		Score **2** points
M	Multilobar CXR involvement		Score **1** point
A	Albumin <35 g/L		Score **1** point
R	Resp rate—age-adjusted cut-offs:		Score **1** point
	Age:	≤50 years	>50 years
	RR:	≥25/min	≥30/min
T	Tachycardia ≥125/min		Score **1** point
C	Confusion (new onset)		Score **1** point
O	Oxygen low—age-adjusted cut-offs:		Score **2** points
	Age:	≤50 years	>50 years
	PaO_2:	<70 mmHg	<60 mmHg
	or SaO_2:	≤93%	≤90%
	or (if on O_2) PaO_2/FiO_2:	<333	<250
P	Arterial pH <7.35		Score **2** points
TOTAL SCORE = (max. 11)			
0–2 points:	Low risk of needing IRVS		
3–4 points:	Moderate (1 in 8) risk of needing IRVS		
5–6 points:	High (1 in 3) risk of needing IRVS		
≥7 points:	Very high (2 in 3) risk of needing IRVS		
IRVS = intensive respiratory or vasopressor support			
A score of 5 or more indicates severe CAP			

Adapted with permission from Charles PG et al. SMART-COP: A tool for predicting the need for intensive respiratory or vasopressor support in community-acquired pneumonia. *Clin Infect Dis* 2008; 47: 375–384.

Table 15.5 CURB-65 score for CAP
1 point for each of: Confusion (new onset) Urea >7mmol/L RR ≥30/min SBP<90 mmHg or DBP<60 mmHg Age ≥65 years.
Score **0–1** points: 30-day mortality 0.6–2.7%. Patients are often treated with PO antibiotics. Score **2** points: 30-day mortality 6.8%. Many patients hospitalised and need IV antibiotics. Score **3–5** points: 30-day mortality 14–27.8%. An HDU/ICU consult is necessary.
Adapted with permission from Lim WS et al. Defining community acquired pneumonia severity on presentation to hospital: An international derivation and validation study. *Thorax* 2003; 58: 377–382.

- Metabolic acidosis or coagulopathy
- Hb <90 g/L.

Antibiotic therapy

- Better outcomes are associated with early administration of antibiotics that cover the suspected causative organism.
- The choice of antimicrobial agent should be based on the rapidity of progression, the severity of pneumonia, the presence of comorbid conditions and knowledge of local aetiological organisms and resistance patterns.
- **Mild CAP:**
  - Give amoxycillin 1 g PO 8-hourly for 5–7 days. If *Mycoplasma pneumoniae*, *Chlamydophila pneumoniae* or *Legionella* infection is suspected, give doxycycline 100 mg PO 12-hourly for 5–7 days instead.
  - If history of immediate hypersensitivity to penicillin, give doxycycline or moxifloxacin 400 mg PO daily, depending on local practice.
  - Patients who fail to improve by 48 hours on amoxycillin PO should have doxycycline added to their regimen.
- **Moderate CAP:**
  - For patients requiring hospital admission, give benzylpenicillin 1.2 g IV 6-hourly until significant improvement, then change to amoxycillin 1 g PO 8-hourly for 7 days, *plus* either doxycycline 100 mg PO 12-hourly for 7 days or clarithromycin 500 mg PO 12-hourly for 7 days (if pregnant).
  - Add gentamicin 5 mg/kg IV daily (assuming normal renal function) if Gram-negative bacilli are identified in blood or sputum. Alternatively, change the benzylpenicillin to ceftriaxone 1 g daily IV.

SECTION C – Common calls

- If the patient has immediate hypersensitivity to penicillin, subsitute ceftriaxone 1 g daily IV for the penicillin or use moxifloxacin 400 mg PO daily monotherapy as a single drug.
- In tropical areas, if the patient has risk factors for melioidosis (see above), give ceftriaxone 2 g daily IV plus gentamicin 5 mg/kg IV as a single dose.
- For patients with moderate and severe CAP who are admitted to hospital, consider use of oseltamivir 75 mg BD PO, particularly in influenza season.
- **Severe CAP (usually with SMART-COP score of 5 or more, or CURB-65 score of 3 or more):**
  - Refer to HDU/ICU.
  - Give ceftriaxone 1 g IV daily *plus* azithromycin 500 mg IV daily.
  - If significant renal impairment or penicillin allergy, give moxifloxacin 400 mg IV daily.
- **Severe tropical pneumonia:**
  - Where *Burkholderia pseudomallei* (melioidosis) or *Acinetobacter baumannii* are prevalent, give meropenem 1 g IV 8-hourly plus azithromycin 500 mg IV daily.
- **Hospital-acquired pneumonia:**
  - Pneumonias developing after 48 hours in hospital may be caused by multiresistant Gram-negative or staphylococcal organisms.
  - Always consult with a microbiology or infectious disease specialist:
    — Amoxycillin–clavulanic acid can be used in mild pneumonia. Ticarcillin–clavulanic acid, ceftriaxone or piperacillin-tazobactam in moderate or severe pneumonia.
    — Add vancomycin if high prevalence of MRSA and consider ciprofloxacin plus azithromycin if *Legionella* suspected.
- **Aspiration pneumonia:**
  - Aspiration pneumonia should be considered in any patient with a decreased level of consciousness or an impaired cough reflex (e.g. alcohol intoxication, stroke, seizure, postsurgery). Minor degrees of aspiration do not require antibiotic therapy.
  - Give benzylpenicillin 1.2 g IV 6-hourly plus metronidazole 500 mg IV 12-hourly when there are clinical signs of infection such as fever, sputum production and leucocytosis.
- **Pneumonia in patients with HIV:**
  - Usually caused by *Pneumocystis jiroveci* or typical organisms.
  - Consult a microbiology or infectious disease specialist when the patient is hypoxic on room air.
  - Organise urgent bronchoscopy, and on recommendation give trimethoprim–sulfamethoxazole 5 + 25 mg/kg PO or IV 8-hourly with prednisolone 40 mg PO 12-hourly.

Asthma

Asthma is an inflammatory condition characterised by reversible bronchial hyperreactivity and airflow obstruction that varies over time. Ask about the current risk profile, any precipitating event and a socioeconomic history:

- **Current risk profile**:
  - Duration of the present episode
  - Peak flow measurements (if performed at home)
  - Use of beta-agonists and response to therapy
  - Use of oral steroid or escalation of preventive inhaler use
  - Previous admission(s) to hospital (particularly in past 4 weeks)
  - Past admission to ICU ever.
- **Precipitating factors:**
  - Viral illness (common)
  - Specific allergies, non-specific irritants
  - Comorbidities (e.g. food allergy, obesity, COPD, heart failure)
  - Recent beta-blocker or aspirin/NSAID administration.
- **Socioeconomic challenges:**
  - Homeless, unemployed, living alone
  - Drug or alcohol use
  - Psychiatric illness.

Differentiate a severe attack (must receive steroids) from a life-threatening attack (needs immediate senior help, an anaesthetist and intensive care).

- **Severe attack**—indicated by any one of the following:
  - Inability to complete sentences in one breath
  - RR ≥25 breaths/min
  - Tachycardia ≥110 beats/min
  - PEFR or FEV_1=33–50% of predicted or known, despite nebuliser therapy.
- **Life-threatening attack with risk of respiratory arrest**—indicated by any one of the following:
  - Silent chest, cyanosis or feeble respiratory effort
  - Bradycardia, arrhythmia or hypotension
  - Altered mental status, with exhaustion or confusion
  - SaO_2 <92%; PaO_2 <60 mmHg or normal or raised $PaCO_2$ >34–45 mmHg on ABG (see later).
  - Remember if precipitate onset to consider anaphylaxis, and look for other features such as urticaria, erythema, pruritus or angio-oedema. Treat as per Chapter 9.

Request a CXR in life-threatening cases or severe cases that fail to respond.
- Look for pneumothorax, focal signs of chest infection, lobar collapse secondary to mucous plugging or pneumomediastinum.

Spirometry and peak expiratory flow rate
- Spirometry provides an objective measurement of the severity of airflow limitation, although patients with critical asthma will be too unwell to perform this.
- Measure the PEFR or the FEV_1 and stratify risk as above.

Arterial blood gases
- ABGs are *rarely* necessary—measure only if the patient has a severe attack that does not respond to treatment, is deteriorating or has life-threatening features.

Management
- Commence high-dose oxygen via a mask maintaining SaO_2 >95%, and attach pulse oximetry monitoring to the patient.
- Give salbutamol 5 mg via an oxygen-driven nebuliser, diluted with 3 mL normal saline. Add ipratropium 500 micrograms to a second dose of salbutamol 5 mg via the nebuliser if there is no response or there is a severe attack.
- Give prednisolone 50 mg PO or hydrocortisone 200 mg IV if unable to swallow.
- Avoid all sedatives, anxiolytics, NSAIDs and histamine-releasers (morphine).
  If the patient's condition does not respond to the above measures:
- Give repeated salbutamol 5 mg nebulisers—up to three doses in first hour.
- Continue regular ipratropium 500 micrograms every 6 hours.
  If the patient's condition is deteriorating or there are severe or life-threatening features:
- Obtain IV access, ensure steroids have been given, perform a CXR and call for senior help.
- Give continuous salbutamol nebulisers.
- Obtain ABGs to check $PaCO_2$, pH and potassium, which may be low secondary to beta-agonist therapy. This does not usually require treatment if >3.0 mmol/L.
- Start bronchodilator infusion IV with ECG monitoring and arrange an ICU bed:
  - Give magnesium sulfate 2.5 g IV (10 mmol) over 20–30 min.
  - Give salbutamol 250–500 micrograms IV over 10 min, followed by an infusion of salbutamol 5 mg in 5% dextrose 500 mL run at 60 mL/h = 10 microgram/min initially. Titrate to response up to 120–240 mL/h or 20–40 microgram/min.

Ventilatory management
The decision to intubate is based on clinical features. It is a complex and dangerous procedure requiring the most senior staff.

Exacerbation of chronic obstructive pulmonary disease
COPD is characterised by airflow limitation that is not fully reversible, usually progressive and associated with an inflammatory

response of the lungs to noxious particles or gases (especially continued smoking).

- Patients have breathlessness, cough, sputum production and wheeze, and are susceptible to infections. Most patients have a smoking history.
- Bronchiectasis is a less common cause of obstructive lung disease with chronic productive cough, and halitosis.
- Chronic bronchitis, emphysema and asthma overlap, as some reversibility is present with COPD and some patients with asthma will develop irreversible components of the disease.
- An exacerbation of COPD can be caused by:
  - Bronchospasm, sputum plugging, pneumothorax, viral illness, pneumonia
  - Right, left or biventricular failure; arrhythmia such as AF
  - ACS
  - PE (commonly seen on autopsy)
  - Development of malignancy
  - Drug non-compliance, inadequate steroid, inappropriate sedation
  - Environmental allergens, weather change.

History
Focus the history on gaining an idea of baseline capacity, and to elicit any of the above causes of an exacerbation:
- Usual and current daily exercise capacity and level of dependence
- Home oxygen use
- Smoking or dust exposure
- New features of cardiac or respiratory disease:
  - Episodes of ischaemic or pleuritic chest pain
  - Increasing sputum production, cough, fever, chills
  - Worsening peripheral oedema or orthopnoea
- Non-compliance with medication, including steroids or diuretics
- Excess sedatives or opioids
- Known cardiac disease.

Clinical examination
- Hyperexpanded, barrel-shaped chest, increased work of breathing
- Fever, wheeze, sputum production
- Cor pulmonale—right heart failure secondary to pulmonary hypertension with cyanosis, ruddy complexion, raised JVP, signs of RVH (parasternal heave, loud P2) and peripheral oedema
- **Perform an ABG** only in a severe episode, if there is no response to treatment or any suggestion of acute or worsening CO_2 retention with altered mental status.
  - Chronic CO_2 retention is indicated by a raised HCO_3^- from metabolic compensation. A pH<7.3 suggests acute respiratory acidosis.
  - Polycythaemia suggests chronic hypoxaemia or sleep apnoea.

SECTION C – Common calls

- *Note*: VBG with reliable pulse oximetry will give similar information as an ABG.
- **Perform a CXR:**
  - CXR is not sensitive for diagnosis of COPD, but may show hyperinflation, chronic fibrosis, bullae, peripheral pruning of vessels and a narrow mediastinum.
  - Acute complications may be demonstrated such as atelectasis, consolidation, pneumothorax, pulmonary oedema or a malignant lung mass.
- **Spirometry and PEFR:**
  - Spirometry during an acute episode is inaccurate and may distress the patient, although it may help quantify the diagnosis in a first episode.
  - FEV_1 is more accurate than PEFR. Perform bedside lung function testing for FEV_1 and FVC to compare with previous respiratory function tests, and to follow the response to treatment.
  - $FEV_1 < 1$ L indicates severe disease.
- **Perform an ECG** looking for:
  - Large P waves (P pulmonale)
  - RVH or strain, multifocal atrial tachycardia or AF
  - Signs of ischaemia with ST and T wave changes.

Management

- Commence controlled oxygen therapy initially at 28% via a Venturi mask if there is evidence of chronic CO_2 retention (raised HCO_3^- or $PaCO_2$). Aim for an oxygen saturation 88–92%.
- Otherwise, use a higher-dose oxygen (40–60%) mask to treat hypoxaemia.
- Attach a cardiac monitor and pulse oximeter to the patient.
- Give salbutamol 5 mg via a nebuliser for bronchospasm and add ipratropium 500 micrograms to the initial three nebulisers, then give both 6-hourly.
- Give prednisolone 50 mg PO, or hydrocortisone 200 mg IV if unable to swallow, for bronchospasm or if on long-term inhaled or oral steroids.
- Treat infection as per local antibiotic guidelines if there is fever or increased sputum volume and increased sputum virulence (change in colour or blood-staining). Amoxicillin 500 mg PO 8-hourly, or doxycycline 200 mg PO once, then 100 mg daily, is suitable.
- Give frusemide 40 mg IV or PO if RV failure with fluid overload is present.
- If no response to above, ongoing hypoxia with SpO_2 <85% despite oxygen therapy, extreme respiratory distress, $PaCO_2$ is rising, patient is becoming exhausted or acidaemia is worsening, commence non-invasive, bilevel (BiPAP) ventilation.

- This requires specialised equipment and trained and experienced staff present to supervise.
- If there is continued deterioration despite the above measures, call the anaesthetist as endotracheal intubation may be necessary.
- This has significant implications for the patient as it may become difficult to impossible to wean the patient off the ventilator, so ideally always try to discuss with the patient, family and intensive care staff *before* the need arises.

Pneumothorax

Simple pneumothorax may be traumatic or spontaneous. In the hospital, a traumatic pneumothorax is usually iatrogenic (e.g. following central line placement or overventilation).

- Spontaneous pneumothorax may occur in healthy people with no lung disease ('primary' pneumothorax), or in the setting of chronic lung diseases such as asthma, COPD and cystic fibrosis ('secondary' pneumothorax).
  - Dyspnoea can range from minimal to significant respiratory distress, where 'significant' is defined as any deterioration in usual exercise tolerance.
  - This depends less on the degree of lung collapse than on the degree of physiological reserve.
  - Chest pain is sudden and pleuritic, and the involved hemithorax is hyperexpanded, hyperresonant and with decreased air entry and breath sounds.
- **Perform a CXR:**
  - Request a standard inspiratory CXR in all cases. Expiratory films are no longer routine, but could be requested if there is doubt on a standard film.
  - CXR will show a collapsed lung with a visible pleural edge and air in the pleural cavity.
  - Assess the size of the pneumothorax on the CXR:
    - 'Small' is a visible air rim <2 cm
    - 'Large' is a visible air rim 2 cm or more around all the lung edge. This represents over 50% of lung volume lost.

Management
- Management is determined by:
  - Cause (traumatic or spontaneous)
  - Size of the pneumothorax (small or large)
  - Presence of chronic lung disease (primary or secondary)
  - Symptomatic (dyspnoeic) or not
  - Need for positive-pressure ventilation (when any pneumothorax is significant).

- **Observation only:**
  - No active management is indicated in patients with a small primary pneumothorax <2 cm and no significant dyspnoea.
  - Repeat the CXR after 6–12 hours and perform simple aspiration if there is any worsening in symptoms or increase in pneumothorax size.
- **Simple aspiration (thoracocentesis):**
  - Symptomatic primary pneumothorax with significant dyspnoea (irrespective of size)
  - Small secondary pneumothorax <2 cm without significant dyspnoea, but must observe carefully for deterioration
  - Small symptomatic pneumothorax complicating CVL insertion.
- **Intercostal catheter (ICC) or tube thoracostomy:**
  - Tension pneumothorax following initial needle thoracocentesis (see below)
  - Traumatic pneumothorax or haemopneumothorax
  - Failed simple aspiration (e.g. with more than just a small residual rim of air around the lung)
  - A secondary pneumothorax causing significant dyspnoea in a patient with underlying lung disease
  - Any pneumothorax prior to anaesthesia or positive-pressure ventilation.

Tension pneumothorax

This is a **medical emergency**, with extreme respiratory distress plus additional circulatory compromise leading to shock (from raised intra-thoracic pressure and decreased venous return).

- The trachea is deviated away from the affected side, neck veins are distended, chest expansion decreased, percussion note hyperresonant and absent or diminished breath sounds on the affected side.
- Treat immediately with needle decompression of the hemithorax:
  - Prepare the skin with antiseptic and infiltrate local anaesthetic to skin, adjacent periosteum and pleura, if the patient's clinical condition allows sufficient time (it may not).
  - Insert a 14G IV cannula over the 3rd rib into the 2nd intercostal space in the midclavicular line on the affected side.
  - Push the cannula gently through the chest wall until it enters the pleural space.
  - Air will escape through the cannula with a 'hiss', followed by rapid improvement in clinical status.
  - Keep the cannula in situ until formal tube thoracostomy is performed. If the diagnosis was in error and no hiss occurred, an ICC is required anyway.

Pleural effusion

Large pleural effusions present with gradually worsening dyspnoea, often associated with chest discomfort or pain.

- They will not cause symptoms or be detectable on CXR until 250–500 mL of pleural fluid is present.
- Pleural effusions with significant dyspnoea require therapeutic drainage and/or diagnostic aspiration in due course (see Box 15.2). This may be able to wait until morning.
- If you decide to aspirate, send pleural fluid for culture, protein and LDH levels, and cytology.
- Definitive treatment of the underlying condition usually prevents the development of further effusions.
- When the underlying cause is not found or not able to be treated, options include recurrent aspirations or pleurodesis using talc, tetracycline or under direct vision on thoracoscopy.

BOX 15.2 Causes of pleural effusion

Common causes of transudates (low pleural fluid protein and LDH):
- Cardiac failure
- Nephrotic syndrome
- Cirrhosis
- Hypothyroidism
- Hypoalbuminaemia.

Common causes of exudates (relatively high pleural fluid protein or LDH, pH <7.3):
- Pneumonia
- Malignancy
- Tuberculosis
- Subphrenic abscess
- Acute pancreatitis
- PE (or can be a transudate).

Haemoptysis

Small amounts of coughed blood are associated with chest infection including bronchiectasis, malignancy, PE, pulmonary hypertension, arteriovenous malformations or local bleeding from the upper respiratory tract, nose or throat. CXR, CT or bronchoscopy is needed for a definitive diagnosis.

- Massive haemoptysis is a life-threatening emergency due to risk of airway obstruction or asphyxiation.
- Apply high-dose oxygen and order an immediate CXR.
- Ensure secure large-bore peripheral IV access and take bloods, including for coagulation studies and cross-match.

- Lie the patient on the affected side if a lateralising source of bleeding is known to prevent blood aspiration on the opposite side.
- Call ICU and anaesthetics. Intubation with a double-lumen tube may be required to stabilise the patient.
- If or once stable, chest CT and bronchoscopy are required.
- Continuing bleeding may be stopped by thermocoagulation or injection of vasoactive agents at bronchoscopy. If unsuccessful, interventional radiology embolisation or emergency thoracotomy may be required.

Hiccups (singultus)

Hiccups lasting for longer than a few hours are often distressing to the patient.

- **Causes of hiccups include:**
  - Usually unknown (and benign relating to stress and anxiety)
  - Postoperative
  - Stomach or oesophageal distension
  - Gastro-oesophageal reflux
  - Diaphragmatic irritation from intrathoracic or an intra-abdominal source
  - Chemotherapy
  - Associated with CNS disease, alcohol, drugs or metabolic disorders such as uraemia.

If physical examination of the chest and abdomen is normal, and the patient has no other associated symptoms, no further investigations are required initially.

- **Therapies include:**
  - Ice water gargle, or direct stimulation of the posterior pharyngeal wall with a suction catheter or cotton-tipped applicator
  - Medication (e.g. metoclopramide 10 mg PO; chlorpromazine 12.5–25 mg IV with 500 mL saline preload; baclofen 5 mg PO QID; lignocaine 2% viscous PO; empirical therapy of gastro-oesophageal reflux with antacid preparations or proton-pump inhibitors)
  - Hiccups lasting for more than 24 hours require at least a CXR, FBC, U&E, LFTs, lipase to investigate an underlying organic cause.

16

Chest pain

Coronary artery disease (CAD) is the leading cause of death in developed countries. A patient with CAD may present critically ill with an arrhythmia, heart failure or hypotension (cardiogenic shock), or may be stable and appear deceptively well, yet still be at risk of sudden death. Thus, when a patient complains of 'chest pain', a cardiac cause due to acute coronary syndrome (ACS), which includes the spectrum from acute myocardial infarction (AMI) to angina, must be considered first.

There are several other equally serious causes of chest pain, such as PE or aortic dissection, that may go undiagnosed if they are not also specifically looked for. The history is the most important aspect in the differential diagnosis of chest pain.

Phone call

Questions

1. What is the character of the pain? Does it change with breathing?
2. Where is the pain maximal and does it radiate?
3. How severe is the pain?
4. What are the vital signs?
5. What was the reason for admission?
6. Does the patient have a history of ischaemic heart disease? If 'Yes', is the pain similar to their usual angina or a previous MI?

Instructions

If you suspect AMI or angina (heavy, crushing, tight pain radiating to jaw or left or right arm):
- Ask the nurse to stay by the patient's bedside and call for additional nursing staff if necessary.
- Give oxygen if hypoxic or shocked to maintain saturation >94%, after attaching a pulse oximeter and cardiac monitor to the patient.
- Request an urgent 12-lead ECG.
- Give aspirin 150–300 mg PO unless contraindicated by hypersensitivity.

- Administer GTN SL (0.6 mg tablets or 0.4 mg spray) and repeat every 5–10 minutes if the pain persists, provided SBP remains >90 mmHg.
- Request an IV trolley for the patient's bedside, with a range of cannulae ready for insertion.

Prioritisation

Attend any patient with chest pain immediately, especially those with abnormal vital signs, particularly an arrhythmia or hypotension.

Corridor thoughts

What causes chest pain? (* = major threat to life)
- **Cardiac**
  - Acute coronary syndrome (ACS)*
  - Acute aortic dissection (AAD)*
  - Pericarditis
- **Respiratory**
  - Pulmonary embolism (PE)*
  - Pleurisy
  - Pneumonia
  - Pneumothorax
  - Pneumomediastinum
- **Gastrointestinal tract**
  - Oesophagitis
  - Oesophageal spasm
  - Ruptured oesophagus*, including Boerhaave's syndrome due to vomiting
  - Hiatus hernia
  - Peptic ulcer disease
  - Biliary colic/cholecystitis
  - Subdiaphragmatic irritation
- **Musculoskeletal**
  - Costochondritis
  - Muscular pain
  - Fractured rib
  - Referred pain from spinal crush fracture or spinal disc disease
  - Herpes zoster or postherpetic neuralgia
- **Psychiatric**
  - Anxiety and panic disorders

Major threat to life

- **Acute coronary syndrome (ACS)**, including ST-elevation myocardial infarction (STEMI), non-ST-elevation myocardial infarction (NSTEMI) and unstable angina (UA).

- Heart failure, cardiogenic shock or ventricular or supraventricular arrhythmias may occur suddenly as a result of ACS, which can be fatal.
- **Acute aortic dissection (AAD)** may cause acute aortic incompetence, pericardial tamponade or aortic rupture, and involve other organs such as the CNS, renal and GI tracts by acute vascular occlusion (which can be intermittent).
- **Pulmonary embolus (PE)** causes hypoxia and, potentially acute right ventricular failure with obstructive shock and sudden death.

Bedside

Quick-look test

Does the patient look well (comfortable), sick (uncomfortable or distressed) or critical (about to die)?
- Patients with chest pain from ACS may look anxious and pale, or are shocked, breathless and clearly unwell.
- Patients with aortic dissection have severe pain and are restless and agitated.
- Patients with PE, pericarditis or pneumothorax are dyspnoeic and breathe with shallow, painful respirations (pleuritic pain).
- However, even if patients look well and appear comfortable at rest, they may still have a life-threatening underlying cause such as ACS, aortic dissection or PE.
- Oesophagitis, or a musculoskeletal cause such as costochondritis, is a diagnosis of exclusion, and is *only* made when all potentially life-threatening causes of chest pain have been considered and actively excluded.

Airway and vital signs

What is the blood pressure?
- Most patients with chest pain have a normal BP. Take the BP in both arms if the pain is suspicious of aortic dissection (sudden onset, sharp, tearing or migratory), and look for a difference of >15 mmHg.
- Hypotension occurs in ACS, massive PE and AAD with cardiac tamponade.
- Hypertension in association with ACS or aortic dissection should be treated urgently in a monitored resuscitation area (see Chapter 19).

What is the heart rate?
- If the HR is >150 beats/min or <40 beats/min, obtain a 12-lead ECG or rhythm strip to help diagnose the arrhythmia.
- Sinus tachycardia may result from chest pain of any cause. A heart rate >140 beats/min raises the possibility of atrial fibrillation or ventricular tachycardia, which require urgent cardioversion,

especially if associated with chest pain and or hypotension ('symptomatic' arrhythmias).
- Bradycardia with chest pain may represent sinus or atrioventricular (AV) nodal ischaemia associated with ACS, or a drug effect such as calcium-channel blocker or beta-blocker use.
- Immediate treatment of bradycardia is not required unless the patient is hypotensive or syncopal and/or the rate is extremely slow (<40 beats/min).

What is the respiratory rate?
- Tachypnoea may accompany any type of chest pain.
- Shallow, painful breathing suggests a pleuritic or musculoskeletal cause.
- Dyspnoea from increased work of breathing occurs with respiratory causes of chest pain or acute LVF, and may lead to respiratory failure.

What does the ECG show? (see Chapter 35)
- Review the ECG immediately after assessing the vital signs. Compare with an old tracing if possible.
- ST-segment elevation or depression, T wave changes and the presence of new Q waves suggest myocardial ischaemia from ACS.
  - Only 50% of patients with ACS will have a diagnostic ECG, with non-specific or no initial ECG changes in the remainder (the diagnosis is then made on a rise in cardiac biomarker levels such as troponin).
- The most common ECG finding in a patient with PE is a sinus tachycardia. Additional changes of right-axis deviation, right bundle branch block, atrial fibrillation with rapid ventricular response or the SI QIII TIII phenomenon should be looked for.
  - *Note:* SI QIII TIII is well known, but is neither sensitive nor specific for PE!
- The ECG in a patient with pericarditis shows diffuse, concave ST-segment elevation with PR depression.
- Left ventricular hypertrophy with R wave and S wave in V1 >35 mm may give a clue to long-standing hypertension, which is a risk factor for aortic dissection in particular, as well as ACS.
- A normal initial ECG does *not* rule out sinister pathology.
  - If the first ECG is non-diagnostic, repeat after 15 minutes if the chest pain is continuing to exclude evolving changes.
  - Repeat the ECG whenever the chest pain recurs, stops or changes in severity or character, as well as after 6–8 hours with repeat cardiac biomarkers (troponin) to rule out ACS.
  - Accelerated chest pain rule-out protocols now include repeat ECG and troponin testing within 2–3 hours. Check your local process.

If the patient has normal vital signs, the chest pain has resolved and the ECG is normal or only has non-specific changes, proceed to further history and examination.

Management

Immediate management

- If the patient still has chest pain or has respiratory distress, hypotension or an altered mental state:
  - Attach continuous non-invasive ECG, BP and pulse oximeter monitoring to the patient.
  - Commence oxygen if hypoxic or shocked to maintain oxygen saturation >94%. Give high-dose 40–60% oxygen unless there is a prior history of obstructive airways disease, in which case give 28% oxygen via a Venturi mask.
  - Establish IV access with two cannulae in peripheral veins. Draw and send bloods for FBC, U&E, cardiac biomarkers (troponin I or T) and coagulation profile.
  - Request a portable CXR.
- If the patient has chest pain and SBP >90 mmHg:
  - Give a second dose of GTN 300–600 micrograms SL, and a third after an additional 5 minutes if pain is still present.
  - Give morphine 2.5–5 mg IV with metoclopramide 10–20 mg IV for nausea, if pain persists despite two to three doses of GTN.
    - *Note*: morphine may also cause hypotension, as well as respiratory depression and drowsiness. Monitor the patient's BP and respiratory rate carefully after each dose administered.
  - Maintain SBP >100 mmHg and avoid excessive hypotension.
- If the patient has chest pain and SBP <90 mmHg:
  - Check that the lung bases are clear to auscultation and give a bolus of 125–250 mL IV normal saline.
  - However, if the patient has signs of pulmonary oedema, with an S_3 gallop, tachypnoea and basal crackles, treat as cardiogenic shock (see Chapter 11).
- Call senior staff immediately, especially if there is:
  - Persistent hypoxia, hypotension or altered mental status despite the above measures.
  - HR >150 beats/min or <40 beats/min associated with hypotension, as cardioversion or pacing may be required.
  - Persistent pain and ST-segment changes on ECG, as urgent treatment for ACS is required (see below).

Selective history and chart review

A careful history of the pain is essential if the initial ECG is non-diagnostic.

How did the chest pain evolve?
- Crescendo, build-up of pain suggests ACS.
- Sudden, precipitate onset suggests PE, aortic dissection or oesophageal rupture.

SECTION C – Common calls

- Onset of pain with physical exertion or emotional stress suggests ACS.
- Onset with coughing suggests a pneumothorax or a mechanical cause of pain (see Chapter 15).
- Sudden pain following vomiting suggests oesophageal rupture (Boerhaave's syndrome).

How does the patient describe the pain?
- Determine the degree of discomfort for the patient (e.g. score the pain out of 10, with zero being no pain at all and 10 being the worst pain the patient has ever experienced). This allows ongoing evaluation of the chest pain to determine the response to treatment.
- If the patient recognises the current discomfort as usual angina pain, assume this is correct.
- Crushing, vice-like or squeezing pain is characteristic of ACS, but note that 'atypical' pain still due to ACS occurs in women, elderly people and those with diabetes and renal impairment.
- Tearing or ripping pain is characteristic of an AAD. Likewise, severe pain that is poorly relieved by large doses of morphine suggests an aortic dissection or an oesophageal rupture.
- Sharp, well-localised pain suggests a pleuritic or musculoskeletal origin, but may occasionally occur with ACS or PE.

Where is the pain? Does the pain radiate?
- Central, retrosternal chest pain indicates a mediastinal or gastrointestinal origin.
- Lateral pain suggests lung, pleura, chest wall or neurological referred pain.
- Radiation of the pain to the jaw, shoulders or arms is suggestive of ACS.
- Radiation of the pain to the back suggests ACS, or less commonly an AAD distal to the left subclavian artery.
- Dissection proximal to the left subclavian artery more characteristically causes non-radiating anterior chest pain.
- Burning retrosternal chest pain radiating to the neck and throat suggests oesophageal reflux, but ACS must always be excluded first (mistaking ACS chest pain for indigestion is a common error in both patients and medical staff).

Are there any related symptoms?
- Nausea, sweating and light-headedness are non-specific but must be taken seriously.
- Collapse, or a syncopal episode, can indicate a sinister cause such as ACS, PE or AAD—again this must be taken seriously.
- Dyspnoea is usually related to a cardiorespiratory cause of pain or a resultant metabolic acidosis (such as a lactic acidosis in shock).

Does anything make the pain worse or better?
- Is the chest pain worse on coughing or deep breathing? Pleuritic chest pain suggests pneumothorax, pericarditis, PE, pneumonia, pleurisy, rib fracture or costochondritis.
- Pain worse on deep inspiration, when lying flat or when raising both legs (increases venous return) is suggestive of pericarditis.
- Pain worse with swallowing suggests an oesophageal source or pericarditis.
- Pain worse on particular movements, especially when muscular actions are resisted, suggests musculoskeletal pain or sometimes pneumothorax from rib injury.
- Relief of pain with antacids or GTN does *not* aid in the differential diagnosis. These should not be used as diagnostic tests, but as specific therapy once you have a working diagnosis.

Review past medical history and risk factors

Confirm a risk-factor profile or past medical history that may increase the likelihood (pre-test probability) of a particular cause of the chest pain:
- **ACS** is more likely with prior known ischaemic heart disease, increasing age >65 years, diabetes, hypertension, smoking, hyperlipidaemia, a family history of premature ischaemic heart disease in first-degree relative under age 50 years, or end-stage renal disease. Cocaine use and HIV are less common risk factors.
- **Aortic dissection** occurs in patients aged 60–80 years, usually males with chronic hypertension, or in younger patients with a connective tissue disorder, such as Marfan's or Ehlers–Danlos syndrome, or a family history.
- **PE** is more likely with recent surgery, immobilisation, malignancy, prior thromboembolic episode (PE or DVT) or history of first-degree relative with thromboembolism, malignancy or chronic cardiorespiratory disease. Thus, a PE is common in hospital patients, with the possible exception of the paediatric ward.

Check the medication list
- Confirm prescribed antianginal medications have been given.
- Check for thromboembolic prophylaxis in immobilised or postoperative patients.
- Check for corticosteroids or NSAIDs as a possible cause of gastritis or oesophagitis.

Selective physical examination

Vitals	Repeat now
Appearance	Does the patient look Marfanoid? A tall, thin patient with long limbs and arachnodactyly ('spider fingers') may have a connective tissue disorder predisposing to aortic dissection
HEENT	Xanthelasma around the eyelids (may indicate hypercholesterolaemia, especially if familial)
	White exudate in oral cavity or pharynx (thrush with possible oesophageal candidiasis)
Resp	Asymmetrical expansion of the chest (pneumothorax, large pleural effusion or massive haemothorax)
	Tracheal deviation:
	Pushed *away* from large pneumothorax, large effusion and large haemothorax
	Pulled *towards* by collapse and consolidation
	Percussion:
	Hyperresonance (pneumothorax)
	Dullness to percussion (pleural effusion, haemothorax and consolidation)
	Auscultation:
	Diminished breath sounds (on the side of a pneumothorax)
	Crackles and/or wheezes (pulmonary oedema, PE or pneumonia)
	Pleural rub (PE or pneumonia)
Chest wall	Tender costal cartilage (costochondritis)
	Note: does not exclude another more serious diagnosis, as a patient with ACS may have chest wall tenderness
	Localised rib pain (rib fracture)
CVS	Unequal carotid pulses (aortic dissection)
	Unequal upper limb BP or diminished or absent radial or femoral pulse (aortic dissection)
	Elevated JVP (biventricular failure with CCF; right ventricular failure secondary to PE, tension pneumothorax or cardiac tamponade)
	Left ventricular heave (LVF)
	Right ventricular heave (acute RV failure secondary to PE)
	Displaced apical impulse (away from the side of pneumothorax; COPD)
	Auscultation:
	S_3 gallop (LVF), loud P_2 (acute RV failure secondary to cor pulmonale)
	Muffled heart sounds (cardiac tamponade, pericarditis)

	Systolic murmur:
	Aortic stenosis (angina)
	Mitral regurgitation (acute papillary muscle or chordae tendinae dysfunction secondary to ACS)
	Late (mitral valve prolapse [Barlow's syndrome] associated with systolic click and non-anginal chest pain)
	Diastolic murmur:
	Early (aortic regurgitation associated with proximal aortic root dissection)
	Pericardial rub—biphasic systolic and diastolic scratching 'squeaky new leather' sound that varies with position (pericarditis)
GIT	Guarding, rigid abdomen (perforated peptic ulcer)
	Epigastric tenderness (PUD)
	Generalised abdominal pain (mesenteric infarction from aortic dissection)
CNS	Hemiplegia or paraparesis (aortic dissection involving carotid or spinal arteries)
Skin	Unilateral, vesicular maculopapular rash, dermatomal distribution (herpes zoster)

Investigations
Laboratory
- Take blood for FBC, coags, BSL, U&E, LFTs and cardiac enzymes (troponin I or T). Send a D-dimer only for low pre-test probability PE (see Chapter 15).
- Anaemia may be associated with angina.
- BSL, U&E, LFTs will show evidence of diabetes and chronic renal disease (risk of ACS) and may be abnormal in cholecystitis.
- Cardiac biomarkers to rule out ACS—these *must* be repeated after 6–8 hours. Never send just one sample for troponin testing following chest pain.
  - Accelerated chest pain rule-out protocols now include repeat ECG and troponin testing within 2–3 hours. Check your local process.

Chest X-ray
Review the CXR as soon as possible (see Chapter 36). The CXR is apparently normal in many conditions, such as uncomplicated ACS, PE and pericarditis. However, abnormal findings may include:
- LVF with upper lobe pulmonary venous congestion, bat-wing peri-hilar haze, Kerley B lines (complicating ACS).
- Aortic dissection—widened mediastinum or prominent aortic knuckle with a 'double calcium' shadow >6 mm.

- Pneumothorax—peripheral hyperlucent area indicating free air in the pleural cavity, with partial or complete collapse of the affected lung.
- Pericarditis—if significant fluid (>250 mL) has accumulated, the cardiac silhouette may be symmetrically enlarged.
- Pneumonia—lobar or diffuse infiltrate changes.
- Pulmonary embolism—blunted costophrenic angle, raised hemidiaphragm, linear atelectasis or infarction, or an area of oligaemia.

Specific management
Acute coronary syndrome

- Classic features of the pain of ACS and its complications are described above.
- However, some patients have atypical pain, especially women, elderly people and those with diabetes and renal disease.
- ACS may also present with dyspnoea, orthopnoea or paroxysmal nocturnal dyspnoea (PND), lethargy, an arrhythmia or confusion (delirium, especially in the elderly), rather than chest pain.
- If the patient has chest pain and the ECG does not demonstrate significant ST elevation (≥1 mm in two or more contiguous limb leads or ≥2 mm in two or more contiguous chest leads):
  - Administer oxygen if shocked or hypoxic with saturation <93%, and give aspirin 300 mg PO.
  - Try to relieve the pain with GTN SL (0.6 mg tablets or 0.4 mg spray). Do not administer GTN if SBP <90 mmHg.
  - Give morphine if the pain continues despite 2–3 doses of GTN. Administer morphine IV in 2.5–5 mg aliquots until the pain is relieved.
  - Send blood for a cardiac troponin level immediately, and after 6–8 hours. Accelerated protocols now allow repeat troponin testing after 2–3 hours.
  - Perform serial ECGs immediately and after 6–8 hours, or every 15 minutes if the pain is continuing. Accelerated protocols now allow repeat ECG testing after 2–3 hours.
  - Determine the patient's disposition and further management. This is based on their ACS risk-profile stratification.

High-risk features
- The patient has:
  - Repetitive or prolonged (>10 min) ongoing chest pain.
  - Elevated troponin level on initial or repeat testing.
  - Persistent or dynamic ECG changes (ST depression or T wave inversion).

- Haemodynamic compromise with SBP <90 mmHg, heart failure, ventricular tachycardia, syncope or new-onset mitral regurgitation.
- Recent PCI (within last 6 months) or prior coronary bypass grafting (CABG).
- Diabetes, or chronic renal impairment (eGFR <60 mL/min) with 'typical' chest pain.
- Commence high-flow oxygen if shocked or hypoxic, give aspirin 300 mg PO and clopidogrel 300 mg PO.
- Contact your senior doctor immediately, then the cardiology registrar. Organise for transfer to CCU for consideration of angiography within next 48 hours.
- *Note*: chest pain with ST elevation on ECG indicates a STEMI and requires immediate reperfusion therapy—see later.

Intermediate-risk features
- The patient has:
  - Resolved chest pain consistent with ACS that occurred at rest, was prolonged (>10 min) or was not controlled with GTN (i.e. not their usual angina).
  - Age >65 years.
  - Known previous AMI or significant coronary artery stenosis >50%. Regular aspirin use.
  - Two or more of cardiac risk factors (hypertension, smoking, hyperlipidaemia or significant family history).
  - 'Atypical' chest pain in a patient with diabetes or chronic renal impairment (eGFR <60 mL/min).
  - First episode of chest pain.
- Give aspirin 300 mg PO as above, call your senior doctor and refer to the inpatient medical registrar. These patients should ideally have continuous ECG monitoring in the CCU (if available), or at least a repeat ECG and troponin in 6–8 hours.
  - Accelerated protocols now allow repeat troponin testing after 2–3 hours.
- If still negative, they then require exercise stress testing (EST), ideally within 72 hours, to further categorise them as high-risk (EST positive) or low-risk (EST negative). An alternative test such as a myocardial perfusion scan, stress echo or even a CT coronary angiogram is indicated in those unable to do an EST.

Low-risk features
- The patient has:
  - Chest pain consistent with ACS and no high-risk or intermediate-risk features.
  - A known diagnosis of angina and the current symptoms resolve promptly with 1–3 GTN doses.

- Review the precipitating cause and ECG, and determine if the threshold for angina has decreased or the severity of pain increased. Consult with your senior, as adjustment to antianginal medication may be all that is required.
- However, if this episode of pain was more prolonged, was worse or occurred with a lower threshold than normal with no easily remediable precipitant, send blood for cardiac biomarkers and repeat them and the ECG at 6–8 hours.
  - Accelerated protocols now allow repeat ECG and troponin testing after 2–3 hours.
- If both are negative, organise an outpatient cardiology or usual physician referral.

ST-elevation myocardial infarction

A patient with chest pain and ST elevation on ECG must be assessed urgently with a view to immediate reperfusion therapy with thrombolysis or PCI.

- Call your senior doctor and obtain an urgent cardiology consult, as the outcome is optimised if reperfusion occurs within 30 minutes (thrombolysis) or 60 minutes (PCI).
- Evaluate the ECG changes in comparison with previous ECGs.
- Check if there are any contraindications to thrombolysis (see Table 16.1) before the decision on which type of reperfusion therapy is made.
- Indications for reperfusion:
  - Typical chest pain (or equivalent) in preceding 12 hours **and**
  - Persistent ST elevation >2 mm in two contiguous chest leads or >1 mm in two contiguous limb leads, or new onset of left bundle branch block (LBBB).
- Commence high-flow oxygen, give aspirin 300 mg PO and clopidogrel 300–600 mg PO or prasugrel 60 mg PO.
  - Give LMWH or IV heparin on discussion with the cardiologist and in the light of which reperfusion therapy is to be used.

Aortic dissection

Predisposed to by hypertension, especially males over 60 years, bicuspid aortic valve, coarctation or iatrogenic (i.e. cardiac catheterisation). When younger than 40 years consider Marfan's or Ehlers–Danlos syndrome. Ask about a family history or a previous dissection.

- There is sudden onset of severe pain that is sharp or tearing in nature, retrosternal to interscapular and may migrate. Patients with dissection typically have pain that is out of proportion to other clinical findings and difficult to relieve, even with large doses of IV opioid.

Table 16.1 **Contraindications to thrombolysis**	
Absolute contraindications	**Relative contraindications**
↑ Risk of bleeding	↑ Risk of bleeding
Active bleeding or bleeding diathesis (excluding menses) Significant closed head injury or facial trauma within past 3 months Suspected aortic dissection (including new neurological symptoms)	Current use of anticoagulants—the higher the INR, the higher the risk of bleeding Non-compressible vascular puncture sites Recent major surgery (<3 weeks) Traumatic or prolonged CPR (>10 min) Recent (<4 weeks) internal bleeding (e.g. GI bleed or urinary tract haemorrhage) Active peptic ulcer Pregnancy
↑ Risk of intracranial haemorrhage	↑ Risk of intracranial haemorrhage
Any previous intracranial haemorrhage Ischaemic stroke in previous 3 months Known structural cerebral vascular lesion (e.g. arteriovenous malformation [AVM]) Known malignant intracranial neoplasm (primary or metastatic)	History of chronic, severe, poorly controlled hypertension Severe uncontrolled hypertension on presentation (SBP >180 mmHg, DBP >110 mmHg) Ischaemic stroke >3 months ago, dementia or known intracranial abnormality not covered in contraindications

- Look for unequal or absent pulses, a difference of >20 mmHg BP between arms or other complications such as aortic incompetence, pleural effusion or any new focal neurology.
- Call your senior doctor if you suspect an aortic dissection, and investigate and treat urgently:
  - Give oxygen to maintain saturation >95%.
  - Insert two large IV cannulae (14–16G) and send blood for an immediate cross-match of six units packed RBCs.
  - Relieve pain with titrated IV morphine 2.5–5 mg repeated as needed.
- Review the CXR (see Figure 16.1)—if suggestive of dissection or if the clinical suspicion is still high:
  - Arrange for an urgent helical CT angiogram (CTA) of the chest, a transoesophageal echocardiogram (TOE) if expertise is available or, in their absence, a transthoracic echo, which may demonstrate some of the complications of a dissection, such as cardiac tamponade or acute aortic regurgitation.
  - Arrange admission to ICU and contact the cardiothoracic or vascular surgical team.

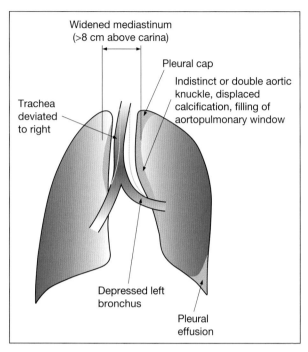

Figure 16.1 Aortic dissection on CXR.

- Give an IV beta-blocker such as esmolol or metoprolol slowly until the pulse is <60 beats/min or the SBP is <120 mmHg.
- If the BP is not controlled at this level, despite a pulse <60 beats/min, add sodium nitroprusside or a GTN infusion until the SBP is 100–120 mmHg. Start these in an intensive care area with intra-arterial BP monitoring.
- Prepare the patient for an operation if the CTA or TOE confirms an ascending AAD (type A). If there is a descending acute aortic dissection (type B), the patient should be managed in ICU with careful control of BP and observation for complications.
- Endovascular stent repair is becoming more common, particularly in descending acute aortic dissection.

Pericarditis

Pericarditis may be postviral (coxsackievirus, echovirus, adenovirus, influenza, mumps, herpes virus); associated with AMI or 2–6 weeks post-MI (Dressler's syndrome), uraemia, malignancy or a connective tissue disorder (SLE, RA, scleroderma or polyarteritis nodosa [PAN]); TB; or follow trauma, radiation therapy or cardiac surgery; and occurs in AAD. There is no discernible cause in 10–20% of cases.

- The pain is sharp, retrosternal and radiates to the back; is worse on inspiration, swallowing or lying down; and is relieved by sitting up.
- A pericardial rub is best heard along the left sternal edge in expiration with the patient sitting up, but may be transient.
- Pericarditis related to TB, uraemia or neoplastic disease is usually more insidious and pain is often mild or absent, with the patient presenting with insidious pericardial tamponade.
- Most patients with pericarditis do not have a haemodynamically significant pericardial effusion or myocardial inflammation. The main issue is control of pain.

Diagnosis and management:
- Attach a cardiac monitor and pulse oximeter to the patient.
- Send blood for FBC, U&E, LFTs, troponin and viral serology.
- Perform an ECG, which may show sinus tachycardia alone, widespread concave ST elevation or PR-segment depression.
  - Late in the course T waves may flatten or become symmetrically inverted, sometimes permanently. Decreased voltages are suggestive of a pericardial effusion, and electrical alternans (components of the ECG such as the QRS axis alternate between beats) is a rare finding in pericardial effusion.
- *Note*: distinguishing pericarditis from STEMI is critical, as thrombolysis is contraindicated in pericarditis due to the risk of bleeding from haemorrhagic transformation.
- Request a CXR, which is usually normal even when a pericardial effusion is present. Apparent cardiomegaly only occurs once 250 mL of pericardial fluid have accumulated.
- Give an NSAID as the drug of choice. If there are contraindications to NSAIDs, colchicine 0.5 mg BD may be used.
- Prednisolone 50 mg PO or dexamethasone 4 mg PO or IV may be tried if intolerant of NSAIDs, or diarrhoea with colchicine.
- Arrange an urgent echocardiogram followed by pericardiocentesis if signs of cardiac tamponade such as tachycardia, hypotension, pulsus paradoxus and a raised JVP that rises on inspiration (known as Kussmaul's sign) occur.
- Otherwise, echocardiography may be organised electively for a stable patient suspected of an effusion.

Pleuritic causes of chest pain

Pleuritic pain is a sharp, well-localised pain that is worse with inspiration. Often patients cannot take a deep breath in because it 'catches' and prevents full inspiration. Radiation to the shoulder or abdomen occurs with diaphragmatic involvement.
- Important causes of pleuritic pain include:
  - Pericarditis (see above)
  - Pneumothorax

- Pneumomediastinum
- Pneumonia
- Pulmonary embolus with a pulmonary infarction
- Autoimmune disorders (SLE, RA)
- Malignancy
- Musculoskeletal pain.
- 'Pleurisy' is a diagnosis of exclusion when none of the above can be identified. It may be due to viruses, such as enteroviruses, including epidemic myalgia (Bornholm's disease) due to coxsackie B virus.
- Examine the patient for features suggestive of an underlying cause such as fever and bronchial breathing in pneumonia etc. Listen to the chest for a pleural rub, although a rub may be inaudible if pain limits deep breathing, and disappears as an effusion develops.
- Perform an ECG, which should be normal, but may show non-diagnostic abnormalities in PE.
- Request a CXR, which may suggest an underlying cause or show non-specific basal atelectasis that may occur in any patient with restricted inspiration. A normal-looking CXR is more likely with PE.
- If no significant underlying cause is found:
  - Give oxygen to maintain oxygen saturation >95%
  - Give NSAIDs (e.g. ibuprofen 400 mg PO TDS) plus paracetamol 1 g PO 4-hourly.

Pneumomediastinum

A patient with a spontaneous pneumomediastinum presents with sudden onset of chest, neck or throat pain. The CXR shows mediastinal air as a dark line outlining a heart border. The pathogenesis is similar to spontaneous pneumothorax and includes inhalational drug use. Most patients remain systemically well and can be treated with oral analgesia alone.

Gastrointestinal causes of chest pain

Suggested by heartburn, burning retrosternal or epigastric pain, worse on stooping or lying flat, exacerbated by swallowing, hot drinks or food and relieved by antacids.

Oesophagitis or oesophageal spasm may mimic cardiac pain and be relieved by sublingual GTN. ACS must always be excluded first if there is any doubt about the diagnosis.

- The pain of oesophagitis, gastro-oesophageal reflux, gastritis or peptic ulcer may be temporarily relieved with oral antacids, but requires acid suppression therapy:
  - Give an antacid 15–20 mL every 2 hours in the acute phase, then TDS after meals and once before bedtime.

- Prescribe a proton-pump inhibitor such as omeprazole 20–40 mg PO daily or an H_2-receptor blocker such as ranitidine 150 mg PO BD.
- Advise lifestyle modification such as stopping smoking, reducing alcohol consumption, omitting hot or spicy food from the diet, eating small meals regularly during the day and not eating immediately before sleep.
- Refer for endoscopic evaluation and *Helicobacter pylori* testing.
- Immunocompromised patients may experience severe chest pain from **oesophageal candidiasis** that does not respond to antacids. Diagnosis should be confirmed by endoscopy. Fluconazole 100 mg PO daily is the treatment of choice.

Oesophageal rupture is associated with sudden onset of severe chest pain, which may follow vomiting (Boerhaave's syndrome). It can also occur after endoscopy, foreign body impaction, caustic ingestion or trauma. Pain is persistent and difficult to relieve, and often associated with dyspnoea, diaphoresis, tachycardia and shock.

- The patient looks unwell and may have palpable subcutaneous emphysema or crunching sounds on auscultation of the heart (Hamman's crunch due to pneuomediastinum).
- ECG may be normal or have non-specific changes.
- CXR shows mediastinal air, left pleural effusion or left-sided pneumothorax.
- Call your senior regarding further investigation—usually by water-soluble gastrografin contrast oesophagram, CT scan or endoscopy.
- If oesophageal rupture is confirmed, obtain large-bore IV access, commence fluid resuscitation and titrated opioid analgesia and broad-spectrum antibiotics. Admit to ICU and arrange immediate cardiothoracic or general surgical consult.

Musculoskeletal causes of chest pain

- Musculoskeletal disorders cause pain that is worse not only with breathing but also with movement. There may have been a preceding bout of coughing, strenuous exercise or a history of minor trauma.
- Palpate and compress the chest wall to identify a tender muscle, fractured rib(s) or tender costochondral junction. Palpate and gently percuss the spine to identify a crush fracture, which may be causing referred dermatomal pain.
- The ECG is normal and other investigations are unhelpful.
- Treat musculoskeletal causes of pain with an NSAID, such as ibuprofen 400 mg PO TDS or naproxen 250–500 mg PO TDS.

Herpes zoster

- Unilateral chest pain in a dermatomal distribution may precede the typical skin lesions of herpes zoster ('shingles') by 2 or 3 days.

The rash begins as a reddened, maculopapular area that rapidly evolves into vesicular lesions.

- Give opioid analgesia to patients with severe pain and commence famciclovir 250 mg or valaciclovir 1 g given orally 8-hourly for 7 days, if seen within 72 hours of vesicle eruption. Combining antiviral therapy with steroids (e.g. prednisolone 50 mg PO daily for 3 days) may provide added pain relief.
- Postherpetic neuralgia occurs after the acute episode and is difficult to treat. Potential therapies include anticonvulsant, antidepressant or antiarrhythmic drugs. Specialist input is required, arranged by the usual medical care team.

Panic and anxiety disorders

Panic attacks are discrete periods of intense fear or discomfort associated with the abrupt onset of four or more symptoms that include palpitations, sweating, trembling, sensation of shortness of breath or choking, chest pain or discomfort, dizziness, weakness. Hyperventilation causes perioral, hand or feet parasthesiae or muscular spasm related to acute hypocalcaemia from a respiratory alkalosis, even lightheadedness to the point of unconsciousness.

Due to the possibility of a life-threatening cause of chest pain, panic and anxiety disorders are *always* a diagnosis of exclusion. Discuss the patient with your senior.

Attempt to control the hyperventilation by reassurance. Alternatively, ask the patient to re-breathe into a paper bag or mask to control the ventilatory loss of CO_2. Give diazepam 2–5 mg PO or lorazepam 1–2 mg SL acutely if there is no response to initial treatment or the attack recurs.

Heart rate and rhythm disorders

Three abnormalities in heart rate or rhythm you will be asked to assess on call are pulses that are too fast, too slow or irregular. The main purpose of the HR is to keep the cardiac output sufficient to perfuse the vital organs, the heart, brain and kidneys. Your task is to identify the rhythm disturbance, determine the potential cause and treat the problem, ideally before it causes hypoperfusion and thus becomes symptomatic.

TACHYARRHYTHMIAS

Phone call

Questions

1. **How fast is the heart rate?**
2. **Is the rhythm regular or irregular?**
3. **What is the blood pressure?** Tachycardia with hypotension signifies an unstable arrhythmia and mandates urgent medical review. Hypotension may be the cause or the result of a tachycardia that does not allow adequate LV diastolic filling time to maintain CO.
4. **Does the patient have chest pain, shortness of breath or an altered mental status?** Unstable arrhythmias are associated with hypoxia, hypotension, tachypnoea, pulmonary oedema and cerebral hypoperfusion. A rapid HR may be the result of myocardial ischaemia, PE or CCF. Conversely, a rapid HR may precipitate myocardial ischaemia or CCF.
5. **Is there a history of illicit drug use?** Cocaine or amphetamine use may precipitate an arrhythmia.
6. **What is the temperature?** Tachycardia proportional to the temperature elevation is expected in a febrile patient. However, examine the patient to ensure that there is no other cause for the rapid HR.
7. **What was the reason for admission?**

Instructions

If the patient has chest pain, SOB, SBP <90 mmHg or altered mental status:

* Ask the nurse to stay by the patient's bedside and get help from additional nursing staff.
* Give oxygen by mask to maintain saturation >94% and attach a pulse oximeter and cardiac monitor to the patient.
* Request an urgent ECG.
* Request an IV trolley for the patient's bedside with two cannulae ready for insertion.
* Request that the cardiac arrest trolley with defibrillator and resuscitation equipment be brought to the patient's bedside.

Prioritisation

See any patient with tachycardia and signs of circulatory compromise such as chest pain, SOB, hypotension or an altered mental status immediately; or if the HR >140 beats/min, as this will trigger a MET call.

Corridor thoughts

What causes a rapid heart rate? (* = major threat to life)
* **Rapid regular heart rate**
  * Sinus tachycardia (see Figure 17.1)
  * Atrial flutter (with constant AV conduction 2:1 or 3:1 etc) (see Figure 17.2)
  * Supraventricular tachycardia (see Figure 17.3)
  * Paroxysmal atrial tachycardia
  * Junctional tachycardia
  * Ventricular tachycardia (monomorphic) (see Figure 17.4)*
* **Rapid irregular heart rate**
  * Atrial fibrillation with rapid ventricular response ('rapid AF') (see Figure 17.5)

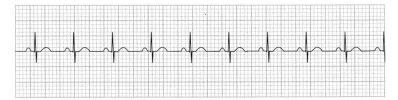

Figure 17.1 Sinus tachycardia. Copyright Tor Ercleve.

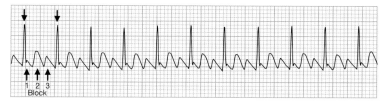

Figure 17.2 Atrial flutter. Copyright Tor Ercleve.

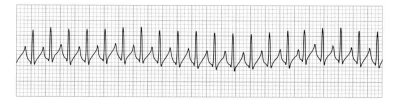

Figure 17.3 Supraventricular tachycardia. Copyright Tor Ercleve.

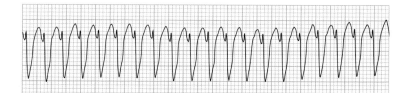

Figure 17.4 Ventricular tachycardia. Copyright Tor Ercleve.

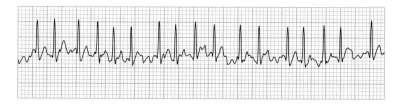

Figure 17.5 Atrial fibrillation. Copyright Tor Ercleve.

- Atrial flutter with variable AV conduction (flutter with variable block) (see Figure 17.6)
- Multifocal atrial tachycardia (see Figure 17.7)
- Sinus tachycardia with atrial ectopic beats (see Figure 17.8) or ventricular ectopic beats (see Figure 17.9)
- Polymorphic ventricular tachycardia, that includes torsades de pointes from a prolonged resting QT interval*

SECTION C – Common calls

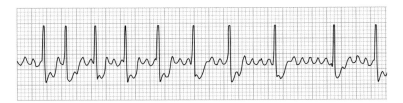

Figure 17.6 Atrial flutter with variable block. Copyright Tor Ercleve.

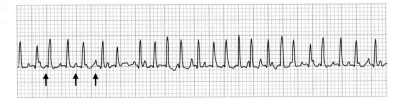

Figure 17.7 Multifocal atrial tachycardia. Copyright Tor Ercleve.

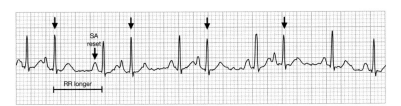

Figure 17.8 Sinus tachycardia with premature atrial contractions. Copyright Tor Ercleve.

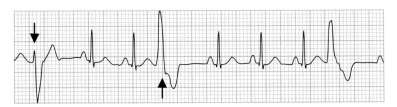

Figure 17.9 Sinus tachycardia with premature ventricular contractions. Copyright Tor Ercleve.

Major threat to life

- Pulseless ventricular tachycardia (pVT) causing cardiac arrest.
- Hypotension resulting in hypoperfusion with shock, confusion and collapse.
- Angina, progressing to MI.
- Acute pulmonary oedema, leading to hypoxia and progressive hypotension.

Bedside

Quick-look test

Does the patient look well (comfortable), sick (uncomfortable or distressed) or critical (about to die)?

- Patients with tachycardia that is sufficiently severe to cause hypotension, angina or pulmonary oedema look sick or critical, with pale, clammy peripheries, cyanosis, agitation or confusion.
- Patients who are normotensive with a tachycardia or arrhythmia may look deceptively well, even occasionally those with a VT.

Airway and vital signs

What is the heart rate?

- Assess the HR by taking the patient's pulse, listening to the apex beat or reading the ECG rhythm strip.
- Does the ECG or monitor also demonstrate acute ischaemic changes such as ST depression or T wave inversion, or a cardiac arrhythmia?
- Feel for the volume of the pulse and its regularity.

Is the rhythm regular or irregular?

- Irregular rhythms are usually caused by AF with rapid ventricular response or atrial flutter. Alternatively, they may be caused by premature atrial or ventricular contractions.

If the rhythm is regular, is the QRS complex narrow or broad?

- Narrow complexes are supraventricular in origin and include:
  - Sinus tachycardia (normal P waves)
  - Atrial tachycardia (abnormal P waves)
  - SVT (no P waves)
  - Atrial flutter (flutter waves visible; or suspect atrial flutter with 2:1 block if the ventricular rate is 150 beats/min).
- Regular broad complexes are VT until proven otherwise.
  - A broad-complex regular tachycardia (e.g. Figure 17.4) may represent VT or an SVT with aberrant conduction (abnormal ventricular depolarisation).
  - Broad-complex tachycardia in an older patient, or in any patient with known prior myocardial ischaemia, is probably VT and should be treated as such.

- Do not assume that a broad-complex tachycardia is an SVT with aberrancy just because the patient is not distressed, or is young.
- It may well be VT, which is made worse by incorrectly treating as an SVT, rapidly leading to VF and even death.

What is the blood pressure?
- This is the most important consideration of all.
- If the patient is hypotensive (SBP <90 mmHg), determine whether the hypotension is related to hypovolaemia (i.e. is it a compensatory tachycardia?) or a result of the tachycardia.
- Hypotension with a compensatory tachycardia:
  - A compensatory tachycardia occurs in any acute illness causing hypotension, whether from fluid or blood loss, internal (concealed) or external (revealed).
  - A sinus tachycardia is most common, but a patient already in chronic AF will accelerate an irregular HR.
  - If the hypotension is left untreated, a sinus tachycardia will deteriorate into an abnormal cardiac rhythm secondary to resultant hypoxia with myocardial ischaemia.
- Tachycardia causing hypotension:
  - The three most common rhythms that cause inadequate diastolic filling leading to a low CO with hypotension are VT, AF with rapid ventricular response and SVT.
  - Early recognition of these primary arrhythmias is essential for prompt and appropriate treatment.

What is the respiratory rate?
- A patient with tachypnoea may have acute pulmonary oedema, indicating a potentially unstable arrhythmia in need of prompt treatment, or from a metabolic lactic acidosis due to hypoxia and hypotension.

Management

Immediate management

Tachycardia in a haemodynamically unstable patient with hypotension, chest pain, SOB and/or altered mental status:
- Call for senior help.
- Apply high-flow oxygen by mask, and gain IV access.
- Attach an ECG monitor/defibrillator to the patient.
- Confirm the cardiac rhythm with a 12-lead ECG (do not try to diagnose the rhythm without a formal 12-lead ECG, except in a dire emergency).
- Prepare procedural sedation, such as propofol 200 mg in 20 mL IV, and keep readily available. Call an anaesthetist, as cardioversion will be required.

- A patient who is haemodynamically unstable and has VT, AF with rapid ventricular response or SVT requires emergency synchronised DC cardioversion (see Chapter 64):
  - Unless the patient is in cardiac arrest (in which case an immediate non-synchronised shock is given), always wait for senior staff to attend. *Never* administer procedural sedation and proceed to electrical DC cardioversion alone.
  - One doctor must attend to the airway, while the other operates the defibrillator and coordinates the cardiac care.
  - Start with 120–150 J biphasic and repeat up to three times, with stepwise increases in joules.
- *Note:* if the patient is hypotensive and the rhythm is sinus tachycardia, the most likely cause is underlying hypotension.
  - Look for and urgently treat any cause(s) for this, such as hypovolaemia, hypoxia, fever etc, and consider other precipitants of the tachycardia, such as anaemia or pain.

Selective history and chart review

Perform a focused history and chart review if the patient is stable or immediate management has been commenced and help is on its way. This helps guide selective management and disposition.

How and when did the palpitations start?
- Sudden onset suggests a new, acute arrhythmia.
- Gradual onset may indicate a worsening of a chronic arrhythmia such as AF.
- Recurrent intermittent episodes suggest a paroxysmal arrhythmia or ectopic beats.
- Onset following chest pain may indicate ischaemia as the cause. Palpitations followed by pain indicate ischaemia secondary to the arrhythmia.

Are there any related symptoms?
- Sweating, light-headedness, chest pain, dyspnoea and syncope indicate circulatory compromise.

Review the patient's past cardiac history
- Enquire about any previous episodes, investigations, treatment given and its success (e.g. a patient with SVT may have undergone a vagal manoeuvre, or been successfully given adenosine in the past).
- Ask about predisposing factors to palpitations:
  - Previous episodes of chest pain, dizzy spell or collapse
  - Known ischaemic heart disease, or atherosclerosis risk factors such as smoking, hypertension, hypercholesterolaemia, diabetes, renal disease or a positive family history
  - Pericarditis
  - Structural heart disease such as valvular disease, cardiomyopathy, congenital heart disease (e.g. atrial septal defect) or recent cardiac surgery

- Thyroid disease
- Illicit drug use such as cocaine or amphetamines.
- Review the patient's family history
  - **Is there a family history of palpitations, syncope or sudden cardiac death?**
    - Premature sudden death in a family member is suspicious of a lethal arrhythmia associated with Wolff–Parkinson–White (WPW) syndrome, Brugada syndrome, long QT syndrome or hypertrophic cardiomyopathy (HCM).

Check the patient's chart

- Previous ECGs may demonstrate a conduction abnormality, prolonged QT interval, QRS widening or a delta wave or tall R wave in lead V1 from ventricular pre-excitation (WPW).
- Previous electrophysiological testing may give a definitive diagnosis.
- Echocardiography:
  - A documented LV ejection fraction <30% is associated with VT and higher risk of sudden death.
  - Atrial diameters >4.5 cm are associated with atrial arrhythmias.
- Medications may cause tachycardia (e.g. salbutamol, terbutaline, pseudoephedrine or anticholinergics).

Selective physical examination

Vitals	Repeat now
HEENT	Exophthalmos, lid lag, lid retraction (hyperthyroidism)
CVS	Murmur of mitral regurgitation or mitral stenosis (mitral valve disease)
	S_3 gallop (LV failure)
Resp	Tachypnoea, cyanosis, wheezing, pleural effusion (LV failure, PE)
MSS	Swelling, thigh or leg tenderness or oedema (DVT)
	Tremor, brisk deep tendon reflexes (hyperthyroidism).

Specific management
Atrial fibrillation

- AF is the most common sustained arrhythmia. The ECG shows an irregularly irregular ventricular rhythm with fibrillatory atrial activity.
- Factors predisposing to the development of AF include chronic alcohol use, ischaemic heart disease, hypertension, cardiomyopathy, congenital heart disease and valvular lesions secondary to rheumatic fever.

- Any acute illness may also precipitate AF:
  - Myocardial ischaemia, pericarditis or myocarditis
  - Hypoxaemia and acute lung disease such as PE, pneumonia or COPD
  - Electrolyte disturbance such as hypokalaemia
  - Thyrotoxicosis
  - Sepsis
  - Cardiac surgery.
- Recent alcohol binge ('holiday heart syndrome').

Unstable atrial fibrillation
AF and hypotension, altered mental state, chest pain (angina) or SOB (LV failure):

- The treatment of choice is synchronised DC cardioversion, beginning with 120–150 J (biphasic)—provided that the AF is of recent onset (<48 h).
  - *Note*: a patient on digoxin therapy may require temporary transcutaneous pacing, as asystole can follow DC reversion.

Stable atrial fibrillation
AF with ventricular rate >120 beats/min, but without evidence of haemodynamic compromise, can undergo rhythm control (duration <48 hours) or rate control (duration >48 hours or unknown):

- **Duration of AF <48 hours:**
  Rhythm control with drugs or electrical cardioversion is indicated.
  - Correct hypokalaemia with 20 mmol potassium in 500 mL 5% dextrose over 30 minutes.
  - Correct hypomagnesaemia (particularly in alcoholics) with magnesium sulfate 10 mmol (2.5 g) IV.
  - Give amiodarone 300 mg IV over 30 minutes, followed by an infusion of amiodarone 900 mg over 24 hours. This is effective in up to 75% of patients. Continuous ECG monitoring is required.
    - *Note:* although flecainide and sotalol are more effective than amiodarone, they have dangerous side effects, including hypotension, and mandate senior advice before use.
  - Commence heparinisation with a LMWH such as enoxaparin 1 mg/kg SC 12-hourly, or UFH 5000 U IV as a bolus, followed by an infusion commencing at 1000 U/h.
  - There may be atrial stunning after reversion to sinus rhythm and an increased likelihood of clot formation in the atria, although this risk is minimal with recent-onset AF.
  - Perform electrical cardioversion if the above measures are unsuccessful, using brief procedural sedation such as propofol with careful airway supervision by an anaesthetist (see Chapter 64).

SECTION C – Common calls

- *Note:* 50–60% of patients will spontaneously revert within 24 hours anyway, so observation may be all that is needed when the AF has been present for fewer than 12 hours.
- **Duration of AF >48 hours or the time duration is unclear: Rate control** only is indicated.
  - Do not attempt to cardiovert with drugs or elective DC reversion, as they are contraindicated prior to full anticoagulation.
  - Commence heparinisation with LMWH such as enoxaparin, or UFH as above.
  - Perform rate control using PO or IV beta-blocker, digoxin, diltiazem or magnesium:
    - The decision to give these agents PO or IV depends on the patient's symptoms, AF duration, availability of monitoring and the patient's comorbidities.
  - Continuous ECG monitoring is required when any agent is given IV, usually necessitating CCU care.
  - If the patient is completely asymptomatic or the AF has been present for several days, rate control with an oral agent is appropriate.
  - Provided the patient has normal LV function (no past history or current evidence of LV failure and no reduced ejection fraction measured on echocardiography), give:
    - Metoprolol 2.5 mg slow IV boluses up to a total of 10 mg. The PO dose is 25–50 mg twice a day thereafter.
  - If the patient has documented or suspected depressed LV function, give:
    - Digoxin 0.5 mg slowly IV or PO, repeated in 8 hours, followed by 0.125–0.25 mg PO daily thereafter.
- **Atrial fibrillation with ventricular rate of <100 beats/min:**
  - AF <100 beats/min in an untreated patient suggests underlying AV nodal dysfunction. These patients do not require immediate rate or rhythm control unless haemodynamically compromised (e.g. hypotension, chest pain or LV failure).
  - The patient should start on anticoagulation, if there is no active contraindication.

Atrial flutter

- The ECG demonstrates a regular narrow-complex tachycardia with sawtooth atrial activity at a rate of 300 beats/min, and with AV conduction varying between 2:1 (gives a ventricular rate of 150 beats/min), 3:1 (rate of 100 beats/min) and 4:1 (rate of 75 beats/min).
- If the diagnosis is unclear, perform a vagal manoeuvre (see below) to increase the degree of AV block and reveal the flutter waves.
- The causes and treatment of atrial flutter are similar to those of AF, although treatment of atrial flutter sometimes causes AF.

- Electrical cardioversion is the most effective treatment if the patient is haemodynamically unstable or the duration is <48 hours.
- If the patient's condition is stable or the duration is >48 hours, use rate control only with a calcium-channel blocker such as diltiazem, a beta-blocker or digoxin (as with AF).
- The indications for anticoagulation are similar to those for AF.

Supraventricular tachycardia

- Paroxysmal SVT results from a re-entry circuit, either in the AV node or via an accessory pathway as in WPW syndrome.
- Re-entrant SVTs are rarely associated with either acquired structural cardiac disease or other illness. The ECG usually shows a narrow-complex regular tachycardia, with absent or retrograde P waves.
- Treatment of a narrow-complex SVT is the same, irrespective of whether WPW is present, unlike a wide-complex SVT with aberrant conduction, where the presence of an accessory pathway in WPW makes a critical difference.

Unstable supraventricular tachycardia
SVT with hypotension, chest pain (angina), SOB (LV failure) or an altered mental state:
- Call for senior help.
- Apply high-flow oxygen by mask and gain IV access
- Attach the ECG monitor/defibrillator to the patient. Confirm the rhythm.
- Prepare procedural sedation such as propofol 200 mg in 20 mL IV and call an anaesthetist.
- Once senior assistance is present, the treatment of choice is synchronised DC cardioversion, beginning with 70–120 J (biphasic) repeated up to three times.

Stable supraventricular tachycardia
Use a vagal manoeuvre to convert the rhythm when the patient is haemodynamically stable:
- **Valsalva manoeuvre**
  - Place the patient in the Trendelenburg (foot-of-the-bed up) position on a trolley.
  - Ask the patient to blow into the nozzle end of a 20 mL syringe for 10 seconds to try to force the plunger halfway up, then release suddenly. Alternatively, ask the patient to hold a breath and to 'bear down' as if having a bowel movement, then suddenly release.
- **Carotid sinus massage**
  - This should always be performed with IV atropine 600 micrograms available and continuous ECG monitoring,

both for safety (some patients develop asystole) and to document the result.

- Carotid sinus massage (CSM) has resulted in cerebral embolisation of an atherosclerotic plaque from carotid artery compression. Always listen over each carotid artery for a bruit and do *not* perform CSM if there is a:
  - carotid bruit, or known carotid stenosis >50%
  - history in preceding 3 months of TIA, stroke or AMI
  - history of symptomatic bradyarrhythmias.

  If there are no contraindications to the procedure, turn the patient's head to the left. Locate the carotid sinus just anterior to the sternocleidomastoid muscle at the level of the top of the thyroid cartilage (see Figure 17.10).
  - Feel the carotid pulsation at this point and apply steady pressure to the carotid artery with two fingers for 10–15 seconds. Try the right side, and if this is not effective, try the left side.
  - Simultaneous bilateral massage of the carotid sinus should *never* be done, as this will effectively cut off the cerebral blood flow and lead to syncope, stroke or even a cardiac arrest.

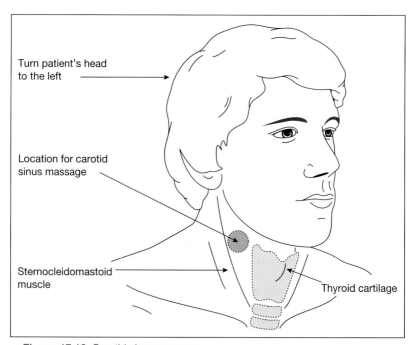

Turn patient's head to the left

Location for carotid sinus massage

Sternocleidomastoid muscle

Thyroid cartilage

Figure 17.10 Carotid sinus massage.

Drug therapy

- **Adenosine**
  - If vagal manoeuvres do not succeed, give adenosine under ECG monitoring.
  - The dose is 6 mg as a *rapid* IV bolus, followed by a 20 mL saline flush. If this is ineffective, increase to adenosine 12 mg IV push, and repeat this after 1–2 min if still no response.
  - Use IV adenosine with caution in patients with COPD and asthma, as it may precipitate wheeze, and reduce the dose in patients on dipyridamole.
  - Side effects are common, but transient. However, warn the patient about these as they are often poorly tolerated— particularly the feeling of impending doom, also facial flushing, dyspnoea and chest pressure.
- **Verapamil**
  - If the adenosine was unsuccessful or poorly tolerated, give verapamil 2.5–5 mg IV over 1–2 minutes repeated every 5–10 minutes to a total dose of 15 mg. Verapamil may cause hypotension if injected too rapidly, so give slowly, particularly in the elderly.
  - Verapamil is a negative inotropic agent and may precipitate hypotension in a patient predisposed to LV failure.
  - *Note*: never give verapamil after a beta-blocker, when digoxin toxicity is suspected or if the patient has a wide-complex tachycardia as it may cause fatal bradyasystole.
- If SVT still persists following verapamil, repeat the vagal manoeuvres.

A patient whose condition is stable, but in whom none of the above measures has worked, should be transferred to CCU for emergency cardioversion.

Ectopic atrial tachycardias and junctional tachycardia

- **Multifocal atrial tachycardia:**
  - Narrow-complex, irregular, with three or more atrial foci, rate >100 beats/min, and variable P–P, P–R and R–R intervals. Frequent PAC may precede the development of multifocal atrial tachycardia, which in turn can be a forerunner of AF.
- **Paroxysmal atrial tachycardia:**
  - Narrow-complex, regular, rate >100 beats/min, usually with abnormal P waves or long P–R interval.
- **Junctional tachycardia:**
  - Narrow-complex, regular with absent P waves, rate usually <150 beats/min.
  - Atrial and junctional tachycardias are commonly secondary to pulmonary disease (especially COPD, PE), cardiac ischaemia, hypokalaemia, hypomagnesaemia, CCF, theophylline or digoxin toxicity, or caffeine, tobacco and alcohol use.

- Treat the underlying cause. If no cause can be found, give
  verapamil 80–120 mg PO TDS or diltiazem 30–90 mg PO QDS
  for rate control and to diminish the frequency of
  ectopic beats.
- Beta-blockers are contraindicated in patients with underlying
  bronchospasm.

Sinus tachycardia

- Sinus tachycardia occurs under the influence of the autonomic
  nervous system. The ECG confirms a regular sinus rhythm with a
  rate >100 beats/min (see Figure 17.1).
- The most common causes of persistent sinus tachycardia in a
  hospitalised patient are:
  - Hypovolaemia
  - Hypoxia of any cause (pulmonary oedema, PE, pneumonia,
    bronchospasm)
  - LV failure
  - Fever or infection
  - Hyperthyroidism
  - Anaemia
  - Sympathomimetic or anticholinergic drugs
  - Pain or anxiety.
- There is no specific drug treatment needed for a sinus tachycardia.
  Attempts at slowing the HR will potentially worsen the
  underlying cause when it is hypovolaemia, hypoxia, LV failure or
  anaemia.
- Instead, search for and treat the underlying cause.

Sinus tachycardia with premature ventricular contractions

- Sinus tachycardia with PVCs frequently presents as palpitations.
  Certain features of the PVCs are described as significant or
  'malignant'. Malignant features include:
  - R-on-T phenomenon (see Figure 17.11)
  - Multifocal PVCs
  - Couplets or salvos with three or more PVCs in a row
    (non-sustained VT)
  - Frequent PVCs (>5/min).

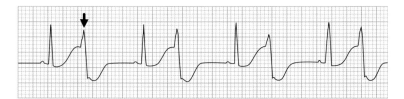

Figure 17.11 R-on-T phenomenon. Copyright Tor Ercleve.

- More importantly, PVCs can be a clue to significant underlying pathology. Look for and treat the common causes of PVCs:
  - Hypoxia
  - Myocardial ischaemia (symptoms or signs of angina or MI)
  - Hypokalaemia (see Chapter 43)
  - Acid–base imbalance. Acidosis and alkalosis are both associated with increased frequency of PVCs
  - Cardiomyopathy and mitral valve prolapse
  - Drugs such as digoxin and other antiarrhythmic agents
  - Hyperthyroidism.
- Transfer the patient to a telemetry ward or CCU for further investigation and continuous ECG monitoring, if there is myocardial ischaemia or frequent runs of non-sustained VT.

Ventricular tachycardia

- The most common cause of VT is myocardial ischaemia or myocardial scarring following acute MI. Other causes include dilated cardiomyopathy, drug toxicity, electrolyte disturbances and congenital.
- A broad-complex SVT with aberrancy from ventricular pre-excitation such as in WPW is treated the same as VT.

Unstable ventricular tachycardia
- **No recordable BP and no palpable pulse (pVT):**
  - Call for the cardiac arrest trolley immediately and proceed with CPR.
  - Early defibrillation is the priority.
- **VT with hypotension, angina, LVF or impaired mental status:**
  - Call for senior help.
  - Apply high-flow oxygen by mask and gain IV access.
  - Attach the ECG monitor/defibrillator to the patient. Confirm the rhythm.
  - Prepare procedural sedation such as propofol 200 mg in 20 mL IV and call an anaesthetist.
  - Once senior assistance is present, the treatment of choice is synchronised DC cardioversion. Start with 120–150 J biphasic and repeat up to three times, with stepwise increases in joules.

Stable ventricular tachycardia
- **Take precautions if the patient is stable, as deterioration can be rapid:**
  - Call for cardiac arrest equipment and senior assistance.
  - Give the patient 100% O_2 by mask.
  - Attach an ECG monitor to the patient.
  - Make sure that an IV line is in place.
  - Obtain a 12-lead ECG. Review QRS complexes and determine if the VT is monomorphic or polymorphic.

Monomorphic ventricular tachycardia
- ECG shows a broad-complex QRS, regular rhythm, rate >100 beats/min, with constant QRS axis.
- **Left ventricular function unknown or impaired:**
  - Give amiodarone 300 mg IV bolus over 20–60 minutes, followed by an infusion of 900 mg over 24 hours.
- **Left ventricular function is known to be normal:**
  - Administer amiodarone as above.
- Prepare for synchronised cardioversion, if amiodarone is unsuccessful or the patient's condition deteriorates.
  - Transfer the patient to the ICU/CCU for continuous ECG monitoring.
  - Look for the precipitating cause of the VT, such as myocardial ischaemia, electrolyte abnormality (hypokalaemia, hypomagnesaemia, hypocalcaemia) or drug toxicity (antiarrhythmic and other sodium-channel blocking drugs, especially tricyclic antidepressants).

Polymorphic ventricular tachycardia
- ECG shows a broad-complex QRS, regular rhythm, rate >100 beats/min, but with a variable and changing axis.
- Review the baseline 12-lead ECG.
- **Normal baseline QT interval:**
  - Give IV amiodarone as for monomorphic VT.
- **Baseline QT interval is prolonged, 'torsades de pointes':**
  - Causes include electrolyte abnormality (e.g. hypokalaemia, hypomagnesaemia, hypocalcaemia), drug toxicity (e.g. quinidine, phenothiazines, tricyclic antidepressants), drug interactions or a congenital disorder. These predispose to torsades de pointes ('twisting of the points').
- Torsades de pointes resembles a corkscrew pattern on the ECG rhythm strip, with complexes rotating above and below the baseline (see Figure 17.12). Torsades may be transient, or can be prolonged and degenerate into VF:
  - Give magnesium sulfate 2 g (8 mmol or 4 mL of 49.3% solution) IV over 1–2 min.
  - Correct any underlying metabolic disorder, particularly hypokalaemia.

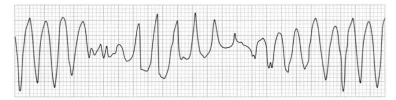

Figure 17.12 Torsades de pointes. Copyright Tor Ercleve.

- DC cardioversion is essential for critical hypotension, but the torsades rhythm often recurs and may require several shocks until it is brought under control.
- Overdrive pacing in CCU may be necessary in resistant torsades.

BRADYARRHYTHMIAS

Phone call

Questions

1. How slow is the heart rate?
2. What is the blood pressure?
3. Is the patient on digoxin, a beta-blocker, a calcium-channel blocker or other antiarrhythmic drug? These drugs have both sinus and AV nodal suppressant properties and may result in profound sinus bradycardia or heart block. Other antiarrhythmics possessing beta-blocking properties such as sotalol or amiodarone may also cause bradycardia.
4. What was the reason for admission?

Instructions

If the patient has a HR <40 beats/min, an SBP <90 mmHg or features of circulatory compromise:

- Give oxygen by mask to maintain saturation >94% and attach a pulse oximeter and cardiac monitor to the patient.
- Ask the nurse to temporarily place the patient in the Trendelenburg position (foot-of-the-bed up) if the patient is hypotensive (SBP <90 mmHg).
  - This theoretically achieves an 'auto-transfusion' of 200–300 mL of blood, but hard evidence is lacking, any beneficial effect is transitory and harm may follow from hypoventilation, aspiration and raised intracranial pressure.
- Request an urgent 12-lead ECG.
- Ask for an IV trolley at the patient's bedside, with two cannulae, ready for your arrival.
- Request the cardiac arrest trolley with defibrillator, pacer and resuscitation equipment be brought to the patient's bedside, and atropine 1 mg drawn up ready.

Prioritisation

See any patient with a bradycardia and signs of circulatory compromise such as chest pain, SOB, hypotension or an altered mental status immediately; or if the HR <40 beats/min, as this will trigger a MET call.

Corridor thoughts

What arrhythmias cause a slow heart rate? (* = major threat to life)
- Sinus bradycardia
- Junctional bradycardia
- First-degree AV block
- Second-degree AV block:
  - Type I (Wenckebach) with an increasingly prolonged PR interval until a beat is dropped (see Figure 17.13)
  - Type II with a normal or short PR interval (see Figure 17.14)*
- Third-degree (complete) AV block (see Figure 17.15)*
- AF with slow ventricular rate ('slow AF')*

What causes a bradyarrhythmia?
  The most common causes are drugs and cardiac disease.
- Drugs:
  - Antiarrhythmic agents such as beta-blockers, calcium-channel blockers, digoxin, amiodarone, sotalol

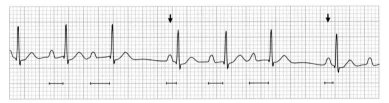

Figure 17.13 Second-degree atrioventricular block (type I). Copyright Tor Ercleve.

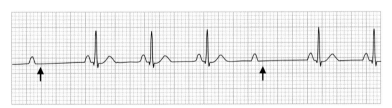

Figure 17.14 Second-degree atrioventricular block (type II). Copyright Tor Ercleve.

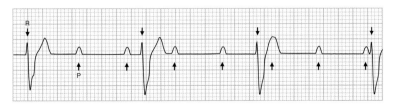

Figure 17.15 Third-degree atrioventricular block. Copyright Tor Ercleve.

- Cardiac disease:
  - Acute MI (usually inferior wall)
  - Sick sinus syndrome
- Other causes:
  - Vasovagal attack (neurocardiogenic syncope)
  - Healthy young athletes
  - Hypothermia
  - Hypothyroidism
  - Increased ICP in association with hypertension (Cushing's reflex)

Major threat to life

- Hypotension
- Agitation or confusion from cerebral hypoperfusion
- Myocardial ischaemia and acute myocardial infarction
  - If the bradycardia is associated with an acute MI, the patient is prone to more ominous arrhythmias such as asystole, VT or VF.

Bedside

Quick-look test

Does the patient look well (comfortable), sick (uncomfortable or distressed) or critical (about to die?)
- Ask the nurse to bring the cardiac arrest trolley to the bedside if the patient looks sick or critical and attach an ECG monitor to the patient.
- This provides an immediate diagnosis of the patient's rhythm and allows continuous monitoring.

Airway and vital signs

What is the heart rate?
Read the ECG or palpate the patient's pulse to identify the rate.
What is the heart rhythm?
Read the ECG to ascertain the type of slow rhythm occurring.
- Look for any association between the P waves and the QRS complexes, to determine whether there is a sinus bradycardia or an AV block.
- Consider a junctional bradycardia if the rhythm is regular but with no visible P waves, or slow AF if it is irregular with no P waves.
What is the blood pressure?
- Most causes of hypotension are accompanied by a compensatory reflex tachycardia, although bradycardia does occur paradoxically in 5–10% of cases of acute haemorrhagic shock.
- Otherwise, the bradyarrhythmia is likely to be responsible for the hypotension.

What is the temperature?

Hypothermia may be associated with a bradyarrhythmia, as well as hypothyroidism.

Management

Immediate management

HR <40 beats/min and SBP <90 mmHg or features of circulatory compromise:

- Call for senior help.
- Apply high-flow oxygen by mask and gain IV access.
- Attach an ECG monitor/defibrillator to the patient and confirm the rhythm.
- Elevate the patient's legs temporarily in the Trendelenburg position.
- Give atropine 0.5–0.6 mg IV. If there is no response after a couple of minutes, give an additional dose about every 3 minutes, up to a total dose of 0.04 mg/kg (approx 3 mg for average adult).
- Organise transthoracic pacing (see Chapter 65) if there is still no improvement and the patient is symptomatic. Small increments of midazolam 1.25–2.5 mg or diazepam 2.5 mg IV will be needed as transthoracic pacing is uncomfortable for the patient.
- If pacing is unavailable, start a low-dose adrenaline infusion. Put adrenaline 1 mg (1 mL of 1:1000) in 100 mL of normal saline and administer IV at 60–120 mL/h (10–20 microgram/min) titrated to response. The patient *must* be on an ECG monitor.
  - Adrenaline 50 microgram IV slow boluses every 2–3 minutes may be used as an alternative.
- Alternatively, use fist pacing if the patient loses consciousness (similar to a praecordial thump, but over the left lower edge of the sternum) at a rate of 50–70/min.
  - If there is no response to this, commence CPR and give 1 mg adrenaline IV.
- Transfer the patient to the ICU/CCU for further monitoring and transvenous pacemaker insertion, either temporary or as a permanent device.

Selective history and chart review

The history and chart evaluation focus on looking for any underlying cause(s) of the bradycardia.

Review the patient's medical history

- Has there been previous bradycardia or heart block?
- Does the patient have any cardiac risk factors such as smoking, hypertension, hypercholesterolaemia, diabetes, renal impairment or a family history?
- Is there a history of angina or previous acute MI?

- Have there been any recent symptoms suggestive of an ischaemic event such as chest pain, SOB, nausea or vomiting?

Review the medication chart
- Look for drugs that might cause bradycardia, including antiarrhythmic agents such as beta-blockers, calcium-channel blockers, digoxin, amiodarone or sotalol.

Selective physical examination

Vitals	Bradypnoea (hypothermia, hypothyroidism)
	Hypothermia (hypothyroidism)
	Hypertension (risk factor for CAD)
HEENT	Coarse facial features (hypothyroidism)
	Loss of lateral third of eyebrows (hypothyroidism)
	Periorbital xanthomas (CAD)
	Fundi with hypertensive or diabetic changes (CAD)
CVS	Mitral regurgitant murmur (recent acute MI)
GIT	Renal, aortic or femoral bruits (CAD and atherosclerosis elsewhere)
Neuro	Delayed return phase of deep tendon reflexes (hypothyroidism).

Specific management
Sinus bradycardia
- No immediate treatment is required if the patient is not hypotensive.
- If the patient is on digoxin with a HR <60 beats/min, withhold further digoxin doses until the HR is >60 beats/min.
- If the patient is on medication that depresses conduction, withhold the next dose until the HR is >60 beats/min.

Atrial fibrillation with slow ventricular response
- This arrhythmia also does not require treatment unless the patient is hypotensive or has symptoms of vital organ hypoperfusion such as syncope, confusion, angina or LVF.
- Definitive treatment includes discontinuation of any drug that depresses cardiac conduction and in some cases transfer to the CCU/ICU for temporary or permanent pacemaker placement.

Atrioventricular block
The patient may be asymptomatic, or present with syncopal episodes without warning (Stokes–Adams attack).
- First-degree AV block:
  - PR interval duration >200 ms.

- Usually asymptomatic, but it can progress to higher grades of AV block if associated with left or right axis and a RBBB, indicating a trifascicular block.
- Second-degree AV block:
  - Mobitz type I—progressive lengthening of the PR interval until an atrial impulse is dropped. Usually benign from high vagal tone. It may progress to complete heart block (CHB), requiring temporary pacing, so continued monitoring is needed in the setting of ACS or drug toxicity.
  - Mobitz type II—constant PR interval with regular, intermittent failure of P wave conduction. This commonly progresses to CHB and requires temporary or permanent pacing.
- Third-degree AV block (complete heart block):
  - The ECG shows regular P waves and regular QRS complexes at an escape rate of 20–50/min, but with complete AV dissociation.

Management of second- and third-degree AV block

- If the patient's condition is stable, transfer to CCU for continuous ECG monitoring.
- Seek and treat any underlying reversible cause(s). Cease medications known to prolong AV conduction and exclude underlying myocardial ischaemia by cardiac biomarker testing.
- Temporary pacing may be required while reversible causes are addressed.
- Insertion of a permanent pacemaker is indicated if no reversible cause is found.

Hypotension

Nursing staff may call you to assess a patient with low BP. Remember that it is the threat to end-organ function that dictates the need for intervention, rather than the absolute BP level. The priority is to assess for tissue hypoperfusion, which indicates shock (see also Chapter 11).

- Not all patients with hypotension have shock, and conversely compensatory changes will maintain the SBP in early shock. Although you may be called to see many patients with hypotension, shock requires evidence of inadequate tissue perfusion.
- Thus, some healthy patients normally have a SBP of 80–100 mmHg, especially thin, young females.
- Conversely, a patient with chronic, severe heart failure has to function with a SBP of 80–90 mmHg. A higher BP precipitates an increased cardiac workload, leading to angina and worsening heart failure; lower pressures lead to light-headedness and decreasing renal function. Reviewing these patients is complex and requires senior assistance.
- Other patients with chronic hypertension require a higher-than-normal perfusing pressure, so a BP of 120/80 mmHg may actually be associated with significant tissue hypoperfusion.

Phone call

Questions

1. **What is the BP?**
2. **What is the HR?**
3. **What is the RR?**
4. **What is the patient's mental status?**
5. **Is the patient clammy or pale?**
6. **Does the patient have dyspnoea or chest pain?** (septic or cardiogenic shock)
7. **Is there evidence of bleeding?** (haemorrhagic shock)
8. **What is the temperature?** (septic shock)
9. **Has the patient been given medication in the last hour?** (anaphylaxis)

10. **Does the patient have a rash?** (anaphylaxis or septicaemia)
11. **What was the reason for admission?**

Instructions

- If there is a possibility of shock:
  - Administer at least 6 L/min oxygen by mask and attach pulse oximetry to the patient.
- Request an IV trolley at the patient's bedside with two large-bore 14–16G cannulae ready for insertion, if an IV is not in place.
  - Give 20 mL/kg normal saline IV as rapidly as possible, unless the patient is SOB and may have pulmonary oedema with cardiogenic shock.
  - Request an ECG immediately and commence continuous cardiac monitoring.
- Organise cross-matching of at least four units of packed RBCs if the admission diagnosis was a GI bleed, or if there is external evidence of blood loss.
- Request 1:1000 adrenaline 0.01 mg/kg up to 0.5 mg (0.5 mL) be drawn up ready for IM injection into the upper lateral thigh if you suspect anaphylaxis.
- Arrange a portable CXR immediately if the patient has dyspnoea or chest pain.

Prioritisation

See every patient with hypotension and suspected shock immediately.

Corridor thoughts

What are the causes of hypotension? (* = major threat to life)
- Shock*:
  - Hypovolaemic, cardiogenic, distributive or obstructive (see Chapter 11)
- Medications (often postural hypotension):
  - Antihypertensives, nitrates, sedatives, analgesics
- Autonomic neuropathy:
  - Diabetes, Parkinson's disease, multiple system atrophy (MSA)
- Vasovagal attack (also known as neurocardiogenic syncope)
- Constitutional:
  - Some patients have a low BP normally

Major threat to life

- **Shock**
  - Progressive hypotension leads to circulatory failure and results in hypoxia, anaerobic metabolism with metabolic lactic acidosis,

organ hypoperfusion and tissue ischaemia that further worsen the cardiovascular status.
- **Underlying cause**
  - Hypotension may be secondary to a life-threatening condition such as ACS, cardiac arrhythmia, hypovolaemia, anaphylaxis, sepsis, massive PE, tension pneumothorax or cardiac tamponade that must be looked for and treated (see also Chapter 11).

Bedside

The immediate bedside review is aimed at quickly determining whether shock is present, rapidly isolating the potential cause(s) and instituting appropriate early management.

Quick-look test

Does the patient look well (comfortable), sick (uncomfortable or distressed) or critical (about to die)?

A patient with hypotension but adequate tissue perfusion usually looks well and has a normal mental status. Once perfusion of vital organs is compromised, the patient looks pale, agitated and sweaty. Patients who are seriously volume-depleted appear haggard, drawn and exhausted.

Airway and vital signs

Is the airway clear?
- If the patient has a depressed conscious level and the airway cannot be protected or maintained, endotracheal intubation will be required.
- Roll the patient onto the left lateral decubitus position to avoid aspiration, and remove loose-fitting dentures.
- Contact your senior urgently, as well as an anaesthetist and the ICU.

What is the respiratory rate/pattern?
- Tachypnoea is a compensatory sign commonly associated with hypotension and shock. Tachypnoea may indicate lactic acidosis secondary to tissue hypoperfusion, acute LVF or an underlying PE, pneumothorax or cardiac tamponade.
- The increased RR serves to increase the thoracic pumping effect, improves venous return and partially compensates for tissue acidosis by blowing off CO_2.

What is the blood pressure?
- Measure the patient's supine BP in both arms.
  - SBP <90 mmHg is usually associated with inadequate tissue perfusion, especially if this is markedly lower than the patient's normal readings.
  - Do not be fooled by an apparently acceptable automated non-invasive blood pressure (NIBP) measurement if the patient

looks sick. The NIBP is notoriously inaccurate at low readings. Retake the BP manually.

- What is the pulse pressure?
  - A narrow pulse pressure (raised DBP from peripheral vasoconstriction as a compensatory mechanism) indicates a low LV stroke volume and shock.
  - A wider pulse pressure (lowered DBP from vasodilation) may be present in anaphylaxis or early septicaemia (i.e. 'warm shock').
- The hypotension may have been caused by a vasovagal episode or orthostatic hypotension if the patient's BP has now returned to normal.
  - If hypotension is not severe and the patient appears well, examine for postural vital sign changes. This is not indicated if the patient is hypotensive when supine.
  - Ask for assistance if the patient is unable to stand alone, or have the patient sit up and dangle the legs over the side of the bed.
  - Repeat the HR and BP after the patient sits or stands for at least 2 minutes. Ask the patient if they feel unwell or light-headed.
    - An increase in HR of >20 beats/min, or the patient reporting light-headedness, is an indicator of inadequate intravascular volume.
    - A fall in SBP of >20 mmHg or any fall in DBP is less specific, as patients with autonomic dysfunction (e.g. beta-blockers, diabetic neuropathy, MSA) may also have a pronounced postural fall in BP without being hypovolaemic and will not have a compensatory rise in HR.

What is the heart rate?

- Low volume or impalpable peripheral pulses indicate hypoperfusion.
- Most causes of hypotension are accompanied by a compensatory reflex sinus tachycardia.
- Look at the ECG or rhythm strip. HR <50 beats/min or >150 beats/min, especially if not in sinus rhythm, could be the cause of shock (cardiogenic).
  - If the resting HR is <50 beats/min in the presence of hypotension, suspect a vasovagal episode, autonomic neuropathy, rate-slowing drugs or bradyarrhythmia. Haemorrhagic shock can cause a relative bradycardia in 10% of cases.
  - If the HR is >150 beats/min and there is any evidence of VT, rapid AF or SVT, emergency electrical cardioversion should be considered (see Chapters 17 and 64).
  - Look for ECG changes suggestive of ACS as a cause of hypotension (cardiogenic shock). ECG changes of diffuse

myocardial ischaemia, such as widespread T inversion and/or ST-segment depression, suggest myocardial hypoperfusion.

* ECG abnormalities can also indicate drug toxicity or electrolyte disorders—or they may be a secondary effect of the hypotension itself.

What is the temperature?
* An elevated (>38°C) or low (<36°C) temperature suggest sepsis. However, sepsis may occur with a normal temperature in some patients, especially the elderly or immunosuppressed.
* Hypothermia will also develop in the later stages of shock because of metabolic changes from tissue hypoperfusion, exposure or fluid resuscitation (particularly cold blood).

Selective physical examination I
Is the patient in shock?

Vitals	Repeat now; pay particular attention to HR and BP
Skin	Cool, mottled and clammy (decreased perfusion)
	Warm and pink (adequate perfusion, or possibly distributive shock)
	Poor turgor, lack of sweating (decreased perfusion)
	Purpura (septicaemia) or urticaria/erythema (anaphylaxis)
CVS	Small pulse volume and slow capillary refill > 2 sec (hypoperfusion)
	Non-visible JVP, flat neck veins (hypovolaemic or distributive shock)
	Elevated JVP, distended neck veins (cardiogenic or obstructive shock)
	Kussmaul's JVP sign rises on inspiration (cardiac tamponade or RV failure)
Resp	Stridor (anaphylaxis)
	Respiratory distress with unilateral hyperexpansion, tracheal deviation to opposite side and hyperresonnance (tension pneumothorax)
	Crackles on chest auscultation (chest sepsis or cardiogenic shock)
	Tachypnoea (acidotic breathing)
GIT	Check for tenderness or a pulsatile mass (AAA)
	Generalised abdominal tenderness with peritonism (bowel infarction, intraperitoneal haemorrhage from ectopic pregnancy or pancreatitis with third-space fluid loss)
CNS	Alert, orientated (maintaining cerebral perfusion)
	Apprehensive, confused, agitated, delirious (decreased cerebral perfusion)
Urine	Urine output >0.5 mL/kg/h, or >30 mL/h (adequate renal perfusion)
	Urine output <0.5 mL/kg/h, or <30 mL/h (decreased renal perfusion)

- Individually, these signs have many causes, but taken together they give an effective rapid overview of intravascular volume status and end-organ perfusion.
- *Note*: the urine output correlates with the renal blood flow, which in turn is dependent on cardiac output. It is an important measure of the adequacy of systemic perfusion, although placement of an IDC should not take priority over resuscitation measures.

Management

Immediate management

Commence resuscitation while taking a focused history and performing a selective physical examination to identify the underlying cause in every patient with clinical features of shock.

- Call your senior immediately.
- Specific management of the various shock conditions is detailed later.
- **Monitor vital signs**
  - Attach continuous non-invasive ECG, BP and pulse oximeter to the patient.
  - Commence oxygen therapy to maintain saturation >94%.
  - Shocked patients require high-flow, high-concentration oxygen and may need assistance with ventilation if consciousness is depressed.
- **Obtain adequate IV access**
  - Insert two large-bore (14–16G) cannulae in large peripheral veins. Antecubital veins are preferred.
  - Send blood for FBC, U&E, coagulation profile, and a troponin if the ECG is abnormal. In the meantime, check a venous blood gas including a lactate. Request an immediate cross-match of 2–6 units of packed RBCs if haemorrhage is suspected.
  - Send two separate sets of paired blood cultures if septic shock is possible. If pregnancy has not been excluded, request a urinary or blood beta-hCG.
- **Resuscitate intravascular depletion**
  - Give 20 mL/kg normal saline IV over 10 minutes if the patient is hypotensive, the JVP is low and there are no crackles on chest auscultation. Elevate or squeeze the IV bag, or use IV pressure cuffs to increase the rate as necessary.
  - Observe the effect of this fluid challenge by monitoring response in HR, BP, JVP, peripheral perfusion, basal lung crackles and urine output, and repeat 20 mL/kg as clinically indicated.

- Titrate fluid resuscitation carefully in a patient with a history of cardiac failure and commence with a smaller fluid bolus of 5 mL/kg.
- Ensure all shocked patients who are bleeding maintain a Hb >90–100 g/L. Search for the site of blood loss.
- **Treat any immediately apparent cause**
  - Give adrenaline 0.3–0.5 mg (0.3–0.5 mL 1:1000) IM for anaphylaxis.
  - Decompress a tension pneumothorax using needle thoracostomy.
  - Give broad-spectrum antibiotics for septicaemia.
- **Insert an IDC to monitor urine output**
  - A urine output of 0.5–1 mL/kg/h indicates restoration of adequate renal perfusion.
- **Perform a 12-lead ECG and review the rhythm strip**
  - Give IV atropine bolus (0.5–1.0 mg) if the HR <50 beats/min.
  - Follow with adrenaline 1:10,000 boluses IV (50 micrograms or 0.5 mL) or by infusion, or transcutaneous or transvenous pacing if the HR remains inappropriately low (see Chapters 17 and 65). Continuous ECG monitoring is essential.
  - Perform electrical DC cardioversion with appropriate sedation (see Chapters 17 and 66) if the HR >150 beats/min with hypotension and evidence of VT, rapid AF or SVT.
- **Request a portable CXR.**

Selective history and chart review

- Determine whether a presenting problem or past medical history is a cause of the hypotension and quickly review the chart for recent trends or medication changes.

Does the patient have any risk factors for hypovolaemic or distributive shock?

- Bleeding (e.g. major epistaxis, haematemesis, melaena, bright-red rectal blood, menorrhagia), concealed bleeding such as AAA or ectopic pregnancy (beta-hCG positive), pelvic or long-bone fracture.
- Vomiting and/or diarrhoea.
- Bowel obstruction, ileus or pancreatitis, which lead to severe fluid sequestration in the abdomen, 'third spacing'.
- Burns or generalised erythroderma, which cause skin surface loss of fluids.
- Fever, rigors, malaise, recent contact with meningococcal disease, which may be associated with sepsis.
  - Ask every female patient about abdominal pain with vaginal bleeding (ectopic pregnancy), and the use of tampons (toxic shock syndrome).

Does the patient have any risk factors for cardiogenic or obstructive shock?

- Chest pain, dyspnoea, orthopnoea, previous ACS or cardiac interventions are associated with cardiogenic shock.
- Diabetes or chronic renal impairment may be associated with 'silent' myocardial ischaemia and cardiogenic shock.
- Pleuritic chest pain, whole-leg swelling, known malignancy or renal failure may be associated with PE or pericardial tamponade.

Check the observation chart

- Check previous BP measurements. Confirm that this episode is abnormally low for the patient. See whether there has been a slow deterioration or sudden change.
- Check the temperature chart for fever.
- Look for a change in weight. A loss of several kilograms since admission may indicate significant fluid loss, related to severe dehydration (>5–10% body weight loss).

Check the fluid balance chart

- Look for evidence of hypovolaemia:
  - Reduced PO or IV intake
  - Excessive fluid loss from nasogastric or surgical drains or ilesostomies
  - Urine output <30 mL/h.
- Check for recent excessive urinary loss from diuretic medications, osmotic diuresis (hyperglycaemia, mannitol administration, hypertonic IV contrast material), postobstructive renal diuresis, diabetes insipidus, recovery phase of acute tubular necrosis, adrenal insufficiency (with vomiting). See Chapter 30.

Check the medication chart

- Note any recent change in dose or addition of hypotension-inducing medications.
  - Antihypertensive medications and alpha-blockers (including many antipsychotic medications) may lower BP excessively.
  - Beta-blockers, calcium-channel blockers and many other antiarrhythmics cause hypotension and will counter a reflex tachycardia. Diuretics may cause hypovolaemia.
  - Excessive doses of potent analgesics or sedatives cause hypotension.
- Recent administration of radiographic contrast or IV/IM medication may precipitate anaphylaxis.
- NSAIDs and steroids can precipitate GI bleeding and anticoagulants worsen any bleeding.

Selective physical examination II
Are there any immediately obvious clues to the cause of shock?

Vital signs	Recheck HR, BP and peripheral perfusion now to assess for any improvement
HEENT	Dry mouth (hypovolaemia)
CVS	Recheck JVP to assess for any improvement
	Displaced apex beat, S_3 gallop (LVF)
	Muffled heart sounds, impalpable apex beat (pericardial effusion)
Resp	Crackles, pleural effusions (cardiogenic shock)
	Wheezes (anaphylaxis, LVF or PE-related bronchospasm)
GIT	Tender hepatomegaly (heart failure)
Rectal	Melaena or haematochezia (GI bleed)
Skin	Pruritic, urticarial rash with vasodilated peripheries (anaphylaxis)
	Pale skin creases and conjunctivae (occult haemorrhage)
Ext	Sacral or ankle oedema (pre-existing CCF)
	Note: patients with acute cardiogenic shock are not oedematous unless they have previous CCF. Patients with anaphylaxis or sepsis may become oedematous from capillary leakage.
Urine	Reassess urine output.

Investigations
- Check the recent Hb for any trends.
- Generalised tissue hypoperfusion causes lactic acidosis from anaerobic metabolism, with low bicarbonate plus other electrolyte abnormalities such as hyperkalaemia.
- Renal hypoperfusion causes a fall in urine output and a worsening of renal function. Look at the urea-to-creatinine ratio. A ratio >12 (calculated in SI units) is suggestive of volume depletion or a GI bleed.
- Send a urine sample for MCS if dipstick testing indicates potential urosepsis (i.e. was abnormal).
- Review the CXR as soon as possible. An abnormal CXR may be seen with:
  - Acute LVF (pulmonary venous congestion, cardiomegaly, Kerley B lines)
  - Aortic dissection (widened mediastinum)
  - Pulmonary embolism (plate atelectasis, basal effusion)
  - Pneumonia (consolidation, diffuse alveolar changes)
  - Tension pneumothorax (CXR *not* usually indicated).

- Bedside ultrasound will diagnose the presence of an aortic aneurysm, pericardial tamponade or ectopic pregnancy. Arrange this urgently.
- Echocardiography is used to determine volume status, myocardial or valvular dysfunction; it will confirm pericardial tamponade, right ventricular strain of PE, and occasionally may diagnose aortic dissection. It is harder to organise after-hours.

Specific management
Cardiogenic shock

Cardiogenic shock has a mortality of 50–70% and is clinically manifest by hypotension, elevated JVP and pulmonary oedema. Patients with acute pulmonary oedema alone will often have poor peripheral perfusion and elevated filling pressures, but they are frequently hypertensive and lowering their BP by decreasing preload (e.g. with GTN or CPAP) improves them.

- Treat ACS-related causes, such as STEMI or NSTEMI.
  - After giving aspirin, heparin and clopidogrel or prasugrel, refer for immediate PCI.
  - *Note*: fibrinolytic therapy does not substantially improve the outcome in cardiogenic shock.
  - Exclude other causes of hypotension with raised JVP.
    – Arrange an urgent echocardiogram to distinguish myocardial dysfunction from pericardial tamponade, PE, acute valvular lesion or a septal perforation.
  - The patient with a new murmur requires echocardiography urgently, as valve repair may be required to save the patient's life.
- Confirm RV infarction in an inferior STEMI by performing right-sided chest leads on the ECG.
  - V4R, V5R, V6R electrodes are placed in the same chest position, but on the right hemithorax.
  - ST-segment elevation indicates RV infarction.
  - These patients are dependent on preload for their cardiac output, so avoid dropping preload with GTN, morphine or diuretics.
  - They are less likely to develop pulmonary oedema; try small aliquots of normal saline at 2 mL/kg.
- Exclude aortic dissection causing shock from tamponade or severe aortic incompetence.
  - Arrange a CT chest scan with IV contrast (CT angiography) or transoesophageal echocardiography (TOE) to best distinguish aortic dissection from ACS.
- Otherwise, general principles of shock management apply.

- Give maximal oxygenation, careful fluid management and consider inotrope infusions such as noradrenaline with or without dobutamine in the ICU.
- If these measures are unsuccessful, intra-aortic balloon pump, left ventricular assist device (LVAD) or circulatory bypass are required if a reversible pathological feature is present and the expertise is available.

Hypovolaemic shock
- Take measures to control external bleeding. Compress or pack any external haemorrhage such as epistaxis or an open wound.
- Consult a surgeon immediately if there is suspicion of acute blood loss causing hypotension (e.g. GI bleed, ruptured AAA, ectopic pregnancy).
- If massive bleeding is occurring, order uncross-matched blood and consider other blood products such as fresh frozen plasma (FFP) and platelets.
- Notify the blood bank that a 'massive transfusion' may be necessary. Some blood banks will then routinely provide additional FFP and platelets as part of this.
- Excess fluid losses via vomiting, diarrhoea, sweating, polyuria, extreme diuretic therapy and third-space losses (e.g. pancreatitis, bowel obstruction, peritonitis) will respond to intravascular volume expansion (resuscitation) with normal saline.
  - Give 20–40 mL/kg to restore the circulation.
  - Then gradually correct the dehydration (rehydration), and include daily maintenance amounts.
  - Search for the underlying cause.

Anaphylaxis
- Treat immediately with adrenaline 0.3–0.5 mg (0.3–0.5 mL of 1:1000 solution) IM plus normal saline 20 mL/kg (see Chapter 9).

Septic shock
- This is defined as a suspected infection (from two or more systemic inflammatory response syndrome [SIRS] criteria— temperature >38°C or <36°C; HR >90 beats/min; RR >20 breaths/min or $PaCO_2$ <32 mmHg; and peripheral leucocyte count >12 or <4, or >10% immature bands) or a documented infection; plus organ dysfunction or tissue hypoperfusion with hypoxia, hypotension, oliguria, confusion or a raised lactate that persist despite adequate fluid resuscitation (>30 mL/kg).
- More than 85% cases originate from the chest, abdominal or genitourinary systems, skin and vascular access.

SECTION C – Common calls

- Arrange a CXR and urinalysis/MSU as initial screens. Make sure at least two sets of paired blood cultures from two different sites have been sent.
- Remember to examine all areas of the skin, looking for a source or entry site of infection, including between the toes (tinea), skin folds (intertrigo), perineum and axillae (abscess), and the ear, nose and throat for localised infections.
  - Consider toxic shock syndrome in any hypotensive premenopausal female, particularly with blanching erythema like sunburn, and ask about tampon use. If the patient is obtunded, perform a pelvic examination and remove a tampon if present (now a rare cause).
- Intravascular fluid resuscitation requires large volumes—up to 50–100 mL/kg—before adequate volume repletion. Ensure Hb is maintained between 70 and 90 g/L.
- Patients who are neutropenic from chemotherapy, diabetic, have HIV or are otherwise immunosuppressed show few signs of sepsis. They demonstrate few focal features and have non-specific inflammatory changes on blood tests.
  - Give a neutropenic patient empiric broad-spectrum antibiotics such as piperacillin 4 g with tazobactam 0.5 g IV plus gentamicin 4–7 mg/kg stat. Add vancomycin 1.5 g IV 12-hourly if line sepsis is possible.
  - Otherwise, give broad-spectrum antibiotics as per hospital guidelines to cover likely pathogens depending on the presumed focus as soon as possible, certainly within 1 hr of the onset of hypotension.
  - Continuing hypotension despite intravascular volume repletion requires admission to ICU.
  - Vasopressor support (adrenaline or noradrenaline infusion) will be needed since vasodilation and increased vascular permeability are common in severe sepsis.

Other causes of hypotension

- **Tension pneumothorax**
  - Causes extreme dyspnoea with elevated JVP and hypotension due to positive intrathoracic pressure decreasing venous return to the heart. Look for unilateral hyperresonance and decreased air entry, with tracheal shift away from the involved side.
  - Do not wait for X-ray confirmation in an unstable patient. Call for senior assistance and get a 14–16G cannula ready to insert into the second intercostal space in the midclavicular line on the affected side.
  - Once inserted into the pleural space, trapped air will be released with immediate improvement in blood pressure. This is followed by formal insertion of a chest tube (see Chapter 59).

- **Cardiac tamponade**
  - Elevated JVP, hypotension and soft heart sounds (Beck's triad) with agitation related to intracerebral venous congestion.
  - Urgent bedside ultrasound now best confirms the diagnosis.
  - Most commonly follows penetrating trauma, or is non-traumatic in a patient with chronic renal impairment, malignancy, connective tissue disorders etc.
    - Traumatic cardiac tamponade requires immediate surgery.
    - Pericardiocentesis with insertion of a catheter into the pericardial sac and aspiration of fluid should result in immediate improvement in non-traumatic causes.
- **Massive pulmonary embolus**
  - Sudden hypotension, elevated JVP and cyanosis accompanied by additional evidence of acute RV overload such as RV heave, loud P_2, right-sided S_3 or murmur of tricuspid insufficiency.
  - If PE is suspected, treat as outlined in Chapter 15.
- **Drug toxicity**
  - Common causes of hypotension are GTN, vasodilators, opioids, sedatives, antiarrhythmics, beta-blockers, calcium-channel blockers and ACE inhibitors. However, hypotension is seldom accompanied by evidence of inadequate tissue perfusion.
  - Place the patient flat, elevate the legs and give 5–10 mL/kg IV of normal saline to support the BP until the effect of the drug wears off.
  - Bradycardia and hypotension from excessive narcotic are reversed by naloxone hydrochloride 0.1–0.2 mg IV, SC or IM every 5 minutes repeated until alert. Beware of precipitating an acutely agitated withdrawal state in an opioid-dependent patient.
  - Following stabilisation of the patient, reduce the dose or alter the schedule of the opioid.
- **Vasovagal syncope**
  - The patient is usually normotensive by the time you arrive, having been laid flat, but will still feel nauseated and miserable. Warn the patient of continuing to feel faint for several hours afterwards.
  - Look for a precipitating stimulus such as pain or exposure to blood, with prodromal light-headedness and sweating.
  - There is no specific treatment, but ensure there was no underlying exacerbating factor such as dehydration, infection, medications that cause orthostatic hypotension, ectopic pregnancy or a ruptured AAA.
  - A vasovagal attack alone is uncommon in elderly patients so more sinister causes of transient hypotension must be considered.

Post-shock complications

After successfully resuscitating a hypotensive patient, watch out during the next few days for:

- Multiorgan failure—a combination of lung, renal, cardiac, coagulation, bowel and other dysfunction requiring high-level ICU care. Translocation of gut bacteria into the portal and then systemic circulation is a prominent mechanism behind multiorgan dysfunction.
- Brain—thrombotic stroke or watershed cortical infarction with sudden blindness.
- Heart—diffuse myocardial injury with elevated troponin.
- Kidney—acute tubular necrosis with oliguria, and rising urea and creatinine.
- Centrilobular hepatic necrosis with jaundice and elevated liver enzymes.
- Bowel ischaemia or infarction with the onset of bloody diarrhoea and deteriorating metabolic acidosis.

Hypertension

Nursing staff may call you to assess a patient with high BP. Remember, it is the threat to organ dysfunction that dictates the need for intervention, not the absolute BP level.

The priority is to exclude acute end-organ damage (hypertensive emergency).

Phone call

Questions

1. **How high is the BP and what has it been previously?**
2. **What was the reason for admission?**
3. **Is the patient pregnant?** Hypertension in a pregnant patient may be due to preeclampsia and must be assessed immediately prior to the development of eclampsia with tonic–clonic seizures.
4. **Does the patient have symptoms suggestive of a hypertensive emergency?** Sudden-onset chest or back pain (aortic dissection); chest pain, arrhythmia or dyspnoea (myocardial ischaemia and or acute pulmonary oedema); sudden headache, vomiting, confusion, seizure (SAH or hypertensive encephalopathy).
5. **What antihypertensive medication has the patient been taking?**
6. **Is the patient taking a MAOI antidepressant?**

Instructions

If the patient has any features of a hypertensive emergency or is pregnant:
- Ask the nurse to stay by the patient's bedside and get help from additional nursing staff.
- Administer oxygen to maintain saturation >94%.
- Attach ECG and pulse oximetry monitoring to the patient.
- Request an IV trolley at the patient's bedside with a selection of cannulae ready for insertion, if an IV is not in place.
- If the patient is asymptomatic and has no abnormal clinical signs, ask the nurse to check the BP again in 10 minutes and call you back with the result.

- Ensure that the patient's regular antihypertensive medication has not been missed recently.

Prioritisation

- See any patient with hypertension associated with acute end-organ damage immediately, as this is a hypertensive emergency.
- Hypertension in an asymptomatic patient does not need to be assessed immediately, irrespective of how high the BP is. The BP may be safely brought under control over the following hours or days.

Corridor thoughts

What are the causes of high blood pressure? (* = major threat to life)
- 'Essential' hypertension (≥90% of cases):
  - No direct aetiology identified, though relationship to sedentary lifestyle, obesity, increasing age, family history etc
- 'Secondary' hypertension (2–10%):
  - Obstructive uropathy, renal artery stenosis, chronic pyelonephritis
  - Glomerulonephritis, diabetic renal disease, polycystic kidney disease
  - Endocrine disease such as Cushing's syndrome, Conn's syndrome, acromegaly, thyrotoxicosis, myxoedema
  - Autoimmune disease such as SLE or scleroderma
- Medications:
  - Corticosteroids, oral contraceptive pill, NSAIDs
- Catecholamine-related:
  - Phaeochromocytoma*
  - Drug overdose
    - Cocaine, amphetamines, ecstasy*
  - Medication withdrawal
    - Abrupt withdrawal from a beta-blocker, clonidine or ACE inhibitor resulting in a rebound hypertensive crisis*
  - Drug interaction
    - MAOI antidepressant in combination with a sympathomimetic or other psychoactive drug, or a food containing tyramine (found in cheese or wine)*
- Neurogenic:
  - Anxiety
    - 'White-coat hypertension', unexpected/distressing hospital admission
  - Raised intracranial pressure
    - Cushing's reflex of hypertension and bradycardia*
  - Cerebral ischaemia (e.g. stroke)*
    - Auto-preservation of cerebral perfusion to the ischaemic brain

- Other:
  - Preeclampsia (from 20 weeks' gestation onwards, usually third trimester)*
  - Coarctation of aorta
  - Polycythaemia
  - Hypercalcaemia
  - Hyperparathyroidism
  - Sleep apnoea
- *Note:* pain, bladder distension, alcohol or nicotine withdrawal, agitation and anxiety can cause transient increases in BP.

Major threat to life

The following conditions associated with a marked increase in BP may be life-threatening:
- Aortic dissection
- Myocardial infarction
- Acute pulmonary oedema
- Subarachnoid haemorrhage
- Preeclampsia/eclampsia
- Hypertensive encephalopathy
- Catecholamine crisis
- Acute renal failure.

Bedside

Quick-look test

Does the patient look well (comfortable), sick (uncomfortable or distressed) or critical (about to die)?
- Unless the patient has chest pain, a seizure (eclampsia, hypertensive encephalopathy) or is markedly short of breath (acute pulmonary oedema), the initial appearance often belies the severity of the situation.
- Even the patient with hypertensive encephalopathy may look deceptively well.

Airway and vital signs

What is the blood pressure?
- Retake the BP in both arms.
- A lower pressure in one arm may be a clue to thoracic aortic dissection or an aortic coarctation.

What is the heart rate?
- Bradycardia and hypertension in a patient not receiving beta-blockers may indicate increasing ICP.

- Tachycardia and hypertension suggest a catecholamine-related cause.

What is the respiratory rate?
- Dyspnoea may indicate pulmonary oedema with acute LVF. Listen at the lung bases for confirmatory basal crackles.

Management

Immediate management

If the patient is acutely symptomatic or may have a serious cause as above:
- Ensure the patient is on oxygen to maintain the saturation >94%.
- Attach cardiac monitoring and pulse oximeter to the patient.
- Establish IV access.
- Call for senior help.
- Acute lowering of the BP may be required, but only when a critical hypertensive emergency is diagnosed.
- The choice of antihypertensive agent otherwise depends on the cause of the hypertension, the patient's age and the patient's medical history.
- Treat specific acute pathologies as they are identified (see below).
- Proceed to further history and examination if the patient has asymptomatic hypertension, with no other acute clinical features.

Selective history and chart review

Does the patient have any symptoms suggestive of a hypertensive emergency? (see Table 19.1)
- Sudden onset, tearing chest or back pain (aortic dissection)
- Focal weakness or sensory symptoms (aortic dissection)
- Shortness of breath, orthopnoea (pulmonary oedema)
- Chest pain (myocardial ischaemia)
- Sudden headache, confusion (SAH)
- Headache, nausea and vomiting, confusion, blurred vision (hypertensive encephalopathy)

Does the patient have a history of hypertension or any risk factors for hypertension?
- Ask specifically about previously diagnosed renal, autoimmune or endocrine disease, amphetamine or cocaine use, steroid therapy or progressive uraemia (renal hypertension).

Was the patient taking antihypertensive medications prior to coming into hospital?
- Ask about prescribed antihypertensive agents. Remember, too, over-the-counter remedies containing ephedrine, liquorice, St John's wort etc

Table 19.1 Signs of end-organ damage indicating a hypertensive emergency	
Target organ/system	**Associated findings**
Cardiovascular	Myocardial ischaemia/infarction
	Aortic regurgitation (aortic dissection)
	Absent pulse (aortic dissection)
Respiratory	Pulmonary oedema (LVF)
Central nervous system	Mental status changes (e.g. agitation, confusion)
	Hyperreflexia
	Seizures
	Coma
Eye/retina	Papilloedema
	Haemorrhages (flame)
	Exudates (yellow)
	Retinal ischaemia ('cotton-wool' spots)

- Check the medication chart to ensure the patient's normal antihypertensive medications have been charted.
  - Discontinuation of an antihypertensive medication is often an oversight at the time of admission, and may be responsible for the patient's poor BP control. Look back in the chart or for a GP's letter.

Check the nursing observation chart
- Check previous BP measurements. Confirm that this episode is abnormally high for the patient. Decide whether there has been a sudden or a slow change.
- Check the HR to determine whether the hypertension is associated with a tachycardia or bradycardia.

Review the patient's medication chart for prescribed agents that cause hypertension
- Corticosteroid
- Amphetamine derivative (for appetite suppression or narcolepsy)
- NSAID
- Nasal decongestant
- Oral contraceptive pill
- MAOI

Selective physical examination
Does the patient have evidence of a hypertensive emergency? (see Table 19.1)

Vitals	Repeat now
	Check BP both arms
Mental	Agitation, confusion (increased ICP, SAH, hypertensive encephalopathy)
HEENT	**Fundoscopy:**
	Assess the fundi for hypertensive changes (arteriolar narrowing, flame-shaped haemorrhages near the disc, exudates and ischaemic changes, 'cotton-wool spots')
	Papilloedema is ominous in a hypertensive crisis, suggesting hypertensive encephalopathy with cerebral oedema
	Note: severe hypertension may occur without marked encephalopathy or papilloedema, but retinal haemorrhages and exudates are almost always seen
Resp	Tachypnoea, crackles, pleural effusion (acute pulmonary oedema)
CVS	S_3 gallop, elevated JVP (left ventricular and biventricular heart failure)
	Absent pulse, new murmur (aortic dissection)
Neuro	Hyperreflexia, clonus, headache and visual disturbances (preeclampsia, hypertensive encephalopathy)
	Focal neurological deficits (aortic dissection, later in hypertensive encephalopathy)

Investigations

Patients with significant but isolated hypertension:
- FBC (polycythaemia, anaemia with chronic renal disease)
- U&E to determine renal function (cause or effect of hypertension)
- LFTs including urate (preeclampsia)
- Urinalysis
  - Urinary beta-hCG in women of childbearing age (preeclampsia)
  - Proteinuria (preeclampsia, nephrotic syndrome, glomerulonephritis)
  - Haematuria (renal hypertension, glomerulonephritis, nephritic syndrome)
- ECG (myocardial ischaemia, chronic hypertension with left ventricular hypertrophy)
- CXR
  - Cardiomegaly
  - Evidence of heart failure
  - Widened mediastinum (aortic dissection).

Patients with other associated pathological features should have investigations directed to the specific condition suspected (see below).

Specific management

Elevated BP is most often an isolated finding in an asymptomatic patient known to have hypertension.

Although long-term control of hypertension in such patients is of proven benefit, rapid lowering of the BP is associated with avoidable yet serious complications, because of the inability to autoregulate cerebral blood flow.

Overly aggressive treatment may cause syncope, cortical blindness with occipital stroke, myocardial ischaemia, even death.

- Do not treat the BP reading. Only treat the complication(s) associated with it.
- Severe hypertension (SBP >180 mmHg) is common in hospitalised patients and usually has no features of a hypertensive emergency. A high reading alone does *not* require urgent treatment.
- Conversely, a 'near-normal' BP such as a BP of 130/85 mmHg may be associated with a hypertensive emergency in a pregnant patient with preeclampsia, or a BP of 140/90 mmHg in a young patient with an acute aortic dissection.

Isolated hypertension

- Exclude end-organ dysfunction:
  - History, examination, urinalysis, ECG, renal function.
- Identify precipitating cause:
  - Non-compliance, incorrect dose, drug interaction
  - Secondary cause (as outlined earlier).
- Gain control gradually over 48 hours or more using oral antihypertensive medications:
  - Review the patient's current antihypertensive treatment, and consider an increase in dose or one-off dose. Make a clear note in the patient's chart.
  - A decision to use a new agent can usually await the patient's regular medical care team. Drug choice will depend on the patient's age, comorbidities, known side effects, dosing schedule and compliance, as well as cost. Commonly used antihypertensives include:
    — Beta-blocker
    — Diuretic
    — ACE inhibitor
    — Angiotensin-receptor blocker (ARB)
    — Calcium-channel blocker.

Aortic dissection (see Chapter 16)

Confirm an acute aortic dissection according to local policy with an urgent helical CT angiogram of the chest (CTA), or a transoesophageal echocardiogram (TOE) if expertise is available, or even a transthoracic echocardiogram in their absence, which may demonstrate some of the complications of a dissection such as cardiac tamponade or acute aortic regurgitation.

- Call your senior doctor and proceed to:
  - Give oxygen to maintain saturation >94%.
  - Insert two large IV cannulae (14–16G) and send blood for an immediate cross-match of six units packed RBCs.
  - Relieve pain with titrated IV morphine 2.5–5 mg repeated as needed.
  - Arrange admission to ICU and contact the cardiothoracic or vascular surgical team.
  - Give an IV beta-blocker such as esmolol or metoprolol slowly until the pulse is <60 beats/min or the SBP is <120 mmHg.
  - If the BP is not controlled at this level, despite a pulse <60 beats/min, add sodium nitroprusside or a GTN infusion until the SBP is 100–120 mmHg. Start these in an intensive care area with intra-arterial BP monitoring.
- Patients with type A dissection (involving the ascending aorta) should be prepared for theatre. Type B dissections that commence at the subclavian artery and involve the descending aorta are usually managed non-operatively in ICU with careful control of BP and observation for complications.
- Endovascular stent repair is becoming more common, particularly in descending aortic dissection.

Hypertensive acute pulmonary oedema or myocardial ischaemia

Treat these patients urgently by reducing pre-load and hence arterial hypertension:

- Administer GTN SL (0.6 mg tablets or 0.4 mg spray) and repeat every 5–10 minutes while awaiting transfer to a monitored area.
- Titrate IV morphine in small boluses 1.25–2.5 mg for chest pain and anxiety, but take care not to depress respirations.
- Transfer the patient to the ICU or CCU urgently for continuous ECG and intra-arterial BP monitoring.
- Start a GTN infusion IV once in a monitored intensive care area.
- Further specific treatment is described in Chapter 15.

Subarachnoid haemorrhage

- Confirm with a CT brain scan. Aim to decrease the SBP to 160 mmHg, which can be initiated with titrated IV morphine plus an antiemetic, as many of these patients have severe pain.
- If this is insufficient, consult your senior or a neurosurgeon for the choice of antihypertensive agent.

Hypertensive encephalopathy

- The DBP is usually >140 mmHg associated with headache, lethargy, confusion, vomiting and blurred vision. Focal neurological signs, fits and coma develop later, especially if the patient is untreated.
- Arrange an urgent CT brain scan to exclude alternative causes of confusion such as a SAH, space-occupying lesion, intracranial infection or stroke. Also consider postictal state or non-convulsive status epilepticus.
- Look for evidence of renal disease. Check for proteinuria on urinalysis. Send a urine sample for microscopy—RBC casts, granular casts or dysmorphic RBCs (>70%) are suggestive of renal disease.
- Look for retinal haemorrhages, exudates or papilloedema on fundoscopy. If present with confusion, the BP should be carefully lowered over the next 2–4 hours. Call for senior help.
- Aim to initially reduce mean arterial pressure (MAP) by 25%, or for a DBP of 100–110 mmHg within the first 24 hours:
  - Start oral therapy such as atenolol 50 mg, labetalol 100 mg, amlodipine 5–10 mg or felodipine sustained-release 5–10 mg.
  - If unsuccessful, give hydralazine 5–10 mg slow IV boluses every 15–30 minutes.
  - If still unsuccessful, arrange for admission to the ICU. In ICU, start sodium nitroprusside 0.25–10 microgram/kg/min IV with intra-arterial BP monitoring.
- Once BP control is achieved, the usual medical team can continue appropriate oral therapy to maintain satisfactory BP control.

Preeclampsia and eclampsia

Hypertension at any level between 20 weeks' gestation and 2 weeks' postpartum, associated with proteinuria (>0.3 g/24 h) plus or minus pathological oedema, indicates preeclampsia. Complications of preeclampsia include headache, visual disturbances, abdominal pain, oliguria, DIC, cerebral haemorrhage, placental insufficiency, haemolysis and thrombocytopenia (HELLP syndrome with haemolysis, elevated liver enzymes and low platelets). Once seizures occur it is termed eclampsia.

- The treatment of choice near term is immediate delivery of the baby and magnesium sulfate IV. Call for senior help including the obstetric team, and commence magnesium for any complications:
  - Give magnesium sulfate 4 g IV over 10–15 minutes, followed by maintenance infusion 1 g/hour continued for at least 24 hours after delivery.
  - Magnesium sulfate does not significantly lower the BP. Therefore, other drugs such as hydralazine or labetalol are given according to local practice.

- Diuretics are *avoided* as the patient is already volume-depleted from an activated renin–angiotensin system, despite being hypertensive.

Catecholamine crisis

- **Phaeochromocytoma**, an exceedingly rare neuroendocrine adrenal tumour associated with paroxysmal pallor, palpitations and perspiration, leads to intermittent and alarmingly high BP. Diagnosis is by measurement of plasma or urinary catecholamines.
- If suspected, call your senior and transfer the patient to the ICU/CCU for ECG and intra-arterial BP monitoring followed by alpha-adrenergic blockade.
- Other presentations associated with sudden hypertension, headache, diaphoresis, anxiety, palpitations, nausea or abdominal pain, which are more likely than a phaeo include:
  - Cocaine, ecstasy and amphetamine misuse
  - Abrupt antihypertensive medication withdrawal (clonidine)
  - Interaction between MAOI and tyramine-containing foods (found in cheese or wine) and/or sympathomimetic or other psychoactive drugs.
    - Call your senior and transfer the patient to the ICU/CCU. Phentolamine or nitroprusside may be used, but beta-blockers should be avoided because of the risk of unopposed alpha stimulation causing increased BP.
    - In cocaine-induced hypertension, use high-dose titrated benzodiazepines such as diazepam 0.1–0.2 mg/kg or midazolam 0.1 mg/kg IV. Check the ECG and measure a troponin to exclude myocardial damage.

Hypertensive renal failure

Lower the BP over a few hours by using an oral ACE inhibitor, provided **renal artery stenosis** has first been excluded, as inadvertent ACE inhibitor use will cause rapid renal failure with uraemia in these patients.

Arrange CT renal arteriography, renal ultrasound or MRI to exclude renal artery stenosis, which is suspected by finding a high-pitched epigastric bruit, hypokalaemia (from secondary hyperaldosteronism) and evidence of vascular insufficiency in other organs, such as leg claudication or a previous stroke.

Altered mental status

An acute confusional state is a common problem among hospitalised patients, especially elderly patients. Unfortunately, the terms 'confusion', 'delirium', 'toxic psychosis' and 'acute brain syndrome' are used interchangeably to refer to any cause of an acute confusional state.

'Altered mental status' is a more precise term as it encompasses both alteration in cognition and alteration in the state of awareness.

Altered cognition of organic cause is termed a delirium (acute), and with progressive intellectual decline it is termed a dementia (chronic).

Delirium refers to transient clouding of consciousness, inattention and failure of recent memory. The result is an acute fluctuating confusional state, with restless and even aggressive behaviour, and non-auditory hallucinations.

Dementia is a chronic, progressive state of irreversible memory loss with global cognitive deficit.

Delirium and dementia have features in common, such as disorientation, abnormal behaviour, memory loss and the inability to maintain attention. However, delirium is characterised by clouding of consciousness, whereas dementia is not.

Psychiatric conditions such as depression and psychosis also cause altered thinking, often with delusions, but there is no disorientation and no clouding of consciousness.

Agitated or aggressive behaviour may result from any of these conditions. Clinicians must be alert to this risk at all times.

Phone call

Questions
1. In what way is the patient acutely confused?
2. Is there a depressed level of consciousness? (See Chapter 12)
3. What are the other vital signs?
4. How old is the patient?
5. What was the reason for admission?
6. Have there been previous similar episodes?
7. Is there an obvious reason for the patient's behaviour?
8. Is the patient aggressive?

9. What measures have been tried to reason or calm the patient?
10. Are staff or patients at risk of harm, or actually injured?
11. What additional hospital personnel are there to help now?

Instructions

- Check the patient's airway, breathing and circulation if the patient becomes unresponsive, and attach a pulse oximeter.
- Combative or aggressive patients may injure others or themselves. Ensure the safety of the nursing staff and patient:
  - Call security personnel if the patient is aggressive, confused or irrational.
  - Check a fingerprick glucose test.
- Ask the nurse to try to give diazepam 5–10 mg PO, or olanzapine 5–10 mg PO.
- Request an IV trolley for the patient's bedside. Ask for 10 mg midazolam or 10 mg diazepam in a 10 mL syringe, and 10 mg haloperidol also in a 10 mL syringe to be drawn up ready.

Prioritisation

- Immediately see any patient with confusion associated with abnormal vital signs, a decreased level of consciousness, agitation or aggressive behaviour.
- Your role is not to rush to the ward to help restrain the patient, but to determine the cause of the patient's behaviour and to organise appropriate support and medical treatment.

Corridor thoughts

What causes acute confusion and/or an altered level of consciousness? (* = major threat to life: these disorders may start with confusion, and progress to a reduced conscious level, even coma)

- CNS causes
  - Infection: meningitis*, encephalitis*, abscess*
  - Stroke: CVA*, SAH*
  - Tumour: secondary or primary; malignant or benign
  - Head trauma: subdural or extradural haematoma*
  - Seizures: post-ictal state*, complex partial seizures*
  - Cerebral vasculitis*: SLE, polyarteritis nodosa
  - Wernicke's encephalopathy: thiamine deficiency
  - Vitamin B12 deficiency
  - Hypertensive encephalopathy*
  - Progressive dementias: Alzheimer's disease, vascular dementia, Lewy body dementia, Parkinson's disease

- **Drugs**
  - Alcohol–confusion may occur when the patient is intoxicated, or during early withdrawal, or later as part of delirium tremens (DT)*
  - Narcotic and sedative drug excess* or withdrawal–even 'standard' doses of these drugs cause confusion in the elderly
  - Psychotropic medications* (tricyclic antidepressants, lithium, phenothiazines, MAOIs, benzodiazepines, SSRIs)
  - Miscellaneous (steroids, antihistamines, anticholinergics, levodopa)
  - Poisoning (carbon monoxide, heavy metals, toxic alcohols, salicylism)
- **Organ failure**
  - Respiratory failure* (hypoxia, hypercapnoea)
  - Congestive heart failure* (hypoxia)
  - Renal failure* (uraemic encephalopathy)
  - Liver failure* (hepatic encephalopathy)
- **Metabolic**
  - Hyperglycaemia*, hypoglycaemia*
  - Hypernatraemia, hyponatraemia*
  - Hypercalcaemia*
- **Endocrine**
  - Hyperthyroidism or hypothyroidism*
  - Cushing's disease
  - Addison's disease
- **Septicaemia**
  - UTI*, biliary tract*, meningococcaemia* or malaria*
- **Environmental**
  - Hyperthermia* or hypothermia*
- **Psychiatric disorder**
  - Mania, depression, schizophrenia–altered behaviour
  - Personality disorders or traits–aggressive behaviour
- **Elderly patients**
  - Elderly patients with limited cerebral reserve become disorientated, even delirious, with relatively 'minor' insults such as:
    - Pain, cold
    - Urinary retention, faecal impaction
    - Decrease in vision or hearing (including missing aids)
    - Unfamiliar surroundings (e.g. being admitted to hospital)
    - Bereavement/separation

What are the causes of aggressive behaviour?

Any of the above 'organic' causes may lead to aggressive behaviour, including:

- A young person who is intoxicated, feels frustrated and overwhelmed by an illness, or is psychotic

- An elderly person delirious from an acute medical illness
- Or simply a person with an antisocial or borderline personality, without any psychiatric or medical illness. Alcohol or illicit drug use may be a precipitant.

Major threat to life

- **Hypoxia** (from respiratory failure, or coma leading to airway obstruction)
- **Hypotension** (shock—see Chapter 11)
- **Sepsis**
  - Septicaemia, including meningitis, must be recognised early for optimal antibiotic effect
- **Intracranial mass lesion**
  - An expanding intracranial mass lesion (e.g. subdural or extradural haematoma) may initially present as confusion, followed by rapid deterioration
- **Seizures**
  - Recurrent seizures, status epilepticus
- **Risk of physical injury**
  - Patients who are agitated or confused may forcibly remove an oxygen mask, IV lines, NGT, CVL or bladder catheter.
  - These patients are also at risk of injury from attempting to crawl out of bed or over bed rails, and may threaten or attack staff.

Bedside

Quick-look test

Does the patient look well (comfortable), sick (uncomfortable or distressed) or critical (about to die)?
- Assess the situation rapidly, and call for senior help early.

Is the patient unresponsive?
- Assess the airway for obstruction, and ensure adequate respiratory effort. Administer oxygen and attach a pulse oximeter to the patient. Check the blood glucose level.
  - Cyanosis or increased work of breathing may signify hypoxia or hypercapnoea.
  - *Note*: critical hypercapnoea may be present despite normal oxygen saturation, if the patient is on supplemental oxygen.
- Pallor or cold peripheries may indicate circulatory failure or blood loss. Gain IV access, send bloods and start fluids.
- Assess the pupils—constriction may indicate narcosis, and dilation critical hypoxia.

What is the patient's general appearance?
- Look for external bruising or bleeding (coagulopathy).
- Subtle facial twitching may indicate ongoing seizure activity (non-convulsive status).

Is the patient aggressive?
- Decide from a safe distance how dangerous the patient is and what immediate measures are required to calm the situation.
- Any signs of escalating aggressive behaviour—call for help.

Airway and vital signs

What is the temperature?
- Raised temperature suggests infection, drug withdrawal or an adverse drug reaction including a hyperpyrexia syndrome, such as neuroleptic malignant or serotonin syndrome (see Chapter 32).
- Hypothermia occurs in myxoedema, alcohol or sedative drug ingestion (unusual once in hospital).

What is the respiratory rate?
- Confusion in association with tachypnoea suggests hypoxia or sepsis.
- A patient with bradypnoea and pinpoint pupils may be narcotised by excessive opioid analgesia, or have suffered a brainstem catastrophe.
- Patients with COPD receiving inappropriate high-flow oxygen (>28%) lose their hypoxic respiratory drive, resulting in confusion due to hypercapnoea.

What is the heart rate?
- Tachycardia is associated with hypoglycaemia, hypoxia, hypotension, sepsis, alcohol withdrawal and hyperthyroidism.
- Bradycardia occurs in raised intracranial pressure, myxoedema or preterminal hypoxia.

What is the blood pressure?
- Confusion in association with SBP <90 mmHg may be due to impaired cerebral perfusion in shock.
- Consider the differential diagnosis of shock including hypovolaemic, cardiogenic, distributive and obstructive (see Chapter 11).
- Hypertension may be associated with intracranial haemorrhage, stimulant drug intoxication or alcohol withdrawal.

What is the blood glucose result?
- Hypoglycaemia is a frequent cause of rapid-onset confusion and coma.
- It is most commonly seen in diabetic patients due to excessive insulin, inadequate food intake or excessive exertion. It may also occur with liver failure, alcohol excess or sulfonylurea overdose in the non-diabetic patient.

Management

Immediate management

The patient is unresponsive:
- Commence immediate management of DRS ABCDE and call for urgent senior help (see Chapter 7).
  - Commence CPR if there are no signs of life.
  - Maintain spinal immobilisation if head trauma has occurred.
- Commence high-dose oxygen via reservoir mask to maintain oxygen saturation >94%. Attach cardiac monitoring and pulse oximeter to the patient.
- Open the airway, insert an oropharyngeal device and assist ventilation with bag-valve-mask if required. Call for senior anaesthetic assistance for endotracheal intubation.
- Obtain IV access and take blood for FBC, U&E, LFTs, blood glucose and a venous or arterial blood gas.
- Give a 20 mL/kg bolus of normal saline if BP <90 mmHg.
- Give 50 mL of 50% glucose IV if fingerprick glucose <2.5 mmol/L.
  - Give thiamine 250 mg IV first to prevent Wernicke's encephalopathy if the patient is alcoholic or malnourished.
- Give naloxone 200 microgram boluses IV every 5 minutes if the patient has evidence of opioid toxicity, but beware precipitating a withdrawal state.
- Start immediate treatment for bacterial meningitis, such as ceftriaxone 2 g IV, if the patient has meningism and fever.
- Organise an urgent CT head scan if the patient has headache, possible head trauma, is on warfarin or a NOAC, or has lateralising neurological signs. Contact the neurosurgeon immediately if there is an intracranial abnormality.

The patient is agitated and aggressive:
- Reassure the patient, and ensure the physical safety of yourself and your staff.
  - Some patients calm down simply because 'the doctor' has arrived. They feel less helpless and more in control with the doctor there.
  - You will be able to judge within the first 30 seconds whether this is the case.
- **Verbal de-escalation:**
  - Define acceptable and unacceptable behaviour and their likely consequences. Speak firmly with courtesy and respect.
  - Try to address immediate concerns.
  - Explain what is happening at all times, reassure the patient and avoid confrontation.

- **Physical restraint:**
  - A 'show of force' with, ideally, five security personnel aims to encourage the patient to accept your reasoning.
  - Have at least one person per limb plus one controlling the head.
  - If the patient continues to threaten you or your staff, security personnel should restrain the patient, after a clear verbal warning.
  - Never tackle a patient alone, however small or frail-looking. You will get hurt or cause harm. Await the arrival of security staff.
- **Rapid tranquilisation:**
  - If the patient has already been given a benzodiazepine and is still out of control, try to convince the patient to have further oral sedation. Give another dose of midazolam 5 mg PO or diazepam 5–10 mg PO.
  - Or move on to a different oral agent such as an olanzapine wafer 10 mg PO.
  - Using temporary physical restraint, insert an IV cannula if still agitated.
  - Give midazolam 2.5–5 mg IV boluses, titrated to effect (smaller amounts in the elderly).
  - Add haloperidol 1–2 mg IV boluses up to 10 mg, if the midazolam is wearing off too quickly.
  - Once the patient is sedated, continuous bedside monitoring with pulse oximetry is essential, ideally with one-on-one nursing, until the patient wakes and is able to protect the airway.
  - Explain to any relatives what has happened. Reassure them that restraint is a temporary measure to protect the patient and others.

Selective history and chart review

The patient's history is unreliable, as with an altered mental status he or she may be unable to describe current symptoms or detail past medical conditions.

- Gain a collateral history from relatives or ward staff, particularly of any precipitating event such as a seizure or a fall out of bed.
- Review the patient's chart and note the presenting problem plus past medical history, and whether they may be related to the cause of the altered mental status, including:
  - History of head trauma, recent febrile illness, travel abroad, etc.
  - History of alcohol or drug misuse. Ask when was the patient's last alcoholic drink? Withdrawal symptoms present within the first 72 hours of hospitalisation and are unlikely after >1 week of abstinence.
  - Previous episodes of confusion. History of dementia.
  - Previous psychiatric history.
  - **Has the patient had recent surgery?**
    - Postoperative patients are at risk of confusion secondary to the residual effects of anaesthetic and analgesic medication, fluid

and electrolyte disturbance, urinary infection (particularly with an IDC), chest infection (including atelectasis in the first 24–48 hours) and/or PE (later, next few days).

Review the observation chart

- A sudden change in vital signs may be caused by drug toxicity or an acute intracranial catastrophe (haemorrhage).
- A gradual onset suggests a preceding or ongoing systemic medical disorder.

Review the medication chart

- Look for newly prescribed medication and potential drug interactions.
- Look at the list of medications normally taken at home. Has an important medication been omitted such as an antihypertensive?
- Even 'normal' doses of some drugs cause confusion in the elderly due to reduced intestinal, renal or hepatic blood flow, altered protein binding or changes in body fluid compartments.

Selective physical examination

Vitals	Repeat now
Mental status	Record a formal GCS score for level of consciousness
	If no depressed level of consciousness, perform a Quick Confusion Scale, which is more rapid than a formal Mini-Mental Status Examination, as it does not require the patient to read, write or draw (see Table 20.1).
HEENT	Nuchal rigidity, neck stiffness, photophobia (meningitis, subarachnoid haemorrhage)
	Pupil size and symmetry:
	Pinpoint pupils occur with opioids, clonidine, brainstem stroke or instillation of constricting eye drops such as pilocarpine for glaucoma
	Dilated pupils suggest sympathomimetic or anticholinergic effect, hypoxia, raised ICP
	Fundoscopy:
	Papilloedema (hypercapnoea, raised ICP or hypertensive encephalopathy)
	Diabetic retinopathy (dot and blot haemorrhages, exudates, neovascularisation)
	Hypertensive retinopathy (silver wiring, AV nipping, cotton-wool exudates and haemorrhage)
	Haemotympanum or blood in the ear canal (basal skull fracture)
	Lacerated tongue or cheek (postictal)

Resp	Cyanosis (hypoxia)
	Barrel chest, wheeze, prolonged expiration and increased work of breathing (COPD with predominant hypoxia 'pink puffer', or with hypercapnoea 'blue-bloater')
	Basal crackles (LVF, pneumonia)
CVS	Elevated JVP, S_3 gallop, pitting oedema (CCF)
Abdo	Costovertebral angle tenderness (pyelonephritis)
	Guarding, rebound tenderness (intra-abdominal haemorrhage or peritonism)
	Jaundice, hepatomegaly, bruising, flap, encephalopathy (liver failure) and/or ascites with splenomegaly (portal hypertension)
Neuro	Bilateral upgoing plantars (encephalopathies, raised ICP, postictal state, non-convulsive status epilepticus, brainstem stroke)
	Asterixis or flap (liver failure, renal failure, hypercapnoea)
	Tremor (DT, Parkinson's disease, hyperthyroidism)

Table 20.1 **Quick Confusion Scale**

Item	Points	× (weight)	Final score
'What year is it now?'	0 or 1	×2	**2** if correct
			0 if incorrect
'What month is it?'	0 or 1	×2	**2** if correct
			0 if incorrect
Present memory phrase:'Repeat this phrase after me and remember it: <u>James</u> <u>Smith</u>, <u>42</u> <u>Garden Road</u>, <u>Melbourne</u>'			
'About what time is it?'	0 or 1	×2	**2** if correct (within 1 hour)
			0 if incorrect
'Count backwards from 20 to 1'	0, 1 or 2	×1	**2** if correctly performed
			1 if one error
			0 if two or more errors
'Say the months in reverse'	0, 1 or 2	×1	**2** if correctly performed
			1 if one error
			0 if two or more errors
'Repeat the memory phrase'	0,1,2,3,4 or 5	×1	**1** for each underlined portion correct, up to 5 points
Final score **11** or less represents clinically significant cognitive impairment			

Investigations

- Exclude hyper- and hypoglycaemia and hypoxia:
  - Check a BGL and pulse oximetry.
- Send blood for FBC, U&E, LFTs:
  - FBC may reveal a leucocytosis indicating infection, or a macrocytosis suggesting alcohol use, folate or vitamin B12 deficiency, or reticulocytes (haemolysis)
  - U&E to identify renal failure and electrolyte abnormalities such as hyponatraemia, hypernatraemia, hypercalcaemia
  - LFTs for evidence of hepatic dysfunction—if abnormal, send a coagulation screen.
- Request a CXR, take two sets of paired blood cultures and send urine for MCS if sepsis is possible.
- Perform other investigations based on the suspected aetiology:
  - Thyroid function tests (myxoedema, thyrotoxicosis)
  - Drug levels (digoxin, lithium, anticonvulsants)
  - Antinuclear antibody, rheumatoid factor, erythrocyte sedimentation rate (raised), complement C3, C4 (reduced) in autoimmune disease etc
  - CT head scan if suspect head trauma, meningism, focal neurological signs, raised ICP (papilloedema, hypertension and bradycardia); seizures
  - Lumbar puncture *after* CT if suspect SAH or meningitis/ encephalitis
  - EEG if non-convulsive status epilepticus is considered (usually only available in the ICU).

Specific management

- **Hypoxia**—see Chapter 10.
- **Hypotension**—see Chapters 11 and 18.
- **CNS disorders including seizures**—see Chapter 23.
- **Drug intoxication or side effects**
  - Stop the medication if the confusion is secondary to drugs.
  - Reverse opioid intoxication—give naloxone 0.1–0.2 mg IV, SC or IM every 5 minutes repeated until alert. Beware precipitating an agitated withdrawal state in an opioid-dependent patient, or re-sedation as the naloxone wears off.
  - Following stabilisation of the patient, reduce the dose or alter the schedule of the opioid.
- **Drug withdrawal**
  - **Alcohol withdrawal syndrome**
    - This usually commences within 12–48 hours of abstinence and may last up to 1 week; characterised by agitation, irritability, fine tremor, sweats and tachycardia.
    - Start the patient on an Alcohol Withdrawal Chart. Commence diazepam 5–20 mg PO regularly until the

patient is comfortable, plus thiamine 250 mg IV daily. Give IV fluids and electrolyte replacement as required.

- **Delirium tremens (DT)**
  - DT is uncommon and usually occurs later at 72 hours after abstinence. There is clouding of consciousness, terrifying visual hallucinations, gross tremor, autonomic hyperactivity with tachycardia and cardiac arrhythmias, dilated pupils, fever, sweating, dehydration and grand mal seizures that may be prolonged (status epilepticus).
  - Give midazolam or diazepam 5–10 mg IV as a bolus every 5–15 minutes until the patient is sedated (i.e. drowsy but rouses when stimulated).
  - Refer to ICU, who will need to rule out other causes of status epilepticus such as head injury or meningitis.
- **Renal and hepatic failure**
  - Ensure that end-stage kidney and liver failure have not been worsened by nephrotoxic or hepatotoxic medications. Aggressive treatment of the kidney failure (dialysis) or liver failure (lactulose, coagulopathy, raised ICP) may be needed. Get senior help.
- **Depressed consciousness of unclear cause**
  - Some patients may have a depressed conscious level with no cause evident on history, physical examination or routine tests, including CT scan and lumbar puncture.
  - Check nothing was overlooked. Consider less likely or frankly unusual causes that may not show in early testing.
  - Intoxication or poisoning with:
    - Anticonvulsant medication (may have ataxia or nystagmus)
    - New-generation antipsychotics
    - Partial-agonist opioids
    - Long-acting benzodiazepines (e.g. clonazepam)
    - Gamma-hydroxybutyrate (GHB)
    - 'Other' alcohols, including methanol, ethylene glycol, isopropanol. Check for a metabolic acidosis with raised anion and osmolar gaps, and renal function.
  - Brainstem stroke
    - May have pinpoint pupils, generalised hyperreflexia and bilateral upgoing plantars.
  - Non-convulsive status epilepticus or prolonged postictal phase
    - Obtain urgent EEG if possible or give therapeutic trial of benzodiazepine to abort suspected seizure activity.
  - Cerebral vasculitis
    - CT or MR angiography will be needed, plus an immunology or rheumatology opinion.
- **Dementia**
  - Stable dementia may acutely decompensate to cause, or follow, hospital admission.

- Manage as for acute delirium after looking for a precipitating cause:
  - Quiet environment
  - Set routines
  - Calendars, clocks and staff continuity for environmental re-orientation
  - Risperidone PO or SL to control agitation.

Psychiatric evaluation

When there is a normal level of consciousness, normal vital signs, normal investigations and no remaining confusion, but the patient has altered mental behaviour, perform a rapid psychiatric evaluation. Discuss any abnormalities with the acute psychiatry service:

- **General appearance**—grooming, posture, eye contact, motor activity, attitude
- **Speech**—rate, volume, spontaneity, articulation, pressure, neologisms
- **Mood** (the patient's subjective experience of the emotional state)—elevated, happy, sad, angry, depressed
- **Affect** (the observer's assessment of the patient's emotional state)—dull, inappropriate, disinhibited
- **Thought process**—quality, relevance, blocking
- **Thought content**—suicidal, delusions, preoccupations, phobias, depersonalisation, ideas of reference, thought disorders
- **Perceptual disorders**—illusions, hallucinations
- **Cognition**
  - Level of consciousness and orientation
  - Memory—remote, recent, immediate (phrase or object recall)
  - Concentration—serial 7s or equivalent
  - Intelligence—vocabulary, general knowledge
  - Judgement—ability to form rational opinions and choices
  - Insight—awareness of situation.

Collapse, syncope and mechanical falls

Patients may collapse as the result of a transient loss of consciousness (syncope), dizziness, seizure or a mechanical fall.

This chapter describes collapses with full and rapid neurological recovery, and includes syncope and mechanical falls. These episodes may be difficult to distinguish from a seizure or acute vertigo, so an eyewitness account is vital.

Seizures and episodes with residual neurological deficit are described in Chapters 23 and 24, respectively.

* **Syncope** is transient loss of consciousness and postural tone from reduced cerebral perfusion, followed by spontaneous and full recovery.
* **Presyncope** refers to a reduction in cerebral perfusion resulting in a sensation of impending loss of consciousness, although the patient does not actually pass out. Presyncope and syncope represent different degrees of the same disorder.

Phone call

Questions

1. Was the collapse witnessed?
2. Was the patient lying, sitting or standing when the episode occurred? Syncope while lying down is potentially cardiac in origin and cannot, by definition, be postural hypotension.
3. Did the patient actually lose consciousness?
4. Was any seizure-like activity observed?
5. What are the vital signs now, including GCS score?
6. Did the patient sustain any injury?
7. What is the blood glucose level?
8. What was the reason for admission?

Instructions

When there is no evidence of head, neck or lower limb injury and the vital signs are stable:

- Ask the nurse to slowly raise the patient to a seated position, then standing position. Place the patient back into bed to remain there until you arrive.
- Request an ECG and attach non-invasive monitoring to the patient if syncope was the cause of collapse. Request a fingerprick BGL.
- Obtain a lying and standing HR and BP. Ask the nurse to wait at least 2 minutes after standing the patient up before taking the observations, then repeat the vital signs every 15 minutes until you arrive at the bedside.
- Ask the nurse to call you back immediately if there is deterioration in the level of consciousness or any cardiorespiratory instability.

Prioritisation

- Attend immediately if the patient remains unconscious and/or the HR or BP are abnormal.
- If the patient is alert and conscious with normal vital signs, or following an uncomplicated fall with no injury, there is no immediate urgency to attend.

Corridor thoughts

What are the causes of collapse?
Differentiate between syncope or a mechanical fall, and the alternative conditions such as dizziness (see Chapter 24), seizure (see Chapter 23) and altered mental status (see Chapter 20).

What causes syncope? (* = major threat to life)
- **Cardiac 'central' vascular:**
  - Bradyarrhythmia (Stokes-Adams attack):
    - Sinus arrest*
    - Second- and third-degree (complete) AV block*
    - Sick sinus syndrome (SSS)*
    - Pacemaker malfunction*
  - Tachyarrhythmia:
    - VT (may be in setting of ACS)*
    - Rapid AF or flutter (often with associated WPW)*
    - Rapid PSVT (often with associated WPW)*
    - Torsades de pointes (usually with prolonged QT)*
  - Obstructive lesions or 'low-flow' conditions, sometimes precipitated by exertion:
    - Aortic stenosis*
    - Pulmonary stenosis (rare)*
    - Hypertrophic cardiomyopathy (HCM, which is also associated with sudden VT or VF)*

  – Pulmonary embolism*
  – Aortic dissection*
- **Peripheral vascular orthostatic (postural) hypotension:**
  - Drug induced
    – Nitrates, hydralazine, prazosin, ACE inhibitors, antipsychotics, levodopa
  - Volume depletion
    – GI bleed*, ruptured AAA*, ectopic pregnancy*, dehydration
  - Autonomic failure
    – Diabetes, Parkinson's disease–multiple system atrophy (MSA)
- **Vasovagal syncope:**
  - Also called neurocardiogenic, neurally mediated syncope, vasodepressor or reflex-mediated syncope
  - Excessive vagal tone associated with standing, emotion, fear, pain, stress, hunger
- **Situational syncope:**
  - Raised intrathoracic pressure from coughing, micturition, swallowing, defecation, sneezing
- **Carotid sinus hypersensitivity**–syncope on turning head
- **Cerebrovascular:**
  - Subarachnoid haemorrhage*
  - Vertebrobasillar insufficiency–brainstem TIA (*not* other types of TIA)
  - Subclavian steal–extremity exercise leading to vertebrobasilar insufficiency
- **Psychogenic:**
  - Hyperventilation
  - Psychogenic collapse–diagnoses of exclusion only; look for underlying organic basis first

What causes mechanical falls?
Older people are prone to falls from a combination of environmental hazards, poor vision, diminished muscular strength and impaired proprioception. Additional underlying medical causes of a fall that must be looked for include:
- **Neurological**
  - Dementia resulting in poor safety awareness
  - Confusion and cognitive impairment
  - Pre-existing weakness
  - Parkinson's disease, or other movement disorders including normal pressure hydrocephalus
  - Cerebellar lesions with ataxia
- **Metabolic disorder**
  - Electrolyte abnormality such as hyponatraemia, hypokalaemia, hypoglycaemia, hyperglycaemia
  - Dehydration, renal failure (multifactorial), hepatic failure

- **Drugs**
  - Narcotics, sedatives, tranquilisers
- **Sensory impairment**
  - Cataracts, age-related macular degeneration, glaucoma
  - Impaired balance and proprioception
- **Musculoskeletal**
  - Arthritis, obesity and physical inactivity
- **Environmental**
  - Wet floor
  - Unsafe clothing or inappropriate footwear
  - Physical
    - Bed rails, IV pole, bed height, edge of a carpet, poor lighting or no handrails.

Major threat to life

- **Cardiac cause of syncope (Stokes–Adams attack) such as complete heart block, VT (remember underlying ACS). Also critical aortic stenosis, PE, SAH.**
  - Ensure an ECG is done in every case, and early cardiac monitoring if a potentially fatal cardiac arrhythmia is present.
- **Hypovolaemia precipitating syncope, especially occult bleeding (ruptured AAA, ectopic pregnancy, GI bleed).**
- **Head, spine or other injuries resulting from the fall.**
  - *Note:* collapse causing secondary mechanical injury such as an intracranial bleed may not result in a rapid recovery from the LOC. See Chapter 12.

Bedside

Quick-look test

Does the patient look well (comfortable), sick (uncomfortable or distressed) or critical (about to die)?
- Patients with a cardiac arrhythmia, poor cerebral perfusion or unstable vital signs who look sick require immediate intervention.
- Pallor followed by flushing occurs in cardiac syncope, whereas persistent pallor may indicate occult bleeding or another cause of poor peripheral perfusion. Cyanosis is a sign of hypoxia.
- However, most patients who have had a simple mechanical fall or an episode of syncope regain normal consciousness and look perfectly well.

Airway and vital signs

What is the heart rate?
- Tachycardia, bradycardia or irregular rhythm may indicate an arrhythmia as the primary cause of the collapse. Perform an ECG and attach a cardiac monitor to the patient.

- Cardiac causes of collapse must be identified as they have an increased mortality risk.

What is the blood pressure?
- Persistent hypotension is a sign of shock.
- A postural fall in BP together with a postural rise in HR (>20 beats/min) suggests intravascular volume depletion.
- A drop in BP without a change in HR, or one that corrects on standing, suggests autonomic dysfunction.
- Hypertension may be associated with SAH or brainstem TIA. Other neurological findings are then expected.

What is the temperature?
- Fever is not a feature of syncope, and is usually an incidental finding.

Management

Immediate management
- Recovery from syncope will be delayed if the patient is kept upright and not placed supine until symptoms resolve. Gradually sit the patient up over a few minutes as tolerated.
- A cardiac arrhythmia should be confirmed with a 12-lead ECG and treated immediately. Transient or intermittent arrhythmias require ECG monitoring, or arrangements for a Holter monitor.
- Obtain IV access and give normal saline 10–20 mL/kg IV rapidly if BP <90 mmHg and does not quickly improve with recumbency.
- Check for head or neck injury, as spinal immobilisation may be needed.
- Move onto selective history and examination if the patient has fully recovered from the syncopal episode, has a normal ECG and normal vital signs.

Selective history and chart review
Has the patient had a previous syncopal episode?
- Ask if the patient has ever had a previous syncopal episode.
- Ask whether these previous episodes, if any, have been documented, investigated or diagnosed.

What does the patient (or a witness) recall about the time immediately before the syncope?
- Try to determine preceding symptoms or obvious precipitant to the collapse.
- Sudden collapse with no warning, syncope lying down, associated palpitations or syncope on exertion suggests a cardiac cause known as a Stokes-Adams attack. This must be carefully assessed.
- Syncope on rising from a supine position suggests orthostatic or postural hypotension.

- Emotion or a noxious stimulus such as IV line insertion or painful wound dressing change may cause collapse secondary to a vasovagal episode.
  - Preceding nausea, sweating, distant hearing and light-headedness are common with a vasovagal episode.
- Syncope during or immediately after coughing, micturition, straining at stool or sneezing, known as situational syncope, is due to transient reduction of venous return to the right atrium plus a neurally mediated reflex bradycardia (Valsalva effect).
- Syncope after turning the head to one side (especially if wearing a tight collar) or while shaving may indicate carotid sinus syncope, often in elderly men.
- Syncope occurring during arm exercise suggests subclavian steal syndrome.
- Numbness and tingling in the hands and feet are common just before presyncope or syncope caused by hyperventilation.
- Events immediately prior will determine if this was in fact simply a trip or fall.

Confirm any presenting problem or past medical history that may have caused the collapse

- Previous episodes of collapse or falls with or without a known diagnosis
- Evidence of LV failure or a documented reduced LV ejection fraction <30%
- Known cerebrovascular disease
- Autonomic neuropathy
- Positive family history of collapse or sudden death may be due to underlying HCM, WPW syndrome, long QT syndrome or Brugada's syndrome (RBBB with ST elevation in leads V1–3 of the ECG).

Check the observation chart

- Check the vital signs to determine whether this is an acute change or if there were long-standing abnormalities in postural BP (autonomic neuropathy).
- Check for signs of hypovolaemia such as tachycardia, narrowing pulse pressure.
- Check for adequate fluid intake and look at the fluid balance chart.

Check the medication list

- Nitrates, vasodilator antihypertensives, diuretics, antiarrhythmics, tricyclic antidepressants, antipsychotics, levodopa and sildenafil (Viagra) cause postural hypotension.
- Beta-blockers (including eye drops), calcium-channel blockers, digoxin and amiodarone may cause bradycardia.

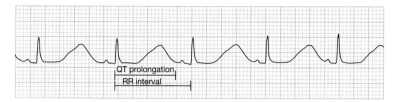

Figure 21.1A Prolonged QT. Copyright Tor Ercleve.

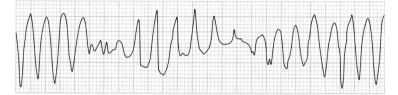

Figure 21.1B Torsades de pointes. Copyright Tor Ercleve.

- Any CNS depressant increases the risk of falls.
- Oral hypoglycaemic agents and insulin may cause hypoglycaemic seizures or syncope related to activity, food intake, drug interaction or associated systemic disease such as liver failure.
- Quinidine, procainamide, disopyramide, sotalol, amiodarone, tricyclic antidepressants, antipsychotics and some of the 'non-sedating' antihistamines prolong the QT interval (see Figure 21.1A). This may lead to polymorphic ventricular tachycardia or torsades de pointes (see Figure 21.1B). See also Chapter 17.

Selective physical examination

Focus the examination on the potentially sinister causes of collapse, especially hypotension (including postural), a cardiac murmur, an abdominal mass or tenderness, and look for any resulting injury.

Vitals	Repeat now, then take the BP in both arms. A difference >20 mmHg may indicate aortic dissection or subclavian steal syndrome
HEENT	Bitten tongue or cheek (seizure disorder)
	Neck stiffness (meningitis causing a seizure, SAH)
	Haemotympanum (fractured base of skull)
Resp	Crackles, wheezes (LVF, or aspiration during syncope)
CVS	Pacemaker (pacemaker syncope)

Continued

	Flat JVP (volume depletion)
	Focal features of right heart failure, such as a raised JVP and parasternal heave with dyspnoea suggesting PE
	Atrial fibrillation (vertebrobasilar embolism)
	Systolic murmur (aortic stenosis, HCM, pulmonary stenosis)
	Supra- or subclavicular bruit (subclavian steal syndrome)
Abdo	Abdominal mass (ruptured AAA)
	Rectal blood or melaena (GI bleed)
	Pelvic tenderness, vaginal bleeding (ectopic pregnancy)
GU	Urinary incontinence (seizure disorder)
Neuro	Residual localising signs such as unsteadiness or cranial nerve abnormalities such as diplopia, nystagmus, facial paralysis, vertigo, dysphagia and dysarthria occur in brainstem (vertebrobasilar) TIA
	Note: a completed stroke is not a cause of syncope, as rapid early recovery is unusual
MSS	Check passive ROM of the limbs and for evidence of a fracture if the patient fell
Skin	Contusions, abrasions and lacerations from injury

Investigations

- Check a fingerprick glucose for hypo- or hyperglycaemia.
- ECG in all patients. Look for:
  - Bradyarrhythmia, tachyarrhythmia, evidence of ACS or previous MI
  - Conduction defects, WPW, prolonged QT, LVH in HCM, or Brugada's syndrome (RBBB with raised ST in V1–3).
- Urinary beta-hCG in women of reproductive years.
- Other tests should only be done according to the clinical indications:
  - FBC (bleeding, anaemia)
  - U&E, troponin (if a recent AMI is suspected—*never* 'routine')
  - CXR (cardiomegaly, heart failure)
  - Echocardiography, Holter monitoring and exercise testing to elucidate a cardiac cause
  - CT if possible neurological cause such as SAH, vertebrobasilar insufficiency (VBI) (usually less than 2% causes of syncope).

Specific management

Decide from the history, physical findings and initial investigations what the most likely cause of the syncope is and arrange further investigation as necessary.

The majority of diagnoses are made by clinical assessment and simple tests alone, although more than 35% of patients with syncope never have a definitive diagnosis.

Cardiac causes

The patient aged >60 years, with a cardiac history (especially heart failure), abnormal cardiac examination or abnormal ECG has a high risk of cardiac syncope, with a 12-month mortality of 20%.

* Arrange continuous ECG monitoring if you suspect a cardiac cause for syncope such as an arrhythmia, valvular or a pacemaker problem.
* Exclude MI with resultant AV block, VT or VF as the cause by ECG analysis and troponin.
* Arrange for an echocardiogram in the morning to document a suspected cardiac lesion, and organise a cardiology consultation if aortic stenosis, hypertrophic cardiomyopathy or an arrhythmia is suspected.
* Pacemaker syncope requires a cardiology consultation for reprogramming of the pacing rate, output or mode, or for an upgrade to AV sequential pacing.
* Otherwise, arrange an outpatient 24-hour Holter ECG in younger patients with no overt evidence of heart disease.

Orthostatic hypotension

Syncope caused by volume depletion is managed initially with IV fluid replacement. Ensure that occult bleeding is identified and treated promptly, by an urgent abdominal USS for ruptured AAA or ectopic pregnancy.

* Drug-induced orthostatic hypotension and autonomic failure are complex to treat. As long as the patient's volume status is normal, they can be addressed electively in the morning.
* Instruct patients that if they need to get out of bed during the night, they must ask the nurse for assistance and should move slowly from supine to sitting, dangle their legs for 2 minutes and then move slowly again from sitting to standing.

Neurological causes

* Arrange a CT head scan for a suspected brainstem TIA (with contrast) or SAH (non-contrast). Consult with your senior.

Vasovagal syncope

This is more common in children and young adults, and is often associated with a family history. It can be recurrent with known stressors such as while standing, and is preceded by warmth, nausea, lightheadedness and visual 'grey-out'.

Bradycardia and hypotension are found initially, with rapid recovery of consciousness on lying supine. Nausea and malaise persist for longer. Exclude pregnancy in females.

Situational syncope

Most situational causes of syncope have a well-defined vagal precipitant. Usually no specific therapy is required other than explanation (e.g. advise men to micturate sitting down).

Refer a patient with suspected carotid sinus syncope to a cardiologist for investigation. Pacemaker insertion may be required if recurrent collapses occur.

Hyperventilation

Reassure the patient with presyncope due to hyperventilation or anxiety. Instruct the patient to breathe into a paper bag when the anxiety presyncopal feeling begins. This will correct the hypocapnia from hyperventilation.

Administer a benzodiazepine if resistant, but remember to explore the underlying precipitating trigger.

Falls

The cause is often multifactorial, such as diuretic-induced nocturia making an elderly patient under the influence of night sedation struggle to the bathroom in an unfamiliar, dimly lit hospital room!

- **Correct the reversible factors:**
  - Postural hypotension from volume depletion and unnecessary drug therapy in the elderly.
  - Nocturia—many elderly patients who fall out of bed at night are going to the bathroom. Make sure that the nocturia is not iatrogenic (e.g. cancel an evening diuretic order or unnecessary IV infusion) and the evening's fluid intake is limited.
  - Disorientation—ensure that the call bell is easily accessible and a nightlight is left on. The use of physical restraints (e.g. bedrails) may contribute to falls, so lower the bed height.
- **Check for complications:**

These may be subtle, such as a stroke patient dislocating a shoulder or fracturing a hip on the paralysed side during the fall.

  - An anticoagulated patient may develop a serious, delayed traumatic intracranial haemorrhage, so leave a message for the usual medical team to re-examine these patients frequently.
  - Common fractures include Colles', femoral neck, pubic rami, spinal crush, rib and humeral neck.
  - Fear, loss of confidence and independence, loss of mobility. Arrange a physiotherapy and occupational therapy consultation in the morning.

22

Headache

Headache is common in hospital. The aim on call is to determine whether the headache is sinister and a symptom of a serious underlying problem, or benign, or a recurrence of the patient's usual headache and of no urgent concern.

The history is vital as physical signs may be minimal or lacking, even in the serious group. Evaluate carefully every new headache or a change in the quality of a usual one, especially in a patient aged over 50 years.

Phone call

Questions

1. **Was the onset sudden or gradual?** Sudden onset of a severe headache is a SAH until proven otherwise.
2. **How bad is the headache?**
3. **What are the vital signs?**
4. **Is there an altered level of consciousness?**
5. **Are there any associated symptoms?** Fever is associated with meningitis, vomiting with raised ICP and phonophobia plus photophobia with migraine headache.
6. **Does the patient regularly suffer from headaches?** Do the features of this headache differ from previous headaches?
7. **Has the patient had a recent LP?** Post-LP headache occurs in 10–30% patients.
8. **What was the reason for admission?**

Instructions

- Ask the nurse to take a full set of vital signs and to assess the patient's neurological status.
- Request medication that has relieved the headache in the past, or prescribe a non-narcotic analgesic such as paracetamol 1 g PO or aspirin 300 mg with codeine 8 mg two tablets PO.

- Give metoclopramide 10–20 mg IV, together with dispersible aspirin 300 mg three tablets (900 mg) PO if migraine is likely. Metoclopramide reduces the pain of migraine in addition to its antiemetic effect.
- Ask the nurse to call back in 1 hour if a headache without concerning features has not been relieved by the medication.

Prioritisation

- A sudden severe headache and a headache associated with fever, vomiting or a decreased level of consciousness mandate seeing the patient immediately.
- A patient with a chronic or recurrent headache should have analgesia prescribed and be reviewed non-urgently.

Corridor thoughts

What are the important causes of headache? (* = major threat to life)

- **'Secondary headaches':**
  - **Intracranial**
    - Haemorrhage (subarachnoid, intracerebral, subdural)*
    - Infection (abscess, meningitis, encephalitis)*
    - Posttraumatic (subdural, extradural, cerebral contusion)*
    - Cerebral space-occupying lesion (secondary metastasis, primary benign or malignant tumour, abscess, tuberculoma)*
    - Cerebral venous sinus thrombosis
    - Idiopathic (benign) intracranial hypertension
    - Cerebral vasculitis such as SLE, RA, PAN, Wegener's granulomatosis*
    - Post-LP
  - **Local**
    - Glaucoma (*always* examine for a painful red eye, with a cloudy cornea and ovoid, fixed pupil)
    - Temporal arteritis
    - Vertebral artery dissection*
    - Neuralgia (greater occipital, glossopharyngeal, trigeminal)
    - Sinusitis, otitis media, mastoiditis
    - Dental caries, tooth abscess
    - TMJ dysfunction
    - Cervical osteoarthritis
  - **Systemic**
    - Severe hypertension*
    - Systemic infection*
    - Hypercapnia*
    - Preeclampsia (is the patient pregnant?)*

- **Drugs**
  - Nitrates
  - Calcium-channel blockers
  - NSAIDs
  - Medication overuse headache
- **'Primary headaches':**
  - Tension headache
  - Migraine
  - Cluster headache

Major threat to life

- **Subarachnoid haemorrhage (SAH)** has an overall fatality rate of 50%, and significant morbidity from the initial bleed or subsequent re-bleeding. Sudden onset, severe headache is typical.
- **Bacterial meningitis** must be suspected with fever, vomiting, confusion and photophobia. It needs urgent treatment with IV antibiotics.
- **Intracranial herniation from a space-occupying lesion.** Any intracranial mass lesion (e.g. infection, blood or tumour) can cause herniation (see Table 22.1).
- **Hypertensive encephalopathy.** See Chapter 19.

Table 22.1 **Presenting signs of intracranial herniation**

Stage of herniation	Signs
Early	Ipsilateral pupillary dilation (uncal herniation) Respiratory pattern changes (Cheyne–Stokes breathing) Progressive decrease in level of consciousness (GCS)
Ongoing	Bilateral pupillary constriction, but reactive Hyperventilation Decorticate flexor posturing
Advanced	Irregular respiration (Biot breathing) Decerebrate extensor posturing Fixed dilated pupils (tonsillar herniation 'coning') Sudden death

Bedside

Quick-look test

Does the patient look well (comfortable), sick (uncomfortable or distressed) or critical (about to die)?

Patients with SAH, meningitis or intracranial herniation look sick, are often in significant pain and frequently have altered mental status.

SECTION C – Common calls

Patients with migraine are also distressed and sick, but remain fully conscious. Most patients, including those with recurrence of a chronic headache, look well.

Airway and vital signs
What is the blood pressure?
* Severe hypertension (may include papilloedema and altered mental status) is associated with SBP >180 mmHg and DBP >120 mmHg.
* Otherwise, headache is *not* a symptom of hypertension unless there has been a sudden increase in BP or an associated intracranial bleed.

What is the heart rate?
* Hypertension in association with bradycardia occurs with increasing ICP.

What is the temperature?
* Fever associated with a headache requires immediate blood cultures, IV antibiotics, CT scan and LP if no contraindication.

Selective physical examination I
Does the patient have signs of raised ICP or meningitis?

HEENT	Nuchal rigidity (meningitis, SAH)
	Fundoscopy:
	Absent venous pulsations (earliest sign of raised ICP)
	Papilloedema (established raised ICP)
	Retinal haemorrhages (hypertension, SAH)
Mental status	Abnormal mental status, drowsiness, yawning and inattentiveness with headache are ominous
Neuro	Test for Kernig's sign and Brudzinski's sign (meningitis, SAH) (see Figure 22.1), despite being somewhat unreliable and inconsistent.
	Unequal pupils with a decreased level of consciousness represent a life-threatening situation. Call for senior help and arrange for endotracheal intubation, a CT head scan and an urgent neurosurgical consult.
Skin	Maculopapular rash (early), petechiae or purpura (later) indicate meningococcaemia. Call for senior help, take blood cultures immediately and give benzylpenicillin 2.4 g IV, or ceftriaxone 2 g IV if penicillin hypersensitive.

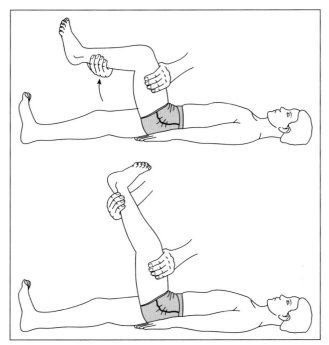

Figure 22.1A Kernig's sign. The test result is positive when pain or resistance is elicited by passive knee extension from the 90-degree hip–knee flexion position.

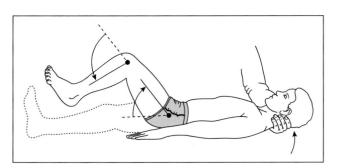

Figure 22.1B Brudzinski's sign. The test result is positive when the patient actively flexes the hips and knees in response to passive neck flexion by the examiner.

SECTION C – Common calls

Management

Immediate general management

- Attach continuous non-invasive ECG, BP and pulse oximeter monitoring to the patient.
- Commence oxygen therapy to maintain oxygen saturation >94%.
- Obtain IV access with large-bore (14–16G) peripheral cannulae. Draw and send blood samples for FBC, coagulation profile, U&E, LFTs, G&H and two sets of paired blood cultures, if infection is possible.
- Give antibiotics for suspected meningitis, and titrate morphine 2.5 mg IV boluses with metoclopramide 10 mg IV for SAH.
- Request an immediate CT head scan if a secondary intracranial cause is suspected. LP is contraindicated when there is papilloedema, focal neurology including an altered conscious level, immunosuppression or coagulopathy, because of the risk of brain herniation or local spinal bleeding.

Immediate specific management

- Suspect **bacterial meningitis** if the patient appears unwell with fever, altered mental status, nuchal rigidity or photophobia (see later).
  - Give normal saline to support a low BP.
  - Give dexamethasone 0.15 mg/kg IV with ceftriaxone 4 g IV as soon as the diagnosis is suspected. *Never* delay the initial treatment while awaiting an LP, especially at night.
  - If there is altered behaviour, speech disorder or focal neurology, or the CSF result shows an atypical leucocytosis (predominantly monocytes) or a negative Gram stain for bacteria, commence aciclovir 10 mg/kg IV for herpes simplex encephalitis.
- Call neurosurgery immediately if the patient appears unwell with fever and there is a subdural empyema, brain abscess or suspected infected ventriculoperitoneal shunt.
- Consider a **SAH** if the patient has severe headache, confusion or an altered conscious level, nuchal rigidity but no fever.
  - Request an urgent non-contrast CT head scan.
- Suspect **migraine headache** if the patient has a typical aura and no fever, no nuchal rigidity, no confusion and no papilloedema. Vomiting with photophobia and phonophobia is common, plus a past history of migraine. *Never* make a 'first' diagnosis of migraine without a definite history of previous similar attacks.
  - Give metoclopramide 10–20 mg IV plus an NSAID, such as aspirin 300 mg three tablets (900 mg) PO and commence IV normal saline at 500 mL/h if volume depleted.

Selective history and chart review

The most important features that signify a sinister headache are in the history, and include the onset, severity and associated symptoms.

Was the onset sudden or insidious?
- Sudden onset of pain suggests a vascular cause such as subarachnoid or intracerebral haemorrhage, cerebral venous sinus thrombosis, or vertebral or carotid artery dissection.

How severe is the headache?
- A sudden-onset 'worst headache ever' is a SAH until proven otherwise.
- Migraine headache causes pain bad enough to interfere with normal daily function.
- Muscle contraction headaches are band-like, mild and rarely incapacitating.

Where is the main site of pain?
- Unilateral throbbing headache is characteristic of migraine. A tight band around the head or ache across the forehead is typical of tension headache, and lancinating or 'electric-shock' pains suggest a neuralgia.
- Cluster headaches cause extreme facial or eye pain in short, recurring bouts, often many months apart.
- *Note:* retro-orbital pain may also be caused by orbital lesions including glaucoma (always examine for a hazy cornea, with an ovoid semi-dilated pupil), cavernous sinus venous thrombosis, berry aneurysm and SAH, and sphenoid or ethmoid sinusitis.

How does posture affect headache severity?
- Muscle contraction headache is improved by lying down and resting.
- Headache made worse by lying or bending down suggests raised ICP.
- Headache made worse by standing up (orthostatic) may indicate a low-pressure syndrome such as post-LP headache or, occasionally, a spontaneous CSF leak.

Are there other associated symptoms?
- Visual aura such as scintillations, zigzag lines, migratory scotomata and tunnel or blurred vision precede a 'classic migraine' headache and are helpful in suggesting the diagnosis. However, an aura is absent in 'common migraine'.
- Cluster headaches are associated with unilateral parasympathetic signs such as conjunctival injection, lacrimation, rhinorrhoea, ptosis and miosis on the same side as the pain.
- Clicking or popping when opening or closing the jaw indicates TMJ dysfunction.
- Hearing loss is associated with otitis media and mastoiditis.

SECTION C – Common calls

Is there a past history of chronic, recurring headaches and what is their pattern?
- Tension headache is generally mild in the morning and becomes more severe over the day. Headache from raised ICP is worse on wakening, with effortless vomiting.
- Migraine headache is commonly unilateral, pulsating or throbbing in nature, is aggravated by movement and is associated with nausea and/or vomiting, photophobia or phonophobia.

Is there a history of recent head trauma?
- Arrange a CT head scan if there has been any recent head trauma, especially in an elderly patient or if on warfarin or a NOAC.

Has the patient been generally unwell for weeks or months?
- Malaise, scalp tenderness or hyperaesthesiae, jaw claudication, weight loss and shoulder girdle ache suggest temporal (giant cell) arteritis ± polymyalgia rheumatica (PMR) in patients older than 50 years.
  - Send blood for an ESR, and if raised >50 mm/h start prednisone 60 mg PO immediately.
- Acute angle-closure glaucoma may be precipitated by pupil dilation. The patient complains of a severe unilateral headache located over the brow and may develop nausea, vomiting and abdominal pain that can be mistaken for an acute abdomen.

What medication is the patient taking?
- Nitrates, calcium-channel blockers, oral contraceptives and NSAIDs can cause headache.
- Anticoagulant therapy (e.g. warfarin or a NOAC) should raise the suspicion of an intracranial haemorrhage. Obtain an urgent CT head scan and seek senior help to reverse the anticoagulation (see Chapter 46).
  - A low threshold for investigation should also be maintained in elderly patients taking aspirin or clopidogrel, particularly following a fall.
- *Note:* relief of pain with analgesia does not aid diagnosis. Do not discount the seriousness of a headache just because it has responded to analgesia, as it can still be a SAH.

Selective physical examination II

Vitals	Repeat now
HEENT	Red eye (acute angle-closure glaucoma, cluster headache)
	Tender, raised temporal artery (temporal arteritis)
	Tenderness on percussion over the frontal or maxillary sinuses (sinusitis)
	Inability to fully open the jaw and tenderness over the TMJ (TMJ dysfunction)

Evidence of recent head trauma (subdural or extradural haematoma)

Haemotympanum or blood in the ear canal, raccoon eyes (basal skull fracture)

Palpate the scalp muscles for evidence of tenderness or contraction (tension headache, occipital neuralgia)

Tenderness at the apex of the suboccipital triangle that exacerbates the pain (greater occipital neuralgia).

Neuro	Perform a complete neurological examination
	Unequal pupils, or abnormality of conscious level, visual fields, eye movements, limbs, tone, reflexes or plantar responses suggests structural brain disease. Make certain an urgent CT head scan has been arranged and you have called your senior.

Investigations
- FBC may be unhelpful, as a proportion of patients with meningitis will have a normal WCC and differential.
- Arrange an ESR in patients aged over 50 years with suspected temporal arteritis (>50 mm/h is consistent).
- Check the coagulation profile if the patient is on anticoagulants, or is septic with DIC (disseminated intravascular coagulation or 'consumptive coagulopathy').
- Arrange an urgent CT head scan for:
  - Sudden-onset 'thunderclap' headache (SAH)
  - Neurological deficits (other than migrainous aura), altered mental status, papilloedema, nuchal rigidity or seizures (space-occupying lesions [SOLs], haemorrhage, abscess, vasculitis etc)
  - Recent head trauma (subdural, extradural or intracranial blood)
  - Anticoagulation medication (subdural or intracranial bleed).
- Then proceed to LP and CSF analysis in suspected meningoencephalitis, SAH or benign intracranial hypertension.
- Reserve cranial MRI/MRA for suspected cerebral venous sinus thrombosis, vasculitis or vertebral or carotid artery dissection if CT scan is inconclusive.

Specific management
Meningoencephalitis
Generalised headache, fever and vomiting with altered mental status, irritability and drowsiness progressing to coma, neck stiffness and photophobia.
- Most often caused by viruses, or if bacterial *Neisseria meningitidis*, *Streptococcus pneumoniae*, *Haemophilus influenzae* (non-vaccinated) and *Listeria monocytogenes*.

- Viral infection usually causes less severe headache, and may have a typical prodrome, but always do an LP if in any doubt.
- Suspect herpes simplex virus (HSV) encephalitis if altered level of consciousness, behavioural disturbance, focal neurological deficits or seizures.
- Immunosuppressed patients are at increased risk of HSV, varicella zoster virus and CMV encephalitis, *S. pneumoniae, L. monocytogenes,* aerobic Gram-negative bacilli and cryptococcal meningitis.
- Commence antibiotics and/or antiviral therapy as soon as two sets of paired blood cultures have been drawn. Do *not* delay by waiting for a CT scan or LP, especially at night.
- Perform a non-contrast CT head scan before an LP to exclude SAH or unexpected focal mass lesion such as a cerebral abscess.

Subarachnoid haemorrhage

Sudden or 'thunderclap', severe, 'worst-ever' headache, sometimes following exertion or straining, with nausea, vomiting, altered conscious state and meningism.

Oculomotor palsy or other focal findings are common. Less typical presentations include acute confusion, sudden collapse or coma. Mild cases can mimic migraine and even respond to analgesia.

- Give the patient oxygen and nurse head upwards. Aim for an oxygen saturation >94%.
- Gain IV access and send blood for FBC, coagulation profile, U&E, blood glucose and G&H.
- Attach a cardiac monitor and pulse oximeter to the patient.
- Give paracetamol 500 mg and codeine phosphate 8 mg or rarely morphine 2.5–5 mg IV boluses for pain relief, and avoid any NSAIDs. Call your senior.
- Control agitation or a seizure with benzodiazepine IV.
- Perform an ECG; request a CXR and an urgent non-contrast CT head scan.
- If the CT head scan is normal, proceed to LP after at least 10–12 hours after the headache onset. This is therefore usually the following morning. Send CSF for microscopy, culture, glucose, protein and xanthochromia studies in every case.
- Refer to neurosurgery if the diagnosis is confirmed by red cells with xanthochromia, or if the CSF analysis for xanthochromia was equivocal.

Space-occupying lesion

Headaches become progressively more frequent and severe, worse in the mornings and exacerbated by coughing, bending or straining. Vomiting without nausea and focal neurological signs develop, including subtle personality change, changes in concentration or even disinhibited behaviour.

Papilloedema may occur. The earliest signs on fundoscopy are loss of spontaneous venous pulsation in the central retinal vein and blurring of the optic disc margin with filling in of the optic cup.

- Arrange an immediate CT head scan and perform a CXR to look for a primary tumour.
- Refer a patient with a confirmed mass lesion to the neurosurgical team.

Temporal arteritis

Occurs in patients aged >50 years, with diffuse or bitemporal headache associated with a history of malaise, weight loss and myalgia plus shoulder girdle weakness from associated polymyalgia rheumatica. Occasionally, there is pain on chewing (jaw claudication). Look for localised scalp tenderness and hyperaesthesia with temporal artery tenderness.

- Send blood for an ESR, and give prednisone 60 mg PO immediately to prevent permanent visual loss from ophthalmic artery involvement associated with anterior ischaemic optic neuropathy (AION).
- Arrange for a temporal artery biopsy within the next 7 days.

Migraine

- Ask the patient what is usually taken for the migraine and prescribe this immediately. Alternatively, give an oral analgesic such as aspirin 300 mg three tablets (900 mg) PO, ibuprofen 600 mg PO or paracetamol 1 g.
- Add metoclopramide 10–20 mg IV and avoid inappropriate opioid analgesia.
- If oral analgesia plus metoclopramide fail, give chlorpromazine 12.5–25 mg IV diluted in 500 mL normal saline over 30 minutes and keep the patient in bed (risk of postural hypotension).
- *Note:* if you consider a triptan such as sumatriptan 6 mg SC for a resistant headache, make certain there is no risk of coronary artery disease and no ergotamine has been given in the last 24 hours.

Cluster headache

Cluster headaches are difficult to treat. Most last less than 45 minutes, and oral treatment has minimal effect. Discuss with your senior and try:

- High-flow oxygen by non-rebreather mask as early as possible to abort an attack
- Intranasal local anaesthetic spray (e.g. 5% lignocaine bilaterally)
- Sumatriptan 6 mg SC.

Avoid giving morphine.

SECTION C – Common calls

Post-lumbar puncture headache

Low-pressure headache on standing up, within 48 hours of LP, is most often secondary to continuing dural CSF leak.

- Treat with strict bed rest (no toilet privileges), oral or IV fluids and regular paracetamol 500 mg with codeine phosphate 8 mg two tablets PO.
- If this is unsuccessful, arrange for the regular medical care team to refer the patient to an anaesthetist for an epidural blood patch.

Muscle contraction (tension) headache

Most common overall type of headache. Pain comes on gradually, is bilateral, dull, constant and band-like, and usually does not affect daily function.

- Treat with oral analgesics such as paracetamol 500 mg with codeine phosphate 8 mg (two tablets 6-hourly PO) or ibuprofen (400 mg 6-hourly PO).
- Arrange for the regular medical care team to discuss a long-term management plan.

23

Seizures

A seizure is one of the more dramatic events you may witness while on call. *Remain calm:* most seizures resolve spontaneously within 1–2 minutes.

The causes of a seizure are similar to those for altered mental status (see Chapter 20), but remember that other conditions can mimic a seizure (see Box 23.1).

'Status epilepticus' is a medical emergency. Generalised convulsive status epilepticus (GCSE) is defined as two or more tonic–clonic seizures without full recovery of consciousness in between, or prolonged tonic–clonic seizure activity for more than 5 minutes.

BOX 23.1 Conditions that mimic a seizure or postictal state

- Pseudoseizure
- Syncopal episode
- Narcolepsy, cataplexy (including following laughter)
- Movement disorder (e.g. hemiballismus, choreo-athetosis, tics, Tourette's syndrome, myoclonic jerks)
- Complicated migraine
- Dystonic reaction
- Carpopedal spasm from hyperventilation

Phone call

Questions

1. **Is the patient still having a seizure and how long has it lasted?** Patients who are actively having seizures are at risk of hypoxia, aspiration, metabolic acidosis, hyperpyrexia and cerebral oedema, ultimately leading to irreversible cellular damage.
2. **What type of seizure was it?** Was the seizure generalised tonic–clonic, or focal?
3. **What is the patient's current level of consciousness?**
4. **Has there been any secondary damage such as a head injury or bitten tongue?**

5. What was the reason for admission?
6. Is the patient pregnant (eclampsia)?

Instructions

If the patient is still having a seizure:
- Ask the nurse to place the patient in the lateral decubitus position to reduce the risk of aspiration of gastric contents, without trying to prise open the patient's mouth.
- Give high-flow oxygen by mask and attach pulse oximetry to the patient.
- Request a fingerprick BGL.
- Ask the nurse to assemble the following at the bedside:
  - Oropharyngeal and nasopharyngeal airway
  - Yankauer sucker with suction equipment
  - IV trolley with 1000 mL normal saline run through a giving set
  - 10 mg diazepam or 10 mg midazolam drawn up in 10 mL saline
  - 50% dextrose 50 mL if the BGL is low.

If the patient has stopped seizing and is postictal:
- Ask the nurse to remove any loose dentures, suction the oropharynx, insert an oral airway if tolerated and observe seizure precautions (see Box 23.2) until medical review.

BOX 23.2   Seizure precautions

- Place the bed in the lowest position.
- Keep the side rails up and pad with a rolled-up towel or blanket.
- Provide a firm pillow, commence oxygen and keep suction handy.
- Keep the patient in bed until reviewed medically, in the lateral position to avoid aspiration.

Prioritisation

See the patient with a seizure immediately, even if the patient has recovered.

Corridor thoughts

What causes seizures? (* = major threat to life, as most likely to progress to status epilepticus with refractory seizures)
- **Idiopathic (patient with known epilepsy):**
  - Inadequate anticonvulsant therapy (usually stopped or forgotten); rarely, anticonvulsant excess or toxicity
  - Hypoglycaemia*

- Alcohol excess or withdrawal*
- Intercurrent infection (e.g. meningitis)*
- Head injury*
- Sleep deprivation or social stressors—5–10% of epileptic patients have recurrent seizures with no obvious precipitating event despite optimal medical therapy
- **Acute symptomatic or secondary seizure (non-epileptic patient, or with known epilepsy):**
  - CNS disorder
    - Infection* (e.g. meningitis, encephalitis, brain abscess)
    - Head injury*
    - Space-occupying lesion* (e.g. tumour)
    - Cerebral ischaemia/infarction/vasculitis*
    - Subarachnoid* or intracerebral haemorrhage*
    - Hypertensive encephalopathy
  - Endocrine and metabolic disorder
    - Hypoglycaemia*
    - Hyponatraemia*
    - Hypocalcaemia
    - Hypomagnesaemia
    - Uraemia
  - Systemic disorder
    - Hypoxia* (cause or effect)
    - Hypotension causing reduced cerebral perfusion
    - Sepsis from renal tract, respiratory or skin infection
    - Hyperthermia* (cause or effect)
    - Eclampsia* (pregnancy)
  - Drug-related toxicity
    - Alcohol*, cocaine, amphetamine, ecstasy
    - Tricyclic antidepressants*; other sodium-channel blockers
    - Theophylline*
    - Isoniazid*
  - Drug-related withdrawal
    - Alcohol*, benzodiazepine, barbiturate or anticonvulsants
  - Psychiatric disorder
    - Pseudoseizures* (mimic true seizures, and are most common in patients with known epilepsy. May ultimately require EEG monitoring to differentiate)

Major threat to life

- **Hypoxia including aspiration**
- **Serious underlying cause such as meningitis**
- **Hyperthermia**
- **Cerebral oedema** if seizures continue more than 30 minutes

SECTION C – Common calls

Bedside

Quick-look test

Don't panic! A seizure is disturbing to witness and causes anxiety in others, particularly relatives. Remember most seizures are self-limited and will resolve in 1–2 minutes.

Airway, vital signs and blood glucose level

Position the patient appropriately, clear the airway and administer oxygen as outlined below.

What is the blood pressure?
Palpate for the femoral pulse, which if present indicates a SBP of at least 70 mmHg.

What is the fingerprick blood glucose result?
Hypoglycaemia must be detected and treated immediately.

Management

Immediate management

- Call your senior for assistance.
- Place the patient in the lateral decubitus position to prevent aspiration of gastric contents.
- Clear the oropharynx and suction the airway, but *never* attempt to wedge the teeth open. Gently insert a nasopharyngeal airway if an airway adjunct is required in the presence of trismus.
- Give high-flow oxygen by mask.
- Attach pulse oximetry to the patient.
- Establish IV access. One or two assistants may need to hold the arm still. Take blood for blood glucose, U&E and other tests as indicated clinically.
- Give 50 mL of 50% glucose IV if the fingerprick BGL is <3.0 mmol/L.
- Give thiamine 250 mg IV by slow injection if the patient is alcoholic or malnourished (risk of glucose precipitating Wernicke's encephalopathy).

The seizure may have stopped by now, but if not:

- Give midazolam 0.05–0.1 mg/kg up to 10 mg IV, or diazepam 0.1–0.2 mg/kg up to 20 mg IV.
- Once the seizure has stopped, follow immediately with phenytoin IV to prevent relapse of the seizure once the midazolam (or diazepam) wears off.
- Insert a second IV line, as phenytoin is incompatible with diazepam or glucose-containing solutions.
- Infuse phenytoin 15–20 mg/kg IV in 250 mL normal saline (*never* dextrose) over at least 30 minutes under ECG monitoring. Do not exceed the maximum infusion rate of 50 mg/min.

- Flush the IV line with normal saline to reduce local venous irritation.
- If the patient is already on phenytoin therapy, but has a subtherapeutic level (or the level is unknown), give half the IV loading dose.
- Repeat the midazolam or diazepam boluses if seizures recur despite phenytoin loading, or they recur before the phenytoin infusion has been completed.
- Start looking for a reversible precipitating cause:
  - Look for evidence of head injury, bruising, IV drug use or cytotoxic use (underlying intracranial haematoma, liver disease or anticoagulant use, infection, malignancy with brain secondary).
  - Consider sepsis, especially meningoencephalitis, and give antibiotics and antivirals (aciclovir) if in doubt.
  - Look at the serum sodium and calcium results.
- Treat as per refractory seizures (status epilepticus) if seizures recur (see later).

ONCE THE SEIZURES HAVE STOPPED

Bedside

Quick-look test

Does the patient look well (comfortable), sick (uncomfortable or distressed) or critical (about to die)?
Assess the level of consciousness. Immediately following a generalised tonic–clonic seizure, the patient is usually semiconscious ('postictal' state). Persistent cyanosis suggests aspiration and/or hypoxia as a cause or effect of the seizure.

What are the pulse rate and blood pressure?
- Sinus tachycardia and hypertension are common and usually settle over 10–30 minutes.
- Eclampsia is likely if the patient is pregnant and hypertensive.

What is the respiratory rate?
- Increased RR is normal in the postictal state as the patient recovers.

What is the temperature?
- A mildly raised temperature is usual in the immediate postictal period, but should settle rapidly.
- A persistent temperature >38°C mandates a search for a potential infective precipitant. Perform blood cultures, CXR, MSU, CT, then LP.
- A temperature >39.5°C indicates hyperthermia, which may be the cause or the effect of seizures. Urgent tepid sponge and fan cooling is necessary.

What is the fingerprick glucose result?
* Hypoglycaemia must be treated to prevent further seizures.

Management

Immediate management of the postictal patient
* Observe seizure precautions (see Box 23.2) until the postictal period passes and the patient's mental status returns to normal.
* Make sure the patient is in the lateral decubitus position to keep the airway clear. Remove any loose dentures and suction the airway. Insert an oral or nasopharyngeal airway if the patient is still drowsy and the airway is not being spontaneously maintained.
* Administer oxygen via mask or nasal prongs.
* Ensure the patient has reliable IV access and draw blood for investigations if not already done.
* Consider a phenytoin infusion of 15–20 mg/kg in 250 mL normal saline (*never* dextrose) over at least 30 minutes under ECG monitoring.
  * Give phenytoin if further seizures are anticipated, such as a patient with known epilepsy who is non-compliant with regular medication, or following repeat seizures.
  * A brief, first, single seizure with no obvious precipitant or a precipitant that has been identified and treated does *not* require further anticonvulsant therapy.

Selective history and chart review
* An eyewitness account is crucial to confirm the diagnosis of an epileptic seizure rather than a faint (vasovagal syncope), fall or episode of vertigo.
* Ask any witnesses the following details about the episode:
  * What was the duration of the seizure?
  * Was the seizure generalised or focal in onset?
  * Was there a preceding aura or postictal drowsiness?
  * Were any injuries incurred during the seizure (head injury, tongue biting, musculoskeletal)?
  * Was the patient incontinent of urine?
* Check for any presenting problem or past medical history that may be relevant to the cause of the seizure:
  * Epilepsy, alcohol or sedative withdrawal, head injury (e.g. recent fall prior to, or in, hospital), stroke, CNS tumour (secondary or primary), diabetes mellitus or immunosuppression.
* Look at the observation chart:
  * Abnormal vital signs (fever, hypoxia, tachycardia) prior to the seizure may indicate an acute illness as a possible precipitant.

- Check the medication list for:
  - Medications that may induce seizures (see *Corridor thoughts*)
  - Missed anticonvulsant therapy.
- Review recent laboratory results for evidence of electrolyte disturbances such as hyponatraemia, hypocalcaemia or hypomagnesaemia.

Selective physical examination

Look specifically for a potential focus of infection and for residual focal neurology.

Vital signs	Repeat now
Mental status	Assess level of consciousness
HEENT	Examine for mouth lacerations, chipped teeth, tongue laceration and facial fracture
	Assess for neck stiffness and signs of meningism
Resp	Look for tachypnoea or hypoxia from aspiration or pneumonia
Neuro	Perform as complete a neurological examination as possible, looking for focal neurology such as asymmetry of pupils, motor power, reflexes or plantar responses
	Note: unilateral partial or complete weakness in the postictal period that resolves within 1–36 hours, average 15 hours, is likely to be a Todd paralysis.
MSS	Assess for injuries secondary to seizure activity, such as:
	Dislocations, especially posterior dislocation of shoulder
	Fractures, including spinal crush fractures or femoral neck fracture following a fall
	Lacerations, contusions and abrasions

Investigations
Laboratory

- Take blood for FBC, U&E, LFTs and serum glucose in every patient. Request other tests as clinically indicated:
  - Beta-hCG to exclude pregnancy in all women of childbearing age
  - Anticonvulsant medication levels
  - Blood cultures if sepsis suspected
  - ESR and autoantibody screen if vasculitis suspected (*not* routine!).

CT head scan

- Every patient with a new, first or undiagnosed seizure should have a scan to look for:
  - Traumatic injury (cause or effect)
  - Underlying intracranial tumour, haemorrhage, infection

SECTION C – Common calls

- Unusual lesions in the immunosuppressed or known HIV patient, such as primary lymphoma or cryptococcal abscess.

Lumbar puncture (only *after* the CT scan)
- If intracranial infection or SAH is suspected.

General management
- Always look for an underlying cause—consider a seizure as a sign, not a diagnosis.
- Treat suspected meningoencephalitis with IV antibiotics and antivirals (see Chapter 22).
- Maintain seizure awareness for at least the next 24 hours.
- Many seizures are self-limiting single events and do not require long-term anticonvulsant medications.
- If the patient normally takes anticonvulsant medication, check levels and adjust dose accordingly to regain the therapeutic range.
- Commence phenytoin 300 mg PO once daily for a recurrent seizure, or a seizure in a patient with a structural CNS abnormality, then according to the blood level.
- Continue 4-hourly neurological observations overnight, or more frequently according to the vital signs. Intensive care may be necessary.

Specific management
Refractory seizures—'status epilepticus'
- Permanent neuronal damage from systemic consequences such as hyperthermia, acidosis and hypoxaemia occurs with status epilepticus lasting more than 30 minutes.
- Contact your senior, the anaesthetist and intensive care registrar on call if the patient is still having seizures despite the measures outlined above.
- Organise for transfer to the ICU for endotracheal intubation and mechanical ventilation, plus IV antiepileptic drugs such as thiopentone, phenobarbitone or propofol.
- Continuous EEG monitoring may be required as brain seizure activity can persist in the paralysed or heavily sedated patient with no overt signs.

Prolonged postictal state
Consider the following underlying causes when a patient fails to regain consciousness, despite the seizures stopping:
- **Medical consequences of the seizure**
  - Hypoxia
  - Hypo- or hyperglycaemia
  - Hypotension

- Hyperpyrexia
- Cerebral oedema
- Lactic acidosis
- Iatrogenic over-sedation
- **Progression of any underlying cause**
  - Meningitis or encephalitis
  - Head injury or stroke
  - Cerebral hypoxia
  - Drug toxicity (e.g. theophylline)
- **Unrecognised continuing non-convulsive status epilepticus**
  - Subtle generalised convulsive status epilepticus (with just flickering of the eyelids)
  - Complex–partial (temporal lobe) status
  - Absence (petit mal) status.

Pseudoseizure

Pseudoseizures are most common in patients with pre-existing epilepsy, or in patients with personality or psychiatric disorders.

The following unusual features favour a diagnosis of pseudoseizure, rather than a true seizure:

- Eyes held shut, normal pupils, absence of nystagmus
- Normal oxygen saturations
- Side-to-side head turning
- Arching the back, pelvic thrusting
- Talking or ability to follow commands during the attack
- Avoidance behaviour in response to noxious stimuli by corneal reflex or nose tickling with cotton wool
- Seizure activity that ceases with suggestion
- Absent postictal period with recollection of the event.

Note: tongue biting and urinary incontinence **can** occur in pseudoseizures!

Seizures related to pregnancy

Eclampsia can occur from gestational week 20 to 3–4 weeks postpartum.

- Check urinary beta-hCG.
- Check for hypertension, proteinuria with or without pathological oedema.
- Call the O&G team urgently.
- Ensure the patient is in the left lateral decubitus position to avoid compression of the IVC when lying supine or on the right side (supine hypotension syndrome from IVC compression by the gravid uterus).
- Give a loading bolus dose of magnesium 4 g IV followed by an additional 2 g if seizures recur, supplemented if necessary with an IV benzodiazepine such as diazepam 0.1–0.2 mg/kg.
- Control BP with hydralazine 5 mg IV boluses. See Chapter 19.

SECTION C – Common calls

Drug toxicity-related seizures

- Sodium-channel blockers (tricyclic antidepressants, antiarrhythmics, antimalarials)–treat with benzodiazepines IV and sodium bicarbonate 50 mmol boluses IV until the QRS interval normalises on ECG or seizures stop. Admit to ICU.
- Alcohol-induced seizures–usually stop spontaneously, but may require benzodiazepines. Avoid phenytoin and remember thiamine.
- Cocaine or amphetamine–benzodiazepines are the drugs of choice and large doses may be required (e.g. titrated boluses of up to 20 mg IV of diazepam). Check the ECG for signs of ischaemia (see Chapter 19).

24

Weakness and dizziness

These two common symptoms are highly subjective, difficult to describe and often even harder to interpret. Patients use vague terms such as 'feeling light-headed', 'unbalanced', 'wobbly', 'lethargic' and 'drained'.

- **Weakness** is defined as the inability to carry out a movement with normal force because of a reduction in muscle strength. This must be differentiated from fatigue, in which repetitive actions cause diminished strength, either real or perceived.
- **Dizziness** is usually a descriptor of light-headedness, vertigo or imbalance.
- **Vertigo** is the sense of disorientation in space with a sensation of motion where none exists. The sensation may be swaying, tilting or rotational in character.

Phone call

Questions

1. Is the mental status normal?
2. What are the vital signs?
3. What is the pattern of weakness and is it progressing?
4. Is there an associated speech disturbance, sensory disturbance or headache?
5. What does the patient mean by dizziness?
6. Is the patient vomiting?
7. What was the reason for admission?

Instructions

If the vital signs are stable and the patient has normal mental status:
- Request that the patient remains under supervision until you are able to assess the problem.
- Keep the patient NBM if there is speech disturbance or difficulty swallowing.
- Request a fingerprick BGL.
- Request an ECG.

- Prescribe prochlorperazine 12.5 mg IM if the patient has dizziness and vomiting.

Prioritisation

The following patients must be seen immediately: those with sudden onset of hemiplegia, rapidly progressive weakness, weakness associated with a headache or depressed consciousness, or bilateral lower-limb weakness associated with numbness.

Other patients with weakness, dizziness or fatigue with normal mental status and vital signs do not need such urgent review.

Corridor thoughts

What are the causes of weakness? (* = major threat to life)
- **Upper motor neuron (UMN) lesion*:**
  - Cerebral cortex, subcortical or brainstem stroke, demyelination or space-occupying lesion such as tumour, abscess or haematoma
  - Spinal cord trauma, infarct, transverse myelitis, spinal epidural or subdural collection (abscess, haematoma), central disc herniation, tumour or demyelination *above* the level of L1 (where the cord ends and becomes the cauda equina)
- **Lower motor neuron (LMN) lesion:**
  - Neuromuscular junction/motor neurons (e.g. myasthenia gravis*, motor neuron disease*, organophosphate poisoning*, snake envenomation* and botulism*)
  - Myopathy (e.g. polymyositis, alcohol-induced, steroid-related, muscular dystrophy*, hypokalaemia and thyroid disease)
  - Ascending polyneuropathy from Guillain–Barré syndrome*
  - Peripheral neuropathy from diabetes, carcinoma, alcohol, vitamin B1 or B12 deficiency, drugs such as isoniazid, nitrofurantoin and phenytoin
  - Spinal nerve root compression from lumbar spinal stenosis, tumour, an epidural abscess or a disc herniation below L1/2
- **Episodic:**
  - Transient ischaemic attack (TIA), migraine aura, seizure followed by Todd paralysis (temporary), periodic paralysis syndromes
  - 'Drop attacks', most commonly carotid sinus hypersensitivity but multiple other causes including syncopal, seizure-related, Ménière's disease, joint disease etc and narcolepsy
- **Non-organic:**
  - Somatisation or anxiety (diagnosis of exclusion *only*)

What are the causes of dizziness?
- **Vertigo** (a subjective sensation of rotational movement):
  - Peripheral—vestibular neuronitis, benign paroxysmal positional vertigo (BPPV), acute labyrinthitis, Ménière's disease, cholesteatoma, otosclerosis and ototoxic drugs such as gentamicin and high-dose frusemide
  - Central—brainstem or cerebellar stroke, tumour, demyelination, vertebrobasilar TIA, cerebellopontine angle mass such as acoustic neuroma, alcohol or basilar migraine
- Light-headedness or pre-syncope
- Non-specific dizziness:
  - Adverse drug reaction, anxiety, somatisation

What are the causes of fatigue?
- Anaemia
- Chronic angina
- Cardiac or respiratory failure
- Thyroid disease (myxoedema or hyperthyroidism)
- Dehydration or electrolyte disturbance
- Sepsis
- Malignancy
- Drugs (many)
- Depression
- Chronic fatigue syndrome and fibromyalgia

Major threat to life

- **Guillain–Barré syndrome (GBS)**
- **Myasthenia gravis (MG)**
- **Intracranial lesion** such as posterior fossa tumour or stroke; extradural or subdural haemorrhage.

Rapidly progressive weakness due to GBS or MG may cause hypoxia secondary to respiratory failure. An expanding cerebral mass lesion may cause brain herniation, with the development of coma and death.

Bedside

Quick-look test

Does the patient look well (comfortable), sick (uncomfortable or distressed) or critical (about to die)?

Stridor, tachypnoea, paradoxical breathing, cyanosis, exhaustion or unresponsiveness are associated with airway or respiratory compromise.

Vomiting may be caused by an intracranial space-occupying lesion, or a central or peripheral vestibular lesion.

Airway and vital signs

Assess the airway and breathing for airway or respiratory muscle paralysis.

What is the heart rate?
- Tachycardia occurs with hypoxia.
- Bradycardia may suggest an intracranial space-occupying lesion.
- An irregular rhythm may indicate AF as a cause of stroke.

What is the blood pressure?
- Hypertension may be associated with stroke.
- Hypotension may be a cause of the weakness (or stroke).

What is the temperature?
- A febrile illness may cause generalised weakness/malaise.

What is the blood glucose level?
- Hypoglycaemia can cause a focal neurological deficit.

What does the ECG show?
- Consider whether myocardial ischaemia is a cause of weakness (ST or T wave depression, Q waves), and identify AF if a stroke is present.

Management

Immediate management

Airway compromise or depressed level of consciousness:
- Apply high-flow oxygen to maintain saturation >94%.
- Assist ventilation if ineffective with a bag-mask device such as a Laerdal or Ambu bag.
- Contact an anaesthetist to provide airway support, including endotracheal intubation to maintain airway patency and prevent aspiration.
- Obtain IV access.

Rapidly progressive weakness present:
- Assess ventilatory function by performing spirometry. Hypoxia or a FVC <10 mL/kg due to neuromuscular weakness require urgent senior review, as intubation and mechanical ventilation may be needed.
- Assemble airway equipment and call your senior and an anaesthetist urgently.
- If the patient does not have rapidly progressive weakness or cardiorespiratory compromise, and no sinister systemic cause is suspected, proceed to selective history and examination to determine an anatomical site for the weakness.

Selective history and chart review

When did the symptoms commence?
- Sudden onset suggests a stroke or other vascular cause.
- Acute onset over hours to days occurs with polyneuropathy, myelopathy, myopathy and neuromuscular junction disorders.

What is the pattern of weakness?
- Unilateral weakness suggests a CNS or spinal cord lesion.
- Generalised or predominantly proximal weakness suggests myasthenia gravis, myopathy or muscular dystrophy.
- Predominantly distal weakness +/− sensory changes suggests a polyneuropathy.
- Bilateral oculomotor and facial weakness suggest GBS or an NMJ disorder.
- Bilateral limb weakness associated with a sensory level suggests a spinal cord lesion.
- Weakness confined to certain movements or functions suggests radicular or peripheral nerve lesion.

What activities are affected by type of weakness?
- Bulbar: slurred, nasal speech; drooling; difficulty whistling or smiling; difficulty swallowing.
- Proximal lower limb weakness: difficulty climbing stairs, arising from a chair, getting out of a car or off the toilet.
- Proximal upper limb muscles: difficulty in reaching for cupboards, shaving or combing hair.
- Distal lower limb weakness: tripping while walking.
- Extraocular muscles: diplopia, ptosis.

Are there any related symptoms?
- Muscle pain occurs with a myopathy.
- Sensory dysfunction occurs in peripheral neuropathy, but not in NMJ disorders or myopathies.
- Headache worse on waking or stooping with vomiting suggests an intracranial space-occupying lesion.
- Bladder or bowel dysfunction occurs with a cauda equina lesion.
- Review the past medical history for risk factors:
  - Cardiovascular (risks for stroke)
  - Recent viral illness (risk for polyneuropathy)
  - Diabetes (risk for stroke, peripheral neuropathy, myopathy)
  - Alcohol misuse (risk for myopathy, peripheral neuropathy, cerebellar degeneration, head trauma with cerebral mass lesion).

Selective physical examination

An altered conscious level (intracranial lesion or systemic illness) or rapidly progressing weakness (GBS, MG, botulism) requires urgent assessment.
- Differentiating UMN and LMN lesions is critical to localising the cause of weakness, and planning further investigation.
  Check the motor and sensory function to determine the pattern of weakness and hence the possible underlying cause:
- **Mixed UMN and LMN:**
  - Consider motor neuron disease, vitamin B12 deficiency, Friedreich's ataxia.

SECTION C – Common calls

- **Anatomically disparate:**
  - Consider multiple sclerosis or mononeuritis multiplex.
- **Bilateral UMN:**
  - Large bilateral cerebral or brainstem lesion if altered mental status.
  - Spinal cord lesion if normal mental status. The sensory level and level of weakness determine the anatomical site of the lesion.
- **Unilateral UMN:**
  - Contralateral cortical, subcortical or brainstem lesion, rarely a spinal cord hemisection (Brown–Séquard syndrome). Cortical lesions have ipsilateral limb and facial signs.
  - Anterior cerebral artery (ACA) stroke syndrome–leg greater than arm weakness, personality change, oculomotor palsy, urinary incontinence.
  - Middle cerebral artery (MCA) stroke syndrome–arm greater than leg weakness, dysphasia, dyspraxias, agnosias, neglect, poor two-point discrimination, dysgraphaesthesia.
  - Posterior cerebral artery (PCA) stroke syndrome–visual disturbance.
  - Subcortical lacunar stroke syndrome–pure motor strokes, dense ipsilateral hemiplegia and hemi-anaesthesia.
  - Brainstem stroke syndrome–crossed abnormalities in facial and limb distributions.
- **Bilateral LMN:**
  - Proximal LMN weakness with normal sensation is probably a myopathy.
  - Distal LMN weakness with decreased reflexes and some sensory involvement is probably a polyneuropathy.
  - Diffuse LMN weakness (including oculomotor and facial muscles) with normal reflexes and normal sensation is probably a NMJ disorder.
- **Unilateral LMN:**
  - Radiculopathy (dermatomal or myotomal distribution).
  - Plexopathy (involvement of more than one spinal or peripheral nerve), usually lumbar or brachial.
  - Peripheral neuropathy.

Investigations

- Dictated by clinical findings:
  - FBC, U&E, serum glucose, LFT, TFT, CK and ECG are indicated in all patients with weakness.
  - Spirometry for respiratory muscle weakness.
  - CXR if suspect malignancy (primary or secondary).
  - Urgent CT indicated in unilateral UMN lesion weakness.
  - Urgent MRI indicated if suspected spinal cord compression (seek senior advice first).

- Brainstem, posterior fossa and spinal cord lesions are best imaged by MRI if CT scan is normal or unhelpful.

Specific management
Transient ischaemic attack

TIAs are episodes of sudden transient focal neurological deficit caused by ischaemia, typically lasting less than one hour, without acute infarction. However, they are associated with a high early risk of stroke (5–10% at 30 days).

- Commonly thrombotic from cerebrovascular disease, hypoperfusion, hypercoagulation state or vasculitis; or embolic from a carotid plaque, or intracardiac thrombus from AF or valvular disease.
- Present as a transient stroke syndrome, or as amaurosis fugax (transient monocular blindness from ophthalmic artery occlusion).
- Progressive or persistent symptoms suggest a stroke.
- Examine the pulse rhythm, heart sounds for murmurs and BP; listen for a carotid bruit.
- Perform a full neurological assessment to look for any residual deficits that distinguish a stroke from a TIA (neurologically go back to normal).
- Perform a fingerprick BGL as hypoglycaemia may cause focal neurological features and mimic a TIA.
- Send blood for FBC, ESR if patient is aged >50 years, coagulation profile, U&E and a lipid profile.
- Perform an ECG and request a CXR.
- Request a CT scan to exclude intracranial haemorrhage, space-occupying lesion and arteriovenous malformation.
- Quantify early risk into 'high' or 'low' according to ABCD^2 score (see Table 24.1).
- Carotid ultrasound and cardiac echocardiography (if suggestion of cardiac disease) are organised according to the risk profile. High risk, as soon as possible; low risk, less urgent but within days.
- Patients at highest risk of stroke have crescendo TIAs with increasing frequency or duration of neurological deficits, embolic TIA despite anticoagulation, DBP >100 mmHg, high-grade carotid stenosis or new or poorly controlled diabetes.

Management of transient ischaemic attack

- Give aspirin 300 mg PO, then 75–150 mg PO once daily after haemorrhage excluded on CT scan. An alternative is clopidogrel 75 mg PO, if aspirin is contraindicated.
- Change to an aspirin–dipyridamole combination (25/200 mg) introduced over 1–2 weeks (to reduce early risk of headache from dipyridamole).
- Commence heparin followed by warfarin or a NOAC alone, if there is a cardioembolic source or AF.

SECTION C – Common calls

Table 24.1 **ABCD² score for early risk stratification in TIA**	
Risk factor	**Points**
Age ≥60 years	1
Blood pressure ≥140 mmHg (SBP) and/or ≥90 mmHg (DBP)	1
Clinical signs	
Unilateral weakness	2
Speech disturbance *without* weakness	1
Other	0
Duration	
>60 min	2
10–60 min	1
<10 min	0
Diabetes	1
Total	/7
High risk ≥4 points: with a 7-day risk of completed stroke of 5.9–11.7%.	
Low risk 0–3 points: with a 7-day risk of completed stroke of 1.2%.	
Adapted with permission from Johnston SC et al. *Lancet* 2007; 369: 283–292.	

- Ensure reversible vascular risk factors are treated (diabetes, hypertension, raised lipids).
- Refer the patient for carotid endarterectomy if there is high-grade carotid stenosis on Doppler ultrasound.

Cerebrovascular accident (stroke)

Most CVAs (80–90%) are caused by cerebral ischaemia from thrombosis or embolism, some of which may have been preceded by a TIA.

- Other CVAs are caused by an intracerebral haemorrhage associated with hypertension, intracranial tumour or bleeding disorder; or a SAH from a berry aneurysm, trauma or an arteriovenous malformation.
- Haemorrhagic CVA is suggested by severe headache, vomiting or coma, although a CT scan is essential to confirm the diagnosis.
  - SAH is typically a sudden-onset, severe 'worst headache ever' and may cause transient LOC or persisting confusion.

The following 'mimic' a CVA, and must be differentiated:

- Hypoglycaemia (check BGL in every patient with altered conscious level or focal neurology)
- Migraine—hemiplegic aura
- Todd paralysis following an epileptic seizure (transient)
- Encephalitis; hypertensive, metabolic or toxic encephalopathy (altered mental status)
- Aortic dissection (sudden onset of neurological symptoms associated with chest pain)

- Multiple sclerosis
- Brown–Séquard syndrome.

Initial management priorities

- Maintain the airway by positioning, oropharyngeal airway and placing the patient in the recovery position if the patient is unconscious (see Figures 9.1 and 9.2).
- Arrange endotracheal intubation if there is respiratory depression, deteriorating neurological status and/or signs of raised ICP. Assemble equipment and contact the anaesthetist.
- Otherwise, keep NBM until swallowing has been formally assessed.
- Gain IV access and send blood for FBC, ESR, coagulation profile, U&E, LFTs, lipid profile and BGL.
- Attach a cardiac monitor and pulse oximeter to the patient.
- Make certain a bedside blood glucose test strip has been done and give 50% dextrose 50 mL IV if it is low. Otherwise avoid glucose administration as hyperglycaemia worsens neurological outcome.
- Never rapidly reduce a raised BP unless aortic dissection or hypertensive encephalopathy are suspected, as cerebral autoregulation is impaired following a CVA.
- Get senior help if SBP >220 mmHg or DBP >140 mmHg.
- If BP is to be lowered, do not lower it by more than 25% of the original value.
- Catheterise the bladder.
- Obtain an ECG and CXR, and arrange an urgent CT head scan, which may initially be normal with a cerebral infarct.
- Maintain normothermia.

Following CT

- Call your senior urgently to discuss thrombolysis if the CT brain scan excludes haemorrhage or a non-vascular cause in a patient >18 years with symptom onset <4.5 hours, in whom there is a measurable and clinically significant deficit on NIH Stroke Scale examination.
- If the CT scan shows a posterior fossa haemorrhage, intraventricular haemorrhage with hydrocephalus or the patient has features of raised ICP, call neurosurgery urgently.
- Otherwise, commence aspirin within 48 hours for an ischaemic CVA, but withold for 24 hours in those receiving thrombolysis.
- Leave the decision when to start warfarin or a NOAC following an AF-associated embolism to the usual medical team.
- Other patients should have usual thromboembolic prophylaxis with LMWH.
- Multidisciplinary stroke care improves survival and neurological recovery. Important aspects include:
  - Removing bladder catheter earlier to prevent urosepsis
  - Early mobilisation to prevent thromboembolic complications and chest infection

- Thorough speech and swallowing assessment to prevent aspiration
- Early physiotherapy and occupational therapy to improve function.

Guillain-Barré syndrome (acute inflammatory demyelinating polyneuropathy)

Ascending paralysis with absent reflexes is typical. Sensory symptoms or predominant cranial nerve involvement with loss of ocular movements are possible.

- 60% of cases follow a history of respiratory or gastrointestinal infection, especially with *Campylobacter jejuni*, CMV or Epstein–Barr virus.
- Obtain spirometry, get senior help and call intensive care early, as death may follow respiratory failure.

Facial nerve palsy

LMN paralysis causes weakness of the whole side of the face, including the forehead muscles.

UMN paralysis spares the forehead muscles, and has associated findings such as hemiplegia.

Causes of LMN facial nerve palsy include:

- Bell's palsy with an abrupt onset, sometimes associated with postauricular pain, hyperacusis and abnormal taste in the anterior two-thirds of the tongue.
  - Give prednisolone 50 mg PO daily for 5 days if a Bell's palsy is seen within 3 days of onset.
- Trauma to the temporal bone or a facial laceration in the parotid area.
- Tumours, such as an acoustic neuroma or parotid malignancy.
- Infection, such as acute otitis media, chronic otitis media with cholesteatoma or geniculate herpes zoster (Ramsay Hunt syndrome).
- Cranial GBS, sarcoidosis (Heerfordt syndrome), diabetes and hypertension. These will often give multiple cranial nerve deficits.
- Provide all patients with ocular lubricant and protection (pad or tape eye at night), as the eye does not close normally and corneal drying with ulceration may occur.

Remember: facial nerve palsy does not cause ptosis (which is caused by a third nerve palsy, sympathetic palsy such as a Horner's syndrome from apical lung tumour, myopathy or is congenital).

Peripheral neuropathy

- LMN, usually symmetrical, distal weakness with arreflexia and/or distal sensory changes ('glove and stocking').

- Causes include diabetes, alcohol, vitamin B1 or B12 deficiency, drugs such as fluoroquinolones, isoniazid, nitrofurantoin, phenytoin and vincristine, uraemia, malignancy, autoimmune disorders such as SLE, HIV, heavy metals etc.
- Thus, begin by looking for and addressing the underlying cause. In particular, alcoholic neuropathy, especially if motor-dominant and acutely progressive, may respond to thiamine (vitamin B1).

Spinal cord compression

Usually presents with bilateral lower-limb weakness, a sensory level and associated back pain depending on the cause. However, motor and sensory deficits may be patchy if there is an incomplete pathological feature.
- Causes include:
  - Intramedullary or extramedullary tumour, secondary (85%) or primary
  - Central disc prolapse
  - Epidural abscess or haematoma.
- Other causes of acute-onset paraplegia:
  - Transverse myelitis
  - Spinal artery thrombosis
  - Vasculitis (e.g. SLE)
  - Paraneoplastic syndrome
  - Cauda equina syndrome—LMN condition with weakness in both legs, arreflexia, associated sensory disturbance, especially in the perineum, and loss of bowel or bladder function with retention or incontinence.
  - GBS (LMN).
- Management:
  - Arrange an urgent MRI to establish the diagnosis and an immediate neurosurgical opinion.
  - Cord compression and partial cord syndromes may respond to dexamethasone 10 mg IV if there is associated oedema, otherwise operative decompression may be required.

Vertigo

Once dizziness has been defined as being due to vertigo, the next thing to determine is whether it is central or peripheral, as this will dictate the likely underlying cause (see earlier).
- **Central vertigo**
  - Onset is usually gradual (except for a posterior fossa vascular event) with persistent vertigo associated with nystagmus and other neurological findings. The patient may feel as if being pushed or tilted, and often cannot walk.
  - Request an urgent CT scan.

SECTION C – Common calls

- **Peripheral vertigo**
  - Usually sudden in onset, episodic, worse with changes in posture, often with associated auditory features and nystagmus, which is horizontal but with a rotatory component.
  - It may be associated with deafness, nausea, profuse vomiting and sweating.
  - Control the vomiting if required with prochlorperazine 12.5 mg IV or IM, or use a general sedative such as low-dose midazolam 2.5 mg or diazepam 2.5 mg IV titrated to effect for incapacitating symptoms.
  - Once the symptoms are controlled, establish whether it is BPPV by performing a provocation test (Dix–Hallpike manoeuvre).
  - If that is positive, contact ENT to perform a canalith repositioning manoeuvre, such as the Epley manoeuvre, that removes debris from the semicircular canals and deposits it in the utricle, where hair cells are not stimulated.
  - If the provocation test is negative, the diagnosis is most likely Ménière's disease (tinnitus, hearing loss and pressure in the head) or vestibular neuronitis (usually viral in the young and ischaemic in older people).
  - Ménière's disease responds to vestibular suppressants such as prochlorperazine, diazepam or betahistine.

Psychogenic weakness

Suspect this if there is initial effort then sudden collapse of the limb ('giveway weakness'), or if an apparently paralysed arm dropped over the face keeps missing (true weakness will cause the face to be hit).

- Proceed no further and get senior help, to avoid prolonged or unnecessary investigations or treatments.

25

Abdominal pain

Abdominal pain is a common complaint. It is essential to distinguish an acute abdominal emergency from the non-emergency or benign recurrent pain.

The former requires urgent surgical or medical intervention, whereas the latter may be investigated at leisure.

Phone call

Questions
1. What is the character of the pain?
2. How severe is the pain?
3. Where is the main site of pain; is it localised or generalised?
4. Are there changes in vital signs such as fever, tachycardia or hypotension?
5. Are there associated symptoms such as vomiting, distension, constipation or dysuria?
6. Has the patient had past or recent abdominal surgery?
7. What was the reason for admission?
8. Is the patient on steroids or immunosuppressed? Steroids and immunosuppression may mask the pain and fever of an inflammatory process, leading to underestimation of the nature or severity of the pain. Even mild abdominal pain should be assessed early in an immunosuppressed patient.
9. Is this a new problem? Has it occurred before?

Prioritisation
- See any patient with abdominal pain associated with hypotension immediately, as there are potentially life-threatening causes. Also see immediately any patient with fever, or severe acute pain of recent onset.
- Mild recurrent abdominal pain is a less urgent problem and may be reviewed later.

Corridor thoughts

What are the causes of abdominal pain? (* = major threat to life)
- These may be broadly thought of as:
  - **Surgical**—general surgical, gynaecological, urological or vascular

BOX 25.1 'Medical' disorders presenting with acute abdominal pain

- Thoracic origin
  - MI, pericarditis
  - PE, pleurisy, pneumonia
  - Aortic dissection
- Abdominal origin
  - Hepatitis, right heart failure
  - Infection, including gastroenteritis, pyelonephritis, cystitis, bacterial colitis and primary peritonitis
  - Intestinal ischaemia from atheroma, vasculitis, Henoch–Schönlein purpura or sickle cell disease
  - Reflux, peptic ulcer disease, inflammatory bowel disease
- Endocrine and metabolic origin
  - DKA
  - Addison's disease
  - Hypercalcaemia
  - Lead poisoning, paracetamol or iron poisoning
- Neurogenic origin
  - Herpes zoster
  - Radiculitis from spinal cord degeneration or malignancy
  - Tabes dorsalis
- Thoracolumbar spine origin
  - Collapsed vertebra from osteoporosis, neoplasm or infection (e.g. TB)

- **Medical**—related to respiratory, cardiac*, GI, renal, endocrine*, metabolic, skeletal, neurogenic and toxic* causes (see Box 25.1).
- Figure 25.1 shows the differential diagnosis by site of pain.

Surgical causes of abdominal pain include:

- **Gastrointestinal**
  - Oesophagus: cancer
  - Stomach: cancer
  - Gallbladder: biliary colic, acute cholecystitis, ascending cholangitis*
  - Pancreas: pancreatitis*
  - Liver: subphrenic abscess, hepatic abscess
  - Spleen: rupture*, abscess
  - Small intestine: intussusception*, obstruction, perforation*, ischaemia
  - Large intestine: obstruction (cancer, volvulus, hernia), perforation*, diverticulitis, ischaemic colitis*
  - Appendix: appendicitis, appendix abscess (+ Meckel diverticulum)

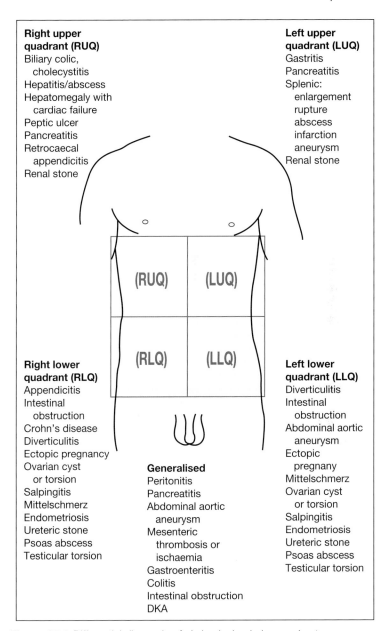

Right upper quadrant (RUQ)
Biliary colic, cholecystitis
Hepatitis/abscess
Hepatomegaly with cardiac failure
Peptic ulcer
Pancreatitis
Retrocaecal appendicitis
Renal stone

Left upper quadrant (LUQ)
Gastritis
Pancreatitis
Splenic:
enlargement
rupture
abscess
infarction
aneurysm
Renal stone

(RUQ) (LUQ)

(RLQ) (LLQ)

Right lower quadrant (RLQ)
Appendicitis
Intestinal obstruction
Crohn's disease
Diverticulitis
Ectopic pregnancy
Ovarian cyst or torsion
Salpingitis
Mittelschmerz
Endometriosis
Ureteric stone
Psoas abscess
Testicular torsion

Generalised
Peritonitis
Pancreatitis
Abdominal aortic aneurysm
Mesenteric thrombosis or ischaemia
Gastroenteritis
Colitis
Intestinal obstruction
DKA

Left lower quadrant (LLQ)
Diverticulitis
Intestinal obstruction
Abdominal aortic aneurysm
Ectopic pregnany
Mittelschmerz
Ovarian cyst or torsion
Salpingitis
Endometriosis
Ureteric stone
Psoas abscess
Testicular torsion

Figure 25.1 Differential diagnosis of abdominal pain by quadrant.

- Mesentery: mesenteric adenitis (children)
- Hernia: inguinal, femoral, umbilical, paraumbilical, incisional, epigastric, Spigelian (lateral ventral), Richter (one sidewall of bowel): with incarceration (irreducible), obstruction or strangulation*
- **Urological**
  - Renal: renal colic, ureteric colic (but remember AAA)
  - Bladder: urinary retention
  - Testicles: torsion, epididymitis, cancer (seminoma, teratoma)
- **Vascular**
  - AAA—sudden expansion or rupture*
- **Gynaecological**
  - Uterine: bleed into fibroid, pregnancy-related* (placental abruption, uterine rupture)
  - Ovarian: torsion, ruptured cyst, haemorrhage, cancer
  - Fallopian tube: ectopic pregnancy*, pelvic inflammatory disease
  - Mittelschmerz, endometriosis
- **Musculoskeletal**
  - Rectus muscle haematoma or tear

Note: constipation is a symptom *not* a diagnosis—look for the underlying cause(s) that need treating in their own right (see Chapter 26).

Major threat to life

- **Exsanguinating haemorrhage with hypovolaemic shock**
  - Caused by a leaking AAA, ruptured ectopic pregnancy or splenic rupture; occasionally it may be iatrogenic following a liver or renal biopsy, or a misdirected thoracocentesis.
- **Perforated viscus**
  - A rigid abdomen with severe pain is associated with bowel perforation. It may result in septic shock from bacterial peritonitis or hypovolaemic shock from third-space losses.
- **Necrosis of viscus**
  - Severe pancreatitis, intussusception, volvulus, strangulated hernia or ischaemic colitis can rapidly cause hypovolaemic or septic shock, and electrolyte and acid–base disturbances.
- **Intraperitoneal septic focus**
  - Infection from a localised site such as ascending cholangitis or an infected obstructed kidney may progress to generalised septic shock within hours.
- **Extra-abdominal causes**
  - Patients with AMI, thoracic aortic dissection and/or DKA may present with acute abdominal pain, usually without localising abdominal signs.

Bedside

Quick-look test

Does the patient look well (comfortable), sick (uncomfortable or distressed) or critical (about to die)?

- Look for signs of shock if the patient is pale, lethargic, drowsy or diaphoretic.
- Patients with severe colic are often restless and writhing in discomfort, whereas those with peritonitis lie still avoiding any movement.

Airway and vital signs

What is the heart rate and blood pressure?

- Look for tachycardia (HR >120 beats/min) and hypovolaemia (SBP <90 mmHg) associated with shock.
  - Sudden abdominal pain associated with hypotension is an ominous sign: consider inferior MI (do an ECG), pancreatitis (measure lipase), ruptured AAA or ectopic pregnancy (urgent USS) and mesenteric infarction (bloody diarrhoea with a metabolic acidosis and raised lactate).
  - More gradual onset abdominal pain progressing to hypotension suggests peritonitis, perforation or urosepsis.
- Recheck the BP and HR with the patient standing if the supine BP is normal. A drop in BP associated with an increased HR (>20 beats/min) indicates underlying hypovolaemia.

What is the respiratory rate?

- Shallow, rapid breathing may be associated with generalised abdominal pain, peritonitis or subdiaphragmatic irritation.
- Sustained tachypnoea is associated with sepsis, metabolic acidosis, anaemia, pneumonia and CCF.

What is the temperature?

- Fever associated with abdominal pain suggests infection or inflammation.
- Temperature is less reliably raised in elderly or immunocompromised patients, who may remain afebrile despite a perforation and sepsis.

Selective history and chart review

An accurate diagnosis depends on careful history taking:

- The onset, nature, character and duration of the pain
- Associated symptoms
- Relevant previous operations and illnesses
- Present medication.

Did the pain develop gradually or suddenly?

- Acute onset of pain suggests perforation of a viscus, ruptured ectopic pregnancy, torsion of an ovarian cyst or a leaking AAA.
- Severe pain in waves that develops over minutes to hours suggests colic (renal, biliary or intestinal).

SECTION C – Common calls

What is the character of the pain?
- There are classic descriptions of pain associated with certain conditions (e.g. severe or mild, burning or knife-like, constant or waxing and waning).
- Peptic ulcer pain tends to be burning, whereas that of a perforated ulcer is sudden, constant and severe.
- Biliary colic is sharp and constricting ('takes one's breath away'), whereas acute pancreatitis is deep and agonising, eased by sitting forwards.
- Bowel obstruction pain is gripping, with intermittent exacerbations.
- Peritonitis pain is relentless and worsened on coughing or moving; the patient prefers to lie still. A patient with ureteric colic rolls around trying to get comfy.

Is the pain localised?
- The location of the pain's maximum intensity provides a clue to the site of origin (see Figure 25.1), although the old, young or confused may not be able to indicate the exact site.
- Although a patient may complain of diffuse abdominal pain, careful examination can localise any area of specific tenderness.

Has the pain changed since its onset?
- A ruptured viscus is initially associated with localised pain that subsequently shifts or becomes generalised.

Does the pain radiate? (see Figure 25.2)
- Pain radiates to the dermatome or cutaneous area supplied by the same sensory cortical cells as the deep-seated structure.
- The diaphragm is supplied by cervical roots C3, C4 and C5. Thus upper abdominal or lower thoracic conditions that cause irritation of the diaphragm lead to referred pain in the cutaneous supply of C3, C4 and C5, which is the shoulder and neck.
- The liver and gallbladder derive innervation from the right 7th and 8th thoracic segments, thus biliary colic frequently causes pain referred to the inferior angle of the right scapula.
- The pain of pancreatitis may radiate to the mid-back or scapula.

Are there any aggravating or relieving factors?
- Duodenal ulcer pain is often relieved by the ingestion of food.
- Pancreatitis pain is worsened after eating and may be relieved by sitting up or leaning forwards.
- Pain that increases with inspiration suggests biliary origin, peritonitis or pleurisy.
- Pain associated with frequency and dysuria aggravated by micturition suggests a urological cause.
- Pain worse with movement such as coughing is usually secondary to localised or generalised peritonitis (e.g. appendicitis).
- Pain relieved by movement or that makes the patient restless is more often colicky in nature (e.g. ureteric colic).

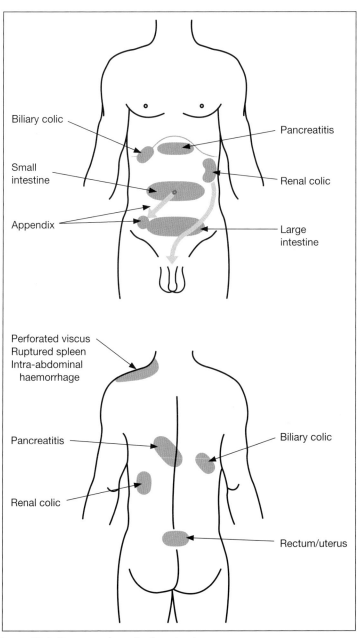

Figure 25.2 Common sites of referred pain.

Associated symptoms

Is there nausea or vomiting?
- Pain tends to precede nausea and vomiting in the surgical acute abdomen, whereas it follows it in gastritis or gastroenteritis.
- Vomiting that occurs at the onset of pain occurs with peritoneal irritation, perforation of a viscus, acute pancreatitis or a high intestinal obstruction.
- Vomiting many hours after the onset of abdominal pain may be caused by lower intestinal obstruction or ileus.

What is the vomitus like?
- Clear fluid indicates obstruction proximal to the sphincter of Oddi in the second part of the duodenum, whereas bilious vomit indicates a more distal obstruction.
- Faeculent vomiting suggests distal intestinal obstruction, or a gastrocolic fistula.
- Frank blood is indicative of an upper GI bleed (see Chapter 27).
- Vomiting food after fasting is associated with gastric stasis or gastric outlet obstruction.

What is the frequency and character of stool?
- Bloody diarrhoea with abdominal pain occurs with invasive enteritis such as *Shigella* and *Salmonella,* ischaemic colitis and inflammatory bowel disease (IBD), such as Crohn's disease and ulcerative colitis.
- Diarrhoea can be associated with appendicitis, partial small bowel obstruction and viral gastroenteritis.
- Diarrhoea alternating with constipation is characteristic of diverticular disease, but may signify a colonic neoplasm.
- Absolute constipation with lack of flatus is caused by a low large bowel obstruction or ileus.

Is there fever or chills?
- Check the temperature record since admission, as fever or chills suggest intra-abdominal infection. Also check the medication sheet for antipyretic or steroid use, which may mask a fever.

Past history and chart review

Does the patient have a past history of abdominal pain?
The most common causes of recurrent abdominal pain include:
- Gastritis or oesophageal reflux
- Peptic ulcer disease
- Alcoholic pancreatitis
- Gallstone disease (cholelithiasis)
- Renal tract stone (ureterolithiasis).

Is there a history of previous abdominal surgery?
- Adhesions are responsible for 70% of mechanical bowel obstructions.

Is there a recent history of blunt trauma to the abdomen?
- Typically, a contained subcapsular haematoma of the spleen may rupture several days later. Rarely, an abnormal spleen in infectious mononucleosis, malaria or a lymphoproliferative disorder can rupture with minimal or even no obvious trauma.

Is there a history of chronic liver disease from alcohol, viral hepatitis or non-alcoholic steatohepatitis (NASH)?
- Spontaneous bacterial peritonitis must be considered in a chronic liver disease patient with ascites and fever.

Is there a history of coronary or peripheral vascular disease?
- This may cause abdominal pain from an inferior MI, leaking AAA, mesenteric infarction or descending aortic dissection (with hypertension).

Could the patient be pregnant?
- All women of reproductive age should have a urinary or serum beta-hCG test, irrespective of whether or not they consider they are pregnant (this avoids an awkward or misleading answer).

What medication is the patient currently prescribed?
- Look specifically for anticoagulants, NSAIDs and steroids.

Selective physical examination

Vitals	Repeat now
HEENT	Jaundiced sclerae (hepatitis, cholangitis, cholelithiasis)
	Spider naevi (chronic liver disease)
CVS	Flat neck veins and JVP (volume depletion)
	New onset of arrhythmia or mitral incompetence murmur (myocardial infarction)
Resp	Shallow respirations with restricted abdominal wall movement (localised or generalised peritoneal inflammation)
	Stony dullness to percussion, decreased breath sounds, decreased tactile vocal fremitus (basal pleural effusion)
	Dullness to percussion, crackles and diminished or bronchial breath sounds (basal pneumonia consolidation)
Skin	Jaundice, spider naevi, palmar erythema, gynaecomastia, bruising (liver failure)
	Caput medusa (portal hypertension with varices)
GIT	Scars, distension, visible peristalsis; hepatomegaly; splenomegaly; tenderness, guarding, rebound (peritonism); distension with increased bowel sounds (obstruction); herniae; bladder enlargement; AAA; renal angle tenderness; colonic mass; pelvic organs (see below)

SECTION C – Common calls

Inspection
- Presence and position of scars (bowel obstruction, hernia).
- Abdominal distension with visible peristalsis (bowel obstruction).
- Bulging flanks (ascites).
- Bruising to flanks or umbilicus (Grey-Turner's or Cullen's sign, respectively, from retroperitoneal haemorrhage).

Palpation
Preparation:
- Before examining the abdomen, make sure the head of the bed is flat and your hands are warm. It may help to relax the abdominal wall by flexing the patient's hips.
- Kneel beside the patient so the palm of your hand is flat on the abdominal surface. Observe the patient's facial response during your abdominal examination.

Technique:
- Start palpation in the quadrants away from the point of maximal pain.
- Palpate gently at first and gradually increase pressure as tolerated, until finally reaching the site of maximal pain.
- Check for **guarding**:
  - Voluntary guarding is the voluntary contraction of abdominal musculature to limit the anticipated pain. Involuntary guarding may be localised or generalised, and is a sign of acute peritonitis.
- Check for **rebound tenderness**:
  - Tenderness elicited over an abdominal region following the rapid release of palpation pressure is termed 'rebound tenderness'. This by itself does not make the diagnosis of peritonitis, but is suggestive. An anxious patient may also have a degree of rebound.
  - As testing for this sign may cause unnecessary pain, it has largely been replaced by eliciting percussion tenderness to determine localised peritonitis.
- Look for the combination of a rigid abdomen, guarding and percussion tenderness (peritonitis).
- Test for shifting dullness and a fluid thrill (ascites).
- Check all hernia orifices, particularly in bowel obstruction (incarcerated or strangulated hernia) (see Figure 25.3).
- Review postoperative wound sites for evidence of infection (erythema, discharge) and/or dehiscence.

Percussion
- Note if it is tympanic (bowel obstruction).

Auscultation
- Also listen out for tinkling bowel sounds (mechanical bowel obstruction).
- Or absent bowel sounds (paralytic ileus or generalised peritonitis).

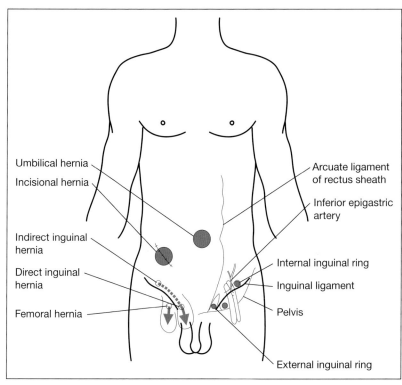

Figure 25.3 Hernial orifices. Copyright Tor Ercleve.

Digital rectal examination (make sure you have a chaperone)

- The purpose is to look for:
  - Anal fissure (sometimes associated with Crohn's disease)
  - Local mass (rectal carcinoma)
  - Prostate (enlargement, cancer, pain in prostatitis)
  - Stool positive for occult blood (colon cancer, ischaemic colitis, intussusception, any GI bleeding).

Pelvic exam

- The purpose is to look for:
  - Adnexal tenderness (ectopic pregnancy, ovarian cyst)
  - Mass (ovarian cyst or tumour)
  - Cervical motion tenderness (PID, cervicitis)
  - Cervical os (miscarriage).

Special-interest signs

- **Murphy's sign**—pain and inspiratory arrest on palpation under the costal margin on the right, as the patient takes a deep breath, seen with cholecystitis, cholangitis and some cholelithiasis.

- **Psoas sign**—abdominal pain in response to passive hip extension, which can also be performed with the patient lying prone or lateral decubitus. May indicate retrocaecal or pelvic appendicitis, or psoas abscess.
- **Obturator sign**—abdominal pain in response to passive flexion and internal rotation of the right hip to 90 degrees with the patient supine. May be present with appendicitis or psoas abscess.
- **Rovsing's sign**—pain felt in the RLQ on palpating the LLQ is seen in appendicitis. Despite being a well-known sign, it is surprisingly unreliable.

Investigations
Bedside investigations
- Urinalysis (in *every* case of abdominal pain):
  - Blood glucose and ketones (DKA)
  - Leucocytes, RBC and positive nitrites (UTI)
  - Macroscopic or microscopic haematuria (ureterolithiasis)
  - Beta-hCG—always rule out pregnancy in any female of reproductive age; urinalysis is the fastest method.
- ECG:
  - In every older patient (may show an unanticipated AMI, and or be needed pre-op).

Laboratory investigations
- FBC (elevated WBC count supports an infectious or inflammatory aetiology, but may still be normal with acute appendicitis).
- U&E (renal function, hydration status, acidosis—low bicarbonate).
- LFTs (raised in hepatitis and biliary tract disease; may show hypercalcaemia)
- Lipase (or amylase) for pancreatitis. May not be raised in chronic pancreatitis.

Radiology
Plain radiographic views
- These can include an erect PA chest and/or AP supine and erect abdomen (AXR).
- AXRs are *never* routine and only indicated to look for specific conditions:
  - Free air under the diaphragm—look for air under the diaphragm on erect CXR, or between the viscera and subcutaneous tissue in the lateral decubitus film (perforated viscus). It is also present after laparoscopy or a laparotomy.
  - Dilated loops of bowel—these occur in small or large bowel obstruction, proximal to the site of obstruction:
    - Small bowel is usually central, with regular transverse bands across the entire diameter (valvulae conniventes)

- Large bowel is peripheral, with irregular haustral folds and faecal mass content
- Toxic megacolon with a diameter >6 cm is due to ulcerative colitis, Crohn's disease, or occasionally pseudomembranous colitis. CT scan gives greater detail and is more accurate. It is a surgical emergency.
- More than five air–fluid levels suggest bowel obstruction or ileus, but are also seen in gastroenteritis.
- Calcification—look for calcified gallstones (cholecystitis or pancreatitis) or renal tract stones. Pancreatic calcification may be a clue to recurrent pancreatitis.

Ultrasound
- Bedside ultrasound is essential to diagnose or rule out suspected AAA, ectopic pregnancy and/or another pelvic cause for the pain (females). Ultrasound is also used in biliary disease, ureterolithiasis and testicular masses.

CT scan
- This is preferred for atypical or uncertain abdominal pain, particularly in older patients, and including undiagnosed masses and/or when diverticulitis, ureteric colic, retroperitoneal nodes or bleeding etc are suspected.
- It should not delay early referral to the duty surgeon in surgical acute abdominal pain. Also make sure analgesia has been given.

Management

Immediate management
The history, examination and investigations so far may not have made a specific diagnosis, but it should be clear whether the patient has shock, peritonitis or other potential life threat.
- Ensure you have given IV fluids, analgesia (this does *not* interfere with the surgical diagnosis), informed your senior and requested a surgical, gynaecological, urological or vascular consult early, particularly in any patient with hypotension.
- Patients with an acute surgical abdomen should be kept fasted (NBM).
- Give any patient with suspected infection, perforation or viscus necrosis 'triple therapy' with IV broad-spectrum antibiotics such as ampicillin 2 g, gentamicin 5 mg/kg and metronidazole 500 mg.

Specific management
Intestinal obstruction
- Small intestine obstruction:
  - Commonly associated with postoperative adhesions, herniae, tumour including lymphoma, intussusception and stricture.

Pain is usually localised to the periumbilical region, or generalised, crampy or colicky in nature. Vomiting is common.

- Examination reveals hyperactive bowel sounds, abdominal distension and generalised tenderness. 'Tinkling' bowel sounds differentiate obstruction from the quiet abdomen of paralytic ileus.
- Large bowel obstruction:
  - Associated with carcinoma, diverticulitis, sigmoid volvulus and stricture (malignant or ischaemic). Pain is gradual in onset, generalised, crampy and intermittent, with associated absolute constipation, nausea and late vomiting.
  - Examination confirms abdominal distension, tympanic percussion and generalised tenderness.
- Keep the patient NBM; insert an NGT if persistent vomiting, commence IV fluid resuscitation and give adequate narcotic analgesia.
- Organise surgical review and abdominal imaging.

Ruptured abdominal aortic aneurysm

Patients are usually elderly and complain of sudden, severe low abdominal, back, flank or groin pain, sometimes associated with syncope. The pain may mimic ureteric colic.

Examination reveals tenderness, a central abdominal mass (expansile pulsation) that may be hard to delineate in the large patient, and progressive signs of haemorrhagic shock.

- Commence fluid resuscitation with small amounts of normal saline or Hartmann's solution (compound sodium lactate), aiming for a SBP of no more than 90–100 mmHg.
  - Avoid the temptation to give massive fluid replacement, as this leads to coagulopathy, hypothermia, increased bleeding and a higher mortality.
- Contact your senior and the vascular surgeon on call urgently.
- Request a rapid bedside USS (if the patient is haemodynamically unstable) to confirm the presence of an abdominal aneurysm, or proceed directly to theatre (if the patient is moribund).
- Ensure that the patient has two large-bore IV cannulae and that blood has been sent for cross-match of 4–6 units of packed RBCs.
- Arrange a CT scan with IV contrast only if the patient's vital signs are stable.
- *Remember:* exclude ruptured AAA in any older patient with apparent ureteric colic.

Ectopic pregnancy

Consider this in all females of reproductive age with sudden-onset sharp, persistent right or left lower quadrant pain. Examination may reveal tenderness or a mass on abdominal or pelvic examination.

- Urgently check urine for a positive beta-hCG (and blood for a quantitative beta-hCG level) and send for a FBC and cross-match.
- Organise an urgent pelvic USS if the patient is not shocked, and contact the O&G team.

Perforated viscus

Intestinal perforation occurs due to a ruptured appendix, diverticulitis, tumour or peptic ulcer disease (PUD). The latter is more common in men on NSAIDs or steroids, and with a history of alcohol or tobacco use.

- The pain is usually sudden in onset, burning or stabbing in nature and localised then generalised, with radiation to the back or shoulder.
- Examination reveals severe tenderness with signs of peritonitis.
- Free air is present under the diaphragm on the upright CXR (>70% cases) or between the viscera and subcutaneous tissue on the lateral decubitus AXR.
- Organise an immediate surgical consultation and keep the patient NBM. Arrange a CT scan to differentiate the underlying cause.

Biliary colic (cholelithiasis) and cholecystitis

- **Biliary colic:**
  - Presents with discrete episodes of colicky RUQ pain, sometimes but not always related to consuming fatty foods.
  - Initial discomfort increases to crescendos of severe pain, which last a short time.
  - Examination reveals RUQ tenderness.
  - Make certain to check a lipase as well as FBC, U&E and LFTs, as gallstones are a common cause of pancreatitis.
  - Request an upper abdominal USS; give IV fluids and IV analgesia such as morphine 0.1 mg/kg IV, with an antiemetic such as metoclopramide 10–20 mg IV if the patient is nauseated or vomiting.
  - Advise the patient to eat a diet low in saturated fat and arrange for a surgical referral.
- **Acute cholecystitis:**
  - Causes acute, constant RUQ pain referred to the scapula, with fever, anorexia, nausea and vomiting.
  - Examination reveals a temperature and localised tenderness, with involuntary guarding and rebound tenderness. Painful splinting of respiration on deep inspiration and RUQ palpation is common (Murphy's sign).
  - Gain IV access, commence IV fluids and give gentamicin 5 mg/kg IV with ampicillin 2 g IV QDS. Give analgesia such as morphine 0.1 mg/kg IV, with an antiemetic such as metoclopramide 10–20 mg IV if the patient is nauseated or vomiting.
  - Confirm with an upper abdominal USS.

SECTION C – Common calls

- **Ascending cholangitis:**
  - This results from biliary obstruction from gallstones, duct stricture or malignancy.
  - It causes fever, rigors, upper abdominal pain and jaundice. Septic shock occurs in severe cases.
  - Look for a raised temperature, jaundice and RUQ tenderness, plus features of shock such as tachycardia, hypotension and confusion.
  - Commence IV fluid resuscitation, analgesia and IV antibiotics (as above), and arrange an immediate surgical consult.

Pancreatitis

Causes of pancreatitis include idiopathic, gallstones, ethanol, trauma, steroids, mumps, autoimmune, scorpion sting (!), hyperlipidaemia/hypercalcaemia, ERCP and drugs (mnemonic I GET SMASHED).

- May be acute, chronic or relapsing. Suspect pancreatitis in any patient with abdominal pain that is deep, constant and progressive, localised to the epigastrium and radiating to the back or both costal margins. It is associated with nausea, vomiting and anorexia.
- An elevated serum lipase or amylase level supports the diagnosis, but a normal level does not exclude it, particularly in chronic pancreatitis.
- Keep the patient NBM, commence IV fluid resuscitation with normal saline and titrate a narcotic analgesic agent such boluses of morphine 0.1 mg/kg IV with an antiemetic such as metoclopramide 10–20 mg IV for nausea or vomiting.
- Arrange an abdominal CT scan if the patient develops fever or shock. A CT scan is diagnostic, prognostic and shows most complications.
- Refer patient to the ICU if severe pancreatitis with sepsis, abscess formation or generalised peritonitis with multiorgan failure.

Intra-abdominal abscess

A patient with a history of diverticulitis or recent abdominal surgery and gradual onset of sharp and constant localised abdominal pain may have a contained intra-abdominal abscess.

- Organise either USS or CT scan, which can wait for the morning provided the patient is otherwise stable.
- Abscesses are treated with ultrasound-guided percutaneous drainage, surgical drainage or antibiotics alone, depending on the circumstance.
- An intra-abdominal abscess that **ruptures** results in acute peritonitis and may progress to septic shock. Arrange urgent surgical consultation and ensure that the patient is kept NBM.

Renal colic

Renal and ureteric calculi cause loin-to-groin pain, haematuria, urinary frequency, obstruction or infection.

- Characteristic symptoms include sudden, severe colicky pain radiating from the loin to the genitalia, restlessness, vomiting and sweating.
- Look for loin tenderness in the costovertebral angle, but remember to exclude a ruptured AAA in men aged over 45 years, especially with a first episode of renal colic, and/or if haematuria is absent.
- Request an urgent non-contrast abdominal CT scan of the renal tract in a patient with acute flank pain to confirm the diagnosis and rule out alternative retroperitoneal pathology.
- Or organise USS if the diagnosis is already known and pain recurs.
- Request a plain AXR (KUB) to later track the course of the calculus.
- Commence IV fluids and give morphine 0.1 mg/kg IV if the pain is intense and incapacitating, adding an antiemetic such as metoclopramide 10–20 mg IV if the patient is nauseated or vomiting. Follow up with indomethacin 100 mg PR BD, which provides excellent longer-lasting analgesia.
- Refer any patient with resistant pain, a stone >6 mm in diameter (unlikely to pass spontaneously), a stone in a unilateral kidney or a patient with *any* evidence of urosepsis (fever, tachycardia, hypotension and leucocytes/bacteria on urinalysis) to the urology team.
- Suspected urosepsis is a surgical emergency requiring *immediate* percutaneous drainage.

Pyelonephritis

Symptom onset is typically rapid and characterised by urinary frequency, dysuria, malaise, nausea, vomiting and sometimes rigors. Raised temperature, renal angle tenderness and vague low abdominal pain are found.

- Dipstick urinalysis shows blood, protein and nitrates. Send an MSU to the lab to look for bacteria, leucocytes and RBCs on microscopy, and for culture.
- Send blood for FBC, ELFTs and two sets of paired blood cultures if shocked.
- Commence IV fluids and give gentamicin 5 mg/kg IV with ampicillin 2 g IV QDS until the specific organism has been identified.
- Otherwise, if the symptoms are mild and consistent with predominant cystitis, commence PO antibiotic, such as cephalexin

500 mg 6-hourly for 10 days, or trimethoprim 300 mg daily for 10 days, depending on local prescribing policy.

Peptic ulcer disease

Patients with suspected PUD or gastro-oesophageal reflux disease (GORD) complain of constant burning or stabbing pain around the epigastrium and radiating to the back. Pain is often abated with food.

- Symptoms are relieved with antacid medication in the short term, then administration of a proton-pump inhibitor (PPI) such as omeprazole 40 mg PO for ongoing treatment.
- A patient with dysphagia, weight loss or symptomatic anaemia (or haematemesis—see Chapter 27) needs urgent endoscopy, which also allows testing for *Helicobacter pylori*.

Special populations

Elderly patient

The investigation and management of abdominal pain in an elderly patient should proceed similarly as for other patient groups. However, the pain may be relatively mild even in the presence of an acute abdomen.

Look for an associated acute confusional state, fever, elevated WCC or metabolic acidosis. Two important conditions more frequent in the elderly are colonic perforation from diverticular disease, and mesenteric ischaemia from atherosclerosis.

Medical disorders

It is rare for non-surgical disorders causing acute abdominal pain to present without other symptoms or signs suggesting their true medical origin. See Box 25.1.

Always remember DKA and perform a urinalysis in *every* patient with abdominal pain. DKA is suggested by glycosuria and ketonuria.

Handy hints

- Always provide analgesia to patients with abdominal pain. Do not withhold analgesia to 'preserve' physical signs. Providing adequate analgesia does not conceal the diagnosis.
- Be wary of diagnosing 'constipation', particularly in the elderly, as it is best thought of as a symptom. There is a high rate of missed diagnoses when the underlying cause of the abdominal pain is not searched for.

26

Altered bowel habit

Calls regarding bowel function are common and, in general, are straight-forward to manage. Many patients have an alteration in bowel habit during their hospital stay, resulting from a change in diet and fluids, decreased mobility, surgery and narcotic analgesia or other medications.

Diarrhoea may require volume replacement therapy while an underlying cause is sought, whereas for constipation the focus is on symptomatic oral treatment as the search for the underlying cause is made.

DIARRHOEA

Diarrhoea, as with constipation, is often best thought of as a symptom of an underlying disorder. Your role on call is to determine the likely cause, whether additional investigations are necessary and if urgent volume replacement therapy is indicated.

Phone call

Questions

1. **What are the vital signs?** Hypotension and tachycardia suggest intravascular volume depletion and shock. Fever may indicate an infectious cause.
2. **Does the patient have a previous history of diarrhoea or related medical problems?** The patient may have a history of gluten or lactose intolerance, inflammatory bowel disease, intestinal malabsorption or short-bowel syndrome.
3. **What is the nature of the stool?** Bloody stools with pus or mucus suggest infection, inflammatory bowel disease or ischaemic colitis.
4. **Does the patient have associated symptoms such as abdominal pain, nausea or vomiting?** Moderate-to-severe abdominal pain is seen in ischaemic colitis, diverticulitis or inflammatory bowel disease.
5. **Has the patient been abroad recently?** Always consider tropical causes including typhoid (which presents *early* with headache, fever, cough and constipation before the diarrhoeal illness with

hepatosplenomegaly develops), amoebiasis, bacillary dysentery or cholera, etc.

6. **Has the patient been in contact with others suffering similar symptoms?** Consider an infectious aetiology from food or poor handwashing technique, isolate the patient and immediately inform public health if confirmed.

7. **Has the patient had recent antibiotics?** Enquire about any antibiotic use in the previous 10 weeks, which predisposes to *Clostridium difficile* associated diarrhoea (CDAD).

8. **Is the patient immunocompromised or HIV positive?** Diarrhoea in patients with HIV may have an opportunistic infection aetiology (viral, bacterial, protozoal or fungal) or be related to antiretroviral therapy.

9. **Is the patient being fed enterally?** Patients being tube-fed often have diarrhoea.

10. **What was the reason for admission?**

Instructions

- Ensure the patient is well hydrated. Ask the nursing staff if the patient can tolerate adequate fluids PO.
- Otherwise, commence IV rehydration in patients with significant dehydration unable to tolerate oral fluids and/or with vomiting.

Prioritisation

- Assess the patient immediately if there is shock with tachycardia and hypotension, or if febrile with a septicaemic illness.
- Otherwise, evaluate the patient as soon as possible if the diarrhoea is frequent, severe or associated with the passage of blood.

Corridor thoughts

What are the causes of diarrhoea? (* = major threat to life)
- **Infectious:**
  - Non-invasive gastroenteritis
    - Viral—rotavirus, norovirus, enteric adenovirus and astrovirus
    - Bacterial—*Escherichia coli* and *Vibrio cholera* produce enterotoxins that cause profuse watery diarrhoea. *Bacillus cereus* (cooked rice) and *Staphylococcus aureus* produce neurotoxins that rapidly induce significant vomiting as well as diarrhoea.
    - Parasitic—*Giardia lamblia* from infected drinking water; *Cryptosporidium* from animals and livestock.
  - Invasive gastroenteritis*
    - *Shigella* spp., *Campylobacter jejuni*, enterohaemorrhagic *E. coli*, *Yersinia enterocolitica*, *Salmonella* spp. and *Entamoeba histolytica*.

- *C. difficile* toxin-related diarrhoea following any recent antibiotic course (even up to 10 weeks prior—see below).
- **Gastrointestinal pathology:**
  - Inflammatory bowel disease:
    - Ulcerative colitis, Crohn's disease, radiation enteritis or colitis
    - Ischaemic colitis secondary to mesenteric thrombosis, vascular embolus, vasculitis or volvulus*
  - Neoplasm:
    - Colon cancer, bowel lymphoma, villous adenoma
  - Malabsorption syndromes:
    - Coeliac disease, short-bowel syndrome, bowel resection
    - Chronic pancreatitis
  - Abdominal surgery:
    - Gastric surgery, cholecystectomy or bowel resection
  - Lactose intolerance
  - Irritable bowel syndrome
  - Faecal impaction 'spurious diarrhoea'. Remember to do a PR exam.
- **Systemic disease:**
  - Hyperthyroidism
  - Medullary thyroid carcinoma
  - Carcinoid
  - Diabetes associated with autonomic neuropathy
- **Medication-related:**
  - Laxatives, stool softeners, magnesium-containing antacids
  - Digoxin, colchicine, quinidine
  - Antibiotic-related diarrhoea can occur with almost any antibiotic and is self-limiting.
  - Antibiotic-associated diarrhoea due to pseudomembranous colitis presents with bloody diarrhoea secondary to *C. difficile* toxin. It is most often related to use of broad-spectrum antibiotics such as clindamycin, quinolones and cephalosporins.
- **Other:**
  - Seafood biotoxins (e.g. diarrhetic shellfish poisoning, scombroid, ciguatera)
  - Heavy metal poisoning such as lead

SECTION C – Common calls

Major threat to life

- **Intravascular volume depletion and hypovolaemic shock**
- **Electrolyte imbalance**
- **Systemic infection**

Bedside

Quick-look test

Does the patient look well (comfortable), sick (uncomfortable or distressed), or critical (about to die)?

Most patients with acute diarrhoea do not look unwell. However, if the diarrhoea is due to an invasive organism such as *Salmonella* or *Shigella* spp. or *Entamoeba histolytica*, the patient may look sick and complain of headache, diffuse myalgia, chills and fever.

Airway and vital signs

What is the blood pressure?
- Resting hypotension suggests significant volume depletion. Examine for postural changes if the supine BP is normal.
- A postural rise in HR >20 beats/min, a fall in SBP >20 mmHg or any fall in DBP indicates orthostatic hypotension and significant hypovolaemia.

What is the heart rate?
- Intravascular volume depletion usually results in tachycardia.
- Tachycardia may also be caused by fever or pain.
- A relative bradycardia despite fever raises the suspicion of *Salmonella typhi* infection.

What is the temperature?
- Fever in a patient with diarrhoea is non-specific, but may occur due to infectious diarrhoea, diverticulitis, inflammatory bowel disease, intestinal lymphoma and tuberculosis.
- Some organisms, such as *Shigella* and *Salmonella* spp., and fulminant amoebiasis cause systemic sepsis.

Selective history and chart review

Has the patient travelled abroad recently?
- *E. coli* enterotoxin is the most common cause of 'traveller's diarrhoea'.
- *Salmonella* spp., *Shigella* spp. and *C. jejuni* cause acute, self-limited traveller's diarrhoea.
- Giardiasis, amoebiasis and tropical sprue usually cause a more chronic condition.

Have any close contacts had a diarrhoeal illness?
- Transmission is common and most often by the faecal–oral route, particularly viral diarrhoea that can cause large outbreaks.

What has the patient eaten recently?
- Ask about ingestion of raw food such as shellfish (*Vibrio* spp.) or reheated rice (*Bacillus cereus*).

Is the patient on any medications that may cause diarrhoea?
- Medications are the most common cause of diarrhoea in the hospital.
- Cease laxative agents, stool softeners and magnesium-containing antacids.

Has the patient received antibiotics recently?
- Many antibiotics cause transient diarrhoea through alteration of the intestinal flora.
- Pseudomembranous colitis caused by C. *difficile* enterotoxin may result in persistent diarrhoea during or after antibiotic use.

Has the patient had previous surgery?
- Resections of the ileum and right colon may result in diarrhoea due to bile acid malabsorption.

Selective physical examination

Physical examination is directed to whether the patient is volume-depleted or septic, and to look for an underlying cause for the diarrhoea.

Vitals	Repeat now
General	Cachexia suggests a chronic process such as carcinoma, malabsorption or AIDS
HEENT	Lymphadenopathy (lymphoma, Whipple's disease, AIDS)
	Enlarged thyroid (hyperthyroidism, medullary carcinoma)
	Aphthous ulcers (Crohn's disease)
CVS	Pulse volume, JVP (flat neck veins in hypovolaemia)
	Skin temperature, colour
Abdo	Surgical scar (gastrectomy, bowel resection)
	Hepatosplenomegaly (*Salmonella* infection)
	RLQ mass or tenderness (Crohn's disease, *Mycobacterium tuberculosis*, giardiasis)
	LLQ mass or tenderness (diverticulitis, tumour, inflammatory bowel disease, ischaemic colitis, faecal impaction)
Rectal	Anal fissure (Crohn's disease)
	Mass (faecal impaction, cancer)
	Fresh blood or stool positive for occult blood (inflammatory bowel disease, invasive gastroenteritis, cancer)
MSS	Arthritis (inflammatory bowel disease, Whipple's disease, Reiter's syndrome secondary to *Yersinia enterocolitica*)
Skin	Dermatitis herpetiformis (coeliac disease)
	Pyoderma gangrenosum, erythema nodosum (inflammatory bowel disease)

Investigations
Laboratory
- Send blood for U&E, LFTs and FBC.
  - Severe diarrhoea is associated with significant fluid loss and electrolyte disturbances such as hypokalaemia, hypernatraemia, hyponatraemia and metabolic acidosis.
  - Raised WCC from infection and inflammation.

Stool sample
- Test for occult blood at bedside.
- **Stool microscopy**
  - Specimens are best evaluated 'fresh' within 6 hours of collection:
    - Faecal leucocytes (infection, inflammatory bowel disease, ischaemia)
    - Ova and parasites (*Giardia, Entamoeba, Cryptospridium*).
- **Stool culture** for patients with fever, abdominal pain and faecal leucocytes; suspected inflammatory cause, or chronic diarrhoea.
  - Use the correct transport medium for specific pathogen cultures. Check with the microbiology laboratory.
- **Stool toxin**
  - *C. difficile* toxin study for antibiotic-associated diarrhoea.

Management

Immediate management
Diarrhoea with significant intravascular depletion or systemic sepsis
- Attach continuous non-invasive ECG, BP and pulse oximeter monitoring.
- Commence oxygen therapy to maintain oxygen saturation >94%.
- Insert a large-bore (14–16G) peripheral cannula and send blood samples to laboratory.
- Commence fluid resuscitation to restore normotension and normovolaemia.
- Give a 20 mL/kg bolus of normal saline. Elevate or squeeze the IV bag, or use IV pressure cuffs to increase the rate if necessary.
- Observe the effect of this fluid challenge on volume status and repeat, but avoid over-aggressive resuscitation in a patient with heart failure.
- Replace potassium as determined by U&E results.

General management
The aim on call is to ensure that the patient is adequately hydrated, does not have a serious electrolyte imbalance and does not have a systemic infection.
- **Fluid and electrolyte replacement**
  - Oral replacement with glucose and electrolyte rehydration solution is preferred in children.
  - Use IV rehydration in patients who have significant volume depletion or do not tolerate oral fluids.
- **Review medications**
  - Discontinue laxatives and stool softeners.

- Withhold magnesium-containing antacids or switch to aluminium-containing preparations.
- Discuss with your senior doctor other medications such as antibiotics or digoxin that may cause diarrhoea prior to discontinuing them, based on a risk–benefit decision.
- **Antidiarrhoeal agents**
  - Use a non-specific antidiarrhoeal agent if the patient's diarrhoea is disabling, provided inflammatory bowel disease, amoebiasis and *C. difficile* are not suspected (risk of precipitating toxic megacolon).
  - **Loperamide:** 4 mg PO stat then 2 mg with each motion until diarrhoea is controlled, to a maximum dose of 16 mg in 24 hours (eight tablets). Side effects are extremely rare, such as abdominal distension, cramping and occasionally nausea.
  - **Diphenoxylate with atropine:** 5 mg PO three or four times a day until diarrhoea is controlled, to a maximum dose of 20 mg in 24 hours. Slower onset of action than loperamide and is contraindicated in patients with hepatic failure or cirrhosis.
    — Respiratory depression may occur when used in combination with phenothiazines, tricyclic antidepressants or barbiturates.
- **Antibiotic therapy**
  - Specific antibiotic therapy should only be implemented in consultation with an infectious disease specialist, guided by stool microscopy and culture results.

Specific management

- **Non-invasive gastroenteritis**
  - Give patients PO or IV rehydration and electrolyte replacement and keep fasted if symptomatic abdominal pain persists.
  - Avoid milk and milk-related products because temporary lactose intolerance may occur.
- **Antibiotic-associated diarrhoea** (pseudomembranous colitis)
  - Send a stool specimen for *C. difficile* toxin study.
  - Discontinue the offending antibiotic, replace lost fluid and electrolytes, and avoid antidiarrhoeal and narcotic medications.
  - Commence metronidazole 400 mg PO or 500 mg IV every 8 hours.
- **Inflammatory bowel disease**
  - Exacerbations of ulcerative colitis and Crohn's disease may present with crampy abdominal pain and fever. The stool is usually watery and blood-stained with faecal leucocytes.
  - Treatment options include bowel rest, rectal or oral steroids, and mesalazine 500 mg PO TDS in consultation with a gastroenterologist.

SECTION C – Common calls

CONSTIPATION

Phone call

Questions

1. **When was the last time the patient passed a bowel motion?** Determine the extent of the problem. If the patient is not passing stool or flatus there may be absolute constipation secondary to mechanical obstruction.
2. **What is the patient's normal bowel function? Does the patient routinely use laxatives?** Normal bowel function varies from three stools a day to one bowel motion a week. Many patients regularly use stimulants or laxatives to maintain regular bowel function.
3. **Are there any associated 'red-flag' symptoms?** Acute-onset abdominal pain, abdominal distension, vomiting and absolute constipation, weight loss and bleeding PR indicate a serious cause for the constipation, which *must* be investigated.
4. **What medication is the patient taking?** Constipation is a side effect of many drugs such as narcotic analgesics, antacids, calcium-channel blockers, anticholinergics and tricyclic antidepressants.
5. **Has the patient had recent surgery?** Do not prescribe a laxative or GI stimulant routinely for postoperative ileus. Instead, wait for GI function to return to normal over 4–5 days.

Prioritisation

- Constipation is not a diagnosis, but a symptom that requires further evaluation.
- Patients with associated 'red-flag' symptoms (see above) or recent surgery need early review. Others can wait for the morning.

Corridor thoughts

What causes constipation? (* = major threat to life)
- **Gastrointestinal disorders**
  - Mechanical obstruction*: cancer, adhesions, hernia (strangulated/incarcerated), intussusception, volvulus, foreign body; rarely, total faecal impaction
  - Ileus: postoperative, electrolyte imbalance, opioids, sepsis*, trauma
  - Neoplasm*: benign or malignant tumours
  - Inflammatory/painful conditions:
    - Diverticulitis, proctitis, Crohn's disease*, ulcerative colitis* (more usually urgency, tenesmus and bloody diarrhoea)
    - Perianal fissure, haemorrhoids

- Colonic dysmotility: spinal injury, MS or autonomic dysfunction
- **Medication-related**
  - Analgesics (e.g. codeine, morphine)
  - Anticholinergic agents (e.g. antihistamines, phenothiazines, antidepressants)
  - Calcium-channel blockers (e.g. verapamil)
  - $5HT_3$-receptor antagonists (ondansetron, granisetron)
  - Iron preparations
  - Antacids containing aluminium hydroxide or calcium carbonate
  - Laxative abuse (causes dysfunctional bowel motility)
- **Other conditions**
  - Diabetes, hypothyroidism, hyperparathyroidism
  - Hypercalcaemia, hypokalaemia
  - Dehydration, hypovolaemia
  - Immobility: associated with decreased ambulation
  - Older age

Bedside

Quick-look test

Does the patient look well (comfortable), sick (uncomfortable or distressed) or critical (about to die)?
Most patients with simple constipation look comfortable at rest.

Airway and vital signs

What are the heart rate and blood pressure?
- Resting hypotension suggests significant volume depletion and dehydration. Examine for postural changes if the supine BP is normal.
- Tachycardia may indicate intravascular depletion, or be a marker of pain, fever or anxiety.

What is the temperature?
- Fever is an alarming feature that suggests an inflammatory cause such as diverticulitis or inflammatory bowel disease.

Selective history and chart review

- Review the nursing observations and fluid balance chart for trends in urine output, fluid intake and weight.
- Look at the stool chart to determine the timing and nature of bowel motions, and confirm the time since the last formed stool was passed.
- Look at the medication chart for specific drugs or combinations of factors that may predispose to constipation.

- Review the patient's history and hospital course, looking specifically for factors that may predispose to constipation (see *Corridor thoughts*).

Selective physical examination

Vital signs	Repeat now
Abdo	Palpate for tenderness, guarding and rebound (peritonism)
	Tender, tense, resonant abdominal distension (mechanical obstruction)
	LLQ mass or tenderness (diverticulitis, cancer, inflammatory bowel disease, faecal impaction)
	RLQ mass or tenderness (Crohn's disease)
	Rigid abdomen (generalised peritonitis, perforated viscus)
	Palpable bladder (urinary retention may be secondary to faecal impaction)
	Scars on abdominal wall (intra-abdominal adhesions)
	Auscultate for bowel sounds: tinkling (mechanical obstruction), absent (ileus)
Rectal	Inspect for external lesions such as a fissure or haemorrhoids
	PR examination: hard stool in the rectum (distal faecal impaction) or blood/mucus (malignancy, polyps, inflammatory bowel disease)

Investigations
Laboratory
- Send blood for FBC, U&E, LFTs and blood glucose if the patient is unwell and/or has any 'red-flag' symptoms (see *Phone call: Questions*).
- Look specifically for evidence of dehydration, hypokalaemia, hypercalcaemia and other metabolic derangements, urea-to-creatinine ratio.
- A low Hb may indicate an underlying benign or malignant tumour, diverticulitis or inflammatory bowel disease.
- Send blood for TFT if history and physical examination suggest hypothyroidism.

Radiology
- Abdominal X-rays:
  - Do *not* order simply to define the extent of faecal loading. They are only indicated for suspected mechanical obstruction, perforated viscus or a volvulus.

- CT scan abdomen:
  - Only to further evaluate complex abdominal pain, mechanical obstruction, a mass or peritonism.

Other

- Perform a bedside bladder scan if you suspect urinary retention related to faecal impaction.

Management

- Management is determined by the underlying cause(s) of the constipation.
- Refer a patient with an acute abdomen to the surgeon.
- All other patients:
  - Discontinue non-essential medications causing the constipation.
  - Use PO or IV rehydration with normal saline to correct dehydration and electrolyte disturbances.
  - Insert an IDC in cases of urinary retention secondary to distal faecal impaction.
  - Consider use of aperients such as laxatives (PO, PR) or a rectal enema.
  - **Oral laxatives**:
    - Indicated for the prevention and treatment of symptomatic constipation in hospitalised patients, provided an acute abdomen or distal faecal impaction have been excluded.
    - **Stool softener** such as Coloxyl (docusate sodium) 1–2 tablets with food BD.
    - **Bulk-forming agents** such as Metamucil (psyllium) 2 teaspoons (6 g) in 200 mL water twice daily.
    - **Osmotic laxatives** such as Movicol (macrogol) 1–2 sachets PO daily, or lactulose 10–15 mL PO up to three times daily.
  - **Rectal laxatives:**
    - **Osmotic laxatives** such as glycerin suppository—onset of action within 30–60 minutes.
    - **Stimulant laxatives** such as bisacodyl suppository 10 mg.
  - **Enemas:**
    - These deliver agents directly into the rectum to assist the patient to evacuate hard stool. Do not use when the patient has nausea, vomiting or abdominal pain.

- **Rectal stool softener** such as Microlax 5 mL (each 5 mL enema contains sodium citrate 450 mg, sodium lauryl sulfoacetate 45 mg, sorbitol 3.125 g).
- **Sodium phosphate hypertonic enema,** such as Fleet enema 60–120 mL given as a single dose, which may be repeated.

- **Digital manual faecal disimpaction:**
  - This is occasionally required when hard stool is trapped in the distal rectum. The patient will need sedation and an analgesic.

Handy hints

- Elderly, immobile patients and patients prescribed narcotic analgesics are particularly prone to reduced bowel transit time and constipation.
- Give prophylactic stool softeners, a high-fibre diet and adequate fluid intake and encourage mobilisation. Provide regular opportunity to use the toilet.

27

Gastrointestinal bleeding

Gastrointestinal bleeding is common in hospitalised patients and can range from minor to life-threatening. The overall mortality rate is around 10%.

Management is aimed at resuscitation, stabilisation and evaluating the underlying cause, looking out particularly for the high-risk patient with oesophageal varices, or aged over 60 years, active fresh and/or recurrent bleeding, shock and comorbid disease.

Phone call

Questions

1. **Where is the blood coming from and what is its colour and consistency?** Haematemesis is vomiting of bright-red blood, altered blood or 'coffee grounds' from an upper GI bleed proximal to the jejunum. Melaena is the passage of black, tarry loose stools from altered blood that originates in the GIT anywhere from the mouth to the caecum.

   Rectal bleeding (haematochezia) is bright-red or maroon bleeding per rectum. It usually indicates a lower GI bleed from the colon, rectum or anus, but in 15% of cases it comes from an upper GI bleed when blood loss is rapid and massive.

2. **How much blood has been lost?** Ask the nurse to estimate the amount of blood lost. Although massive external bleeding will be obvious, an apparently small volume of fresh haematemesis may be followed by a much larger vomit from blood retained in the stomach.

3. **What are the vital signs?** Significant GI haemorrhage is associated with tachycardia, hypotension and haemorrhagic shock.

4. **Has there been a previous GI bleed?** Ask about previous bleeding from varices, peptic ulcer disease, oesophagitis or gastritis, or from the lower GIT such as diverticulitis.

5. **Is there an existing medical condition that causes GI bleeding?** Chronic liver disease with cirrhosis makes oesophageal varices and/or coagulopathy more likely, with more serious bleeding.

6. **What medications is the patient taking?** Patients taking NSAIDs or steroids are more likely to develop PUD. Anticoagulants (e.g. heparin, warfarin or a NOAC) or a thrombolytic agent (e.g. tPA or tenecteplase) must be discontinued immediately and/or reversed in the actively bleeding patient.
7. **What was the reason for admission?**

Instructions

Significant GI bleed with tachycardia, hypotension and other signs of shock:
- Ask the nurse to stay by the patient's bedside and get help from additional staff.
- Administer oxygen to maintain saturation >94% and attach a pulse oximeter and cardiac monitor to the patient.
- Ask for an IV trolley by the patient's bedside with two large-bore (14–16G) cannulae ready for your arrival.
- Commence infusion of normal saline 10–20 mL/kg if the patient already has an IV cannula.

Prioritisation

See immediately any patient with upper or lower GI bleeding associated with tachycardia or hypotension, if varices are possible and/or if the bleeding is fresh or recurrent, particularly in patients aged over 60 years.

Corridor thoughts

What causes GI bleeding? (* = major threat to life)
- **Upper GI bleed:**
  - Peptic ulceration (35–50% of cases)
    - Duodenal ulcer
    - Gastric ulcer (less common)
  - Reflux oesophagitis (20–30%)
  - Gastric erosions or gastritis (10–20%)
    - Alcohol-related
    - Medication-related (e.g. aspirin, NSAIDs, steroids)
  - Oesophageal or gastric varices* (5–12%)
    - Associated with portal hypertension from chronic liver disease with cirrhosis. Most often due to alcohol, hepatitis B, C or D, chronic active hepatitis, haemachromastosis or NASH
  - Mallory–Weiss tear (2–5%)
    - Oesophageal tear following vomiting or retching

- Neoplasm (2–5%)
  - Oesophageal* or gastric*
- Other
  - Angiodysplasia (2–3%)
  - Aorto-enteric fistula* (<1%)–note any past history of an AAA repair
- **Lower GI bleed:**
  - Secondary to rapid upper GI bleeding* (haematochezia)
  - Diverticular disease (>50% of cases)
    - Diverticulosis, occasionally diverticulitis
    - Meckel diverticulum
  - Neoplasm*
    - Colon, rectum or anus, small bowel
  - Colitis
    - Crohn's disease* (any part of GIT)
    - Ulcerative colitis* (colon and distal)
  - Gastroenteritis
    - Infectious (dysenteric), ischaemic*, post-irradiation
  - Arteriovenous malformation and angiodysplasia
  - Intussusception*
  - Polyps and polyposis syndromes
    - Colonic polyps, Peutz–Jeghers syndrome (perioral pigmentation with GI polyps), familial adenomatous polyposis
  - Benign anorectal disease
    - Haemorrhoids, anal fissure, fistula-in-ano (*must* always exclude an additional more sinister cause such as a malignancy with sigmoidoscopy or colonoscopy)
- **Bleeding diathesis:**
  - GI bleeding may occur in the absence of structural pathological features in a patient who is on an anticoagulant, is coagulopathic or has a bleeding tendency, thrombocytopenia or abnormal platelet function.

Major threat to life

- **Variceal bleeding:**
  - Patients with chronic liver disease with portal hypertension and/or known varices are at highest risk of early death.
- **Hypovolaemic shock:**
  - Patients with significant GI haemorrhage deplete the intravascular volume and become hypotensive.
  - Patients aged over 60 years, and those with comorbidity such as heart failure, do not tolerate shock well and so are also at higher risk of dying.

Bedside

Quick-look test

Does the patient look well (comfortable), sick (uncomfortable or distressed) or critical (about to die)?

- Patients with significant GI bleeding are pale, sweaty and apprehensive, and have cold clammy skin with tachycardia and hypotension. Make sure you have called your senior.
- Patients with minor GI bleeding look comfortable, are less concerned and are well perfused.

Airway and vital signs

Is the airway clear?

- Protect the airway as it is common for the debilitated patient to aspirate during ongoing bleeding.
- Consider endotracheal intubation in the presence of shock, diminished mental status, hepatic encephalopathy, massive haematemesis or active variceal haemorrhage. Call your senior and an anaesthetist urgently. Inform the ICU.

What is the blood pressure and heart rate?

- Hypotension and tachycardia in the supine patient indicate significant hypovolaemia. The presence of shock suggests a high risk of rebleeding, surgery and mortality.
- A resting tachycardia alone may still indicate significant bleeding.
- Always check for orthostatic hypotension as evidence of early hypovolaemia in patients without obvious haemodynamic compromise. Check the SBP and HR while the patient is supine and then after at least 2 minutes sitting or standing.
  - A SBP fall of >20 mmHg and HR increase >20 beats/min indicate hypovolaemia from blood loss.

Selective physical examination I

Is the patient in shock?

Vitals	Repeat now; pay particular attention to HR, BP and postural changes
CVS	Assess perfusion; note skin colour and warmth
	Pulse rate and volume, JVP (flat in hypovolaemia)
CNS	Level of consciousness and mental status. Apprehension, confusion and agitation indicate cerebral hypoperfusion and hypoxia from hypovolaemic shock.

- As the BP falls with significant GI bleeding, cerebral perfusion decreases and the patient becomes agitated, confused and lethargic.

- Urine output correlates with the renal blood flow, which in turn is dependent on cardiac output. It is an early indicator of hypovolaemia; however, placement of an IDC does not take priority over other resuscitation measures.

Management

Immediate management
- **Monitor vital signs.**
  - Attach continuous non-invasive ECG, BP and pulse oximeter monitoring to the patient.
  - Commence oxygen therapy to maintain oxygen saturation >94%.
- **Obtain adequate IV access.**
  - Insert at least two large-bore (14–16G) peripheral cannulae in large veins, preferably the antecubital.
  - Draw and send blood for FBC, U&E, LFTs, coagulation profile and cross-matching.
  - Request immediate cross-match of a minimum of two, but as many as four, units of packed RBCs depending on the presumed aetiology and degree of shock.
- **Replenish intravascular depletion.**
  - Commence fluid resuscitation to restore and maintain adequate tissue perfusion, avoiding excessive volumes of fluid.
  - Give a 10–20 mL/kg bolus of normal saline and observe the effect on the vital signs.
  - A patient with known CCF is at high risk of fluid overload with pulmonary oedema. Monitor the respiratory rate, JVP and lung bases for crackles, and consider ICU admission.
- **Insert an IDC to monitor fluid balance.**
  - Urine output is a sensitive measure of end-organ perfusion and volume status.
  - Aim for a urine output of 0.5–1 mL/kg/h.
- **Commence blood transfusion with packed RBCs.**
  - While crystalloid is being given, make certain type-specific or full cross-matched blood is organised.
  - A full cross-match takes ≈ 45 minutes, but if blood is already held, it should be available at the bedside within 30 minutes.
  - Give blood only if the patient remains shocked or the bleeding is continuing.
    - If the Hb drops below 70 g/L, restore to 70–90 g/L.
    - Aim for 100 g/L if active ischaemic heart disease.
- **Correct abnormal coagulation, especially if known chronic liver disease.**
  - Give FFP 4 units and vitamin K 10 mg IV for patients with known liver cell failure, such as in cirrhosis.

SECTION C – Common calls

- **Request an ECG**, particularly for older patients or patients with risk factors for coronary artery disease.
- **Cease antiplatelet and anticoagulant medications.**
- **Keep the patient NBM** for urgent upper GI endoscopy, colonoscopy and, occasionally, surgery. Contact your senior and the admitting surgical team.

Selective history and chart review

Is there an existing medical condition that causes GI bleeding?
Ask about chronic liver disease with cirrhosis or active PUD.
Has there been a previous GI bleed?
Look for prior episodes of GI bleeding and documented causation.
Are there medical comorbidities that increase the general risks from GI bleeding?
Look for evidence of CCF, COPD, renal impairment, altered mental status.
Is the patient on medication that may worsen the situation?

- **NSAIDs** counteract the protective effect of prostaglandins on gastric mucosa and result in gastric erosions or peptic ulceration, especially in older people.
- **Steroids** increase the frequency of ulcer disease.
  - *Note:* most disease processes for which a patient receives steroids preclude their immediate discontinuation.
- **Heparin** prevents clot formation by enhancing the action of antithrombin III, which in turn inactivates thrombin and factor Xa.
- **Warfarin** prevents activation of vitamin K-dependent clotting factors.
- **NOAC agents** act either as a direct thrombin inhibitor or as a factor Xa inhibitor.
- **Antiplatelet agents**—aspirin, clopidogrel, prasugrel, ticagrelor and glycoprotein IIb/IIIa inhibitors (e.g. abciximab, eptifibatide or tirofiban)—interfere with platelet activation, adhesion or aggregation.

Selective physical examination II

Where is the apparent site of bleeding?

HEENT	Epistaxis—exclude this, as swallowed blood may masquerade as a GI bleed
	Jaundice, telangiectasia, parotid gland hypertrophy (liver disease)
Abdo	Hepatosplenomegaly and ascites (liver disease with portal hypertension and varices; or intra-abdominal malignancy)
	Epigastric tenderness (PUD)
	RLQ tenderness or mass (caecal disease such as Crohn's disease, diverticular disease)

	LLQ tenderness (sigmoid cancer, diverticular disease, ischaemic colitis)
Rectal	Rectal mass (>75% rectal cancers are palpable on PR)
	Haemorrhoids, anal fissure (still need exclusion of cancer and other more serious causes)
Skin	Spider naevi, jaundice, palmar erythema, bruising, clubbing, gynaecomastia (chronic liver disease)

Investigations

- Take blood for FBC, U&E, blood glucose, LFTs, clotting studies and cross-matching.
  - *Remember:* Hb level may be normal early in an acute bleed, and drops following fluid resuscitation.
  - LFT may be deranged in chronic liver disease with liver failure, as well as the coagulation profile.

Definitive management

- The goal is to maintain adequate fluid resuscitation with oxygen-carrying capacity (Hb), correct the coagulopathy and identify and treat the underlying cause of the bleeding.
- Endoscopy is diagnostic, therapeutic (sclerotherapy, banding ligation in varices) and prognostic. Discuss the urgency with your senior doctor.

Upper GI bleed

- Commence high-dose oxygen via a mask and maintain the oxygen saturation >94%.
- Begin fluid replacement:
  - Normal saline 10–20 mL/kg, aiming for a urine output of 0.5–1 mL/kg/h.
  - Give cross-matched blood if the patient is shocked or the bleeding is continuing.
- Give a proton-pump inhibitor (e.g. omeprazole 80 mg stat IV followed by an infusion at 8 mg/h) if **peptic ulcer disease** is likely and early endoscopy is not feasible.
  - PPI benefit is proven only post-endoscopy for high-risk non-variceal bleeding with stigmata of recent haemorrhage.
- Give octreotide 50 micrograms IV (a somatostatin analogue that reduces portal pressure), then 50 microgram/h if **varices** are known or are likely from the presence of features of chronic liver disease and portal hypertension.
  - Octreotide reduces rebleeding, the need for transfusion and surgery, but not overall mortality.
  - An alternative is terlipressin 1.7 mg IV 6-hourly (a vasopressin analogue that reduces portal pressure).

SECTION C – Common calls

- Upper GI endoscopy:
  - Organise urgent endoscopy in patients who have suspected varices, continue to bleed, remain haemodynamically unstable and/or are aged over 60 years. Consult your senior immediately.
  - Early endoscopy enables diagnosis, prognosis and immediate therapy.
  - Oesophageal varices are treated with banding and/or sclerotherapy.
  - Gastric or duodenal ulcers with a visible vessel at the base may be treated with electrocoagulation, heater probe therapy or direct injection.
  - Emergency endoscopy can be performed within 24 hours in patients who are otherwise haemodynamically stable with an upper GI bleed that has stopped.
- Surgery may be required if endoscopy fails, and for high risk of rebleed in elderly patients.
- Angiography is performed for severe, persistent bleeding in high-risk patients unsuitable for surgery. May use intra-arterial gelatin, springs or tissue adhesive.
- Balloon tamponade (Sengstaken–Blakemore and Minnesota tubes).
  - Temporising measure for life-threatening variceal bleeds.
  - *Only* use if access to endoscopy is not immediately available and/or the patient needs interhospital transfer.
  - *Must* be inserted by an expert as they are associated with a 25% complication rate and require an ETT.

Lower GI bleed

The colour of the blood is associated with the length of time in the GIT and its origin. Lower GI bleeds occur distal to the ligament of Trietz, at the duodenojejunal flexure.

- In up to 15% of cases, bright-red blood from the rectum may be associated with a proximal upper GI lesion, such as a duodenal bleed, if the transit time through the gut is short.
- Provide resuscitative care as above and continue to monitor the patient's volume status and response to therapy.
- Most cases of lower GI bleeding cease spontaneously and the majority require no further intervention other than initial resuscitation. They can then be scheduled for elective colonoscopy.
- Haemodynamically unstable patients not responsive to fluid and blood resuscitation require urgent surgical review.
- In some institutions, technetium-labelled RBC scanning and angiography may be available, if the origin of bleeding remains unclear on colonoscopy.

- Surgery is reserved for those patients in whom life-threatening bleeding persists despite all measures, and may involve partial colectomy.

Specific management
Oesophageal varices
Chronic liver disease with portal hypertension leads to variceal bleeding from the oesophagus and stomach.
- Look specifically for signs of liver cell failure such as jaundice, bruising, encephalopathy, asterixis, spider naevi, gynaecomastia and ascites.
- Also look for signs of portal hypertension such as splenomegaly, ascites and caput medusae (although the latter is uncommon).
  - Prehepatic causes of portal hypertension include portal vein thrombosis, and posthepatic causes include hepatic vein thrombosis (Budd–Chiari syndrome).
- Management is aimed at resuscitation with blood, correction of coagulopathy and *early* endoscopy.

Diverticular disease
Up to 20% of patients with diverticulosis suffer from lower GI bleeding, with 3–5% having massive haemorrhage. Diverticulitis with inflammation and abscess formation with a risk of perforation is *not* commonly associated with bleeding.
- Haemorrhage stops spontaneously in 80–90% of patients with no intervention required.
- Persistent large-volume bleeds require transfusion and urgent surgical review.

Cancer
Colonic adenocarcinoma and rectal adenocarcinoma usually cause occult bleeding.
- The incidence of massive bleeding due to colorectal carcinoma varies from 5% to 20%.

Non-infectious colitis
Massive haemorrhage from ulcerative colitis (4%), Crohn's disease (1%) or ischaemic colitis is rare but life-threatening. Get early advice from a gastroenterologist.

Angiodysplasia
- Arteriovenous malformations are usually located in the caecum and ascending colon.
- They cause slow, repeated episodes of bleeding. Patients present with anaemia and/or a history of syncope. Infrequently,

angiodysplasia causes an abrupt loss of a large quantity of blood.
- Colonoscopy is necessary to identify angiodysplastic lesions and active bleeding sites, which are treated with electrocoagulation.
- A red cell scan or angiography may be needed when no source is found.

Indications for urgent surgical consultation
- Exsanguinating haemorrhage with hypovolaemic shock.
- Ulcer with a visible vessel at the base on endoscopy, unresponsive to coagulation technique.
- Failed variceal ligation or sclerotherapy.

Patients who refuse blood transfusion
Some patients may refuse blood transfusion for personal or religious reasons (e.g. Jehovah's Witness).

Respect their views (see Chapter 4), call your senior doctor and follow the hints in Box 27.1.

BOX 27.1   Patients who refuse blood transfusion

Call your senior for help and consider:
- Immediate endoscopy, with a view towards therapeutic intervention (e.g. sclerotherapy, heater coagulation, laser therapy), with early surgical consultation.
- Normal saline may be used, but avoid over-aggressive fluid replacement before bleeding is controlled, as this leads to dilutional coagulopathy that inhibits spontaneous haemostasis and causes further bleeding.
- A rule of thumb is to aim for a SBP of 90–100 mmHg in a previously normotensive patient, or 20–30 mmHg below a hypertensive patient's usual SBP. This approach is referred to as 'minimal volume resuscitation'.
- Consider agents such as specific clotting factors (to raise factor VIII and von Willebrand factor and reduce bleeding time), prothrombin complex concentrate (Prothrombinex) or anti-fibrinolytics (e.g. tranexamic acid), which *may* be acceptable to some Jehovah's Witness patients.
- Consult a haematologist for advice and help.

Handy hints

- Always look for signs of chronic liver disease with portal hypertension, which suggest the presence of oesophageal varices until proven otherwise.
- Insertion of an NGT to look for bright-red blood is *not* recommended, as it may miss significant bleeding and cause mucosal artefacts that hamper interpretation of endoscopic findings.
- The patient's volume status is the best indicator of blood loss.

Handy hints—Continued

- Iron supplements and bismuth compounds turn stools black, but they remain *formed*. True melaena is sticky, tar-like and pitch black, with an unpleasant odour.
- An aorto-enteric fistula may present with a sentinel (minor) GI bleed followed by rapid exsanguination.
  - ○ Consider this possibility in *any* patient who has had previous abdominal vascular surgery, and in a patient with a midline abdominal scar who is unable to give that history.
- *Never* attribute a lower GI bleed to haemorrhoids until a colonoscopy or sigmoidoscopy has been arranged to rule out more serious causes such as cancer or polyps.

28

Haematuria

Blood in the urine is abnormal. Generally, gross or macroscopic haematuria will be the reason you are called.

Although haematuria rarely results in significant blood loss, it may be the first manifestation of a bleeding disorder, be associated with clot formation leading to colic or urinary obstruction, or indicate urosepsis.

Phone call

Questions

1. **When did the haematuria start and has it happened before?**
2. **Are there any associated symptoms?** Colicky flank pain suggests a renal tract stone. Dysuria and frequency are associated with UTIs.
3. **Is there a urinary catheter in place? Has this just been inserted?** Traumatic or inexperienced attempts at IDC insertion may lead to bleeding.
4. **Has the patient had recent surgery?** Procedures on the bladder and kidneys are associated with transient bleeding.
5. **Is the patient anticoagulated?** Anticoagulants (e.g. heparin, warfarin or a NOAC) may require reversal in an actively bleeding patient.
6. **What are the vital signs?** Significant blood loss can occasionally be associated with tachycardia and hypotension. Fever may be associated with urosepsis.
7. **What was the reason for admission?**

Instructions

- The patient with significant bleeding and hypotension:
  - Request an IV trolley for the patient's bedside, with two large-bore 14–16G cannulae ready for insertion.
  - Commence infusion of 10 mL/kg normal saline if the patient already has IV access.
- Ask the nurse to flush the urinary catheter with 20–30 mL normal saline to dislodge sediment or clots if an IDC is in place and the patient is anuric.

- Ask for a sample of urine for dipstick analysis and send to the laboratory for MCS.

Prioritisation

- Patients with significant pain, anuria, tachycardia, hypotension or evidence of symptomatic anaemia need urgent assessment.
- Provided that the patient is not in pain and the bleeding is slight, assessment may be delayed if other problems of higher priority exist.

Corridor thoughts

What causes haematuria? (* = major threat to life)

- **Renal tract disorder:**
  - Infection—cystitis, pyelonephritis*, prostatitis (Remember TB, and schistosomiasis with history of travel to Africa, South America, Middle East)
  - Malignancy—transitional cell carcinoma*
  - Stones—calculi in the renal pelvis, ureter or bladder
  - Trauma—blunt (or penetrating) trauma to the abdomen or pelvis*; catheter insertions will commonly cause slight haematuria
  - Benign prostatic hypertrophy (common cause of intermittent gross haematuria)
- **Renal disorder:**
  - Primary renal disease (e.g. glomerulonephritis including IgA-related, membranous, mesangiocapillary, focal and minimal change)
  - Systemic vasculitis* (e.g. SLE, polyarteritis nodosa, Wegener granulomatosis)
  - Malignancy* (e.g. renal cell carcinoma—Wilms tumour)
  - Structural (e.g. polycystic kidney disease)
  - Papillary necrosis (e.g. diabetic nephrosclerosis, pyelonephritis, analgesic nephropathy)
  - Hereditary (e.g. Alport syndrome)
- **Coagulopathy:**
  - Anticoagulation*
  - Inherited defect* (e.g. haemophilia, von Willebrand disease)
  - Acquired defect* (e.g. thrombocytopenia, DIC)
- **Free haemoglobin or myoglobin:**
  - Haemoglobinuria* (intravascular haemolysis)
  - Myoglobinuria* (rhabdomyolysis, crush injury, electrocution)
- **Factitious:**
  - Foods and colourings (e.g. beetroot, rhubarb, blackberries)
  - Drugs (senna, doxorubicin, vitamin B12, rifampicin—dark orange)

Major threat to life

- Hypovolaemic shock
- Renal tract obstruction with urosepsis

Bedside

Quick-look test

Does the patient look well (comfortable), sick (uncomfortable or distressed) or critical (about to die)?

Patients may be agitated if ureteric or urinary obstruction is present, but are usually otherwise well.

Selective history and chart review

What are the vital signs?

- Occasionally hypovolaemia secondary to blood loss causes tachycardia and hypotension.
- Fever and/or hypotension may indicate an infectious cause.
- Acute anaemia causes tachypnoea and restlessness from hypoxia.

Is there a history or family history of bleeding problems or renal disease?

Is there a past history or risk factors for renal tract stones?

- Risk factors for renal tract stones include dehydration, hypercalcaemia, hypercalciuria, hyperoxaluria, cystinuria and recent UTI.

Are there any risk factors for renal tract neoplasm?

- Occupational exposure to aniline dyes or rubbing compounds, cigarette smoking, prior pelvic irradiation, analgesic misuse.

Is the patient on medication that causes bleeding?

- Anticoagulants such as heparin, warfarin or a NOAC.
- Antiplatelet agents such as aspirin, clopidogrel, prasugrel, ticagrelor or glycoprotein IIb/IIIa inhibitors (e.g. abciximab, eptifibatide or tirofiban).
- Recent thrombolysis (e.g. with tenecteplase or tPA).

Does the patient have an indwelling urinary catheter?

- Look for documentation of traumatic or multiple attempts at insertion if the IDC is recent.
- Consider infection if the IDC has been in place for more than 2–3 days.

What are the latest laboratory results?

- Review recent laboratory results and urine output. Note the haemoglobin, platelet count and coagulation profile, U&E plus urine microscopy and culture.

Selective physical examination

Vital signs	Repeat now for evidence of hypoxia or hypovolaemia
Mental status	Confusion, delirium (infection, hypovolaemia)
CVS	Cool, clammy skin (hypovolaemia)
	Tachycardia, hypotension (hypovolaemia, infection)
Resp	Tachypnoea (sepsis, pain)
Abdo	Palpable mass (polycystic kidney disease, tumour, enlarged bladder)
GU	Flank tenderness (pyelonephritis, renal stone, obstruction, sickle cell crisis)
	Urethra—blood at meatus following recent instrumentation
Skin	Bruising, petechiae, telangiectasia may be associated with coagulation disorder, including thrombocytopenia, or vasculitis
	Pallor (anaemia)

Investigations
Urinalysis
- Perform a bedside dipstick urinalysis and send sample for MCS:
  - RBC casts and glomerular-origin RBCs with >70% dysmorphic (glomerulonephritis)
  - WBCs or bacteria (infection)
  - Red discolouration of urine and dipstick positive for blood, but with no RBCs on microscopy, indicates haemoglobinuria from haemolysis, or myoglobinuria (check a CK).

Serum
- Send blood for FBC, U&E and coagulation profile as clinically indicated:
  - Raised WCC associated with infection and inflammation
  - Deranged clotting studies and reduced platelet count associated with bleeding diathesis and/or anticoagulant therapy.

Radiology
- Abdominal X-ray (KUB).
  - Although >80% of renal tract calculi are radiodense, their anatomical renal tract location must still be confirmed.
- CT or ultrasound is indicated to investigate the renal tract, which may be arranged for the morning if the patient is otherwise stable and comfortable.

Management

Immediate management of serious symptoms
- Attach continuous non-invasive ECG, BP and pulse oximeter monitoring to the patient.

SECTION C – Common calls

- Commence oxygen therapy to maintain oxygen saturation >94%.
- Insert a large-bore (14–16G) peripheral cannula, draw and send blood.
- Commence fluid resuscitation to maintain normotension and normovolaemia.
- Commence antibiotics for pyelonephritis such as gentamicin 5 mg/kg once-daily (less in elderly patients) plus ampicillin 2 g IV QID.

Renal colic

- Renal and ureteric calculi cause loin-to-groin pain, haematuria, urinary frequency, ureteric obstruction or infection.
- Although most stones pass spontaneously, commence IV fluids.
- If the pain is significant, give morphine 0.1 mg/kg IV with an antiemetic such as metoclopramide 10 mg IV.
- Follow this with indomethacin 100 mg PR, or an oral NSAID, provided there is no renal impairment, active peptic ulcer disease or asthma.
- Call the urological surgeon immediately if there is evidence of urosepsis with stone disease.
- Otherwise, surgical removal, basket extraction, lithotripsy or stenting may be required if the stone has not passed within a few days, or if it is causing recurring pain or obstruction with hydronephrosis.

Decreased urine output and acute kidney injury

Decreased urine output results from pre-renal, renal or post-renal causes. An assessment of fluid balance, as well as volume status, is necessary to establish the cause.

Phone call

Questions

1. **How much urine has been passed in the past 24 hours?** Oliguria is defined as a urine output of <400 mL/day (<20 mL/h) and may be the earliest sign of impaired renal function. Complete anuria suggests a mechanical obstruction of the bladder outlet, a blocked IDC or an obstructed single kidney.
2. **Is the patient complaining of abdominal pain?** Generalised lower abdominal pain is associated with an acutely distended bladder with urinary retention.
3. **What are the vital signs?**
4. **Does the patient have an indwelling urinary catheter?** The assessment of urine output is most accurate if the patient has an IDC. Blockage of an IDC is an important cause of post-renal oliguria or anuria.
5. **What was the reason for admission?**

Instructions

- If an IDC is in place and the patient is anuric, ask the nurse to flush the catheter with 20–30 mL normal saline to dislodge sediment or clots and restore patency.
- Request blood for FBC, U&E and creatinine:
  - A serum potassium level of >5.5 mmol/L indicates hyperkalaemia (see Chapter 43).
  - Elevated serum urea and creatinine levels and their ratio are a guideline to assessing the degree of renal insufficiency.

Prioritisation

- Urgently assess a patient with painful urinary retention, with a urine output <20 mL/h or daily urine output of <400 mL. Oliguria or anuria may be a sign of acute kidney injury (AKI) [acute renal failure], which can cause dangerous hyperkalaemia and fluid overload.
- Otherwise, the assessment of decreased urine output can wait if problems of a higher priority exist, provided the patient is not in pain and that a recent serum potassium level is not elevated.

Corridor thoughts

What are the causes of a reduced urine output? (* = major threat to life)

Pre-renal

- **Absolute decrease in circulating blood volume**, leading to pre-renal hypoperfusion:
  - Inadequate fluid intake (e.g. after surgery)
  - Increased loss of blood or fluids*
    - Haemorrhage (traumatic and non-traumatic, internal or external)
    - Burns, erythroderma, hyperthermia
    - GI fluid loss: vomiting, diarrhoea, NG suction
    - Renal loss: diuretics, glycosuria
  - Third spacing of fluid* (e.g. pancreatitis, bowel obstruction)
- **Cardiac pump failure:**
  - MI (cardiogenic shock)*, CCF*
- **Effective decrease in blood volume (vasodilation):**
  - Sepsis*, anaphylaxis*, neurogenic
  - Vasodilatory drugs, anaesthetic agents
- **Obstruction to circulation:**
  - Constrictive pericarditis, cardiac tamponade*, PE*
- **Locally reduced renal perfusion:**
  - Renal artery or renal vein occlusion secondary to thrombosis or stenosis
  - Noradrenaline, adrenaline
  - NSAIDs, ACE inhibitors

Renal

- **Acute tubular necrosis (ATN)*:**
  - Usually secondary to pre-renal causes with continuing intravascular depletion, hypotension and renal ischaemia
  - Medications (e.g. aminoglycosides, amphotericin B, IV contrast, chemotherapy)

- Poisons (e.g. ethylene glycol, mercury, carbon tetrachloride)
- Endogenous substances (e.g. myoglobin, Bence–Jones protein, amyloid)
- **Glomerulonephritis (GN)*:**
  - Diabetes mellitus with basement membrane thickening and glomerular sclerosis, neoplasia
  - Connective tissue disease (e.g. scleroderma, SLE)
  - Vasculitis (e.g. polyarteritis nodosa, Wegener granulomatosis)
  - Infection (e.g. post-streptococcal, malaria, hepatitis B, HIV)
  - Medications (e.g. gold, penicillamine)
  - Immune (e.g. IgA nephropathy—Berger's disease, Henoch–Schönlein purpura, Goodpasture's syndrome)
  - Genetic (e.g. Alport's syndrome, with hearing loss)
- **Interstitial nephritis*:**
  - Infection (e.g. pyelonephritis, viral, fungal)
  - Medications (e.g. NSAIDs, penicillins, cephalosporins, sulfonamides, ciprofloxacin, rifampicin)
  - Malignancy (e.g. lymphoma or leukaemia)
  - Systemic disorder (SLE, sarcoidosis, hypercalcaemia)

Post-renal

- **Upper renal tract obstruction (bilateral ureteric obstruction or ureteric obstruction of a single kidney):**
  - Stone, blood clot, sloughed papilla (single kidney)
  - Retroperitoneal fibrosis*, retroperitoneal tumour*
- **Lower urinary tract obstruction (bladder outlet obstruction):**
  - Prostatic hypertrophy, carcinoma of the cervix*
  - Stone, blood clot, urethral stricture
- **Blocked indwelling urinary catheter**

Major threat to life

- **Hypotension and shock**
  - Urine output is one of three clinical indicators of end-organ perfusion, together with mental status and skin colour/temperature.
  - A reduced urine output may be the earliest manifestation of shock; conversely, return of urine output >0.5 mL/kg/h signifies restoration of adequate renal perfusion.
- **Oliguric acute renal failure**
  - Decreased urine output associated with oliguric renal failure may be associated with an acute life threat from hyperkalaemia, hypertension or acute pulmonary oedema.
- **Sequelae of acute renal failure**
  - **Hyperkalaemia** (cardiac arrhythmias, muscle weakness, paralysis)

- **Metabolic acidosis** (Kussmaul's respirations, raised anion gap)
- **Acute hypertension** (see Chapter 19)
- **Pulmonary oedema** secondary to salt and water retention.

Bedside

Quick-look test

Does the patient look well (comfortable), sick (uncomfortable or distressed) or critical (about to die)?
- A sick or critical-looking patient suggests a systemic or renal cause for the reduced urinary output.
- A restless patient with abdominal discomfort, agitation and a sensation of needing to pass urine suggests an acutely distended bladder.
- Occasionally, urinary retention and/or a reduced urine output produce few or no obvious problems.

Airway and vital signs

What is the heart rate and blood pressure?
- Look for evidence of dehydration causing pre-renal hypoperfusion. A rise in heart rate of >20 beats/min, a fall in SBP >20 mmHg or any fall in DBP on standing suggest significant hypovolaemia.
- A resting tachycardia alone may be related to a decreased intravascular volume, the pain of a distended bladder or infection.
- Acute hypertension with oedema may result from acute glomerulonephritis.

What is the temperature?
- Fever suggests sepsis secondary to a UTI, pyelonephritis or systemic bacteraemia.

Selective history and chart review

- Review the patient's history and hospital course, looking for factors that predispose to pre-renal, renal or post-renal causes of decreased urine output with AKI (see *Corridor thoughts*).
- Review the nursing observations and fluid balance chart for fluctuations in fluid intake, urine output and body weight.
- Look carefully at the medication chart in particular:
  - Search for any nephrotoxic drugs, especially in combinations such as an ACE inhibitor with a diuretic and NSAID; an aminoglycoside with amphotericin B; IV contrast material with an ACE inhibitor; or a patient in CCF given a NSAID.

- Does the onset coincide with the commencement of a nephrotoxic drug?
- Potassium supplements will worsen hyperkalaemia.
- Look for recent blood urea and creatinine values:
  - A urea-to-creatinine ratio >20 with urine specific gravity of >1.020 or urine sodium concentration of <20 mmol/L suggest a pre-renal cause.
  - A urea-to-creatinine ratio <10 with urine specific gravity of <1.020 or urine sodium concentration of >20 mmol/L suggest a renal cause, such as ATN.

Selective physical examination

Examine for pre-renal (volume status), renal or post-renal (obstructive) causes of decreased urine output. Remember that more than one cause can be present.

Vital signs	Repeat now
	Skin temperature and colour
	Tachycardia or postural BP changes (dehydration)
	Hypertension
Mental status	Altered mental status (cerebral hypoperfusion, uraemic encephalopathy)
HEENT	Jaundice (hepatorenal syndrome)
	Scleroderma facies
	Dry tongue and mucous membranes (dehydration)
Resp	Basal crepitations, pleural effusions (CCF)
	Tachypnoea (CCF or compensatory hyperventilation in metabolic acidosis)
	Pleuritic chest pain (uraemia, SLE, neoplasm)
CVS	Pulse volume
	JVP (elevated with CCF; flat neck veins with dehydration)
	Pericardial friction rub (uraemia, SLE, neoplasm)
GIT	Enlarged kidneys (hydronephrosis secondary to obstruction, polycystic kidney disease)
	Enlarged bladder (bladder outlet obstruction, blocked IDC, neurogenic bladder)
Rectal	Enlarged prostate gland (bladder outlet obstruction)
Pelvic	Cervical or adnexal masses (ureteric obstruction secondary to cervical, uterine or ovarian cancer)
Skin	Rash (acute interstitial nephritis)
	Livedo reticularis on lower extremities (hypoperfusion, embolic renal failure)
	Pruritic excoriation (uraemia, drug rash)

SECTION C – Common calls

Investigations

- Take blood for FBC, U&E and blood glucose:
  - Urea and electrolytes—look for hyperkalaemia in both acute and chronic renal failure. A normal Hb is consistent with acute renal impairment, and a low Hb with chronic renal impairment (or acute blood loss).
- LFTs, autoantibodies etc—according to suspected underlying causes.
- Check VBG for a raised anion gap metabolic acidosis from uraemia.
- Perform an ECG.
  - Check for signs of hyperkalaemia such as peaked T waves, depressed ST segments, prolonged PR interval, loss of P waves and wide QRS complexes.
  - Look for evidence of MI or the widespread concave elevation of pericarditis.
- Perform a bedside bladder scan to measure the residual bladder volume in obstruction.
- Collect urine for dipstick analysis and send to laboratory for MCS including cells and casts, plus urinary electrolyte testing.
  - **Specific gravity (SG)**
    - SG >1.025: highly concentrated urine associated with dehydration and pre-renal failure
    - SG 1.010: may be associated with chronic renal disease
    - SG <1.005: inability to concentrate urine (ATN, pyelonephritis).
  - **Haematuria** (stone disease, pyelonephritis, GN with >70% dysmorphic RBC)
  - **Proteinuria** (nephrotic syndrome, GN, pyelonephritis, CCF, myeloma)
  - **Leucocytes and nitrites** (UTI, pyelonephritis)
  - **Urine microscopy**
    - Leucocytes, Gram-stained organisms, erythrocytes, epithelial cells
    - RBC casts are diagnostic of GN
    - WBC casts (especially eosinophil casts) are seen in acute interstitial nephritis
    - Pigmented granular casts are seen with ATN
    - Oval fat bodies are suggestive of nephrotic syndrome.

Management

Immediate management
Monitor vital signs and fluid balance

- Commence oxygen therapy to maintain saturation >94%.
- Attach continuous non-invasive ECG, BP and pulse oximeter monitoring to the patient.

- Insert an IDC to accurately monitor fluid balance.
  - Lower urinary tract obstruction is recognised (and treated) by the passage of an IDC.
    - If there has been bladder outlet obstruction, the initial urine volume on catheterisation is usually >400 mL and the patient experiences immediate relief.
    - After catheterisation for urinary retention, watch for a post-obstructive diuresis by measuring urine volumes hourly.
- Flush a blocked IDC with 20–30 mL sterile normal saline. This resolves an intraluminal blockage causing anuria from post-renal obstruction.

Identify and treat life-threatening complications

- **Severe hyperkalaemia** (see Chapter 43)
  - Give 10% calcium chloride 10 mL IV over 2–5 minutes to provide immediate cardioprotection to prevent cardiac arrest.
    - Calcium temporarily relieves the adverse cardiac and neuromuscular effects of hyperkalaemia. It does *not* lower the potassium (K^+) level.
    - The onset of protection is immediate, and its effect lasts up to 1 hour.
  - Reduce the serum potassium level.
    - Give 50 mL of 50% dextrose IV with 10 units of soluble insulin over 20 minutes. This shifts extracellular K^+ intracellularly within 15 minutes, and lasts 1–2 hours.
    - Give salbutamol 5–10 mg nebulised, or 250–500 micrograms salbutamol IV slowly, which temporarily reduces serum K^+ by shifting K^+ intracellularly. Repeat doses may be given.
    - Give 8.4% sodium bicarbonate ($NaHCO_3^-$) 50 mL IV over 5 minutes if the patient is acidotic, provided there is no volume overload. This works best in combination with dextrose/insulin therapy and salbutamol, and its effect lasts 1–2 hours.
    - Follow up with potassium exchange resin: calcium resonium 30 g PO or by enema. Other than diuretics, this is the only drug treatment that actually removes K^+ from the total body pool, but it takes 1–3 hours to take effect.
  - Arrange urgent dialysis if the patient remains hyperkalaemic, severely acidotic and/or volume overloaded.
- **Hypotension and intravascular depletion**
  - Restore the intravascular volume with normal saline in pre-renal failure. Give an IV fluid bolus of 20 mL/kg normal saline, repeated as necessary.
  - Observe the effect of this fluid challenge on the pulse, JVP, BP and urine output, aiming to optimise renal perfusion by reversing hypovolaemia.

- **Acute pulmonary oedema**
  - Sit the patient upright and give 40–60% oxygen.
  - Give GTN 300–600 micrograms SL every 5–10 minutes as required. Remove the tablet if excessive hypotension (SBP <100 mmHg) occurs.
  - Give 40–80 mg frusemide IV, provided pre-renal perfusion is normal.
  - Consider CPAP and/or IV GTN. Consult your senior doctor.
  - Monitor diuresis with hourly urine measures and frequent checks of vital signs.
  - Arrange urgent dialysis if the patient remains volume overloaded, severely acidotic and/or hyperkalaemic.

Further management
Identify and cease all inappropriate medications
These will include:
- Potassium supplements and potassium-sparing diuretics
- NSAIDs, ACE inhibitors
  - Make sure to leave a clear message why in the notes for the usual medical team
- Reduce the dose of renally excreted medications that cannot be stopped immediately (e.g. aminoglycosides).

Consider dialysis (haemodialysis or peritoneal)
Consult your senior and call the ICU for the following indications for dialysis:
- Hyperkalaemia (> 6.5 mmol/L) refractory to conventional therapy
- Severe and symptomatic metabolic acidosis (pH <7.1)
- Fluid overload unresponsive to diuretics
- Uraemic encephalopathy with symptoms of decreased mental status, obtundation and seizures, or uraemic pericarditis.

30

Frequency and polyuria

It is often difficult to differentiate between polyuria and frequency, and in many elderly patients either of these problems may present as incontinence. Increased urine output is an uncommon emergency call alone, but may be described in association with other symptoms.

Phone call

Questions

1. **What problem is present? Polyuria** refers to a urine output >3 L/ day recognised on review of the fluid balance chart. **Frequency** of urination refers to the frequent passage of urine, whether of large or small volume. It may occur with polyuria and/or be associated with dysuria or urinary incontinence.
2. **What are the vital signs?**
3. **Is the patient catheterised?**
4. **What was the reason for admission?**

Instructions

- In a patient with mental state changes, or who is sick:
  - Request insertion of an IDC if one is not already in place.
  - Ask for an IV trolley for the patient's bedside to await your arrival.
  - Check fingerprick BGL.
  - Collect and send serum for FBC, U&E and LFTs.
  - Collect a urine sample, perform bedside urinalysis and prepare sample to send for MCS and urinary electrolyte analysis.
- Commence volume replacement with an initial bolus of 10–20 mL/kg normal saline if the patient has signs of volume depletion.

Prioritisation

- See the patient immediately if there are significant changes in vital signs, mental status or features of dehydration.

- Otherwise a patient with polyuria, frequency or incontinence need not be seen urgently if the vital signs are stable.

Corridor thoughts

What are the potential causes of increased urine output? (* = major threat to life)
- **Polyuria:**
  - **Diabetes mellitus**
    - Glucose is passed in the urine, causing an osmotic diuresis.
  - **Diabetes insipidus (DI)**
    - Caused by either reduced ADH secretion (central DI) or failure of the kidneys to respond to ADH (nephrogenic DI).
    - Both result in inability to reabsorb water in the distal renal tubule, associated with massive urine output of 5–10 L/day.
    - DI is most commonly associated with head trauma*, cerebral oedema* (late finding and/or after treatment), pituitary tumours*, prescribed medication and occasionally after neurosurgical procedures.
    - In up to 25% of cases no cause is found (idiopathic).
  - Drugs
    - Diuretics, mannitol
    - Lithium toxicity, amphotericin B, demeclocycline (nephrogenic DI)
  - Renal disease
    - Diuretic phase of acute tubular necrosis
    - Postobstructive diuresis
    - Salt-losing nephritis
    - Polycystic kidney disease (causes nephrogenic DI)
  - Hypercalcaemia* (nephrogenic DI)
  - Hypokalaemia (nephrogenic DI)
  - Physiological diuresis
    - Follows large volumes of PO or IV fluids during the resolution phase of major illness, or during recovery from major surgery.
  - Primary, psychogenic polydipsia
    - A psychiatric diagnosis after excluding the conditions above, sometimes associated with phenothiazine use.
- **Increased frequency:**
  - Urinary tract infection
  - Partial bladder outlet obstruction (e.g. prostatism)
  - Bladder irritation (tumour, stone, infection)
  - Large fluid intake
  - Psychological

- Incontinence:
  - **Urge incontinence**
    - Caused by UTI, diabetes mellitus, urolithiasis, dementia, stroke, normal pressure hydrocephalus, BPH, pelvic tumour, depression, anxiety.
  - **Stress incontinence**
    - Usually in multiparous women, caused by lax pelvic bladder support. In men, it occurs after prostate surgery.
  - **Overflow incontinence**
    - Caused by bladder outlet obstruction such as BPH, urethral stricture, spinal cord disease, autonomic neuropathy, faecal impaction (*always* do a PR examination).
  - **Iatrogenic factors**
    - Diuretics, sedatives, anticholinergic drugs, alpha-blockers, calcium-channel blockers, ACE inhibitors.
  - **Environmental factors**
    - Inaccessible call bell, poor mobility, obstacles to the bathroom.

Major threat to life

- **Severe hypernatraemia associated with DI** (see Chapter 42)
- **Intravascular volume depletion** leading to hypovolaemic shock
- **Diabetic ketoacidosis**—new diagnosis or in known diabetic patient (see Chapter 41)
- **High-output renal failure**

Bedside

Quick-look test

Does the patient look well (comfortable), sick (uncomfortable or distressed) or critical (about to die)?
- Most patients with polyuria, frequency or incontinence look well. Patients who look sick or critical often have intravascular volume depletion, or may be septic.
- If the patient looks unwell, search for a previously unrecognised condition.
- Similarly, look for a UTI in a patient with frequency or incontinence.

Airway and vital signs

What are the heart rate and blood pressure?
- Look for signs of dehydration with intravascular volume depletion such as a resting tachycardia or hypotension (SBP <90 mmHg).

- Examine for postural changes if the HR and BP are normal at rest. A rise in HR >20 beats/min, a fall in SBP >20 mmHg or any fall in DBP indicates hypovolaemia.

Does the patient have a fever?
- Fever suggests possible UTI.

Management

Immediate management

- Attach continuous non-invasive ECG, BP and pulse oximeter monitoring to the patient.
- Commence oxygen therapy to maintain oxygen saturation >94%.
- Insert a large-bore (14–16G) peripheral cannula; send blood samples for FBC, U&E and calcium. Add blood cultures if suspicious of sepsis.
- Dipstick the urine for sugar and ketones. Send an MSU for microscopy, culture and sensitivity, as well as urinary sodium and osmolarity.
- Commence fluid resuscitation to maintain normotension and normovolaemia.
- Give a 20 mL/kg normal saline bolus for acute volume depletion.
- Observe the effect of this fluid challenge on the BP.
- A patient with significant polyuria will require further IV fluid to balance the urinary losses and maintain normotension.
- Replace potassium according to U&E results.
- Watch for complications, such as pulmonary oedema from excessive fluid resuscitation.

Selective history and chart review

- **Polyuria**
  - Ask about associated symptoms such as polydipsia in diabetes mellitus, DI, hypercalcaemia or compulsive water drinking (primary, psychogenic polydipsia).
  - Review the medication chart for causative medications:
    - Lithium, amphotericin B and demeclocycline (nephrogenic DI).
      Note: in view of its effect on the kidney, demeclocycline is actually used therapeutically to treat hyponatraemia in SIADH.
    - Diuretics.
  - Check for recent laboratory results:
    - Blood glucose and bicarbonate (diabetes mellitus)
    - Hypokalaemia and hypercalcaemia (important reversible causes of nephrogenic DI).

- **Frequency**
  - Ask about associated symptoms:
    - — Fever, dysuria, haematuria and bad-smelling urine suggest UTI.
  - Poor stream, hesitancy, terminal dribbling and nocturia suggest prostatism.
- **Incontinence**
  - Directly question the patient as to when the incontinence occurs (i.e. what type).

Selective physical examination

Vitals	Repeat now; look for signs of tachycardia or postural BP changes (hypovolaemia)
	Fever (UTI, urosepsis)
Mental status	Altered mental status (decreased cerebral perfusion, sepsis, intracranial pathology)
HEENT	Dry mucous membranes and flat neck veins (dehydration)
	Visual field abnormality (pituitary tumour)
	Papilloedema (increased intracranial pressure)
Resp	Kussmaul's breathing (deep, sighing respirations from metabolic acidosis in DKA, or uraemia)
	Ketotic breath (DKA)
Abdo	Enlarged palpable bladder (bladder outlet obstruction with overflow incontinence, neurogenic bladder)
	Suprapubic tenderness (UTI, cystitis)
Rectal	Enlarged prostate or pelvic mass (bladder outlet obstruction)
Neuro	Focal neurological signs
	Perform a complete neurological examination, particularly for altered perineal sensation, abnormal anal tone or (bilateral) leg weakness suggesting a neurogenic bladder
Skin	Perineal skin breakdown (a complication of repeated incontinence and a source of infection)

Investigations
- Send blood for U&E looking for evidence of renal dysfunction (urea and creatinine), hypokalaemia or hypercalcaemia.
- Serum glucose or fingerprick blood glucose testing.
- **Urinalysis:**
  - Urine sodium
    - — >40 mmol/L: acute tubular necrosis
    - — <40 mmol/L: pre-renal failure and dehydration
    - — <10 mmol/L: diabetes insipidus

- Specific gravity (SG)
  - Very low (SG <1.010): diabetes insipidus
  - High (SG >1.020): dehydration
- RBCs associated with UTI or urolithiasis
- Abnormal RBCs >70% dysmorphic (glomerular disease)
- Glucose or ketones.

Specific management

What else needs to be done on call?
- **Polyuria**
  - Once intravascular volume has been restored, ensure adequate continuing replacement fluid (usually IV) estimated by urine output, insensible loss (400–800 mL/day) and other losses such as NG suction, vomiting and diarrhoea.
  - Start a strict fluid balance chart with daily weight.
  - Review serum and urine results:
    - Replace potassium as required and manage hypercalcaemia (see Chapter 44)
    - Manage serum hyperglycaemia (see diabetic ketoacidosis in Chapter 41).
  - Cease all non-essential medications that may be implicated in nephrogenic DI. Check no diuretic is being given in the evenings.
- **Frequency**
  - Commence trimethoprim 300 mg PO once daily or cephalexin 500 mg PO every 6 hours for uncomplicated cystitis (i.e. no evidence of upper UTI, no evidence of prostatitis, no renal disease and no recent urinary tract instrumentation); usually caused by *Escherichia coli* or sometimes *Staphylococcus saprophyticus.*
  - Catheterise the bladder for suspected partial bladder outlet obstruction.
  - Other causes of frequency, such as bladder irritation by stones or tumours, can wait until the morning.
  - Organise an early morning urine specimen.
- **Incontinence**
  - Check for UTI, hyperglycaemia, hypokalaemia and hypercalcaemia if there is also polyuria, as these may present as incontinence in an elderly or bedridden patient.
  - Arrange specialist consult for a neurogenic bladder—urgent if cauda equina compression is suspected.
  - Differentiate overflow caused by bladder outlet obstruction (e.g. BPH, uterine prolapse) from impaired detrusor contraction (e.g. LMN bladder).

- Urge incontinence is the most common cause of incontinence in the elderly population, manifested by involuntary micturition preceded by a warning of a few seconds or minutes only.
- Ensure that there are no physical barriers preventing the patient from reaching the bathroom or commode and check that there is easy access to the call bell.
- Arrange for occupational therapy to address medical disabilities in the morning.
- Consider a temporary IDC or condom catheter to allow skin healing in patients with perineal skin breakdown.

31

Leg pain

Most leg pain originates from the joints, bones, muscles or the vascular supply; however, there are several causes of referred leg pain.

Phone call

Questions
1. Which part of the leg hurts?
2. Is the leg swollen or discoloured?
3. What are the vital signs?
4. Was the pain sudden in onset?
5. Is there a history of prior chronic leg pain?
6. What was the reason for admission?
7. Has there been a recent injury or fracture?
8. Does the patient have a leg cast on? Leg pain after an injury or a fracture, or with a cast, suggests the possibility of compartment syndrome or DVT.

Prioritisation
An acutely pulseless limb, significant pain, new-onset tense swelling, increasing leg pain within 24–48 hours of a cast, associated SOB or fever require immediate assessment.

Corridor thoughts

What causes leg pain? (* = major threat to life)
- Vascular causes:
  - Arterial disease
    - Acute arterial insufficiency* (e.g. embolic, dissection, false aneurysm)
    - Chronic arterial insufficiency (arteriosclerosis obliterans)
    - Buerger's disease (thrombo-angiitis obliterans)
  - Venous disease
    - DVT
    - Superficial thrombophlebitis

- **Bone and joint disease:**
  - Arthritis
    - Septic*: *Staphylococcus aureus, Neisseria gonorrhoeae, Streptococcus pyogenes* and Gram-negative bacilli
    - Inflammatory: gout, pseudogout, RA, SLE
    - Degenerative: osteoarthritis
  - Osteomyelitis
  - Bone or muscle tumour
  - Lumbar disc disease (referred sciatica)
- **Muscle, soft-tissue or nerve pain:**
  - Cellulitis
  - Compartment syndrome*
  - Fasciitis*, pyomyositis*, myonecrosis*
  - Ruptured Baker's cyst (behind the knee; it mimics a DVT, which must be excluded first)
  - Diabetic neuropathy or amyotrophy
  - Reflex sympathetic dystrophy syndrome (Sudeck's dystrophy)
  - Erythema nodosum
  - Benign nocturnal leg cramps (Ekbom's syndrome—'restless legs')

Major threat to life

- **Acute arterial insufficiency with potential loss of limb**
  - Acute arterial occlusion results in gangrene in as little as 6 hours if untreated.
- **PE from DVT**
  - DVT may lead to severe respiratory insufficiency or sudden death if PE occurs.
- **Necrotising fasciitis, pyomyositis and myonecrosis**
  - Rapidly spreading infection may cause septic shock.
- **Septic arthritis**
  - Unrecognised septic arthritis can result in permanent joint damage.
- **Compartment syndrome**
  - Compartment syndrome causes ischaemic muscle damage within hours, leading to permanent contractures.

Bedside

Quick-look test

Does the patient look well (comfortable), sick (uncomfortable or distressed) or critical (about to die)?
A patient with significant leg pain lies still and is reluctant to move the affected limb. Patients with overwhelming local or systemic sepsis look

sick, and patients with ischaemia or DVT look uncomfortable and/or distressed.

Airway and vital signs

Leg pain rarely affects the vital signs. However, abnormal vital signs provide clues to the underlying cause.

What is the heart rate? Is it regular or irregular?
- Pain from any cause may result in tachycardia.
- An irregular rhythm suggests AF, with the possibility of arterial embolism.

What is the blood pressure?
- Pain or anxiety from any cause may raise the BP.
- Hypotension is associated with systemic sepsis, or may precipitate acute arterial insufficiency in a chronically ischaemic leg.

What is the respiratory rate?
- Sudden SOB and tachypnoea suggest a PE from a DVT.

What is the temperature?
- Fever suggests infection such as septic arthritis, fasciitis, pyomyositis or an inflammatory myonecrosis.
- A DVT can cause a low-grade raised temperature.

Selective history and chart review

Perform a systematic inspection in a patient with leg pain, looking for evidence of any of the five major threats that require emergency treatment on call (see *Major threat to life*).

Which part of the leg is painful?
- Sudden-onset severe leg pain may indicate arterial or venous compromise, injury or an acute lumbar disc herniation.
- Pain in a joint may indicate an inflammatory or infectious process.
- Pain in the calf suggests DVT or compartment syndrome.

Are there any associated colour or temperature changes?
- Does the patient have a prior history of leg pain? Is the current pain similar to or worse than previous episodes?
- Patients with atherosclerosis of the leg arteries may have a history of intermittent claudication, or resting leg or foot pain.
- Patients with inflammatory or degenerative conditions often have a history of chronic pain.
- More severe or a new/different pain necessitates re-examination of the leg.

Does the patient have any risk factors for developing DVT? (see Box 31.1)
- Patients who have had a prior DVT are at increased risk of recurrence.
- Patients with a malignancy, cardiorespiratory disease, who are bedridden or have had surgery, are pregnant or have a

BOX 31.1 Predisposing risk factors for deep vein thrombosis (DVT)

Stasis
- Prolonged bed rest
- Immobilisation
- Congestive cardiac failure
- Pregnancy (especially postpartum)
- Recent long-haul travel (>5000 km)

Hypercoagulability
- Malignancy
- Inflammatory bowel disease
- Nephrotic syndrome
- Polycythaemia rubra vera
- Antiphospholipid syndrome
- Deficiencies of antithrombin III, protein C or S
- Factor V Leiden mutation

Vein injury
- Trauma or fracture of lower limbs or pelvis
- Surgery, particularly abdominal, pelvic or leg

Other
- Age >50 years
- Oestrogen therapy (particularly within past 2 weeks)
- Intravascular device (e.g. venous catheter)

pro-coagulant state are also at increased risk of venous thromboembolism.

Does the patient have any significant past medical history?
- A history of underlying cardiac disease (e.g. AF, ventricular aneurysm, prosthetic heart valve) predisposes to arterial embolisation or insufficiency.
- Patients with diabetes mellitus may develop arterial insufficiency, cellulitis, ulcer disease, osteomyelitis and painful peripheral neuropathy.

Review the medication chart
- Check whether the patient has been prescribed thromboprophylaxis, such as LMWH, if confined to bed or postoperative (risk of DVT).
- Check whether the patient is on oestrogen therapy (risk of DVT).

Selective physical examination
The focused examination is directed towards recognising potential life threats, localising the site of leg pain and looking for signs of arterial insufficiency, venous disease, infection and inflammation.

SECTION C – Common calls

Vitals	Repeat now; look for signs of fever (infection or DVT), tachypnoea (sepsis or PE from DVT) and hypotension (shock)
Resp	Listen for a friction rub or evidence of pleural effusion (PE)
CVS	Irregular pulse (AF) and metallic click on auscultation (prosthetic heart valve) increase the risk of arterial embolisation
Limb	Examine both the affected and the unaffected limbs and compare
	Look for localised or generalised swelling
	Measure the girth of the calf and thigh, and compare with the other leg

- Look for erythema, cyanotic changes, pallor and mottling.
- Feel for temperature change, oedema and subcutaneous crepitus (secondary to gas formation in gas gangrene—an extreme emergency).
- Palpate the femoral, popliteal, dorsalis pedis and posterior tibial pulses and record if absent (arterial insufficiency).
- Examine for tenderness, sensory function and motor strength.
- Examine each joint for erythema, swelling or deformity. Feel for warmth and crepitus, and record the amount of active and passive movement in degrees.

Management

Specific management
Acute arterial insufficiency
Selective physical examination
- Look for the **six Ps** that indicate acute arterial occlusion:
  - **P**ain—an early sign of ischaemia, particularly on passive movement
  - **P**allor—also an early sign of ischaemia
  - **P**ulselessness—distant to the site of occlusion; indicates large arterial occlusion
  - **P**araesthesiae—sensory change in the ischaemic region usually associated with reduced light-touch sensation or two-point discrimination
  - **P**aralysis—late finding associated with established ischaemic tissue damage
  - **P**erishing cold (compare other limb).
- Thus, acute arterial embolism causes unilateral pain, pallor, pulselessness, paresthesiae, paralysis and perishing cold.
- Chronic arterial insufficiency caused by arteriosclerosis obliterans (peripheral vascular disease) usually involves both legs with

bilaterally reduced pulses, trophic skin changes, including loss of limb hair, and dependent rubor (redness).
- Fresh thrombosis, as well as a fixed atherosclerotic plaque, may completely obstruct arterial flow, which then results in an acute-on-chronic presentation.

Management
- Acute arterial insufficiency is a vascular surgical emergency:
  - Notify your senior and the vascular surgeon.
  - Administer oxygen and attach a pulse oximeter to the patient.
  - Gain IV access and send blood for FBC, U&E, coagulation profile and G&H.
  - Begin heparin 80 U/kg IV bolus if there are no contraindications, followed by a maintenance infusion of 18 U/kg/h titrated to an aPTT that is 1.5–2.5-fold the control value by 4–6 hours.
  - The patient will require emergency thrombectomy or vessel bypass if limb viability is threatened.
- Give a patient with chronic intermittent claudication and pain at rest a non-narcotic analgesic, such as paracetamol 1 g PO every 6 hours, and place the affected leg more dependent.
- Commence a platelet inhibitor, such as aspirin 150 mg once daily, if not already prescribed. More definitive therapy such as lumbar sympathectomy or direct arterial surgery can be discussed electively with the usual medical team.
- A patient with an acute thrombosis, as well as long-standing arteriosclerosis obliterans, may require direct intra-arterial thrombolysis under the guidance of a vascular surgeon.

Deep vein thrombosis
Ask about predisposing causes (see Box 31.1) and examine for local signs.

Selective physical examination
- Look for unilateral limb oedema, erythema, warmth, superficial venous dilation, increased girth and tenderness along the deep venous system.
- Cellulitis, musculoskeletal injury and varicose vein insufficiency have some similar features, but DVT should be considered first.
- New-onset oedema may be subtle and is best appreciated by measuring and comparing the circumference of both thighs and calves at the same level.
  - Homans' sign of pain in the calf from abrupt dorsiflexion is unreliable, unhelpful and no longer accepted to demonstrate a possible lower-leg DVT.

SECTION C – Common calls

Table 31.1 Estimation of the clinical pre-test probability for suspected deep vein thrombosis (DVT)

Clinical feature*	Score
Active cancer (treatment ongoing or within 6 months or palliative)	1
Calf swelling >3 cm when compared with the asymptomatic leg (at 10 cm below the tibial tuberosity)	1
Collateral superficial veins (non-varicose)	1
Entire leg swollen	1
Localised tenderness along the distribution of the deep venous system	1
Paralysis, paresis or recent plaster immobilisation of the lower extremities	1
Pitting oedema: confined to the symptomatic leg	1
Previously documented DVT	1
Recently bedridden for >3 days, or major surgery within the previous 12 weeks	1
Alternative diagnosis as likely or greater than that of DVT	–2

Pre-test probability	Score	Risk of DVT
Low	≤0	<5%
Moderate	1–2	17%
High	≥3	53%

*In patients with symptoms in both legs, the more symptomatic leg is scored. Adapted from Well PS et al. Does this patient have deep vein thrombosis? *JAMA* 2006;295:199–207.

Investigations

- Determine the clinical pre-test probability of a DVT *before* requesting diagnostic testing (see Table 31.1).
- Send blood for FBC and coagulation profile.
- *Only* request a D-dimer if the pre-test probability is low.
- Perform Doppler USS on all moderate and high pre-test probability patients, and if the D-dimer result was positive.

Management

- Treatment of DVT reduces the risk of PE.
- When the pre-test probability of DVT is high (and awaiting a confirmatory test), or the diagnosis of proximal DVT is confirmed by USS, commence anticoagulant therapy with heparin, provided there are no contraindications.
  - Give LMWH such as enoxaparin 1 mg/kg SC 12-hourly. Measuring the aPTT is not necessary or helpful.
  - Alternatively, commence UFH 80 U/kg IV bolus followed by a maintenance infusion of 18 U/kg/h. Monitor the aPTT every 4–6 hours, aiming for an aPTT that is 1.5–2.5-fold the control level.

- Write up UFH as an infusion with heparin 25,000 U in 50 mL saline (500 U/mL) run at 2 mL/h = 1000 U/h, then according to the aPTT.
- Commence warfarin 10 mg PO on the second day of heparin therapy once the diagnosis of significant proximal DVT has been confirmed. Titrate the dose to achieve a therapeutic INR of 2.0–3.0, which usually takes 4–5 days, by which time heparin can be discontinued.

Necrotising fasciitis, pyomyositis and myonecrosis

These conditions may be life- or limb-threatening, and are caused by a variety of organisms including beta-haemolytic streptococci, staphylococci and anaerobes such as *Clostridium perfringens* (gas gangrene).
- Most are a complication of surgery or a deep traumatic wound, but may follow even a superficial injury such as an abrasion, a cut, an insect bite or a bruise.
- High-risk patients include those with diabetes or peripheral vascular disease, and intravenous drug users.

Selective physical examination

Vitals	Fever, tachycardia and hypotension—may be rapid onset
General	Sick looking
Mental status	Apprehension followed by delirium (clostridial myonecrosis and necrotising fasciitis)
Skin	Local swelling, oedema and erythema around a wound site, often with pain out of all proportion to the clinical findings
	Pale red without distinct borders (early); skin becomes progressively darker, purple and finally black (*late* finding of cutaneous gangrene)
	Woody firmness sometimes with subcutaneous crepitus (gas formation in soft tissues is an **absolute emergency**).

Management
The mortality rate of necrotising fasciitis exceeds 30%. If you think the patient has necrotising fasciitis, pyomyositis or myonecrosis:
- Gain IV access, draw blood samples and send for FBC, ELFTs, lactate, G&H and at least two sets of paired blood cultures.
- Contact your senior and the orthopaedic or general surgical admitting team for *immediate* surgical debridement.
- Commence empirical IV antibiotics including meropenem 1 g 8-hourly plus vancomycin 1.5 g 12-hourly and clindamycin 600 mg 8-hourly.

Septic arthritis

This can lead to systemic sepsis or permanent joint dysfunction. The knee joint is the most commonly affected.

SECTION C – Common calls

- Septic arthritis may follow penetrating trauma or haematogenous spread, in both the previously healthy or the immunocompromised:
  - Non-gonococcal arthritis is usually caused by *Staph. aureus* or *Strep. pyogenes* and may be associated with immunocompromise or joint trauma.
  - Gonococcal arthritis is the most common cause of a septic arthritis in a healthy, sexually active adult.
- Consider predisposing factors:
  - Penetrating trauma, especially with organic matter such as a stick or thorn
  - Recent arthroscopy or intra-articular injection of steroids
  - Joint prosthesis
  - New sexual partner
  - Rheumatoid arthritis
  - Intravenous drug use.

Selective physical examination
- Look for an elevated temperature.
- Examine for a tender, hot, erythematous, swollen joint that is painful or impossible to move.
- To avoid missing the diagnosis, remember that:
  - A single red, swollen, tender joint is considered septic until proven otherwise.
  - In a patient with polyarticular rheumatological disorder, a joint that is acutely inflamed out of proportion to the other joints involved should also be considered infected until proven otherwise.

Diagnosis and management
- Check temperature, HR and BP looking for systemic signs of sepsis.
- Send blood for FBC, ESR, CRP, two sets of paired blood cultures and serum glucose.
  - Take diagnostic samples, including blood cultures and a joint aspirate, before starting empirical antibiotics.
- Call your senior to aspirate the joint, or ask Orthopaedics or Rheumatology to perform this.
- Joint aspiration is vital to diagnosis, as well as to reducing intra-articular pressure and improving the penetration of antibiotics. Send the synovial fluid immediately for:
  - Gram stain
  - WCC and differential
  - Glucose and protein level
  - Aerobic, anaerobic, gonococcal and Chlamydial culture and PCR
  - Polarising microscopy for acute crystal arthropathy such as gout (strongly negative birefringence) and pseudogout (weakly positive birefringence).

- Synovial fluid is usually cloudy or purulent in septic arthritis, with a WCC >50,000/mm^3 with >90% neutrophils. Gram stain may demonstrate microorganisms. Synovial glucose is <50% of serum glucose.
- Give antibiotics as directed by the results of the Gram stain including WCC. When microorganisms are not seen on the synovial fluid sample, administer empirical antibiotics in the presence of a high joint WCC.
  - The choice of antibiotics depends on the clinical setting and local prescribing policies. Discuss with your senior or consult a microbiologist.
- Elevate and splint the joint, and give adequate analgesia.
- Refer to Orthopaedics for surgical drainage in the following:
  - Septic hip joint
  - Prosthetic joint infection
  - Osteomyelitis or joint cartilage infection concomitant with septic arthritis.

Compartment syndrome

Increased pressure within a myofascial sheath interferes with the micro-circulation to the nerves and muscles within that compartment.

- The patient presents with pain particularly on passive movement, altered or diminished sensation and weakness. The anterior compartment of the lower leg is the most commonly affected.
- Predisposing factors include:
  - Recent fracture
  - Tight pressure bandages or a full encircling plaster cast that has not been split
  - Blunt trauma, including pressure from prolonged immobility (i.e. drug overdose)
  - Unaccustomed, vigorous exertion
  - Anticoagulant medication.

Selective physical examination
Look for the following:
- Erythematous, glossy and oedematous overlying skin.
- Pain and tenderness over the involved compartment.
- Pain, particularly on passive stretching of the involved muscle groups, that increases with greater movement.
- Sensory loss and weakness. This will occur particularly over the dorsum of the foot and between the first and the second toes, and with dorsiflexion of the ankles and toes (leading to foot drop), if lower leg compartment syndrome develops.
- *Note:* do *not* be fooled by pulses being present. Compartment syndrome results from loss of capillary perfusion, so pulses may be felt despite progressive muscle and nerve damage within the compartment.

SECTION C – Common calls

- Increasing pain within 24–48 hours of casting the lower leg should be suspected as compartment syndrome, and the plaster removed to properly examine the lower leg and relieve the constriction.
- If the diagnosis is in doubt, or physical examination is impossible (e.g. the unconscious patient), arrange for an invasive measure of the compartment pressures by the orthopaedic team. Various devices are available.

Management

- Gain IV access and give normal saline 20 mL/kg IV to improve any hypoperfusion. Give analgesia such as morphine 2.5 mg titrated to effect.
- Send blood for FBC, U&E and CK; dipstick the urine for myoglobinuria (positive for blood, but RBCs absent on microscopy).
- Perform an ECG for hyperkalaemia.
- Request X-rays to exclude underlying fracture.
- Remove an external constriction such as a tight bandage, pressure dressing or plaster by cutting (or bivalving a cast).
- Place the affected limb at the level of the heart, but avoid excessive elevation that reduces arterial flow and may worsen the ischaemia.
- Refer the patient to the orthopaedic team for urgent decompressing fasciotomy, if symptoms do not resolve rapidly. A delay of >8–12 hours may lead to irreversible muscle necrosis and contracture formation (Volkmann's ischaemic contracture).

Less urgent conditions

Once these five major threats have been excluded, a more leisurely approach to the diagnosis can be taken, looking for other less urgent conditions.

Selective physical examination

Skin	Erythema, swelling and warmth (cellulitis)
	Painful subcutaneous red bruise-like nodules (erythema nodosum)
	Tender superficial vein, surrounding erythema and oedema (superficial thrombophlebitis)
	Erythema, swelling, dysaesthesiae, increased hair growth of one foot (reflex sympathetic dystrophy syndrome)
MSS	Posterior knee joint swelling (Baker's cyst)
	Joint inflammation (OA, RA, SLE, gout, pseudogout)
	Painful hip movement, particularly on external rotation, with decreased range of movement may cause referred leg pain
Neuro	Perform a complete neurological examination to look for lumbar disc disease (e.g. sciatica) or peripheral neuropathy (e.g. diabetes) if no abnormality has been found yet

Management
- **Acute gout**
  - Usually affects the ankle or great toe MTP joint, which may be exquisitely painful, with sudden onset.
  - Although the diagnosis is confirmed on polarising microscopy of synovial fluid showing strongly negative birefringent monosodium urate crystals, often a presumptive clinical diagnosis can be made based on prior attacks.
  - Aim to terminate the acute attack as quickly as possible by giving ibuprofen 600 mg PO then 400 mg 8-hourly, or indomethacin 100 mg PO, followed by 50 mg PO 6-hourly until pain relief occurs.
  - Colchicine or prednisone is an alternative if NSAID-intolerant. Give colchicine 1 mg PO initially, followed by 0.5 mg PO up to 1 hour later; or give prednisone 50 mg PO daily for 3 days.
- **Pseudogout (chondrocalcinosis)**
  - Diagnosis is made by polarising light microscopy demonstrating weakly positive birefringent rods.
  - Give ibuprofen 400 mg 8-hourly, or indomethacin 25–50 mg PO TDS. Intra-articular steroid injection by an expert may also help.
- **Cellulitis**
  - Most often caused by *Staph. aureus* or *Strep. pyogenes*.
  - Treatment should cover both organisms until confirmation or resolution occurs.
  - Cellulitis associated with a skin ulcer should be swabbed for Gram stain, culture and sensitivity.
  - Treat small, localised areas of cellulitis with intact skin with flucloxacillin 500 mg PO QDS. In cases of previous penicillin anaphylaxis, commence clindamycin 450 mg PO TDS.
  - Give flucloxacillin 2 g QDS or clindamycin 600 mg IV if the patient is febrile, the area of cellulitis is extensive or the patient is diabetic.
- **Buerger's disease (thrombo-angiitis obliterans)**
  - The only definitive treatment is complete abstinence from smoking.
- **Erythema nodosum**
  - Erythema nodosum is characterised by tender, red raised nodules appearing over 10–14 days, followed by bruise-like colour changes over the next few weeks.
  - It is usually on the shins related to a drug reaction (oral contraceptives, penicillin, sulfonamides), infection (*Streptococcus*, *Mycoplasma*, *Yersinia*, TB), sarcoidosis, inflammatory bowel disease or cancer.
  - Treatment is of the underlying condition.

SECTION C – Common calls

- **Baker's cyst**
  - Rupture of a Baker's cyst from extension of inflamed synovial tissue into the popliteal space results in pain and swelling behind the knee.
  - This may mimic a calf DVT, so USS is essential to differentiate the two.
  - Treatment is conservative, but drainage of the cyst or surgical synovectomy may be required if it recurs.
- **Benign nocturnal leg cramps**
  - Often occur in the absence of physical findings. The cause is unknown.
  - Although they respond to quinine orally, this has been replaced with sedatives.

32

Febrile patient

It is common to be called about a febrile patient. Most fevers seen in hospitalised patients are caused by infection, and locating the cause requires some detective work. Remember too that there are several important non-infective causes of fever to consider.

Whether the cause of a fever needs immediate treatment depends on the patient's clinical status and premorbid condition, and the suspected underlying cause.

Phone call

Questions

1. **What is the temperature?** A core temperature >38.5 °C is significant.
2. **How long has the patient had a raised temperature?**
3. **What are the other vital signs?**
4. **Are there any associated localising symptoms?**
5. **Is the patient immunosuppressed?**
6. **Has the patient had recent surgery?** Postoperative fever is common and may be caused by atelectasis, pneumonia, PE, wound infection, UTI or an infected IV site.
7. **Has the patient been overseas recently?** Do not forget tropical illnesses, such as malaria, typhoid, typhus, trypanosomiasis and dengue, in the returned traveller.
8. **What was the reason for admission?** Fever may be an integral feature of the admission diagnosis, such as with cholecystitis or pneumonia.

Instructions

If the patient is febrile and hypotensive, give 500 mL of normal saline IV rapidly. Otherwise request paracetamol 1 g PO to reduce patient discomfort.

Prioritisation

An elevated temperature alone is seldom life-threatening, unless there is fever in association with hypotension, meningitic symptoms or immunosuppression.

Corridor thoughts

What causes fever? (* = major threat to life)
Infective causes
- **Infection**
  - Common sites of infection are the lung, urinary tract, a wound and the IV site. See Table 32.1 for useful localising signs.
  - Less common is CNS*, abdominal or pelvic infection
  - Tropical infections, including malaria (particularly *Plasmodium falciparum**), typhoid, typhus, trypanosomiasis and dengue (so remember the travel history)
  - Immunosuppressed patients* are not only predisposed to infection, but also more susceptible to serious complications
- **Postoperative infection**
  - Atelactasis, urinary catheter, wound infection, venous cannula
  - Nosocomial pneumonia (especially if prolonged intubation in the ICU)

Non-infective causes
- **Drug-related fever**
  - Allergic or immune-complex reaction
  - Drug withdrawal—alcohol, including delirium tremens*; benzodiazepines
  - Serotonin syndrome* (SS) (see Box 32.1)
    - Mental confusion, shivering, sweating, muscle twitching and hyperreflexia (legs > arms)
  - Neuroleptic malignant syndrome (NMS)*
    - Newly commenced or increased dose of a neuroleptic agent such as haloperidol, chlorpromazine or risperidone or agents such as metoclopramide and promethazine
    - Or abrupt withdrawal of dopaminergic agents such as levodopa in the treatment of Parkinson's disease
    - Confusion, sweating, muscle rigidity, autonomic lability and raised CK
- **Transfusion reaction**
  - Can range from simple febrile reaction (non-haemolytic) to acute haemolysis* with haemoglobinaemia and haemoglobinuria (see Chapter 34)
- **Neoplasia**
  - May be secondary to intercurrent infection, or the disease process itself (e.g. chronic myeloid leukaemia, renal cell carcinoma, hepatocellular carcinoma, lymphoma)
- **Connective tissue disease**
  - Systemic lupus erythematosus (SLE)
  - Still's disease (juvenile RA)
  - Vasculitis (e.g. polyarteritis nodosa, temporal arteritis)

Table 32.1 Localising clues to infection source

Localising clue	Diagnostic consideration
Recent surgery	Pneumonia, atelectasis, pulmonary embolus Infected surgical wound or biopsy site *Note:* postoperative fever from atelectasis is a diagnosis made after excluding pneumonia
Headache, altered mental status, neck stiffness, seizure	Meningitis
Headache and sinus discomfort	Sinusitis
Toothache, dental caries	Periodontal abscess
Sore throat	Pharyngitis, tonsillitis
Dysphagia, drooling and respiratory distress	Retropharyngeal abscess Epiglottitis (now rare with *Haemophilus influenzae* vaccination) *Note:* both of these are medical emergencies; consult ENT and anaesthetist immediately
SOB with cough	Pneumonia Lung abscess Pulmonary embolus
Cardiac murmur, peripheral embolic lesions including splinter haemorrhages	Infective endocarditis. Send at least three sets of blood cultures before any antibiotics are given (antibiotics can usually wait until morning).
Pleuritic chest pain	Pneumonia Empyema Pulmonary embolus Myocarditis

Continued

Table 32.1 Localising clues to infection source—cont'd

Localising clue	Diagnostic consideration
Flank pain	Pyelonephritis, perinephric abscess Urolithiasis with obstruction
Dysuria, haematuria, frequency	Cystitis, pyelonephritis Note: a urinary catheter predisposes to UTI
Abdominal pain: RUQ	Subphrenic abscess, hepatic abscess, hepatitis, cholecystitis RLL pneumonia Ascending cholangitis: Does the patient have Charcot's triad (fever, jaundice and RUQ pain)?
Abdominal pain: RLQ	Appendicitis Crohn's disease Salpingitis
Abdominal pain: LUQ	Splenic abscess Subphrenic abscess LLL pneumonia
Abdominal pain: LLQ	Diverticular abscess Salpingitis
Ascites	Spontaneous bacterial peritonitis
Diarrhoea and vomiting	Infective gastroenteritis
Swollen, red tender joint	Septic arthritis, bursitis, reactive arthritis Infected prosthesis
Red, tender IV site, particularly any central line	Septic phlebitis—remove the line

> ## BOX 32.1 Drugs implicated in serotonin syndrome
> - Selective serotonin reuptake inhibitors (SSRIs)—fluoxetine, paroxetine, sertraline, fluvoxamine, citalopram, escitalopram
> - Serotonin and noradrenaline reuptake inhibitors (SNRIs)—venlafaxine, bupropion
> - Tricyclic antidepressants—imipramine, amitriptyline, desipramine
> - Monoamine oxidase inhibitors (MAOIs)—phenelzine, moclobemide
> - Lithium
> - Analgesic agents—pethidine, tramadol, fentanyl, dextromethorphan
> - Antiemetics—metoclopramide, ondansetron
> - Anticonvulsants—valproic acid
> - Illicit drugs—amphetamines, methylenedioxymethamphetamine (MDMA; 'ecstasy'), lysergic acid diethylamide (LSD)
> - Dietary supplements and herbal preparations—ginseng, St John's wort (*Hypericum perforatum*)

- **Other medical conditions**
  - PE*, DVT, MI*
  - Thyroid storm*, Addisonian crisis* (both exceedingly rare)
- **Environmental**
  - Heat stroke, which is only seen as an Emergency Department presentation.

Pyrexia of unknown origin (PUO)
- PUO was originally defined as a fever higher than 38.3°C for more than 3 weeks, with no cause found despite at least 1 week of investigations in hospital.
- The term is now often used more indiscriminately to indicate a fever without an apparent cause despite looking for the more common infectious and non-infectious causes (i.e. an undifferentiated febrile illness).

Major threat to life

- **Septicaemia with shock**, with risk of development of multiple system organ failure (MSOF)
- **Other life-threatening infections** related to effects on a specific organ system (e.g. meningitis, meningoencephalitis, pneumonia, cerebral malaria)
- **Drug-induced hyperpyrexia** (SS, NMS)

Bedside

Quick-look test
Does the patient look well (comfortable), sick (uncomfortable or distressed) or critical (about to die)?

Most patients will be comfortable. Ominous signs such as apprehension, agitation or lethargy suggest serious infection.

SECTION C – Common calls

Airway and vital signs

What is the respiratory rate?
- Tachypnoea in the absence of cardiorespiratory disease is an early indicator of septicaemia with metabolic acidosis (Kussmaul breathing).

What is the heart rate?
- Tachycardia, proportionate to the temperature elevation, is an expected finding in a febrile patient, but may equally signify circulatory failure.

What is the blood pressure?
- Fever in association with supine or postural hypotension indicates relative hypovolaemia and severe sepsis.
- Ensure that an IV line is in place and give normal saline 20 mL/kg repeated to correct the intravascular volume deficit.
- Fever in association with an SBP <90 mm Hg that does *not* respond to a fluid bolus of at least 30 mL/kg indicates a serious degree of hypovolaemia with septic shock.

Selective history and chart review

Perform a focused history based on the likely causes of fever (see *Corridor thoughts*) and a selective chart review, looking for localising clues (see Table 32.1), provided the patient is not in septic shock and does not have symptoms or signs of meningitis.
- What was the reason for admission?
- Are there any associated symptoms?
- Has the patient just travelled abroad?
- Has the patient had recent surgery?
- Is there an occupational, sexual, recreational, food and animal contact history?
- Medical history:
  - Evidence of immunodeficiency (e.g. cancer chemotherapy, haematological malignancy, HIV infection, steroid therapy)
  - Other possible reasons for fever (e.g. connective tissue disease, neoplasm)
  - Does the patient have diabetes? Diabetes increases the susceptibility to bacterial and fungal infection.

Observation chart

- Progressive tachycardia with fever and hypotension suggests septicaemia.
- Look at the **temperature pattern:**
  - Fever may be sustained (septicaemia, drug fever) or intermittent (urinary or biliary tract, malaria, lymphoma), although its pattern rarely assists in elucidating the underlying cause.

Medication and fluid charts

Review prescribed medications, especially for any recent changes and potential interactions:

- Newly prescribed medications such as a neuroleptic agent
- Recently discontinued drugs (e.g. levodopa, bromocriptine)
- Potential drug interaction (e.g. combination of an SSRI and a MAOI or pethidine and tramadol causing SS)
- Recent blood product administration (see Chapter 34)
- Allergies
- Prescribed antipyretics, antibiotics or steroids that may modify the fever pattern.

Selective physical examination

Physical examination directed by the focused history will help determine a potential source of infection, or highlight a possible non-infective cause such as a drug-induced or multisystem disorder.

Vitals	Repeat now
Mental status	Delirium, confusion, agitation and mental obtundation (severe sepsis or hypoxia)
HEENT	Neck stiffness and photophobia (meningo-encephalitis)
	Kernig's sign: with the patient supine, flex one hip and knee to 90 degrees, then straighten the knee; pain or resistance in the ipsilateral hamstrings indicates a positive test, suggesting meningeal irritation.
	Brudzinski's sign: with the patient supine, passively flex the neck forwards; flexion of the patient's hips and knees in response to this manoeuvre indicates a positive test result, again suggesting meningeal irritation.
	Note: neither sign is particularly sensitive and may be absent in meningitis.
	Conjunctival or scleral petechiae (meningococcaemia, infective endocarditis)
	Fundi: papilloedema (intracranial mass lesion, such as an abscess, or advanced meningitis), Roth's spots (oval haemorrhage with pale centre: 'a grain of sand on a red velvet cushion') seen in infective endocarditis
	Ears: red tympanic membranes (otitis media)
	Sinuses: tenderness
	Oral cavity: dental caries, tender tooth on tongue blade percussion (periodontal abscess)
	Pharynx: erythema, pharyngeal exudate (pharyngitis, oral candidiasis)

Continued

SECTION C – Common calls

CVS	Pulse volume
	Skin temperature, colour
	New murmur (infective endocarditis)
CNS	Hypertonicity and bradykinesia (NMS)
	Hypertonicity, clonus, hyperreflexia (SS)
Resp	Crackles, friction rub or signs of consolidation (pneumonia, PE)
Abdo	Localised tenderness or evidence of peritonism (acute abdomen—see Chapter 25)
	Fever, jaundice and RUQ tenderness (ascending cholangitis—Charcot's triad)
	Costovertebral angle tenderness (pyelonephritis)
	Ascites (spontaneous bacterial peritonitis)
Rectal	Tenderness or mass (rectal abscess, prostatitis)
MSS	Joint erythema or effusion (septic arthritis, reactive inflammatory arthritis)
Skin	Erythema and tenderness (cellulitis)
	Decubitus ulcer (bedsore)
	Osler's nodes (tender finger nodules); Janeway lesions (non-tender, raised haemorrhagic macules or nodules on the palms or soles from septic emboli); splinter haemorrhages—infective endocarditis
	Petechiae or purpura (meningococcaemia)
	IV sites (cellulitis, phlebitis)
	Any surgical wound for potential dehiscence and infection (take off the dressings)
Pelvis	Perform a pelvic examination if a pelvic source of fever such as endometritis or salpingitis is suspected. You must have a chaperone, and send swabs to microbiology including for *Chlamydia* and gonococcus.

Investigations

Any patient with an unexplained fever >38.5°C (orally) that has developed in hospital should have the following:
- Full blood count
  - An elevated WCC with neutrophilia sometimes with 'shift to the left' (of younger neutrophil precursors) suggests infection.
  - Low WCC may also occur and indicate overwhelming sepsis, a viral infection or neoplasia.
- Blood cultures
  - Obtain a 10 mL (minimum) aliquot of blood from two *different*, sterilised venepuncture sites away from any established IV access site (one for each pair of blood culture bottles). Two sites of puncture reduce the risk of a single false-positive result from a skin contaminant.

- Urinalysis, and urine microscopy and culture (if positive).
- Chest X-ray.

Other, more selective tests depend on the localising clues elicited from the chart review, history and physical examination. They may include:

- Lumbar puncture (headache, fever, altered mental status, neck stiffness/meningism)
- Throat swab for microscopy and/or culture (suspected streptococcal, gonococcal) and/or PCR assay (influenza virus, adenovirus, herpes simplex infection)
- Sputum for Gram stain (suspected staphylococcal pneumonia), culture and/or PCR assay (streptococcal, *Legionella, Mycoplasma* pneumonia).
  - *Note:* if TB is suspected in an elderly, immunosuppressed or immigrant patient, request a Ziehl–Neelsen stain for mycobacteria followed by Lowenstein–Jensen medium culture (*not* performed routinely).
- Joint aspiration
- Swab an infected or draining wound for Gram stain and culture
- Remove any IV line suspected to be infected and replace at a new site. Send the catheter tip to the laboratory for culture.

Management

Immediate management

- Apply supplemental oxygen to maintain saturation >94%.
  - Fever shifts the O_2 dissociation curve to the right, so oxygen has a lower affinity for Hb, thus for any given arterial partial pressure of oxygen (PaO_2) there is a relatively lower saturation of Hb (SaO_2).
- Insert an IV line and commence normal saline at 250–500 mL/h to restore or maintain normotension, replace insensible losses and cover maintenance fluids.
  - Patients with septic shock will also need inotropic support, as well as aggressive fluid resuscitation with normal saline. Call for urgent senior help.

Antibiotic therapy: choice of antibiotics

- Specific antibiotic choices depend on local resistance patterns or known problems (e.g. MRSA).
- Follow your local antibiotic guidelines and/or consult a microbiologist early.

Patients who require empirical broad-spectrum antibiotics

- Febrile patient with hypotension, particularly if unresponsive to a fluid bolus (i.e. septic shock)

- Febrile neutropenia
  - Immunocompromised patients such as a transplant recipient, a patient with AIDS or a patient on high-dose steroids or chemotherapy
- Febrile patient who looks unwell, but with no obvious localising source
- *Note:* always refer to hospital antibiotic guidelines, syndrome-specific protocols and/or an antibiotic choice decision-support aid (if available); plus consult your senior doctor.
- Often, more than one antibiotic is needed. Common choices include a third-generation cephalosporin (e.g. ceftriaxone 2 g IV) **or** extended-spectrum penicillin (e.g. piperacillin/tazobactam 4 + 0.5 g IV) and an aminoglycoside (e.g. gentamicin 4–7 mg/kg once).
- Ensure that the patient is not allergic before ordering any antibiotic.
- Anaerobic cover with metronidazole 500 mg IV is required for deep-tissue, gastrointestinal or female pelvic infections.

Patients who require specific or directed antibiotics

- A patient with fever and localising signs who has had appropriate culture specimens collected and whose condition is currently stable should have 'targeted' antibiotics.
- The initial antibiotic selection is based on the source or site of infection, the most likely causative organism(s) and the likely antibiotic sensitivities (e.g. flucloxacillin 2 g IV for *Staphylococcus aureus* [cellulitis], gentamicin 5 mg/kg plus amoxycillin 2 g IV [pyelonephritis]).

Patients who require no immediate antibiotics

- A patient who does not look sick, is immunologically competent and in whom the source of fever is not readily apparent can delay antibiotics until a specific infective agent has been identified.

Patients with fever already taking antibiotics

- Consider:
  - Inadequate dose or choice of antibiotic
  - Resistance to the antibiotic
  - Antibiotic not getting to the site of infection (e.g. thick-walled abscess requiring surgical drainage instead)
  - Drug fever 'secondary' to the antibiotic itself, *not* the infection
  - The fever being treated is not an infection (e.g. a connective tissue disorder or paraneoplastic syndrome).

Specific management
Drug-induced hyperthermia

Fever may result from the use of a prescription or non-proprietary medication, even such commonly used medications as antibiotics, which can cause a 'drug fever'. This usually occurs within 7 days of beginning the offending medication, which should be stopped if no other cause for the fever is found, usually by the patient's regular medical team.

Serotonin syndrome and neuroleptic malignant syndrome

- Discontinue the offending medication.
- Administer oxygen, commence IV fluids and call your senior.
- Patients with persistent fever >39.5°C with altered mental status may require neuromuscular paralysis, intubation and ventilation to prevent further muscle-generated heat production, rhabdomyolysis and multiorgan failure. Call an anaesthetist and inform intensive care.

Other non-infective causes of fever

- Delirium tremens is a serious cause of fever that is occasionally seen in patients withdrawing from alcohol. It is associated with confusion, including visual hallucinations and delusions, agitation, seizures and signs of autonomic hyperactivity, such as fever, tachycardia and sweating.
- It can be fatal if not treated aggressively with high-dose IV benzodiazepines to stabilise the patient, usually in an HDU or ICU.
- Fever caused by a drug reaction, neoplasm, connective tissue disorder or vasculitis is always a diagnosis made *after* excluding all potential sources of infection, and so is unlikely to be made on call.

SECTION C – Common calls

Handy hints

- High-spiking fever 5–7 days after a surgical procedure may indicate abscess formation.
- Fever is a sign of rejection in a transplant patient.
- Steroids elevate the WCC and suppress the fever response, regardless of the cause.
- Other causes of a raised WCC in the *absence* of infection are vomiting, haemorrhage, seizures and marrow dysplasia, including leukaemia.
- Administering an antipyretic for a fever caused by infection only treats the symptom. The febrile response itself is a positive adaptive mechanism that inhibits bacterial replication and enhances the ability of macrophages to kill bacteria.
- Therefore, observe the fever pattern, and if the fever is not too high (<40°C) and the patient is comfortable, it is *not* necessary to give aspirin or paracetamol (but be certain to explain why not to the nurse or patient).

33

Skin rashes including allergic reactions

You may be called because a rash has appeared abruptly (e.g. drug reaction) or because a patient has been admitted with a rash and nursing staff are concerned it may be infectious (e.g. scabies, lice or even a viral exanthem).

Urticarial rash and angio-oedema are important to recognise, as they may be cutaneous markers of systemic anaphylaxis that requires urgent treatment with adrenaline.

Phone call

Questions

1. **How long has the patient had the rash?** Is this a new rash or an acute exacerbation of a chronic skin condition?
2. **What are the vital signs?**
3. **Is there facial swelling, with stridor and SOB?** These features suggest angio-oedema with the possibility of upper airway obstruction. Pruritus may be absent and full-blown anaphylaxis may develop.
4. **Is there any urticaria (hives)?** Urticaria may be a cutaneous sign of a generalised allergic reaction, along with erythema and/or pruritus. These may herald the onset of anaphylaxis if accompanied by systemic respiratory or cardiovascular features.
5. **Has the patient received any foods, drugs, blood products or IV contrast material within the past few hours?** An acute allergic reaction may occur to any drug, food or biological agent, including IV contrast. In the latter case, the reaction usually occurs within minutes, often when the patient is still in the radiology department.
6. **Does the patient have any known allergy or pre-existing skin condition?**
7. **What was the reason for admission?**

Instructions

If the patient has evidence of angio-oedema or anaphylaxis (stridor, wheezing, SOB or hypotension—see Chapter 9):

- Give high-dose oxygen via mask and at least raise the legs if there is associated hypotension. Do *not* try to lie flat a patient with airway compromise.
- Attach continuous cardiac monitoring and pulse oximetry to the patient.
- Ask that the following be prepared prior to your arrival at the bedside:
  - IV trolley with two large-bore (14–16G) cannulae.
  - Line primed with 1 L normal saline 0.9%.
  - 1:1000 adrenaline (1 mg in 1 mL) prepared: dose up to 0.3–0.5 mg IM (0.3–0.5 mL of 1:1000 solution) into the upper lateral thigh.

Prioritisation

- Evidence of facial angio-oedema or anaphylaxis with stridor, wheezing, SOB or hypotension requires *immediate* attention.
- A generalised rash with no associated systemic symptoms of anaphylaxis can wait, if other problems of higher priority exist.

Corridor thoughts

What are the important skin rashes and their causes? (* = major threat to life)

- Most calls regarding acute-onset skin rashes are non-anaphylactic drug reactions that can have a widely varied morphology.
- They are usually symmetrical and may start on the buttocks. Early drug reactions may be localised or a 'fixed drug eruption' that recurs in the same place each time.
- Potentially serious rashes include acute urticaria*, vesiculobullous*, petechial* and erythroderma*.

Urticaria

Itchy, oedematous, sometimes transient skin swellings, which may occur in crops and last several hours to days. They may be immune-mediated or non-immune.

- **Iatrogenic:**
  - Medications
    - Antibiotics: penicillins, cephalosporins, sulfonamides, tetracyclines
    - Opioids: morphine, codeine
    - Aspirin and other NSAIDs
    - ACE inhibitors (e.g. perindopril, enalapril). *Note:* single most common drug cause of angio-oedema
    - Natural rubber latex

- IV contrast material
- Blood transfusion reaction (see Chapter 34)
- Food allergy:
  - Shellfish, nuts, eggs, strawberries, chocolate, food dyes or preservatives
- **Insect sting, animal bite, parasitic infection**
- **Physical:**
  - Cold, heat, pressure, vibration, exercise
- **Autoimmune disease:**
  - SLE, chronic active hepatitis
- **Systemic illness:**
  - Malignancy, including Hodgkin's lymphoma
  - Vasculitis
  - Viruses, such as hepatitis A or EBV, and serum sickness
- **Pregnancy-related:**
  - Pruritic urticarial papules and plaques of pregnancy (PUPPP), also known as polymorphic eruption of pregnancy

Vesicobullous rashes including erythema multiforme

- **Allergic contact dermatitis**
- **Medications:**
  - Antibiotics (e.g. penicillins, sulfonamides)
  - Anti-inflammatory drugs (e.g. NSAIDs)
  - Anticonvulsants
  - Allopurinol
- **Infection:**
  - Viral (e.g. herpes simplex, herpes zoster)
  - Bacterial (e.g. *Mycoplasma pneumoniae* infection)
  - Bullous impetigo (*Staphylococcus aureus* infection)
- **Autoimmune bullous disease**
  - Pemphigus vulgaris (may be life-threatening, especially in the elderly) and pemphigoid
  - Dermatitis herpetiformis (gluten sensitivity)
  - Bullous eczema, paraneoplastic pemphigus, bullous lupus

Included in the above are erythema multiforme minor with 1–2 cm 'target lesions' only, erythema multiforme major involving one mucous membrane, and the most serious Stevens–Johnson syndrome (SJS) and toxic epidermal necrolysis (TEN).

Erythema multiforme minor and major are commonly associated with a viral infection such as herpes, whereas SJS and TEN are more commonly drug-related. The patient may develop mucosal erosions with blistering and extensive loss of epidermis if the medication is not discontinued. Severe SJS or TEN requires intensive care.

Petechial and purpuric rashes

Non-blanching, cutaneous bleeding that may be non-palpable or palpable.

Causes of non-palpable purpura

- Thrombocytopenia *with* splenomegaly:
  - Normal marrow
    - Liver disease with portal hypertension
    - Myeloproliferative disorders
    - Lymphoproliferative disorders
    - Hypersplenism
  - Abnormal marrow
    - Leukaemia
    - Lymphoma
    - Myeloid metaplasia
- Thrombocytopenia *without* splenomegaly:
  - Normal marrow
    - Immune: ITP, drugs, infections including HIV
    - Non-immune: vasculitis, sepsis, DIC, HUS, TTP
  - Abnormal marrow
    - Cytotoxics
    - Aplasia, fibrosis or infiltration
    - Alcohol, thiazides
- Non-thrombocytopenic:
  - Cutaneous disorders
  - Trauma, sun, steroids, old age
- Systemic disorders
  - Uraemia, scurvy, amyloid
  - von Willebrand's disease

Causes of palpable purpura

- Vasculitis
  - Polyarteritis nodosa
  - Leucocytoclastic (hypersensitivity), Henoch–Schönlein purpura
- Emboli
  - Meningococcaemia
  - Gonococcaemia
  - Other infections—*Staphylococcus*, *Rickettsia* (Rocky Mountain spotted fever), enteroviruses

Erythroderma

Acute erythroderma refers to a generalised exfoliative dermatitis that affects >90% body surface. The scaling exfoliation may be fine or coarse, and can lead to fluid loss, hypoalbuminaemia and secondary infection that may be fatal despite intensive care. Causes include:

SECTION C – Common calls

- Eczema
- Psoriasis
- Drugs, cosmetics, household chemicals
- Toxic shock syndrome
- Staphylococcal scalded skin syndrome
- Streptococcal toxic shock syndrome
- Haematological malignancy, graft-versus-host disease.

Maculopapular rashes

- **Drugs:**
  - Antibiotics—penicillin, cephalosporin, sulfonamides, chloramphenicol
  - Antiretroviral agents—nelfinavir, abacavir, didanosine
  - Antihistamines
  - Antidepressants (e.g. amitriptyline)
  - Diuretics (e.g. thiazides)
  - Oral hypoglycaemics
  - Disease-modifying antirheumatic drugs (e.g. gold)
  - Sedative agents (e.g. barbiturates)
- **Infection:**
  - Measles, rubella, parvovirus B19, dengue
- **Infestation with scabies or lice:**
  - Scabies presents with intensely itchy lesions between the finger webs, on the wrists, waist, axillae, breast areolae, genitalia and feet. It is associated with excoriated papules and is usually worse after a hot shower or bath.
  - Lice may occur anywhere on the body, but particularly on the scalp, genitalia, neck, flanks, waistline and axillae. Look at the patient's clothing for eggs along the seams.

Fixed drug eruption

Certain drugs may produce a skin lesion in a specific area. Repeat drug administration causes the skin lesion in the same location. Lesions are usually dusky-red patches distributed over the trunk or proximal limbs.

Recurrent administration of the offending drug increases the distribution and intensity of the rash, which may become oedematous or even bullous. Causes include:

- Antibiotics (sulfonamides, metronidazole, tetracyclines)
- Oral contraceptive pill
- Paracetamol, NSAIDs
- Anticonvulsants (e.g. phenytoin)
- Sedatives (barbiturates).

Major threat to life

- **Upper airway obstruction due to angio-oedema**
  - Angio-oedema causes facial, lip and tongue swelling progressing to laryngeal oedema with hoarseness and upper airway obstruction. It is also associated with abdominal cramps and diarrhoea (GI mucosa).
- **Erythema, urticaria or generalised pruritus heralding anaphylactic shock or severe bronchospasm**
  - Urticaria may accompany angio-oedema and either may progress to anaphylaxis. In hospital, they are/can be precipitated by medications, IV contrast material and foods.
- **Meningococcal septicaemia**
- **Toxic epidermal necrolysis**
  - Patients are usually febrile and shocked, with reddened desquamating skin. Transfer to the ICU (or a burns unit) immediately and arrange an urgent dermatological opinion.

Bedside

Quick-look test

Does the patient look well (comfortable), sick (uncomfortable or distressed) or critical (about to die)?

- Patients with upper airway obstruction have noisy distressed breathing and sit upright in bed looking frightened. Facial, tongue or pharyngeal angio-oedema may be associated with laryngeal oedema causing airway obstuction.

What is the respiratory rate?

- Tachypnoea associated with audible stridor or wheezing is an ominous sign.
- Inspiratory stridor suggests impending upper airway obstruction. Notify your senior and an anaesthetist immediately.

What is the blood pressure?

- Hypotension with urticaria suggests anaphylactic shock. The patient requires immediate treatment with adrenaline, plus IV fluid (see Chapter 9).
- Hypotension may also be associated with meningococcaemia, toxic shock syndrome, TEN or SJS.

What is the temperature?

- Pyrexia with rash has extensive differential diagnoses.
  - Conditions range from minor viral exanthems such as rubella, to life-threatening such as meningococcal septicaemia, toxic shock syndrome, SJS, TEN and pustular psoriasis. If in doubt, involve your senior doctor immediately.

SECTION C – Common calls

Selective history and chart review
- How long has the rash been present?
- Is it itchy?
- Is this a new or a recurrent problem?
- Which drugs did the patient receive before the rash started?
- Is it already being treated?

Selective physical examination
Where is the rash located?
- Is it generalised, acral (on the hands and feet) or localised?
- *Note:* remember to examine the buttocks, a common site for the onset of a drug eruption. Also inside the mouth for evidence of oral mucosal lesions associated with serious skin diseases such as erythema multiforme major, SJS, TEN and pemphigus vulgaris.

What is the main lesion? (see Figure 33.1)
- **Macule:** circumscribed flat area of skin, different in colour from the surrounding tissue, <0.5 cm in diameter
- **Patch:** large macule >0.5 cm in diameter
- **Papule:** solid, raised lesion <0.5 cm in diameter with variable colour
- **Plaque:** circumscribed elevation of skin >0.5 cm in diameter and with a distinct edge; often a confluence of papules
- **Nodule:** solid, raised and palpable lesion >0.5 cm in diameter. Similar to papule but located deeper in the dermis and subcutaneous tissue
- **Cyst:** abnormal closed membranous sac containing liquid or semisolid substance
- **Vesicle:** raised circumscribed accumulation of clear, serous-like fluid ('blister') within a papule or epidermal layer; diameter <0.5 cm
- **Bulla:** circumscribed, elevated, fluid-filled lesion >0.5 cm in diameter
- **Petechiae:** small red, brown or purple non-blanching macule <0.5 cm in diameter ('flea bite')
- **Purpura:** red, brown or purple non-blanching lesion >0.5 cm in diameter. May be palpable or non-palpable (macule)
- **Hive (wheal):** circumscribed, firm, smooth elevated lesion that changes in colour, appearance and location borders. Usually intensely itchy with central pallor and irregular borders ('nettle rash')

What is the secondary lesion? (see Figure 33.2)
- **Scale:** thin, dry plate of dead epidermal cells produced by abnormal keratinisation (white colour differentiates it from crust)
- **Pustule:** vesicle containing purulent exudate
- **Crust:** dried, yellow exudate of plasma from broken vesicle, bulla or pustule

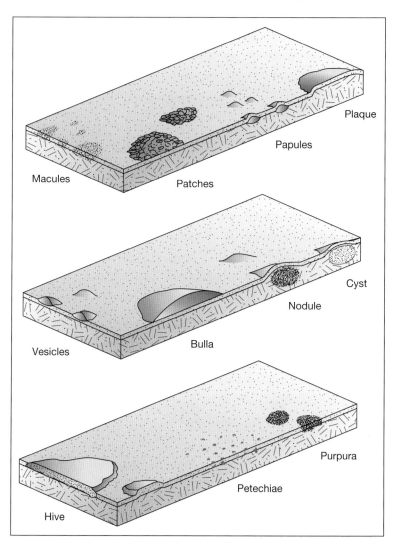

Figure 33.1 Primary skin lesions.

- **Fissure:** linear, epidermal tear
- **Erosion:** focal loss of epidermis, moist and well circumscribed; heals without a scar
- **Ulcer:** focal erosion of epidermis and dermis; heals with a scar
- **Scar:** flat, raised or depressed area of fibrosis
- **Atrophy:** depression in the skin secondary to thinning of the epidermis or dermis
- **Excoriation:** linear or angular erosion secondary to scratching

SECTION C – Common calls

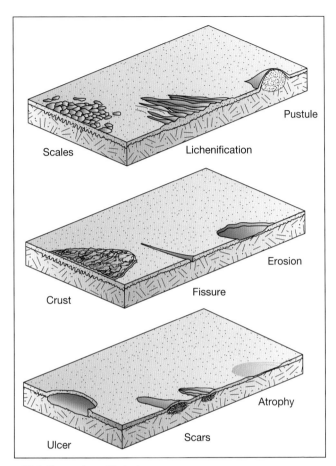

Figure 33.2 Secondary skin lesions.

- **Lichenification:** dry, leathery chronic area of thickened epidermis, often with a shiny surface; secondary to habitual rubbing

What colour is the rash?

- Rashes can be pigmented, depigmented, red, brown to violet or yellow. Try to examine under natural light if possible.

What is the configuration of the rash?

- **Annular:** ring-like or circular
- **Linear:** in lines
- **Arcuate:** in the shape of an arch or a curve
- **Grouped:** local collection of similar lesions, such as the vesicular lesions of herpes zoster or herpes simplex

- **Koebner phenomenon:** Skin lesions along lines of trauma, including scratching in psoriasis, lichen planus and vitiligo

Management

Immediate management
Angio-oedema and anaphylaxis (see Chapter 9)
- Commence high-flow oxygen to maintain saturation >94%.
- Give 1:1000 adrenaline 0.3–0.5 mg (0.3–0.5 mL) IM into the upper outer thigh, repeated as necessary every 3–5 minutes.
- If shock and circulatory collapse are present, give a bolus of normal saline 20–40 mL/kg IV and repeat as necessary.
- Call your senior urgently.
- Give 1:1000 adrenaline 5 mg (5 mL) nebulised with oxygen for respiratory distress while the IM dose is being absorbed.
- Call the anaesthetist. Prepare for surgical airway.
- Second-line measures, only indicated after achieving cardiorespiratory stability:
  - Hydrocortisone 200 mg IV or prednisolone 50 mg PO for severe wheeze
  - H_1 and or H_2 antihistamines such as cetirizine 10 mg PO or fexofenadine 180 mg PO, plus ranitidine 150 mg PO. Their role in anaphylaxis is unproven.
- Remember to enquire about the use of ACE inhibitors, which are the single most common drug cause of angio-oedema.

Urticaria
- Attempt to identify the likely cause from the recent history. Most reactions occur within minutes, but may be delayed for up to 24 hours.
- Consider precipitants such as aspirin, NSAIDs or opioids and loosen any tight clothing or belts (physical urticaria).
- Give the patient a non-sedating H_1 antagonist such as cetirizine 10 mg PO once daily. A sedating agent such as promethazine 10 mg PO TDS may be useful in patients unable to sleep secondary to intense itch (pruritis).
- Add an H_2 antagonist such as ranitidine 150 mg PO BD for all but the mildest of cases, as their combined use is synergistic.
- Observe closely for any multisystem involvement suggesting progression to anaphylaxis or angio-oedema.

SECTION C – Common calls

Erythema multiforme and vesiculobullous rashes

Patients with SJS, TEN, staphylococcal scalded-skin syndrome and pemphigus may die from fluid extravasation, intercurrent infection then multiorgan failure (see Table 33.1 for the spectrum of rashes).

Severe cases:

- Consult your senior and the ICU.
- Gain IV access, administer 20 mL/kg IV normal saline and commence a careful fluid balance chart.
- Administer empiric antibiotics if evidence of secondary infection exists (see below).
- Control pain with systemic opiates such as morphine 2.5 mg IV titrated to effect.
- Avoid corticosteroids in most cases. Their use is controversial as they do not improve the prognosis, and may increase the risk of complications. Seek senior advice.
- Look for the underlying cause. Withdraw any possible causative drug.

Milder cases require symptomatic care only:

- Antihistamine PO such as promethazine 10 mg TDS or chlorpheniramine 4 mg QDS for associated pruritus, with a warning about drowsiness.
- Antibiotics PO such as flucloxacillin 500 mg QDS for secondary staphylococcal infection in herpes zoster, impetigo, insect bites and eczema; or roxithromycin 300 mg once daily for patients allergic to penicillin.
- Antiviral agent PO such as famciclovir 1500 mg for severe herpes simplex, or famciclovir 250 mg TDS for 7 days for severe herpes zoster.
- Topical steroid antiseptic such as 0.1% betamethasone with 3% clioquinol cream TDS for areas of papular urticaria or bullous eczema.

Drug reactions

- Stop any medication implicated, as a minor rash may rapidly progress.
- If the offending medication is essential to the patient's management overnight, choose an alternative.
- Leave a note for the usual medical team to monitor for progression to mucous membrane lesions, blistering and skin sloughing.
- Give an antihistamine for pruritis; apply mild topical steroid such as 0.5% hydrocortisone or moisturising lotions as necessary.

Table 33.1 **Spectrum of rashes**

Condition	Rash	Distribution	Mucous membranes	Epidermal detachment TBSA	Mortality
EM minor	1–2 cm target lesions	Acral—palms, soles, dorsum of hands	Not affected	None	0
EM major	Target lesions Oedematous papules	Acral	One or more mildly affected	<10%	0–1%
SJS	Blistering, purpuric macules	Generalised	Mucosal erosions	10%	5%
TEN	Blistering, purpuric macules	Generalised	Mucosal erosions	30%	30%

EM, erythema multiforme; SJS, Stevens–Johnson syndrome; TEN, toxic epidermal necrolysis; TBSA, total body surface area.

Pruritic urticarial papules and plaques of pregnancy (PUPPP)

- Usually occurs around 36 weeks' gestation, but can be seen postpartum in 1:120 to 1:240 pregnancies.
- Pruritus disrupts sleep and is centred around the abdomen, particularly if striae are present. It may also occur on the trunk and proximal limbs.
- Apply a high-potency topical steroid such as betamethasone, and emollients depending on the severity.

34

Transfusion reactions

Reactions to blood products may vary from mild to severe, even fatal. Types of transfusion reaction include febrile non-haemolytic, acute haemolytic, anaphylactic, pulmonary oedema and bacterial contamination. An organised approach helps sort out the nature of the reaction and what to do about it.

Phone call

Questions

1. **What symptoms does the patient have?** Fever, chills, chest pain, back pain, diaphoresis and SOB can all be manifestations of a transfusion reaction.
2. **What are the vital signs?**
3. **Which blood product is being transfused?**
4. **How long ago was it started?**
5. **What was the reason for admission?**

Instructions

- *Stop* the transfusion immediately and disconnect the IV giving set, if the patient has any of the following:
  - Tachypnoea
  - Hypotension
  - Chest or back pain
  - Symptoms occurring within minutes of the start of the transfusion such as chills, wheeze or urticaria
  - Fever in a patient who has never received a blood transfusion before, or who has never been pregnant, as this may represent an acute haemolytic reaction.
- An acute haemolytic transfusion reaction may cause any of the above symptoms. Such reactions, though rare, are usually due to ABO incompatibility associated with human error. The mortality rate is high and proportional to the volume of blood infused.
  - However, in a previously pregnant or previously transfused patient, fever may simply be a non-haemolytic febrile reaction.

- Give normal saline IV through a fresh giving set.
- Compare the identification tag on the blood with the patient's wristband. Do not dispose of the unit of blood—keep for blood transfusion laboratory analysis.

Prioritisation

Any suspected haemolytic, anaphylactic or other major transfusion reaction requires the patient to be seen immediately.

Corridor thoughts

What causes transfusion reactions? (* = major threat to life)
- **Immune haemolysis:**
    - Acute haemolytic reaction*
        - Errors in identification of the patient or labelling of the blood may result in mismatched RBCs with ABO incompatibility.
    - Delayed haemolytic reaction
        - This occurs following RBC antibody formation from prior exposure to foreign RBC antigens in pregnancy or a previous blood transfusion.
        - Haemolysis occurs 3–14 days after the transfusion, accompanied by fever, jaundice, increasing anaemia and a falling Hb level.
- **Non-immune haemolysis*:**
    - Occurs if the blood has been overheated or undergone trauma. Damage to blood products follows excessive hand squeezing or pumping of an infusion bag during the rapid administration of blood in an emergency, or by forcing through a cannula that is too small.
- **Urticaria and anaphylaxis*:**
    - IgE-mediated immune response to transfused soluble allergens, such as food or drug-related, or other plasma protein allergen.
    - Acute IgG-mediated immune response to transfused IgA antibodies in a previously sensitised, but IgA deficient, patient.
- **Fever:**
    - A non-haemolytic febrile reaction is the most common cause of a transfusion reaction. It does *not* require stopping the transfusion. It is usually seen in a prior multi-transfused or multiparous patient because of a WBC antigen–antibody reaction, or is due to cytokines.

- Fever can also be an early sign of acute haemolytic transfusion reaction* (particularly in patients who have not had prior transfusions or been pregnant) or bacterial contamination*.
- **Pulmonary oedema***:
  - Transfusion-associated circulatory overload (TACO) usually associated with hypertension. Volume overload in a patient with impaired cardiac function as the blood transfusion expands the intravascular volume excessively.
  - Transfusion-related acute lung injury (TRALI). Acute respiratory distress often associated with fever, non-cardiogenic pulmonary oedema and hypotension developing within 6 hours.

Major threat to life

- **Anaphylaxis** causes death due to hypoxia from asphyxia with severe laryngeal oedema or bronchospasm, or by massive peripheral vasodilation with fluid extravasation. It is rare, but potentially fatal.
- **Acute haemolytic reaction** causes hyotension, acute renal failure and disseminated intravascular coagulation (DIC). It is also rare, but potentially fatal.
- **TRALI** causes death from respiratory failure.
- **TACO** causes death from circulatory failure.
- **Bacterial contamination** causes death from septic shock.

Bedside

Quick-look test

Does the patient look well (comfortable), sick (uncomfortable or distressed), or critical (moribund and about to die)?

A patient with anaphylaxis looks unwell and is agitated, restless or short of breath. A patient with acute pulmonary oedema looks sweaty, pale and prefers to sit upright due to severe SOB.

Airway and vital signs

What is the respiratory rate?
- Tachypnoea is a manifestation of volume overload, TRALI or, particularly if associated with stridor or wheezing, anaphylaxis.

What is the blood pressure?
- Hypotension is an ominous sign. It occurs in acute haemolytic reactions, anaphylaxis and with bacterial contamination. Ensure that the transfusion has been stopped.

Selective physical examination

HEENT	Flushed face (anaphylaxis or haemolytic reaction)
	Facial or pharyngeal oedema (anaphylaxis)
Resp	Wheeze or crackles (anaphylaxis, pulmonary oedema)
Neuro	Decreased level of consciousness (anaphylaxis or haemolytic reaction)
Skin	Warmth or redness along the vein being used for the transfusion (haemolytic reaction)
	Oozing from IV sites may be the only obvious sign of haemolysis in an unconscious or anesthetised patient, although DIC is a late manifestation of an acute haemolytic transfusion reaction
Urine	Check the urine colour—free Hb turns urine red or brown and indicates a haemolytic reaction

When there is evidence of anaphylaxis, haemolysis or pulmonary oedema stop the transfusion, call for senior help and immediately begin treatment (see later).

Selective history
Has the patient developed new symptoms since the initial telephone call?
- Fever or chills (non-haemolytic febrile reaction)
- Headache, chest pain, back pain or diaphoresis (haemolytic reaction)
- SOB (pulmonary oedema from TRALI or TACO). These are difficult to distinguish, but initial hypotension suggests TRALI and hypertension TACO. Get an ECG and CXR.

Has the patient had previous transfusion reactions?
- Chills and fever are most common in a patient who has received multiple transfusions or who has had previous pregnancies.

Management

Immediate management
Anaphylaxis
- *Stop* the transfusion and change the IV giving set for another primed with normal saline.
- Administer high-dose oxygen via mask and attach a pulse oximeter.
- Give adrenaline 0.01 mg/kg up to 0.5 mg (0.5 mL of 1:1000 adrenaline) IM into upper outer thigh (see *Anaphylaxis* in Chapter 9).

SECTION C – Common calls

- Administer 20 mL/kg normal saline stat for hypotension.
- Call for senior help.
- Give prednisolone 50 mg PO or hydrocortisone 100 mg by slow IV injection for wheeze (efficacy uncertain).
  - Administer nebulised salbutamol as an adjunctive measure for severe bronchospasm.

Acute haemolytic reaction

- *Stop* the transfusion.
- Exchange the IV giving set for another primed with normal saline.
- Call for senior help.
- Give 10–20 mL/kg normal saline IV rapidly. Continue further IV fluid boluses to maintain a urine output of >100 mL/h.
- Give frusemide 40 mg IV with 20% mannitol 2.5 mL/kg IV over 5 minutes (to promote diuresis).
- Draw 20 mL of the patient's blood and send for repeat cross-matching, direct Coombs' test, free Hb, FBC, coagulation profile and U&E. Contact the blood transfusion laboratory immediately.
- Check the first void urine for haemoglobinuria by dipstick for blood (will be positive), plus microscopy (will be negative for RBCs).
- Send the donor blood back for repeat cross-matching and an indirect Coombs' test.

Pulmonary oedema

- Stop the transfusion, unless the patient is actively bleeding at the same time (difficult problem!).
- Call for senior help immediately.
- See Chapter 15 for the management of circulatory overload (TACO), including stopping the transfusion, nitrates and frusemide.
  - Volume overload with pulmonary oedema should be anticipated in patients with a history of CCF. Pulmonary oedema may be prevented by administering a diuretic such as frusemide 10 mg IV at the start of each unit of blood.
- Patients *without* volume overload (TRALI) need oxygen and admission to the ICU.

Urticaria (hives)

- Do not stop the transfusion for mild urticaria alone as it is rarely serious, unless there is upper airway oedema, wheeze or hypotension, which indicates anaphylaxis.
- Give promethazine 10–25 mg PO or IV for urticaria alone.
- The patient should also be premedicated with promethazine in future transfusions to prevent an urticarial reaction. If that fails,

the patient will need washed RBCs, after consulting the blood transfusion laboratory.

Fever

- Do not stop the transfusion if the patient has fever without other symptoms of an acute haemolytic reaction. Generally no treatment is required.
- Give paracetamol 1 g PO if the fever is high and the patient is distressed.
- Premedication with an antipyretic before subsequent transfusions is indicated if the patient has documented fever with two consecutive blood transfusions. If this step fails to prevent fever, washed RBCs should be given, after consulting the blood transfusion laboratory.

SECTION C – Common calls

Investigations

35

Electrocardiogram

- Ensure that the ECG is from the correct patient, on the correct date with a specified time.
- Check the age and sex of the patient—these will assist in interpreting the ECG.
- Note whether additional information has been added such as 'with chest pain' or 'post-cardioversion'.
- Compare with previous ECGs to determine whether the changes are pre-existing (old).

Electrocardiogram interpretation

Rate

Calculate the rate:

- *Multiply* the number of QRS complexes in the 10-second rhythm strip of a standard 12-lead ECG (paper speed 25 mm/s) by 6 to obtain the rate per minute. This is useful for slow or irregular rhythms. It is easy to calculate and gives the average rate over this period.
- Alternatively, *divide* the number of large squares between consecutive R waves into 300 (see Figure 35.1).
  - Normal (in adults) 60–100 beats/min.
  - Tachycardia >100 beats/min
  - Bradycardia <60 beats/min.

Rhythm

- Check the regularity of the P waves and QRS complexes and the association between them.
- If the regularity is in doubt, use a piece of paper to mark out at least three successive R waves and check the rate is the same further along the rhythm strip (i.e. the marks line up again exactly).

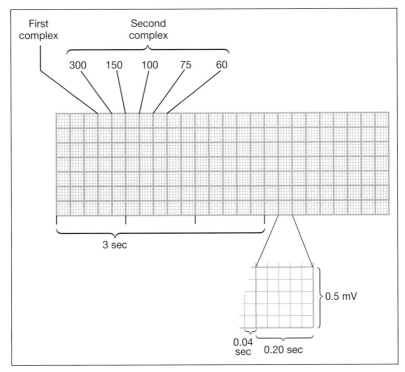

Figure 35.1 Rate.

- Regular rhythm with normal P wave preceding every QRS complex = sinus rhythm.
- Regular rhythm with abnormal P wave preceding each QRS complex = atrial rhythm.
- Irregular rhythm with P waves = multifocal atrial rhythm.
- Regular narrow-complex rhythm with no (or retrograde) P waves = SVT.
- Regular rhythm with visible flutter waves = atrial flutter.
- Irregular rhythm with no P waves = atrial fibrillation or atrial flutter with variable AV conduction block.
- Broad-complex rhythm = ventricular rhythm or supraventricular rhythm with abnormal ventricular depolarisation (bundle branch block).

Axis

To identify a significant deviation in axis, look at the QRS complexes in leads I and aVF (see Figures 35.2 and 35.3 and Table 35.1). Lead I is a left-sided lead, and because aVF is perpendicular to lead I, it can be considered as a right-sided lead.

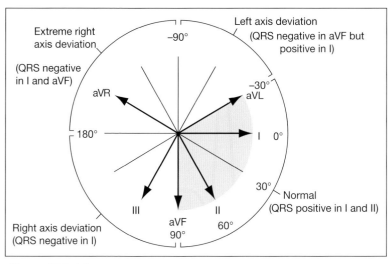

Figure 35.2 Axis.

Table 35.1	Identifying axis deviation	
QRS deflection		
Lead I	aVF	**Axis**
Positive	Positive	Normal
Positive	Negative	LAD
Negative	Positive	RAD
Negative	Negative	Either extreme RAD or extreme LAD

- Both leads I and aVF have mainly positive QRS complexes = normal axis.
- Lead I positive and aVF negative = left axis deviation (LAD).
- Lead I negative and aVF positive = right axis deviation (RAD).
- Both leads negative = extreme RAD or extreme LAD.

P wave morphology

- Normal P wave (see Figure 35.4A) is smooth, upright and 80 msec duration (two small squares).
- Left atrial enlargement (P mitrale) is associated with a prolonged (>120 msec) notched P wave (see Figure 35.4B).
- Right atrial enlargement (P pulmonale) is associated with a high-amplitude P wave (>2.5 mm in inferior leads) (see Figure 35.4C).
- Variable morphology of P waves indicates multifocal atrial ectopy.

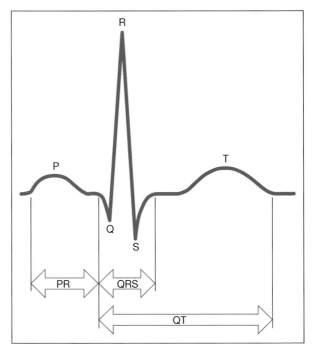

Figure 35.3 Normal ECG parameters.

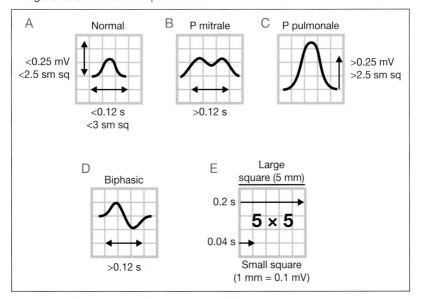

Figure 35.4 P wave configuration in lead II. **A** Normal P wave. **B** Left atrial enlargement. **C** Right atrial enlargement. **D** Biphasic P wave. **E** Standard ECG square. (Copyright Tor Ercleve.)

PR interval and segment

- PR interval is measured from the start of the P wave to the start of the QRS complex.
  - Normal duration is 120–200 msec (3–5 small squares)
  - First-degree AV block if >200 msec.
  - Accessory AV pathway if <120 msec.
- PR segment is measured from the end of the P wave to the start of the QRS complex.
  - Normal duration is 50–120 msec.
  - Depression occurs in pericarditis and atrial ischaemia.

Q waves

- Pathological if >33% of the total QRS complex, or >40 msec (one small square) width—suggests previous myocardial infarction.
- Small Q waves can be normal non-pathological in leads III and V1 from septal depolarisation.

QRS width

- Normal if <120 msec (three small squares).
- Widened QRS complexes may be associated with:
  - RBBB (upright RSR in V1) (see Figure 35.5A)
  - LBBB (upright RSR in V6) (see Figure 35.5B)
  - Depolarisation abnormalities (tricyclic, phenothiazine, local anaesthetic etc. toxicity; electrolyte disturbance such as $\uparrow K$; hypothermia; cardiomyopathy)
  - Ventricular arrhythmias.

QRS height

- Low voltage overall may be caused by body habitus, lung hyperinflation (e.g. COPD), hypothermia, hypothyroidism, pericardial effusion, chronic cardiac ischaemia.
- Left ventricular hypertrophy (LVH) if:
  - S in lead V1 or V2 plus R in V5 >35 mm
  - R in aVL >11 mm
  - ST-segment depression and inverted T waves in left lateral leads (V4–6).
- Right ventricular hypertrophy (RVH) if:
  - R > S in V1
  - Right axis deviation (> +90 degrees)
  - ST-segment depression and inverted T wave in right praecordial leads (V1–2).
- QRS complexes are usually predominantly negative in V1 and become more positive across to V6, being equipotential at V3 or V4.

SECTION D – Investigations

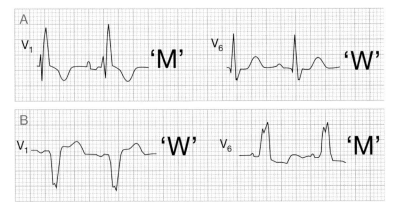

Figure 35.5 A Right bundle branch block. **B** Left bundle branch block.
Copyright Tor Ercleve.

- Loss of R wave progression across the praecordial leads may signify ischaemia with loss of functional LV muscle.

R waves
- Tall R waves in V1 can be associated with:
  - RVH
    - RV strain with pulmonary hypertension (e.g. PE)
    - Left-to-right shunt
    - Persistence of infantile pattern
  - RBBB
  - WPW syndrome type A
  - Posterior AMI (with ST elevation in leads V7, V8 and V9)
  - Hypertrophic cardiomyopathy
  - Lead misplacement
  - Muscular dystrophy
  - Normal variant in children and young adults
  - Dextrocardia.

ST segment
- *Elevation* from acute myocardial infarction, ischaemia, ventricular aneurysm, pericarditis, benign early repolarisation, paced rhythm, Brugada syndrome (sodium channelopathy causing sudden death).
- *Depression* from myocardial ischaemia, infarction (posterior MI), reciprocal change in STEMI (electrically opposite leads), strain, digoxin effect ('reverse tick'), hypokalaemia.

QT interval

- QT interval (measured from the beginning of QRS complex to end of T wave):
  - Normal <450 msec
  - *Prolonged* in sodium-channel blocker toxicity, hypokalaemia, hypomagnesaemia, hypocalcaemia, hypothermia, myocarditis, congenital 'long QT syndrome'.

T waves

- *Peaked* with hyperkalaemia, hyperacute MI.
- *Flat* or *inverted* with cardiac ischaemia, infarction, myocarditis, PE, LVH, adrenergic stress including Takotsubo cardiomyopathy, neurogenic such as SAH, or a normal finding in children plus some young adults (V1–V3).

Other waves

- Delta wave (slurred initial upslope on QRS complex) = ventricular pre-excitation in WPW syndrome.
- J (Osborn wave) notch at junction of QRS and ST segment = hypothermia, hypercalcaemia, vasospastic angina, SAH.
- U wave (occurs after T wave) = hypokalaemia, bradycardia.

Conduction abnormalities

- First-degree block
  - PR interval >200 msec (one large square).
- Second-degree block (occasional absence of QRS and T after a P wave of sinus origin)
  - Type I (Wenckebach)—progressive prolongation of the PR interval before the missed QRS complex
  - Type II—absence of progressive prolongation of the PR interval before the missed QRS complex.
- Third-degree block
  - No relationship between P waves of sinus origin and QRS complexes (AV dissociation).
- Left anterior hemiblock
  - Left axis deviation, Q waves in leads I and aVL, and a small R in lead III, in the absence of LVH.
- Left posterior hemiblock
  - Right axis deviation, a small R in lead I and a small Q in lead III, in the absence of RVH.

SECTION D – Investigations

Myocardial infarction patterns

- Various regional changes may signify myocardial infarction (MI) including:
  - ST-segment elevation (STEMI)
  - ST-depression (NSTEMI)
  - Biphasic, flat or inverted T waves
  - Development of Q waves.

Typical ECG lead patterns suggesting their anatomical location are outlined in Table 35.2.

Table 35.2 Myocardial infarction patterns

Site of infarction	Pattern of changes
Anteroseptal	V1–4
Lateral	V5, V6
High lateral	II, aVL
Inferior	II, III, aVF
Posterior wall	V7, V8, V9 R > S in V1 with positive T in V1 or V2 Q may develop in V6
Right ventricle	II, III, aVF V4R, V5R, V6R

36

Chest X-ray

Standard views

- An erect posteroanterior (PA) inspiratory image is the preferred CXR view (see Figure 36.1). The patient stands in front of a radiographic plate, hands on hips, with the X-ray source 2 m behind.
- A left lateral CXR is also performed with the patient standing (see Figure 36.2). It is used in combination with a PA CXR to localise and further delineate masses, lesions or consolidation, particularly those obscured by the heart or diaphragms.

Alternative views

- An **anteroposterior (AP)** CXR is performed in patients unable to stand for a PA view, and in those who require a portable CXR when it is deemed unsafe to move them to the radiology department.
  - The X-ray is taken from the front with the cassette placed behind the patient. AP films magnify the size of the heart and mediastinum, and are more commonly associated with rotational artefact.
- **Supine AP, lateral decubitus and expiratory films**
  - Occasionally a film taken in full expiration is helpful in defining a small pneumothorax or to determine gas trapping with an inhaled foreign body.

Interpretation

Adopt a systematic approach to CXR interpretation to avoid missing significant pathological changes.
Ownership, adequacy and technical quality of the film:
- Name and date of birth of the patient, and date radiograph was performed.

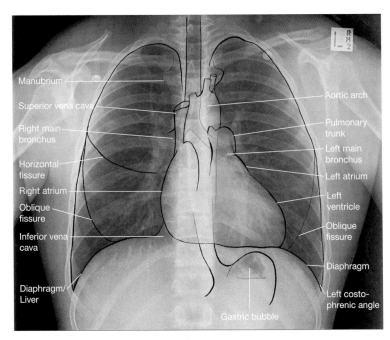

Manubrium

Superior vena cava

Right main
bronchus

Horizontal
fissure

Right atrium

Oblique
fissure

Inferior vena
cava

Diaphragm/
Liver

Aortic arch

Pulmonary
trunk

Left main
bronchus

Left atrium

Left
ventricle

Oblique
fissure

Diaphragm

Left costo-
phrenic angle

Gastric bubble

Figure 36.1 Posteroanterior chest X-ray. Copyright Tor Ercleve.

- Projection (e.g. PA, AP, lateral).
- Posture (e.g. supine or erect).
- Adequacy of exposure. This is determined by easily visible mid-thoracic intervertebral spaces.
- Degree of inspiration. Check the film is taken in full inspiration, with the diaphragm at the level of the 10th or 11th ribs posteriorly and the 6th costal cartilage anteriorly.
- Degree of rotation. A well-centred (non-rotated) film has the spinous processes of the upper thoracic vertebrae located centrally and equidistant from the medial ends of the clavicles.

The key components of the CXR are summarised in Table 36.1 and expanded below.
- **Trachea:** should be central, with slight deviation to the right as it crosses the aortic arch.
  - The trachea may be pushed *away* from an abnormal lung affected by a large pleural effusion, large simple pneumothorax, tension pneumothorax, aortic aneurysm or mediastinal mass.

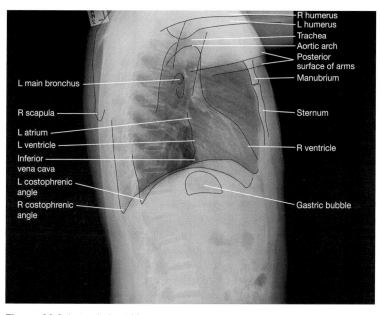

Figure 36.2 Lateral chest X-ray. Copyright Tor Ercleve.

Table 36.1	**Chest X-ray check sheet**	
A	Airway	Check trachea—midline or deviated? Look for paratracheal masses.
B	Bones and soft tissues	Look for fractures, dislocations and lytic lesions involving visible bones and ribs. Identify breast shadows and evidence of surgical emphysema. Do not confuse nipple shadows with coin lesions.
C	Cardiac silhouette	Examine the size, shape and position. Measure the CTR on PA films.
D	Diaphragms	Look for elevation, flattening, rim of free air. Examine the costophrenic angles for blunting. *Note:* right normally higher than left.
E	Equal volume	Compare the two lung fields and count the visible posterior ribs on both sides. Determine loss of volume and mediastinal shift.
F	Fine detail	Trace the outline of the pleura on both sides and examine the lung parenchyma. Examine specifically for the presence of a pneumothorax.
G	Gastric bubble	Look at the position in relation to the left ventricle and diaphragm and the size.
H	Hilum	*Note:* left normally higher than right.
I	Iatrogenic intervention	Look for tubes, lines, drains and foreign bodies.

- The trachea may be pulled *towards* an abnormal lung affected by extensive collapse, consolidation, pulmonary fibrosis, lobectomy or pneumonectomy.
- **Superior mediastinum:** should have a width <8 cm on a PA CXR. A widened mediastinum is associated with:
  - AP CXR view, which magnifies the heart and mediastinal structures
  - Unfolded aortic arch (not pathological)
  - Thoracic aortic aneurysm (always pathological)
  - Ruptured aorta in deceleration trauma from vehicle crash or fall from a height
  - Mediastinal lymphadenopathy, retrosternal thyroid, thymoma (associated with myasthenia gravis), enlarged thymus (in young children)
  - Paravertebral mass, oesophageal dilation (achalasia).
- **Mediastinal emphysema** (abnormal air) secondary to:
  - Asthma, whooping cough, pneumothorax (pneumomediastinum)
  - Penetrating wound ± lacerated lung
  - Perforation of oesophagus or trachea.
- **Hila:** level with the T6–7 intervertebral space on either side of the mediastinum. Are made up of the pulmonary arteries and veins.
  - The left hilum is usually higher and squarer than the V-shaped right hilum.
  - Unilateral or bilateral hilar enlargement is caused by enlarged hilar lymph nodes (e.g. sarcoidosis or infection such as TB, *Mycoplasma*), hilar malignancy (e.g. carcinoma, lymphoma) or vascular disease (e.g. pulmonary hypertension or proximal pulmonary artery aneurysm).
- **Heart:** usually positioned with one-third of its diameter to the right and two-thirds to the left of the thoracic vertebrae spinous processes.
  - The right atrium makes up the right heart border and the left ventricle the left heart border. Loss of distinction of the right heart border suggests consolidation of the right middle lobe, whereas poor distinction of the left heart border suggests lingular consolidation.
  - Obliteration of this normal air–soft-tissue interface is known as the silhouette sign.
- **Cardiothoracic ratio (CTR)**
  - Compares the transverse diameter of the heart to the internal thoracic diameter at its widest point.
  - Should be less than 0.5 (50%) on a PA CXR, but may appear magnified on AP films.

- Abnormally increased CTR occurs with ventricular dilation (usually left), cardiac failure and a pericardial effusion.
- **Diaphragms**
  - The right is usually higher than the left by 1–3 cm.
  - A pleural effusion will blunt the costophrenic angle. Loss of the diaphragmatic outline indicates fluid, consolidation or collapse of adjacent lung (i.e. of the right or left lower lobe).
  - Both hemidiaphragms are flat in COPD such as emphysema.
  - Free gas under a diaphragm on an erect film indicates rupture of an abdominal hollow viscus, such as the duodenum or small or large intestine, but remember it also occurs normally after laparoscopy following the introduction of a pneumoperitoneum.
- **Lung outlines**
  - Trace the outline of the right and left lungs, looking for evidence of pneumothorax, bullae, collapse, consolidation, effusion, masses or pleural changes such as fibrosis (see Table 36.2)
  - Both lung fields should be equally translucent. On the lateral view the lung lucency should increase towards the diaphragms.
  - An abnormal increase in lucency occurs with vessel loss, as in emphysema or pneumothorax, and a decrease results from alveolar or interstitial fluid, effusion or consolidation.

SECTION D – Investigations

Table 36.2		Causes of pulmonary fibrosis
Upper zone	S	Silicosis, sarcoidosis
	C	Coal worker's pneumoconiosis
	A	Aspergillosis, allergic alveolitis, ankylosing spondylitis, amiodarone
	T	TB
Lower zone	B	Bronchiectasis
	R	Rheumatoid arthritis
	A	Asbestosis
	S	Scleroderma
	H	Hamman–Rich syndrome (acute interstitial pneumonitis)
Either zone		Radiation, smoke inhalation, ARDS, drugs

- **Pulmonary nodules** may be diffuse, or solitary 'coin lesion'. Causes of nodules on CXR include:
  - Neoplasia—metastases, primary lung tumour, adenoma, lymphangitis carcinomatosa
  - Infection—miliary TB, varicella (chickenpox) pneumonia, fibrotic lung disease, histoplasmosis
  - Vascular—arteriovenous malformation, hamartoma, pulmonary embolus (with infarction).
- **Cavitating lung disease** (see Table 36.3).

Table 36.3	Cavitating lung disease	
C	Carcinoma	Lung primary—squamous cell carcinoma, small-cell carcinoma and adenocarcinoma Metastasis—breast, colon, prostate, renal, bladder, thyroid, bone, melanoma, squamous cell carcinoma (head and neck)
A	Autoimmune	Wegener granulomatosis, rheumatoid nodules, SLE
V	Vascular	PE with infarction
I	Infection	Gram-positive (e.g. *Staphylococcus aureus*, streptococcal pneumonia [rare]) Gram-negative (e.g. *Klebsiella*, *Pseudomonas*, *Legionella*, *Haemophilus*) Opportunistic (e.g. *Aspergillus*, TB)
T	Trauma	Traumatic lung cyst after haemorrhage
Y	Young	Bronchogenic cyst, diaphragmatic hernia

37

Abdominal X-ray

The two most commonly requested abdominal X-ray (AXR) films are:
- Anteroposterior (AP) supine
- Anteroposterior (AP) erect.

Alternative views

- **Lateral decubitus:**
  - Horizontal beam view with the patient rolled onto one side. A useful alternative to the erect AP view if the patient is unable to sit or stand.
- **Supine lateral:**
  - The beam is shot across the patient.
- **KUB** (kidneys, ureters, bladder):
  - Allows follow-up of the passage of a renal tract calculus.

Indications

Indications for plain AXR differ and are influenced by the availability of CT or USS, which give considerably more information. Thus abdominal X-rays are *only* useful for certain defined pathological features that are known to be visualised, such as 'abnormal gases, masses, bones and stones'. So do not order one unless you are specifically looking for one of the following:
- Undifferentiated abdominal pain with a provisional diagnosis of:
  - Toxic megacolon in acute inflammatory bowel disease (colonic diameter >6 cm)
  - Bowel obstruction (50% sensitive for acute obstruction, although CT may show not only the site but also the cause)
  - Perforation of a viscus with abdominal free air (ask for an erect CXR as well).

- KUB for renal tract calculus: 80–90% sensitivity if radiolucent stone >3 mm diameter. Will still need further imaging such as a non-contrast CT KUB or renal ultrasound to confirm ureteric origin.
- Foreign body—following ingestion (radiodense tablets such as iron; metal objects). Plain AXR has 90% sensitivity for foreign body identification.

There is no evidence that correlates AXR findings with 'constipation', so do *not* use radiography to make this diagnosis (see Chapter 26).

Interpretation

Adopt a systematic approach to AXR interpretation to avoid missing significant pathological changes.

Ownership, adequacy and technical quality of the film:
- Name and date of birth of the patient and date radiograph was performed.
- Projection.
- Posture (e.g. supine or erect).
- Adequacy of exposure.

Look for 'gases, masses, bones and stones', which are known to be visible on an AXR.

Gases

Look for normal or abnormal intraluminal and extraluminal gas distribution.
- **Small bowel**
  - Intraluminal gas is usually modest, centrally located within numerous tight loops of small diameter (2.5–3.5 cm), distinguished by valvulae conniventes (circular folds or valves of Kerckring). These are characteristic mucosal folds that stretch all the way across the small bowel loops (see Figures 37.1 and 37.2).
- **Large bowel**
  - A mixture of gas and faeces located within loops of larger diameter (3–5 cm) around the periphery, with haustra, which are mucosal folds that stretch only partway across the diameter of the large bowel loops (see Figure 37.3).
- **Abnormal findings include:**
  - Dilated loops of small or large bowel—obstruction, ileus or inflammation
  - Air–fluid levels on erect AXR—more than 5 fluid levels, each greater than 2.5 cm in length, is abnormal and associated with obstruction, ileus, ischaemia and gastroenteritis

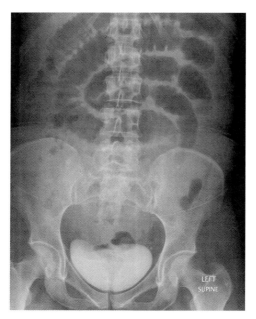

Figure 37.1 Small bowel obstruction (supine view). Note the regular transverse bands (valvulae conniventes) extending across the entire diameter of the bowel.

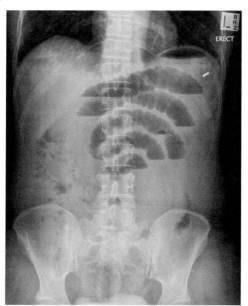

Figure 37.2 Small bowel obstruction (erect view). Note the regular transverse bands (valvulae conniventes) extending across the entire diameter of the bowel.

SECTION D – Investigations

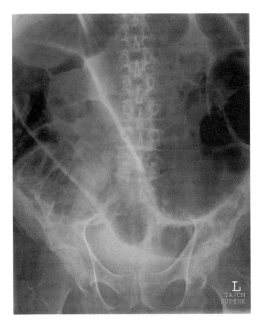

Figure 37.3 Large bowel vovulus (supine view).

- **Intramural gas**–ischaemic colitis
- **Intraperitoneal gas**–perforated viscus (or penetrating abdominal injury)
  - Rigler's sign (double-wall sign) is seen when both sides of the bowel wall are visualised, indicating free intraperitoneal gas. However, the overall sensitivity for detecting perforation on AXR is low, so is best confirmed as subdiaphragmatic air on erect CXR (see Figure 37.4) or by CT scan.
- **Extraperitoneal gas**–within the soft tissues, retroperitoneal structures or chest in infection or trauma.

Masses

- Look for the size and position of the solid organ shadows of the liver, spleen, kidneys and bladder.
- Identify the retroperitoneal shadow of the psoas muscles. Bulging of the lateral margin or obliteration of the psoas shadow may indicate a retroperitoneal pathological feature.
- Look for the dilated, calcified sac of an aortic aneurysm, or for adjacent bony trauma (e.g. transverse process fractures).
- All require a CT scan instead of, or following, AXR.

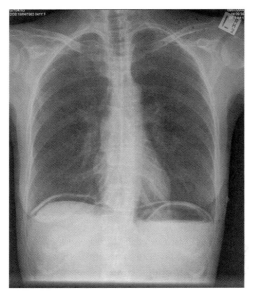

Figure 37.4 Erect CXR showing subdiaphragmatic air from perforated viscus.

Bones

- Look for abnormalities of the visible bones such as the ribs, spine, sacrum and pelvis (e.g. for fracture, scoliosis, degenerative disease, tumours and metastatic deposition).
- These may be incidental or provide additional information on the cause of the abdominal pain.

Stones

- Look for renal, ureteric and bladder stones/calcification. Trace the course of the ureter from the pelvis of the kidney, along the tips of the lumbar spine transverse processes, over the sacroiliac joint, down to the ischial spine and medially to the bladder.
- 80–90% of renal tract stones are radio-opaque, but will still require non-contrast CT or USS to confirm their position within the ureter. *Note:* phleboliths, faecoliths and vascular calcifications mimic renal tract calculi.
- Examine the RUQ and transpyloric plane at the level of L1 for evidence of gallstones (15% radio-opaque) or pancreatic calcification. Again, confirmation with USS or CT is indicated, rather than an AXR.

38

CT head scan

Principles

Fine X-ray beams passed through a subject are absorbed to different degrees by different tissues and the transmitted radiation is measured by a scanning device to give a computed tomography (CT) image.

- The CT head scan is thus a computer-generated series of images from multiple X-rays taken at different levels.
- The degree of absorption of X-rays is proportional to the density of the tissue through which the beam passes. The Hounsfield unit (HU) is used to measure how much of the X-ray beam is absorbed by the tissues at each point in the body.
- The denser the tissue, the more the X-ray beam is attenuated and the higher the number. Units are established on a relative scale with water as the reference point. Water is always 0 HU, bone is approximately 1000 HU and air is −1000 HU (see Table 38.1).

Interpretation

Use a systematic approach to viewing the anatomical structures in the many slices ('cuts') generated by the CT scanner.

- **Orientation:**
  - The CT slice is regarded as being viewed from the patient's feet, so the left side of the picture as you view it is the right side of the patient.
- **General review:**
  - Generate a system to review all of the essential features of the CT head scan (see Table 38.2).
- **Contrast versus non-contrast:**
  - Determine whether scans have been taken with or without IV contrast, as contrast may mimic the presence of blood.
  - IV contrast does not cross the normal blood–brain barrier, and is used if there is a suspicion of tumour, infection (e.g. abscess) or vascular abnormality (e.g. AVM or aneurysm).

Table 38.1	CT number in Hounsfield units for various tissues	
Tissue	CT number (HU)	Greyscale colour
Cortical bone	300–1000	White
Trabecular bone	80–300	
Retracted clot	60–80	
Fresh blood	40–60	
Grey matter (brain)	36–46	
White matter (brain)	22–32	
Cerebrospinal fluid	15	
Water	0	
Fat	(–50)–(–100)	
Air	–1000	Black

Table 38.2	Mnemonic for interpreting CT head scan	
B	*Blood*	Blood
C	*Can*	Cisterns
B	*Be*	Brain
V	*Very*	Ventricles
B	*Bad*	Bone

Blood

- Look for the presence of blood. Clues to the origin of the haemorrhage, its duration and the cause may be indicated by its position and spread.
- Acute haemorrhage absorbs X-rays and appears hyperdense (white) on CT scans. As the clot evolves, it becomes more hyperdense over the first few hours up to 7 days, then isodense with brain over the following 1–4 weeks and finally hypodense compared with brain over the subsequent 4–6 weeks.
- **Extracerebral (-axial) haemorrhage**—within the skull, but outside the brain:
  - **Extradural haemorrhage (EDH)**—biconvex lesion that does not cross suture lines; usually secondary to arterial injury (see Figure 38.1).
  - **Subdural haemorrhage (SDH)**—crescent-shaped blood collection that can cross suture lines; usually secondary to venous disruption of surface and/or bridging vessels (see Figure 38.2).
  - **Subarachnoid haemorrhage (SAH)**—haemorrhage into the CSF and cisterns secondary to a berry aneurysm, arteriovenous malformation or trauma (see Figure 38.3).

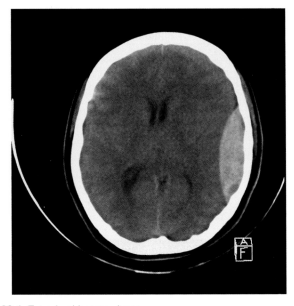

Figure 38.1 Extradural haemorrhage.

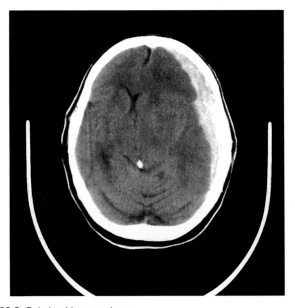

Figure 38.2 Subdural haemorrhage.

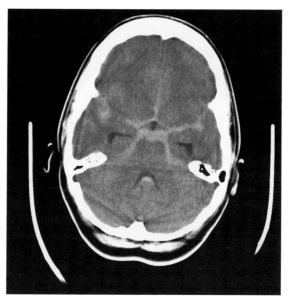

Figure 38.3 Subarachnoid haemorrhage.

- **Intracerebral (-axial) haemorrhage**—within the brain substance itself:
  - **Intracerebral haemorrhage (ICH)**—secondary to hypertension, haemorrhagic stroke and trauma.
  - **Intraventricular haemorrhage (IVH)**—usually associated with significant trauma.

Cisterns

Cisterns are collections of CSF that surround and protect the brain. Examine each for evidence of effacement, asymmetry and the presence of blood.
- **Peri-mesencephalic**—surrounding the midbrain.
- **Suprasellar**—around the circle of Willis.
- **Quadrigeminal**—located at the top of the midbrain.
- **Cerebellomedullary (cisterna magna)**—between the cerebellum and the dorsal surface of the medulla oblongata.

Brain matter

- Compare the sulcal pattern (gyri) for evidence of effacement, and the relative volume of the left and the right sides of the brain for asymmetry. Trace the falx through the series of scans, looking for midline shift secondary to compartmental mass effect.

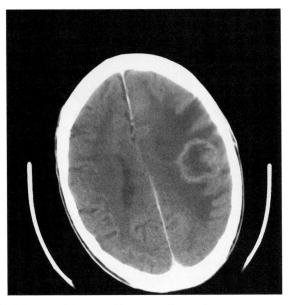

Figure 38.4 Intracranial mass with surrounding oedema.

- Look for inconsistencies in the grey–white differentiation (e.g. evolving embolic stroke).
  - Patients with CVA may have a normal CT head scan on presentation, with subtle oedema beginning at 6–12 hours, hypoattenuation after 24 hours and maximal oedema at 3–5 days.
- Identify hyperdense regions associated with blood, IV contrast or calcification.
- Identify hypodense regions associated with air, fat, ischaemia or tumour (see Figure 38.4).

Ventricles
- Examine the ventricles—two lateral, 3rd and 4th for asymmetry, dilation (hydrocephalus), effacement due to mass effect, and haemorrhage.

Bone
- Cortical bone has the highest density on the CT scan (300–1000 HU) and is best viewed on separate bony windows when looking for evidence of fracture or tumour (osteolytic or osteosclerotic changes).

39

Urinalysis

Urinary analysis or urinalysis (UA) is used as a screening and/or diagnostic test to detect abnormal substances or cellular material in the urine. This aids in determining metabolic disorders such as diabetic ketoacidosis, renal dysfunction causing proteinuria and/or casts, urinary white cells (pyelonephritis or UTI) or urinary red cells (renal tract calculus, trauma).

Substances such as glucose, protein or cells may also be found in the urine before a patient is aware there is a problem, such as glycosuria (diabetes), proteinuria (renal disease) or microscopic haematuria (renal tract malignancy).

Urine can be assessed at the bedside (dipstick) and in the laboratory (microscopy, culture, sensitivity and urinary electrolytes). Urine for laboratory analysis must be transferred rapidly and at the correct temperature to avoid spoiling.

Urinary sample collection

- **Midstream urine (MSU)**
  - A clean-catch, MSU specimen is collected after cleansing the external urethral meatus. The first half of the urine stream is discarded and serves to flush contaminating cells and microbes from the outer urethra. The collection vessel is then introduced into the urinary stream to catch the 'middle' portion.
- **Catheter specimen of urine (CSU)**
  - A per urethral bladder catherisation specimen ('in–out' catheter) should be carried out only in special circumstances (e.g. patient is confused or comatose). The procedure risks introducing infection (rate <1%) or causing urethral trauma with bleeding (haematuria).
- **Suprapubic transabdominal needle aspiration**
  - A suprapubic urine specimen, when performed under ideal conditions, provides the least contaminated sample of bladder urine. It is an accurate method to confirm UTI in infants and small children, ideally using ultrasound guidance.

Urine examination

Direct visualisation
- **Colour:** normal, fresh urine is pale to dark yellow or amber in colour and clear.
- **Transparency:** turbidity or cloudiness is caused by excessive cellular material or protein in the urine; or may develop from crystallisation or precipitation of salts upon standing at room temperature or in the refrigerator.

Urinalysis
Specific gravity
- Specific gravity (SG) of urine is a measure of the amount of solutes dissolved in urine as compared to water (SG 1.000).
- Specific gravity between 1.002 and 1.035 on a random sample is considered normal if kidney function is normal.
- Specific gravity is directly proportional to urine osmolality, which measures solute concentration and the ability of the kidney to concentrate or dilute the urine over that of plasma. The SG of glomerular filtrate in Bowman's space ranges from 1.007 to 1.010. Any measurement below this range indicates overhydration and any measurement above it indicates relative dehydration.
  - **Decreased (<1.005):**
    - Excessive hydration (volume resuscitation with IV fluids).
    - Inability to concentrate urine in nephrogenic diabetes insipidus, acute glomerulonephritis, pyelonephritis or acute tubular necrosis.
    - *Note:* if SG does not rise >1.022 after a 12-hour period without food or water, renal concentrating ability is impaired and the patient has either generalised renal impairment or nephrogenic diabetes insipidus.
    - Falsely low SG can be associated with alkaline urine.
  - **Fixed (1.010):**
    - Occurs in end-stage renal disease, as the SG tends towards 1.010.
    - Indicates chronic renal failure (CRF), chronic glomerulonephritis (GN).
  - **Increased (>1.035):**
    - Indicates a concentrated urine with a large volume of dissolved solutes.
    - Dehydration (fever, vomiting, diarrhoea), SIADH, renal artery stenosis, hepatorenal syndrome, CCF, nephrotic syndrome.
    - SG elevation also occurs with glycosuria (e.g. diabetes mellitus or IV glucose administration), following IV contrast, urine contamination, LMW dextran solutions (colloid).

pH

- The kidneys play an important role in acid–base regulation within the body. They maintain a normal urinary pH range between 5.5 and 6.5, although this may vary from as low as 4.5 to as high as 8.0.
- The glomerular filtrate of blood plasma is usually acidified by renal tubules and collecting ducts from a pH of 7.4 to about 6.0 in the final urine.
- Control of pH is important in the management of several diseases, including bacteriuria, renal calculi and drug therapy.
- **High pH (alkaline urine):**
  - Vegetarian diet, low carbohydrate diet or ingestion of citrus fruit
  - Systemic alkalosis (metabolic or respiratory)
  - Renal tubular acidosis (RTA) type 1–distal, Fanconi's syndrome
  - UTIs (urea-splitting bacteria e.g. *Proteus* sp.)
  - Medications: amphotericin B, carbonic anhydrase inhibitors (acetazolomide), $NaHCO_3^-$, salicylate OD
  - Stale ammoniacal sample (left standing).
- **Low pH (acidic urine):**
  - High-protein diet or fruits such as cranberries
  - Systemic acidosis (metabolic or respiratory)
  - Diabetes mellitus, starvation, diarrhoea, malabsorption
  - Phenylketonuria, alkaptonuria, renal tuberculosis.

Protein

- Normal daily protein excretion should not exceed 150 mg/day (24 hours) or 10 mg/100 mL, mostly consisting of Tamm-Horsfall glycoprotein. Proteinuria is defined by the production of >150 mg/day, and nephrotic syndrome is defined as the production of >3.5 g/day per 1.73 m^2 body surface area.
- Dipstick urinalysis detects protein with bromphenol blue indicator dye. This is most sensitive to albumin and less sensitive to Bence–Jones protein (myeloma) and globulins.
- 'Trace' positive results are equivalent to 10 mg/100 mL or about 150 mg/day (the upper limit of normal). See Table 39.1.
- **Protein elevation:**
  - **Renal:** increased renal tubular secretion, increased glomerular filtration (glomerular disease), nephrotic syndrome, pyelonephritis, glomerulonephritis, severe hypertension
  - **CVS:** benign hypertension, CCF, subacute bacterial endocarditis
  - **Functional proteinuria (albuminuria):** fever, cold exposure, stress, pregnancy, eclampsia, CHF, shock, severe exercise
  - **Other:** orthostatic proteinuria, electric current injury, hypokalaemia, Cushing's syndrome

- **Medications:** aminoglycosides, gold, amphotericin, NSAIDs, sulfonamides, penicillins.
- **False positive:**
  - Concentrated urine (UO <2.5 L/day), alkaline urine (pH >7.5), trace of bleach in container, acetazolamide, cephalosporins, $NaHCO_3$.
- **False negative:**
  - Dilute urine (UO >5.0 L/day) or acidic urine (pH <5).
  - Bence–Jones protein associated with multiple myeloma, lymphoma and Waldenstrom macroglobulinaemia, which is *not* detected by dipstick urinalysis.

Table 39.1   Urine protein levels

Dipstick protein reading	Protein excretion (g/day)	Protein excretion (mg/dL)
Negative	<0.1	<10
Trace	0.1–0.2	15
1+	0.2–0.5	30
2+	0.5–1.5	100
3+	2.0–5.0	300
4+	>5.0	>1000

Leucocytes (white cell count [WCC])

- Determines the presence of whole or lysed white cells in the urine (pyuria) by detecting leucocyte esterase activity.
- A positive leucocyte esterase test correlates well with pyuria (good specificity). However, the diagnosis may be missed in up to 20% of cases if a negative urinalysis dipstick is used to exclude UTI (poor sensitivity) (see Table 39.2).
- **False positive:**
  - Contaminated specimen (especially in females), *Trichomonas vaginalis*, drugs or foods that colour the urine red.
- **False negative:**
  - Intercurrent oxidising antibiotic therapy (gentamicin, nitrofurantoin and cephalosporin), glycosuria, proteinuria, high SG.
  - Low bacteria count UTI (females).

Nitrites

- Nitrates in the urine are converted to nitrites in the presence of Gram-negative bacteria such as *Escherichia coli* and *Klebsiella* spp. A positive nitrite test is thus a surrogate marker of bacteriuria.

Table 39.2	Diagnosing a UTI on dipstick urinalysis or microscopy			
	Sensitivity	**Specificity**	**PPV**	**NPV**
Dipstick				
Leucocyte esterase	75–90	95	50	92
Nitrite	35–85	95	96	27–70
Nitrite and leucocyte esterase	75–90	70	75–93	41–90
Microscopy				
WCC >8 × 10^6	91	50	67	83
Culture				
>10^5 bacteria/L	95	85	88	94
>10^8 bacteria/L	51	59	98	94

PPV, positive predictive value; NPV, negative predictive value, WCC, white cell count.

- A positive test strongly suggests infection (good specificity), but a negative test does not exclude it (poor sensitivity) with a PPV 95% and NPV 25–70%.
- **False positive:**
  - Drugs or foods that colour the urine red.
- **False negative:**
  - Ascorbic acid
  - Certain bacteria such as *Staphylococcus saprophyticus*, *Acinetobacter* spp. and most enterococci, urobilinogen.

Red cells (red blood cell [RBC] count)

- Dipstick urinalysis is able to detect haemolysed and non-haemolysed blood in the urine by the pseudoperoxidase reaction of erythrocytes, or free haemoglobin or myoglobin, which catalyses chromogen oxidation on the dipstick to produce a colour change.
- A positive result is indicative of haematuria from infection, inflammation, infarction, calculi, neoplasia, clotting disorders or chronic infection or trauma (see Chapter 28).
- Positives also result from haemoglobinuria (intravascular haemolysis) and myoglobinuria (crush injury, electrocution, rhabdomyolysis)
  - **False positive:** hypochlorite bleach.

Ketones

- Ketones (acetone, acetoacetic acid, beta-hydroxybutyric acid) are the end-point of incomplete fat metabolism. They accumulate in the plasma and are excreted in urine.

- Ketonuria is associated with a low-carbohydrate (high fat/protein) diet, starvation, diabetes, alcoholism, hyperemesis gravidarum, eclampsia and hyperthyroidism.
- Ketonuria is also associated with overdose of insulin, isoniazid or isopropyl alcohol.
- Most urinalysis reagent tests utilise the nitroprusside test, which is most sensitive to acetoacetic acid, less sensitive to acetone and not sensitive to beta-hydroxybutyric acid (i.e. will miss it).
- **False positive:**
  - Heavily pigmented urine
  - Levodopa, salicylates, phenothiazines.
- **False negative:**
  - Ketonaemia due to increased beta-hydroxybutyric acid concentrations missed by nitroprusside tests.

Glucose

- Glucose is not normally present in the urine. Usually, <0.1% of glucose filtered by the glomerulus appears in urine (<130 mg/day).
- Glycosuria occurs in patients with an elevated serum glucose level (e.g. diabetes mellitus—see Chapter 41) or in the presence of a reduced renal threshold and/or reduced glucose reabsorption in renal tubular disease and pregnancy.
- Glycosuria is also associated with certain drugs, such as cephalosporins, penicillins, nitrofurantoin, methyldopa and tetracycline (false positives), lithium, carbemazepine, phenothiazines, steroids and thiazides (true positives).
- **False positive:**
  - Hydrogen peroxide or bleach in container.
- **False negative:**
  - Ascorbic acid (vitamin C) or fruit juices
  - Some dipsticks are affected by increased SG and ketonuria.

Note: dipsticks that use the glucose oxidase–peroxidase reaction for screening are specific for glucose. They will miss other reducing sugars (e.g. galactose and fructose) and so are not suitable for testing newborn and infant urine. Use a modified Benedict's copper reduction test instead in this group.

Bilirubin

- Bilirubin is not present in the urine of healthy individuals and its presence may be an early indicator of liver disease occurring before clinical signs of jaundice develop.
- Bilirubin is formed as a by-product of RBC degradation in the liver. It is then conjugated with the solubilising sugar glucuronic acid and excreted in bile. Within the intestine, the bilirubin is converted into stercobilin (excreted in faeces and responsible for

the brown colouration) and urobilinogen (excreted by the kidneys and colourless).
- Failure of conjugated bilirubin to reach the intestines (e.g. biliary obstruction) will result in bilirubinuria (dark amber colour).
- Raised conjugated bilirubinaemia (with bilirubinuria) is associated with hepatocellular disease, cirrhosis, viral and drug-induced hepatitis, biliary tract obstruction (e.g. choledocholithiasis), pancreatic causes of obstructive jaundice (e.g. carcinoma of the head of the pancreas) and recurrent idiopathic jaundice of pregnancy.
  - **False positive:** phenothiazines.
  - **False negative:** ascorbic acid (vitamin C), aged sample (conjugated bilirubin hydrolses to unconjugated bilirubin at room temperature), rifampicin and exposure to UV light (converts bilrubin to biliverdin).
- *Note:* only conjugated bilirubin can be excreted as bilirubinuria. A positive test for urine bilirubin confirms conjugated hyperbilirubinaemia (see Table 39.3).

Urobilinogen

- Urobilinogen is normally present in the urine in low concentrations (0.2–1.0 mg/dL or <17 micromol/L). Bilirubin is converted to urobilinogen by intestinal bacteria in the duodenum. Most urobilinogen is then excreted in the faeces or transported back to the liver and converted into bile. The remaining urobilinogen (<1%) is excreted in the urine.
- Urobilinogen is present in increased concentrations in the urine in patients with cirrhosis, infective hepatitis including Epstein-Barr virus, extravascular haemolysis, haemolytic anaemia, pernicious anaemia and malaria.
- Measuring urobilinogen is a sensitive, but non-specific test to determine liver damage, haemolytic disease and severe infections. Urobilinogen levels are decreased or absent in obstructive jaundice and with elevated levels of bilirubinuria.

SECTION D – Investigations

Table 39.3 Urine bilirubin and urobilinogen levels				
Dipstick urinalysis	**Normal**	**Biliary obstruction**	**Hepatic disease**	**Haemolytic disease**
Bilirubin	Negative	Positive	Positive or negative	Negative
Urobilinogen	Positive	Negative/ decreased	Increased	Increased

40

Acid–base disorders

Arterial blood gas (ABG) analysis is used to determine the adequacy of oxygenation and ventilation, assess respiratory function and determine the acid–base balance. These data provide information regarding potential primary and compensatory processes that affect the body's acid–base buffering system (see Table 40.1). Interpret an ABG in a stepwise manner:

Determine the *adequacy of oxygenation* (PaO_2)
- Normal range: 80–100 mmHg (10.6–13.3 kPa)

Determine the *pH status*
- Normal pH range: 7.35–7.45 (H^+ 35–45 nmol/L)
  - pH <7.35: *acidosis* is an abnormal process that increases the serum hydrogen ion concentration, lowers the pH and results in *acidaemia.*
  - pH >7.45: *alkalosis* is an abnormal process that decreases the hydrogen ion concentration and results in *alkalaemia.*

Determine the *respiratory component* ($PaCO_2$)
- Normal $PaCO_2$ range: 35–45 mmHg (4.7–6.0 kPa)
  - $PaCO_2$ >45 mmHg (>6.0 kPa)
    - Primary respiratory acidosis (hypoventilation) if pH <7.35 and HCO_3^- normal.
    - Respiratory compensation for metabolic alkalosis if pH >7.45 and HCO_3^- ($\uparrow$).
  - $PaCO_2$ <35 mmHg (4.7 kPa)
    - Primary respiratory alkalosis (hyperventilation) if pH >7.45 and HCO_3^- normal.
    - Respiratory compensation for metabolic acidosis if pH <7.35 and HCO_3^- ($\downarrow$).

Determine the *metabolic component* (HCO_3^-)
- Normal HCO_3^- range: 22–26 mmol/L
  - HCO_3^- <22 mmol/L
    - Primary metabolic acidosis if pH <7.35
    - Renal compensation for respiratory alkalosis if pH >7.45.
  - HCO_3^- >26 mmol/L
    - Primary metabolic alkalosis if pH >7.45.
    - Renal compensation for respiratory acidosis if pH <7.35.

Table 40.1 **Determining the likely acid–base disorder from the pH, $PaCO_2$ and HCO_3^-**

pH	$PaCO_2$	HCO_3^-	Acid–base disorder
↓	N	↓	**Primary metabolic acidosis**
↓	↓	↓	Metabolic acidosis with respiratory compensation
↓	↑	N	**Primary respiratory acidosis**
↓	↑	↑	Respiratory acidosis with renal compensation
↓	↑	↓	**Mixed metabolic and respiratory acidosis**
↑	↓	N	**Primary respiratory alkalosis**
↑	↓	↓	Respiratory alkalosis with renal compensation
↑	N	↑	**Primary metabolic alkalosis**
↑	↑	↑	Metabolic alkalosis with respiratory compensation
↑	↓	↑	**Mixed metabolic and respiratory alkalosis**

N, normal.
Respiratory compensation by changes in $PaCO_2$ occurs rapidly.
Renal compensation by changes in HCO_3^- occurs more slowly.

- A simple way to calculate the expected HCO_3^- in a respiratory disorder is to use the 1, 2, 4, 5 rule. For every 10 mmHg change in $PaCO_2$ from the normal (40 mmHg), the HCO_3^- changes by a factor of 1, 2, 4 or 5 from the baseline of 24 mmol/L.

Blood gas interpretation helps determine most primary disturbances of acid–base balance. The expected associated renal or respiratory compensatory changes can be calculated using Table 40.2 and are discussed

Table 40.2 **Determining the compensatory changes in $PaCO_2$ and HCO_3^-**

	Metabolic acidosis	
Predicted $PaCO_2$ (mmHg)	$1.5 \times [HCO_3^-] + 8$ mmHg (± 2)	
	Respiratory acidosis	
	Acute	Chronic
Predicted HCO_3^- (mmol/L)	$24 + \dfrac{PaCO_2 - 40}{10}$	$24 + \dfrac{PaCO_2 - 40}{10} \times 4$
	Metabolic alkalosis	
Predicted $PaCO_2$ (mmHg)	$0.7 \times [HCO_3^-] + 20$ mmHg (± 5)	
	Respiratory alkalosis	
	Acute	Chronic
Predicted HCO_3^- (mmol/L)	$24 - \dfrac{40 - PaCO_2}{10} \times 2$	$24 - \dfrac{40 - PaCO_2}{10} \times 5$

SECTION D – Investigations

below. Chronic compensatory changes may return the pH value towards normal, but overcompensation *never* occurs.

Acidaemia

Acidaemia is associated with a primary metabolic acidosis (secondary to acid gain or HCO_3^- loss) or a primary respiratory acidosis (secondary to hypoventilation).

Metabolic acidosis

pH	↓	<7.35
$PaCO_2$	↔	Compensatory changes only (unless mixed picture)
HCO_3^-	↓	<22 mmol/L (primary change)

Metabolic acidosis is an abnormal condition or process that increases the concentration of fixed acids in the blood. Causes are classified as high anion gap or normal anion gap. The anion gap (AG) is calculated from the equation:

$$AG = [Na^+] - ([Cl^-] + [HCO_3^-])$$

The AG is the sum of anions (A–) not routinely measured. The normal range is 8–16 mmol/L and comprises phosphates, sulfates etc.

Causes

High anion gap acidaemia (AG >16)

- Increased acid production
  - Ketoacidosis (e.g. type 1 diabetes, alcohol or starvation)
  - Lactic acidosis (serum lactate >2.5 mmol/L) from tissue hypoxia or hypoperfusion in cardiac arrest, shock, hypoxia or sepsis (type A). Or from impaired carbohydrate metabolism in hepatic or renal failure, lymphoma and drugs such as metformin (type B).
- Decreased acid metabolism or excretion
  - Renal failure, hepatic failure.
- Drugs and toxins
  - Methanol or ethylene glycol metabolites
  - Iron, cyanide and salicylates.
- High-flux dialysis acetate buffer.

Note: in the case of a high anion gap metabolic acidosis, remember to also calculate the osmolar gap to determine if an exogenous ingestant, such as a toxic alcohol, has contributed to the acidaemia.

Normal anion gap metabolic acidosis (AG 8–16)

- Renal loss of HCO_3^-
  - Renal tubular acidosis
  - Carbonic anhydrase inhibitors.

- Gastrointestinal loss of HCO_3^-
  - Severe diarrhoea
  - Small bowel fistula
  - Drainage of pancreatic or biliary secretions
  - High-output ileostomy.
- Other
  - Synthetic amino acid solutions, NH_4Cl and large volume sodium chloride administration
  - Recovery from ketoacidosis.

Compensation

The normal respiratory response to a metabolic acidosis is to hyperventilate, causing a decrease in $PaCO_2$. The expected decrease in $PaCO_2$ in an uncomplicated metabolic acidaemia may be calculated from Table 40.2.

When the $PaCO_2$ is *higher* than expected, the acidosis is only partially compensated, or a dual process with a combined primary metabolic and primary respiratory acidosis should be suspected. Conversely, when the $PaCO_2$ is *lower* than expected, a combined primary metabolic acidosis and primary respiratory alkalosis should be suspected.

Occasionally, the pH may be within *normal* limits, but the presence of a wide AG gives a clue to an underlying compensated metabolic acidaemia.

Clinical features

The symptoms and signs of a metabolic acidosis are non-specific and include the following:

- Hyperventilation (physiological attempt to remove CO_2 to normalise the pH)
- Fatigue
- Confusion, followed by stupor, then coma
- Decreased cardiac contractility
- Peripheral vasodilation leading to hypotension.

Management

- **Mild:**   pH 7.26–7.35
- **Moderate:** pH 7.11–7.25
- **Severe:**   pH <7.10

The best management for a patient presenting with a metabolic acidosis is to correct the underlying cause, and to use specific treatment for potentially dangerous complications. This includes:

- Supportive treatment with oxygen, IV fluids and treating symptomatic hyperkalaemia
- Giving IV fluid and insulin, and replacing potassium for diabetic ketoacidosis

SECTION D – Investigations

- Restoring adequate intravascular volume to improve peripheral perfusion for lactic acidosis
- Antidote therapy in some cases of poisoning, such as ethanol infusion or fomepizole for methanol poisoning
- Haemodialysis in renal failure, and for some poisonings such as methanol.

Most cases of mild-to-moderate metabolic acidosis are treated effectively by reversing the underlying condition. However, in some instances (e.g. chronic renal failure), the condition is not easily reversed and longer-term bicarbonate therapy may be required.

Bicarbonate therapy (NaHCO$_3^-$)

Severe metabolic acidosis from chronic renal failure with volume depletion may be treated with NaHCO$_3^-$ given PO or IV, with care not to precipitate volume overload.

Administration of NaHCO$_3^-$ is reserved for a severe metabolic acidosis (pH <7.10) with hyperkalaemia or cardiac decompensation. Bicarbonate is hypertonic and has a large sodium load. Thus, dangers of bicarbonate therapy include:

- Hyperosmolarity and volume overload
- Hypernatraemia
- Hypokalaemia
- Hypercapnoea and paradoxical CSF acidosis
- *Increased* lactic acidosis
  - Bicarbonate administration removes the acidotic inhibition of glycolysis and results in increased lactate production
  - Left shift of the oxyhaemoglobin dissociation curve leads to impaired peripheral oxygen unloading, tissue hypoxia and a worsening lactic acidosis.

Respiratory acidosis

pH	↓	<7.35
PaCO$_2$	↑	>45 mmHg (6.0 kPa) (primary change)
HCO$_3^-$	↔	Compensatory changes only (unless mixed picture)

Respiratory acidosis is a primary acid–base disorder associated with inadequate alveolar ventilation, respiratory failure and an arterial PaCO$_2$ greater than 45 mmHg (6.0 kPa).

Causes

- **CNS depression**
  - Medications, illicit drugs and poisons (e.g. opioids, sedatives, large amounts of alcohol, anaesthetic agents)
  - Inhibition of the respiratory centre secondary to cerebral trauma, tumour, haemorrhage or stroke

- **Neuromuscular disorders**
  - Guillain–Barré syndrome, myasthenia gravis
  - Hypokalaemia, hypophosphataemia
  - Toxins such as organophosphates and snake venoms
  - Medications (e.g. muscle relaxants inadequately reversed)
- **Respiratory compromise**
  - Acute upper airway obstruction and laryngospasm
  - COPD, restrictive lung disease, critical (imminently fatal) asthma
  - Pulmonary oedema, aspiration, pneumonia or massive pleural effusion
  - Thoracic trauma, pneumothorax and thoracic cage limitation (e.g. constricting burns)
  - High thoracic or cervical cord trauma (transient or permanent, from trauma or a transverse myelitis)
  - Morbid obesity, sleep apnoea syndrome

The compensatory response in acute respiratory acidosis is limited to intracellular buffering. An immediate increase in HCO_3^- occurs because the increase in $PaCO_2$ results in the generation of HCO_3^-, according to the law of mass action:

$$CO_2 + H_2O \rightleftharpoons H^+ + HCO_3^-$$

However, a respiratory acidosis persisting for over 3–4 days stimulates renal tubular preservation of HCO_3^- to buffer the change in pH. To calculate the expected increase in serum bicarbonate in respiratory acidosis, see Table 40.2.

The expected increase in HCO_3^- in acute respiratory acidaemia is $0.1 \times \Delta PaCO_2$ and in chronic respiratory acidaemia is $0.4 \times \Delta PaCO_2$.

When the HCO_3^- is lower than expected, a mixed respiratory and metabolic acidaemia should be suspected. If the HCO_3^- is greater than expected, this suggests a combined respiratory acidaemia and metabolic alkalaemia.

Clinical features

Respiratory acidosis occurs when there is a failure (either acute or chronic) in ventilation. Most clinical features are directly attributable to CO_2 retention and are uncommon with $PaCO_2$ <70 mmHg. However, they are usually overshadowed by the symptoms and signs of any accompanying hypoxia. Classic signs of pure hypercapnoea include:

- Headache and acute confusion progressing to mental obtundation and somnolence
- Warm, flushed, sweaty and tachycardic with 'bounding pulses'
- Papilloedema
- Asterixis or 'flap' (this *may* also occur with liver, cardiac and renal failure).

Management

Mild: pH 7.26–7.35

Look for and correct reversible causes. Obtain repeat ABGs depending on the patient's clinical condition and course. The exception is a patient with an acute asthmatic attack, in whom even a normal (or definitely an elevated) $PaCO_2$ is critical and needs immediate therapy. Call for urgent senior help before respiratory arrest occurs.

Moderate: pH 7.11–7.25

A patient with moderate respiratory acidosis is in a 'grey zone'. A further decrease in pH increases the risk of life-threatening ventricular arrhythmias. The patient can be carefully monitored, if a readily reversible cause is found, while treatment is instituted.

Maintain careful observation by nursing staff and remain at close call. Do not leave the patient alone until there is an improvement in condition and call your senior. Sequential measurement of pH should be guided by the patient's clinical condition and course.

Severe: pH <7.10

This patient is at high risk of respiratory arrest, life-threatening ventricular arrhythmias or both. Call your senior for help now. The patient will probably require transfer to the ICU for non-invasive ventilation or endotracheal intubation and mechanical ventilation with arterial line monitoring, while reversible causes are sought. You may temporarily need to assist ventilation with a bag-valve mask system (Laerdal or Ambu) until senior help arrives.

Alkalaemia

Determine whether the patient has a primary metabolic alkalosis or a primary respiratory alkalosis.

The normal response to respiratory alkalaemia is a decrease in HCO_3^-. An immediate decrease in HCO_3^- occurs because the decrease in $PaCO_2$ results in a reduction of HCO_3^-, according to the law of mass action:

$$CO_2 + H_2O \rightleftharpoons H^+ + HCO_3^-$$

Later, renal tubular loss of HCO_3^- occurs to buffer the change in pH. The expected decrease in HCO_3^- in acute respiratory alkalosis is $0.2 \times \Delta PaCO_2$. The expected decrease in HCO_3^- in chronic respiratory alkalosis is $0.5 \times \Delta PaCO_2$ (see Table 40.2).

When the HCO_3^- is *greater* than expected, a combined respiratory and metabolic alkalosis should be suspected. When the HCO_3^- is *less* than expected, a combined respiratory alkalosis and metabolic acidosis should be suspected.

The normal response to metabolic alkalosis is hypoventilation, with an increase in the $PaCO_2$. If the $PaCO_2$ is *greater* than expected, a combined metabolic alkalosis and respiratory acidosis should be suspected. If the $PaCO_2$ is *less* than expected, a combined metabolic and respiratory alkalosis should be suspected.

Metabolic alkalosis

pH	↑	>7.45
$PaCO_2$	↔	Compensatory changes only (unless mixed picture)
HCO_3^-	↑	>28 mmol/L (primary change)

Causes
Metabolic alkalosis is a primary acid–base disorder that increases the concentration of plasma bicarbonate. The most common causes are vomiting, NG tube drainage and diuretic use:
- **Extracellular volume depletion** (urinary Cl⁻ <10 mmol/L)
  - GI losses
    - Vomiting
    - GI drainage (NGT suction)
    - Chloride-wasting diarrhoea, laxative misuse
    - Villous adenoma of the intestine
  - Renal losses
    - Diuretic therapy
    - Post-hypercapnoea
    - Non-resorbable anions
    - Penicillin, ticarcillin
    - Bartter syndrome (low potassium)
- **Extracellular volume expansion** (urinary Cl⁻ >20 mmol/L)
  - Mineralocorticoid excess
    - Endogenous—hyperaldosteronism (primary—Conn's syndrome, or secondary); Cushing's syndrome
    - Exogenous—glucocorticoids; mineralocorticoids; liquorice excess
  - Alkali ingestion
  - Post-starvation feeding
  - Massive blood transfusion (metabolism of citrate).

Clinical features
There are no specific symptoms or signs of a metabolic alkalosis other than hypoventilation. However, symptoms associated with hypokalaemia (weakness) or hypocalcaemia (tetany) may be present. Severe alkalosis may result in:
- Apathy
- Confusion or stupor.

Management

- **Mild:**   pH 7.45–7.55.
- **Moderate:** pH 7.56–7.69.
- **Severe:**   pH <7.70.

Mild or moderate metabolic alkalosis rarely requires specific treatment beyond correcting the underlying cause.

Metabolic alkalosis associated with extracellular fluid volume depletion responds to infusion of normal saline to restore the intravascular volume, replace chloride and enhance renal HCO_3^- excretion.

If the patient is volume-overloaded and has a metabolic alkalosis, saline therapy is usually ineffective. Acetazolamide 250–500 mg PO or IV 8-hourly may be helpful, as it enhances renal HCO_3^- excretion.

In diuretic-induced alkalosis, administration of KCl at 10–20 mmol/h may improve the alkalosis.

In Bartter's syndrome, the alkalaemia may respond to prostaglandin synthetase inhibitors such as indomethacin.

Note: attention to additional electrolyte disorders is essential, as these associated abnormalities (particularly hypokalaemia) may be a more immediate threat to life than the metabolic alkalosis.

Respiratory alkalosis

pH	↑	>7.45
$PaCO_2$	↓	<35 mmHg (4.7 kPa) (primary change)
HCO_3^-	↔	Compensatory changes only (unless mixed picture)

Causes

- Physiological conditions (pregnancy, high altitude)
- CNS-mediated (anxiety, pain, fever, tumour)
- Drugs (salicylate overdose, nicotine, progesterone)
- Pulmonary disorders (CHF, PE, asthma, pneumonia)
- Hypoxia
- Iatrogenic from excessive artificial ventilation
- Miscellaneous (hepatic failure, hyperthyroidism)

Clinical features

- Light-headedness
- Confusion
- Numbness, tingling, paraesthesiae (perioral, hands, feet)
- Tetany in severe cases

Management

- **Mild:**   pH 7.45–7.55
- **Moderate:** pH 7.56–7.69
- **Severe:**   pH <7.70

Mild respiratory alkalosis is common in physiological conditions (e.g. pregnancy, high altitude) and in these cases requires no treatment.

However, a mild respiratory alkalosis may be the marker of a serious underlying disorder that must be looked for, even though the patient can be treated symptomatically (e.g. a febrile patient with antipyretics, a patient in pain with analgesia and an anxious patient with reassurance or sedation). An underlying serious cause must be considered.

More pronounced degrees of respiratory alkalosis that are definitely anxiety-related can be treated by re-breathing into a paper bag (to raise the inspired CO_2), again provided no serious cause is present. The only effective treatment for other causes listed is to eliminate the underlying condition.

SECTION D – Investigations

41

Glucose disorders

A variety of hormones including insulin and glucagon maintain the blood glucose level within a narrow range, with none excreted in the urine.

Hyperglycaemia develops gradually, and may be asymptomatic, or associated with ketoacidosis or hyperosmolarity. Its clinical features relate to the degree of volume depletion and electrolyte losses, plus or minus acidosis, as well as to the underlying precipitating cause usually, but not always, in a known diabetic.

Hypoglycaemia develops more rapidly and presents with an altered conscious level, seizures or coma. Again it usually occurs in a known diabetic, but is seen in the non-diabetic following poisoning, sepsis, liver disease or even rare tumours.

Hyperglycaemia

Hyperglycaemia occurs in two main settings:
- Patients with documented diabetes mellitus (DM) or impaired glucose tolerance.
- Patients *without* previously known DM.

The underlying precipitant of elevated serum glucose level is the same in both cases, with the exception of dosing regimen-related problems.

Causes

Intercurrent illness, surgery, other drugs and non-compliance with hypoglycaemic medications, including insulins, are the most common causes of hyperglycaemia in a patient with DM. The causes of a raised blood glucose level (BGL) are best divided into known diabetics and not known.
- **Patients *with* previously documented DM (type 1 or 2):**
  - Poor control (usually poor compliance with therapy and/or poor glucose monitoring)
  - Inappropriate diet (high in simple sugars)
  - Reduced exercise
  - Change in insulin or oral hypoglycaemic regimen
    - New medications
    - Non-compliance

- Reduction in insulin dose secondary to illness 'because the patient is not eating' (a common precipitant of diabetic ketoacidosis [DKA])
- Inappropriate insulin dose regimen
- Insulin pump problems (e.g. programming error, pump or alarm malfunction, reservoir problem, infusion set or injection site problem—see Box 41.1).
- **Patients *without* previously documented DM:**
  - New-onset DM
  - Gestational diabetes (glucose intolerance associated with pregnancy)
  - Acute stress
    - Trauma, surgery
    - Acute MI, CVA
    - Severe illness including sepsis
  - Endocrine
    - Cushing's syndrome (endogenous glucocorticoids)
    - Acromegaly (excessive growth hormone)
  - Medications
    - Steroid administration (exogenous glucocorticoids)
    - Thiazide diuretics, beta-blockers, phenytoin
    - Olanzepine, clozapine, antiretrovirals
  - Exogenous glucose load
    - TPN
    - Peritoneal dialysate
  - Pancreatic injury
    - Acute or chronic pancreatitis
  - Factitious (false)
    - Blood taken from a proximal vein containing dextrose
    - Fingerprick BGL from a finger covered in sugar.

BOX 41.1 Using an insulin pump

An insulin pump is a small mechanical device that delivers insulin subcutaneously via an infusion set. The pump is worn outside the body in a pouch or on a belt. The infusion set is a long, thin, plastic tube connected to a flexible plastic cannula that is inserted into the skin at the infusion site, usually in the subcutaneous abdominal tissue. The infusion set remains in place for 2–4 days and is then replaced, using a new location each time.

When a patient with an insulin pump is admitted to the hospital, the pump should remain on the patient at all times, unless other arrangements are made for insulin replacement. These patients have been trained in insulin pump therapy and, in most situations, can help maintain glycaemic control using the pump, together with the diabetes education nurse and the attending doctor. If the patient is unconscious, the pump should be removed and insulin administered by alternative methods.

The insulin pump is not an artificial pancreas. It is a computer-controlled unit that delivers insulin in precise amounts at preprogrammed times. It uses

Continued

> **BOX 41.1 Using an insulin pump—con't**
>
> only short-acting insulin. The pump is not 'automatic'. The patient has to decide how much insulin will be given, based on blood glucose results and the amount of food that will be consumed.
>
> The device contains a small reservoir of insulin (up to 3 mL), a small battery-powered pump and a computer to control its operation. The pump is set to deliver insulin in two ways:
>
> 1. Basal rate—a small, continuous flow of insulin automatically delivered every 15 minutes. The basal rate is programmed by the operator and may vary at different times of the day.
> 2. Bolus dose—designed to cover the food eaten during a meal or to correct elevated BGL. Bolus doses can be programmed at any time, which gives the patient greater flexibility with regard to when and what to eat.

Clinical features
Severe acute hyperglycaemia
- **Type 1 DM with acidosis** (i.e. DKA)
  - Volume depletion/osmotic diuresis
    - Dry skin, tachycardia, ± hypotension
    - Polyuria, polydipsia
  - Acidosis
    - Ketotic breath (sickly sweet, fruity smell)
    - Kussmaul's breathing (rapid, deep, sighing respirations)
  - GIT
    - Anorexia, nausea, vomiting
    - Abdominal pain, gastric dilation, ileus
      Note: this may mimic an acute surgical abdomen, so *always* check the urine for glucose and ketones in these patients.
  - Neurological
    - Delirium, confusion, coma (but remember the possibility of an underlying precipitating infection such as meningitis).
- **Type 2 DM without acidosis** (i.e. hyperosmolar, hyperglycaemic state [HHS]–previously known as HONK)
  - Polyuria, polydipsia
  - Tachycardia, dry mucous membranes
  - Weakness, lethargy, fatigue
  - Confusion, convulsions and coma
  - Focal neurological deficits.

Moderate hyperglycaemia
- Volume depletion (tachycardia ± hypotension)
- Polyuria, polydipsia, thirst
- May be asymptomatic

Mild hyperglycaemia
- Usually asymptomatic
- Polyuria, polydipsia, thirst

Management
Assess the severity

Severity is determined by reviewing the measured BGL in the context of the patient's clinical symptoms.

Diabetic ketoacidosis is defined by pH <7.3 or serum bicarbonate <15 mmol/L, ketonaemia >3.0 mmol/L (or marked ketonuria >2+ on dipstick) and hyperglycaemia with BGL >11 mmol/L.

Note: the absolute elevation of the BGL does not determine the severity of the problem, as a severe ketoacidosis may occur with only a moderately elevated BGL.

Treatment
Severe hyperglycaemia

Prolonged, severe hyperglycaemia requires urgent treatment, which includes giving IV hydration and insulin and temporarily stopping the patient's previous diabetic medications in most cases.

Diabetic ketoacidosis (DKA)
- DKA may occur in a *known* diabetic patient and is usually precipitated by:
  - Inadequate insulin administration including iatrogenic 'because the patient was not eating'
  - Intercurrent illness (e.g. infection, acute MI, pancreatitis)
  - Trauma, or emergency surgery with inadequate preparation.
- Alternatively, DKA may present in a patient without previously diagnosed DM, heralded by a history of polyuria, polydipsia, weight loss, lethargy, abdominal pain or coma.
- The predominant features are from total body depletion of salt, water and potassium, acidosis and a progressive altered level of consciousness (unlike hypoglycaemia, which causes sudden coma).
- **DKA is a medical emergency.** Get expert help and organise:
  - Volume replacement
  - Insulin administration
  - Potassium and occasionally other electrolyte (magnesium) replacement.
    Note: bicarbonate therapy is rarely, if ever, indicated.
- **Correct the volume depletion** (total body deficits of water 100 mL/kg and sodium 7–10 mmol/kg):
  - Restore the intravascular volume rapidly if the patient is shocked. Give 1000 mL normal saline IV bolus to normalise perfusion over the first hour.
  - Continue rehydration with normal saline at 500 mL/h for the following 4 hours, then at 250 mL/h for the next 8 hours, i.e. to give about 5 L over the first 13 hours. The rate of fluid administration is guided by frequent reassessment of volume

status and response to therapy. Do *not* be tempted to go too
fast.

— *Caution:* a patient with a history of CCF, or who weighs
<50 kg, or is elderly, should have a slower fluid replacement
regimen to avoid fluid overload.

- **Start an insulin infusion:**
  - Commence a short-acting insulin such as Actrapid 50 U IV in
    50 mL normal saline via an infusion pump. Begin the insulin
    infusion at 0.1 U/kg/h.
  - *Note:* a bolus dose of insulin is no longer recommended.
  - Titrate the infusion rate to decrease the BGL by around 10%
    per hour, at no more than 5 mmol/L/h.
  - If the BGL drops to under 15 mmol/L, add 10% dextrose at
    125 mL/h and continue the insulin and saline infusions as well,
    until the ketones are cleared.
  - *Remember:* discontinue any standing orders for insulin or oral
    hypoglycaemics before beginning the insulin infusion.
- **Replace potassium** (total body deficit of potassium 3–5 mmol/kg):
  - Patients with DKA *always* have a *total body deficit of potassium,*
    even though most patients will present with an initial high
    serum potassium level related to the acidaemia.
  - Serum potassium levels will fall precipitously with volume
    replacement, insulin therapy and acidosis correction, as the
    glucose is driven intracellularly, taking the extracellular
    potassium with it.
  - After initial fluid bolus resuscitation, if the serum potassium
    level is <5.5 mmol/L and urine is being produced, add
    potassium chloride to all replacement fluids at a rate of
    10–20 mmol/h.
  - *Note:* potassium should not be administered while the:
    — Patient is anuric
    — Serum potassium level is >5.5 mmol/L
    — ECG shows peaked T waves or widening of the QRS complex.
- **Bicarbonate therapy (rarely ever indicated):**
  - Bicarbonate therapy *may* be considered if the pH remains <7.0
    or in the presence of circulatory shock, when cardiac
    contractility is compromised. Be guided by your senior.
  - There is no evidence to support the 'routine' administration of
    sodium bicarbonate in DKA. It does not improve outcome and
    in fact may cause harm and delay recovery.
  - The optimal treatment for the significant metabolic acidosis is
    adequate volume resuscitation, insulin therapy and electrolyte
    replacement.
- **Monitor BGL and serum electrolytes:**
  - Monitor BGL 1–2 hourly. As it falls, the rate of insulin
    infusion can be adjusted (e.g. 0.025–0.05 U/kg/h) to decrease

the BGL by around 10% per hour, at no more than
5 mmol/L/h.
- Continue the insulin infusion until the BGL remains stable at
8–10 mmol/L and the ketones have been cleared. Check the
bedside glucose every 4 hours and add regular SC insulin
6-hourly to keep the BGL between 8 and 10 mmol/L as the
insulin infusion is ceased.
- **Search for and treat the underlying precipitating cause:**
  - Infection (MSU, CXR, blood cultures, even LP if history
  suspicious of meningitis)
  - Pancreatitis (lipase); acute MI (ECG and troponins)
  - Dietary indiscretion—ask diabetes educator or dietitian to speak
  to patient
  - Inadequate insulin dosage. Make sure the patient knows to
  increase daily insulin requirements during illness—ask diabetes
  educator to speak to patient.

Hyperosmolar, hyperglycaemic state (HHS)

HHS is common in more elderly, non-insulin-dependent diabetic patients. It is associated with profound volume depletion resulting from
a sustained hyperglycaemic diuresis without compensatory fluid intake.
- Typically, the patient is 50–70 years old and may have no prior
history of DM. The precipitating event may be a stroke, MI,
urinary or chest infection, pancreatitis or drugs, including steroids
and thiazide diuretics.
- The BGL is often very high (40–50 mmol/L), but ketosis is absent.
- *Note:* the mortality rate is 20–40%, which is much greater than for
DKA at approximately 5%.
- Treatment is similar to that of DKA, but with lower requirements
for insulin and greater for potassium, an increased risk of
pulmonary oedema, and the addition of heparin to reduce the risk
of venous thromboembolism.
- **Monitor BGL and serum electrolytes:**
  - Check baseline electrolytes, urea, creatinine and glucose levels.
  - Repeat the BGL and electrolytes in 2 hours and thereafter as
  required.
  - Replace the potassium at a higher rate than for DKA.
- **Search for the precipitating cause** (see above):
  - Infection, acute MI, CVA
  - Inadequate fluid intake
  - Other drug use such as antipsychotics, steroids, thiazides, some
  antihypertensives and phenytoin.
- **Commence heparin** (assuming there is no active bleeding,
particularly intracerebral):
  - UFH 5000 units IV bolus, then infusion at 800–1000 units/h or
  - LMWH such as Clexane 1.5 mg/kg/day.

Moderate hyperglycaemia

Patients with moderate hyperglycaemia require adjustment of their insulin dosing regimen or oral hypoglycaemic agents. Whenever possible, make adjustments using the same insulin and the same delivery device that the patient is already using.

Example: you are called to review an insulin-dependent diabetic patient with a bedtime fingerprick BGL of 21 mmol/L. Your immediate actions should be to:

- Examine the patient and exclude ketonuria.
- Review the diabetic record for the past 3 days.
- Request a VBG and a laboratory venous glucose to confirm the level.
- Give 5–10 units of short-acting insulin SC now.
- Request a further fingerprick BGL for 03:00 hours. Determining the reason(s) for poor control of blood glucose before breakfast may aid in the adjustment of the patient's insulin regimen:
  - *Hyperglycaemia* documented at 03:00 hours coupled with a pre-breakfast hyperglycaemia is most commonly caused by inadequate insulin coverage overnight (hypoinsulinaemia) or growth hormone secretion. This is correctly managed by increasing the pre-dinner insulin dose.
  - *Hypoglycaemia* documented at 03:00 hours is a complex problem correctly managed by decreasing the patient's evening long-acting insulin (NPH) and by dietary review.

It is not your role to devise a schedule that will achieve perfect blood glucose control for the rest of the patient's hospital stay. Short-term control of the BGL is not shown to alter complications in patients with diabetes.

Instead, when seeing a patient with an elevated BGL at night, your aim is to prevent the development of ketoacidosis (in a patient with type 1 DM) or a hyperosmolar state (in a patient with type 2 DM), without producing symptomatic hypoglycaemia.

Mild, asymptomatic hyperglycaemia

Mild, asymptomatic hyperglycaemia does not require immediate treatment, regardless of whether a patient is taking oral hypoglycaemic medications or an insulin preparation.

If the patient is not known to have diabetes, request a fasting serum glucose to be taken in the morning, and fingerprick BGL before breakfast and at bedtime. A diagnosis of true diabetes is then made by finding:

- Fasting venous glucose >7.0 mmol/L on two or more occasions
- Random venous glucose >11.1 mmol/L on two or more occasions—with symptoms of hyperglycaemia such as polyuria and polydipsia
- Glycated haemoglobin (HbA$_{1c}$) value of ≥6.5%.

Hypoglycaemia

Hypoglycaemia causes an altered conscious level, seizures and coma. It is potentially life-threatening if undiagnosed or untreated. There is individual variation in the BGL required to produce symptoms, but it is generally regarded as <2.5 mmol/L.

Causes (see Box 41.2)

- Patients *with* documented DM:
  - Excess insulin or oral hypoglycaemic administration (sulfonylurea)
  - Increased exercise
  - Decreased kilojoule intake or missed meal or snack.
- Patients *without* previously documented DM:
  - Overdose of insulin or oral hypoglycaemic such as a sulfonylurea
  - Drugs—ethanol + MAOIs, haloperidol, sulfonamides, salicylates, quinine
  - Hepatic failure, sepsis or hypothermia
  - Adrenal insufficiency (Addison's disease)
  - Insulinoma or islet cell hyperplasia
  - *Plasmodium falciparum* malaria (severe).

BOX 41.2 Causes of hypoglycaemia

- **Patient with known diabetes**
  - Medication change or error, particularly with insulin or sulfonylurea oral hypoglycaemic (*very rarely* metformin)
  - Inadequate dietary intake
  - Excessive energy use such as exercise
- **Any patient**
  - Poisoning (usually deliberate) with insulin, sulfonylurea, salicylates, beta-blockers, quinine, chloroquine, valproic acid
  - Ethanol overdose
  - Liver disease
  - Sepsis
  - Malaria (*Plasmodium falciparum*), especially severe infection in children; in pregnancy; quinine-related
  - Starvation, including anorexia nervosa
  - Post-GI surgery 'dumping syndrome'
  - Adrenal insufficiency (Addison's disease)
  - Hypopituitarism
  - Islet cell tumour (insulinoma) or extrapancreatic tumour
  - Tumour-related such as mesenchymal, epithelial or endothelial tumour producing insulin-like factors
  - Congenital metabolic disorders such as glycogen storage disease type I or III.
  - Artefact 'Münchausen's syndrome'

Clinical features

- Catecholamines are released secondary to an absolute decrease in blood glucose. The degree of catecholamine response is inversely proportional to the BGL, not to the rate at which hypoglycaemia develops.
- Adrenergic symptoms usually precede neuroglycopenic symptoms (see below) and provide an 'early warning system' for the patient. They include:
  - Sweating
  - Palpitations
  - Tremulousness
  - Anxiety
  - Hunger.
    Note: these signs and symptoms are masked in a patient on beta blockers.
- Deficient cerebral glucose availability is usually a secondary and slower response than the adrenergic response and occurs over 1–3 hours (neuroglycopenia). Features include:
  - Headache, diplopia
  - Difficulty in concentrating, hallucinations
  - Confusion, irritability
  - Focal neurological deficits (e.g. hemiplegia or dysphasia— always check the BGL *before* requesting a CT brain scan in a patient with a suspected stroke!)
  - Seizures
  - Coma.

  Note: the adrenergic response does not always precede the CNS response. Some patients progress from confusion, or inability to speak, directly to seizures or coma.

Management
Assess the severity

All symptomatic patients with hypoglycaemia require treatment. Symptoms may be precipitated by either a rapid fall in the usual blood glucose or an absolute low level of blood glucose.

Glucose administration

- **Immediate therapy:**
  - Assess the patient and perform bedside fingerprick BGL.
  - In a cooperative, awake patient give oral glucose in the form of sweetened fruit juice.
  - If the patient is unable to take oral fluids or is unconscious, give 50 mL of 50% dextrose (25 g) IV by slow injection. Flush the vein with 50 mL normal saline following dextrose administration, as concentrated dextrose is highly irritating to veins.
  - If there is no IV access in a patient unable to take oral fluids, give 1 mg glucagon SC or IM.

- *Remember:* glucagon may cause vomiting, so the patient must be carefully watched to prevent aspiration.
- **Ongoing therapy:**
  - Begin a maintenance infusion of 10% dextrose IV at a rate of 100 mL/h if hypoglycaemia is persistent or anticipated (e.g. in hepatic failure, seizures or coma).
  - Repeat a fingerprick BGL after 1 hour and reassess the patient. *Note:* hypoglycaemia following excess oral hypoglycaemics may require repeated doses of 50% dextrose because of the slow metabolism and excretion of these drugs. Octreotide 50–100 microgram IV or SC may also be used to prevent further hypoglycaemic episodes in these patients and may avoid the need for further boluses of hypertonic glucose. Seek senior advice.

Further investigations

- When the cause of hypoglycaemia is unclear or obscure, send blood for insulin, C peptide and beta-hydroxybutyrate measurement (*not* routinely).
- Insulin produced endogenously includes the C peptide fragment, whereas commercial preparations of insulin do not.
- Thus, a high insulin level associated with a high C peptide level with hypoglycaemia suggests endogenous production of excess insulin (e.g. an insulinoma—a rare but exciting 'once-in-a-lifetime' diagnosis!).
- Hypoglycaemia together with a high insulin level and a low C peptide level suggest therapeutic (or surreptitious) administration of exogenous insulin.

Examples of insulins available in Australia
Rapid-acting analogues
Humalog (insulin lispro)
NovoRapid (insulin aspart)
Apidra (insulin glulisine)
Short-acting
Humulin R (regular)
Actrapid (human)
Hypurin neutral (bovine)
Intermediate-acting
Humulin NPH
Protophane (human)
Hypurin isophane (bovine)
Long-acting
Levemir (insulin detemir)
Lantus (insulin glargine)
Combinations
Humulin 30/70 (70% NPH, 30% regular)
Humalog Mix25 (75% lispro protamine, 25% insulin lispro)
Humalog Mix50 (50% lispro protamine, 50% insulin lispro)
Pen devices and insulin pumps
Many varieties

42

Sodium disorders

Sodium (Na^+) is the most abundant cation in the extravascular and intravascular spaces. It has a major influence on serum osmolality and determines the volume of the extracellular fluid (ECF).

The clinical manifestations of severe sodium disturbances are mainly neurological, compared to potassium, which has cardiac and neuromuscular effects.

Hypernatraemia

Hypernatraemia is defined as a serum Na^+ level >150 mmol/L. It most often results from ECF depletion caused by vomiting, diarrhoea, an osmotic diuresis or excessive sweating.

Causes
- **Inadequate water intake with normal fluid loss**
  - Inability to communicate water needs (e.g. coma, infants)
  - Disordered thirst perception (e.g. hypothalamic dysfunction)
- **Water loss in excess of salt loss** (hypotonic fluid deficit)
  - Renal losses (impaired salt concentrating ability)
  - Diabetes insipidus (nephrogenic or pituitary)
  - Osmotic diuresis (hyperglycaemia, hypercalcaemia, mannitol administration)
  - Chronic renal disease
- **Extrarenal losses**
  - GI losses (vomiting, NG suction, diarrhoea)
  - Insensible losses (excessive sweating in a hot climate, febrile illness and extensive burns)
- **Excessive sodium load** (Na^+ gain greater than water gain)
  - Primary hyperaldosteronism (Conn's syndrome) or Cushing's syndrome
  - Iatrogenic (e.g. administration of 8.4% $NaHCO_3^-$ (1 mL = 1 mEq Na^+) or hypertonic saline)
  - Ingestion of salt tablets or seawater

Clinical features

The clinical features of hypernatraemia are related to acute cerebral neuronal cell shrinkage resulting from the outward shift of intracellular water, which occurs as a result of increased ECF osmolality. The symptoms and signs are dependent on both the absolute increase in serum osmolality, as well as the rate at which it changes:

- Thirst
- Weakness, fatigue, tremor and irritability
- Altered mental status, ataxia and focal neurological signs
- Seizures and coma
- Respiratory paralysis and death.

Management

- **Assess the severity:**
  - This is determined by the clinical manifestations (see above) particularly seizures, the serum sodium level, serum osmolality and the ECF volume.
  - Although a patient with hypernatraemia can have an accompanying extracellular volume deficit that may compromise vital organ perfusion, most patients have relatively few symptoms and are not at immediate risk of dying.
  - The normal range of serum osmolality is 280–300 mmol/kg. It can be measured in the laboratory or calculated using the equation:

$$\text{Serum osmolality (mmol / kg)} = 2 \times (Na^+[\text{mmol / L}])$$
$$+ \text{urea (mmol / L)} + \text{glucose (mmol / L)}$$

- **Correct the volume and water deficits:**
  - The choice of fluid, route and rate of administration are dependent on the severity of the extracellular volume deficit. Following initial resuscitation, correction of Na^+ and H_2O abnormalities should be gradual and occur over 48 hours to prevent sudden fluid shifts with the development of cerebral oedema. Do *not* reduce serum Na^+ by more than 12 mmol/L/24 hours.
  - **Volume depleted (hypovolaemic) patients:**
    – Give IV isotonic normal saline until the patient is haemodynamically stable.
    – Correct the remaining water deficit with free water PO, or 0.45% saline or 5% dextrose IV.
  - **Non-volume-depleted (euvolaemic) patients:**
    – Give free water PO or hypotonic fluids IV such as 0.45% saline or 5% dextrose.

- **Volume overloaded (hypervolaemic) patients:**
  - Remove the excess Na$^+$ by initiating a diuresis using frusemide 20–40 mg IV.
  - Repeat at intervals of 2–4 hours as necessary.
  - Once the extracellular volume has returned to normal, continue the diuresis if the serum Na$^+$ level is still elevated, by replacing urinary volume losses with 5% dextrose IV until the serum Na$^+$ level is in the normal range again.

Hyponatraemia

Hyponatraemia is defined as a serum Na$^+$ <130 mmol/L. It affects 1% of hospital inpatients and in most cases is stable and requires no treatment.

Causes

- **Pseudohyponatraemia (artefactual)**
  - Laboratory analysis technique
  - Hyponatraemia with normal serum osmolality
    - Hyperlipidaemia, hyperproteinaemia
  - Hyponatraemia with increased serum osmolality
    - Hyperglycaemia, mannitol, excess urea
    - Toxic alcohols (ethanol, methanol, isopropyl alcohol, ethylene glycol)
- **Hyponatraemia with high urinary Na$^+$ (>20 mmol/L)** indicates inappropriate renal wasting of sodium (rather than retention, which should occur in hyponatraemia).
  - **Hypovolaemic**
    - Diuretic excess
    - Diuretic phase of acute tubular necrosis
    - Vomiting, NG suction
    - Hypoaldosteronism, Addison's disease, adrenal insufficiency and spironolactone
    - Cerebral salt wasting
    - Sodium-losing nephropathies
    - Bartter's syndrome (rare inherited defects usually affecting thick ascending limb of loop of Henle leading to hypokalaemia and a metabolic alkalosis)
  - **Euvolaemic** due to syndrome of inappropriate antidiuretic hormone (SIADH)
    - Malignancy: small-cell lung, pancreas, prostate, leukaemia, cervical
    - CNS disorders: brain tumour, meningitis, encephalitis, Guillain–Barré syndrome
    - Pulmonary disorders: tuberculosis, pneumonia, carcinoma of the lung

- GIT: duodenal and pancreatic carcinoma
- Drugs: neuroleptics (e.g. haloperidol), antidepressants (e.g. amitriptyline, SSRIs), antineoplastic drugs (e.g. cyclophosphamide), carbamazepine, narcotics
- **Hypervolaemic**
  - Chronic renal failure
  - Hypothyroidism
- **Hyponatraemia with low urinary Na$^+$ (<20 mmol/L)** indicates appropriate renal conservation of sodium.
  - **Hypovolaemic**
    - Diarrhoea
    - Sweating, burns, pancreatitis
  - **Euvolaemic**
    - Hypotonic postoperative fluids, such as 4% dextrose with 1/5 saline or 5% dextrose (avoid!)
    - Hypotonic irrigation fluids during TURP
    - Psychogenic polydipsia
    - Elderly patient with poor diet ('tea and toast' diet)
    - Large-volume binge beer drinking (beer potomania)
  - **Hypervolaemic**
    - CCF
    - Cirrhosis of the liver
    - Nephrotic syndrome
    - Hypoalbuminaemia

Explanation

The renal response to salt and water loss varies according to the cause of the hyponatraemia. Urinary electrolyte determination helps in identifying the primary cause of hyponatraemia.

- When extrarenal losses of sodium and water occur through the skin (e.g. sweating, burns) or from third-space losses (e.g. pancreatitis), the renal response is to conserve sodium (urinary Na$^+$ <20 mmol/L) and to conserve water through secretion of ADH (high urine osmolality).
- However, if the volume loss is from vomiting or NG suction, acid HCl is primarily lost from the gastric secretions. The kidneys generate and excrete NaHCO$_3$$^-$ to maintain the acid–base balance, resulting in urine with a normal Na$^+$ (>20 mmol/L), but low Cl$^-$ (<20 mmol/L).
- If volume loss is from diarrhoea, NaHCO$_3$$^-$ is primarily lost in the stools. The kidneys generate and excrete NH$_4$Cl to maintain the acid–base balance, and produce urine that is low in Na$^+$, but normal in Cl$^-$.
- Hyponatraemia with ECF excess and oedema may be accompanied by a low urinary Na$^+$ (<20 mmol/L), as in nephrotic syndrome, CHF and cirrhosis of the liver, or normal urinary Na$^+$, as in renal failure.

Clinical features

Clinical symptoms are dependent on the rate of development of hyponatraemia, the absolute decrease in serum osmolality and the patient's volume status. Progressive signs and symptoms of hyponatraemia include:

- Lethargy, weakness and ataxia
- Nausea and vomiting
- Headache
- Confusion
- Seizures and coma.

Thus, if hyponatraemia develops gradually, the patient may tolerate a serum Na^+ of <110 mmol/L, with only moderate lethargy and nausea. However, when the serum Na^+ falls rapidly from 140 to 115 mmol/L, the patient is likely to become obtunded and have a seizure or repeated seizures.

Management

Assess the severity

Severity is determined by the serum sodium level, serum osmolality, the ECF volume and the rapidity of onset of clinical symptoms (see above).

Asymptomatic mild hyponatraemia

- Patients with asymptomatic hyponatraemia and Na^+ ≥120 mmol/L usually have a chronic underlying cause and require no treatment if the level is stable.
- Sodium should be replaced slowly to raise serum sodium by no more than 0.5 mmol/L/h (max. serum sodium change 12 mmol/L/24 h), or fluid restricted to 500–750 mL/24 h in SIADH if treatment is required.

Symptomatic hyponatraemia

- Call for *immediate* senior assistance.
- Patients who are symptomatic with confusion, seizures, coma or signs of brainstem herniation must receive hypertonic saline urgently to correct serum sodium towards normal and to stop any progression of symptoms.
- Aim to replace Na^+ to raise serum sodium by 1–2 mmol/L/h until neurologically stable and then revert to raising the serum sodium by no more than 0.5 mmol/L/h once the patient is seizure-free.
- Hypertonic saline is available in different strength solutions (3%, 7.5% up to 20%). Generally, 1.5 mL/kg (100 mL) of 3% given over 10 minutes is enough to stop seizures or improve neurological status. This must be given by a senior doctor, preferably in an intensive care area, and may be repeated twice more.

- Only ever use hypertonic saline in patients with neurological symptoms, seizures or coma when attempting to correct hyponatraemia, as cerebral neuronal cells try to maintain their volume by losing solutes (e.g. K^+).
- If the serum Na^+ level is corrected too rapidly (i.e. >120–125 mmol/L), the serum may become hypertonic relative to brain cells, resulting in an outward shift of water, with resultant CNS damage from acute brain shrinkage, known as the osmotic demyelination syndrome or central pontine myelinolysis.
- Once the serum Na^+ is >120 mmol/L, many of the symptoms of hyponatraemia resolve. Therefore, aim to initially raise the serum sodium level by no more than 4–6 mmol/L.

Syndrome of inappropriate antidiuretic hormone secretion

The diagnosis of SIADH is made when the following stringent criteria are met:
- Hyponatraemia with normal ECF volume (normovolaemia)
- Urine osmolality > plasma osmolality
  - Serum osmolality <280 mmol/kg (hypotonic hyponatraemia)
  - Urine osmolality >100 mmol/kg (inappropriately concentrated)
- Urinary Na^+ >20 mmol/L
- Normal renal, thyroid and adrenal function
- Patient is *not* on diuretics.

Management
- Look for and correct the underlying cause or contributory factors (e.g. stop any contributory drugs).
- Restrict free water intake between 500 and 750 mL/day in an attempt to maintain a negative fluid balance.
- Frusemide-induced diuresis (1 mg/kg) may be useful in patients with severe symptomatic hyponatraemia (serum Na^+ <115 mmol/L), by maintaining urine output and blocking the secretion of ADH. Remember to replace urinary Na^+ and K^+ losses with normal saline with KCl 20 mmol/L.
- Demeclocycline 300–600 mg PO BD is occasionally useful in patients with chronic symptomatic SIADH, in whom water restriction has been unsuccessful. Demeclocycline takes 1–3 days to work by inhibiting the action of ADH on the kidney, and is available on Special Access Scheme.

Psychogenic polydipsia

'Water intoxication' is an uncommon condition characterised by excessive water intake without physiological stimulus to drink. Classically, the condition is associated with hospitalised major psychosis patients in whom hyponatraemia is exacerbated by the effects of neuroleptic or antidepressant medications.

SECTION D – Investigations

Immediate treatment includes fluid restriction, but this is only temporarily effective if not coupled with ongoing psychiatric management.

Hypovolaemic hyponatraemia

Patients have decreased total body Na^+ stores and are volume-depleted.

Correct the ECF volume using normal saline. The amount of Na^+ required to improve the serum concentration can be calculated using the following the formula:

$$Na^+ \text{ deficit (mmol / L)} =$$
$$[\text{serum } Na^+ \text{ (desired)} - \text{serum } Na^+ \text{ (observed)}] \times$$
$$[\text{body weight (kg)} \times \text{percentage of TBW}]$$

The percentage of TBW should be 0.6 for young men, 0.5 for young women and elderly men, and 0.4 for elderly females.

Example: the amount of sodium required to raise the serum sodium level from 120 to 145 mmol/L in a 70 kg elderly male is:

$$(145 \text{ mmol / L} - 120 \text{ mmol / L}) \times (0.5 \times 70 \text{ L}) = 875 \text{ mmol.}$$

As 1 L of normal saline contains 150 mmol of sodium, approximately 5800 mL of normal saline are required to raise the patient's serum level to 145 mmol/L.

Remember: corrections are made at a rate similar to that at which the abnormality developed. It is safest to correct half the deficit slowly and then reassess the situation.

Hypervolaemic hyponatraemia

Asymptomatic patients with extracellular volume excess and oedema:
- Place on strict water restriction with diuretic therapy and monitor with a fluid balance chart.
- Restrict fluid intake to 50% of estimated maintenance fluid requirements (≈750 mL/day). The daily water intake should be less than the daily urine output to raise the serum sodium.
- The best choice of diuretic agent is spironolactone, provided the patient is not hyperkalaemic—give 25–200 mg PO once daily or in divided doses, as most of these states are accompanied by secondary hyperaldosteronism.

Note: diuretic effect of this drug may be delayed for 3–4 days.

Pseudohyponatraemia

Pseudohyponatraemia is a falsely low serum sodium measurement, most commonly seen in hyperglycaemia. A simple way to correct the sodium for hyperglycaemia is to adjust the serum sodium up by 1 mmol/L for every 3 mmol/L elevation in BGL.

43

Potassium disorders

Potassium (K^+) is predominantly an intracellular ion, with the extracellular K^+ level strictly regulated between 3.5 and 5.0 mmol/L. This level is affected by many processes, including serum pH.

As the pH rises, K^+ is shifted intracellularly and the serum level falls; conversely when serum pH decreases, intracellular K^+ shifts extracellularly into the vascular space and so the serum level increases.

A gradient across the cell membrane is essential to maintain the excitability of nerve and muscle cells, including the myocardium.

Hyperkalaemia

Hyperkalaemia is defined as a serum potassium (K^+) above 5.0 mmol/L.

Causes
- **Excessive intake**
  - K^+ supplements (oral or too rapid intravenously)
  - Transfusion of stored blood
  - High-dose IV therapy with K^+ salts of penicillin such as penicillin G
- **Increased production**
  - Haemolysis
  - Crush injury, rhabdomyolysis
  - Intense physical activity
  - Ischaemia
  - Extensive burns
  - Tumour lysis syndrome (occurs after treatment of cancers such as lymphoma and leukaemia)
- **Shift from intracellular to extracellular fluid**
  - Acidosis (metabolic or respiratory)
  - Insulin deficiency or resistance
  - Hyperglycaemia causing hypertonicity
  - Medications (beta-blockers, digoxin toxicity, suxamethonium)
  - Hyperkalaemic periodic paralysis
- **Decreased excretion**
  - Renal failure (acute or chronic)
  - Distal tubular dysfunction (i.e. RTA type IV)
  - Addison's disease, hypoaldosteronism

- Medications (especially when different groups are given concurrently)
  - K^+-sparing diuretics (e.g. spironolactone, amiloride, triamterene)
  - ACE inhibitors
  - NSAIDs
  - Trimethoprim, cyclosporine, tacrolimus, pentamidine, ketoconazole
- **Artefact**
  - Prolonged tourniquet placement for venepuncture
  - Blood sample haemolysis, massive leucocytosis, thrombocytosis

Clinical features
Cardiac

Hyperkalaemia is the most common electrolyte disturbance to cause cardiac arrest (see Chapter 8).

The ECG changes of hyperkalaemia are usually progressive and determined by the absolute serum K^+ level, as well as its rate of increase:
- Tall, peaked (tented) T waves (see Figure 43.1)
- Decreased amplitude of the R waves
- Prolonged PR interval
- ST-segment depression
- Widened QRS complexes, absent P waves
- Biphasic sinusoidal wave pattern
- Ventricular tachycardia
- Cardiac arrest secondary to ventricular fibrillation, pulseless electrical activity or asystole.

Neuromuscular
- Weakness, paraesthesiae
- Depressed or absent tendon reflexes
- Ascending paralysis
- Respiratory failure

Management

Assess the severity, as determined by the ECG manifestations, the serum K^+ level and whether the underlying cause is immediately

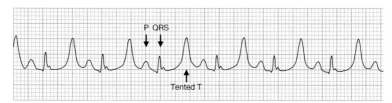

Figure 43.1 Tall, peaked T waves. Copyright Tor Ercleve.

remediable. Fatal ventricular arrhythmias may occur at any time and continuous ECG monitoring is required if the K$^+$ level is >6 mmol/L.

Severe hyperkalaemia

- Serum K$^+$ >6.5 mmol/L.
- Life-threatening ECG changes (widened QRS).
- Call your senior immediately. Cease any exogenous K$^+$ supplementation, gain IV access and commence continuous ECG monitoring.
- If the QRS is widened or there is an arrhythmia, give calcium IV to provide immediate cardioprotection to prevent cardiac arrest:
  - 10% calcium chloride 10 mL IV over 2–5 minutes. Calcium temporarily antagonises the cardiac and neuromuscular effects of the hyperkalaemia. The onset of protection is immediate, and its effect lasts for up to 1 hour. It does *not*, however, lower the K$^+$ level.
    Caution: administration of calcium to a patient on digoxin may precipitate ventricular arrhythmias because of the combined effects of digoxin and calcium, so a pacemaker may be required first.
- Reduce the serum K$^+$ level.
  - Give 50 mL of 50% dextrose IV with 10 units of short-acting insulin IV over 20 minutes. This shifts K$^+$ from the ECF to the ICF, with an onset of action within 15 minutes that lasts 1–2 hours.
    - Measure BGL to determine whether additional doses of insulin are required and to ensure that hypoglycaemia does not occur.
    - Omit the dextrose if the patient is already hyperglycaemic.
  - Give salbutamol 5–10 mg nebulised, or 250–500 micrograms IV slowly. Beta-2-adrenergic agonists temporarily reduce serum K$^+$ by stimulating cyclic AMP and shifting K$^+$ into the ICF from the ECF. Repeat doses can be given.
  - Give 8.4% sodium bicarbonate (NaHCO$_3^-$) 50 mL IV over 5 minutes, particularly when the patient is acidaemic. This also shifts K$^+$ from the ECF to the ICF. Its effect is immediate and lasts 1–2 hours, and works best in combination with dextrose/insulin therapy and salbutamol.
    Caution: take care or avoid NaHCO$_3^-$ solution in patients who are fluid overloaded, as each mL contains 1 mmoL sodium (e.g. 50 mL contains 50 mmoL Na$^+$).
  - Administer a diuretic agent such as frusemide 40–80 mg IV, provided the patient is not anuric. This removes K$^+$ by causing a diuresis.
  - Use a potassium exchange resin, such as calcium resonium, 30 g PO or PR. This is the only drug treatment that actually

removes K^+ from the total body pool, but it takes 1–3 hours for this effect to occur.

- Haemodialysis must be considered urgently if the above measures fail or when the patient is in acute or chronic oliguric renal failure with volume overload.
- Continue to monitor the serum K^+ concentration every 1–2 hours until it is <6 mmol/L, and correct any underlying contributing factors.

Moderate hyperkalaemia

- Serum K^+ 6–6.5 mmol/L.
- ECG shows peaked T waves only.
- Cause is not progressive.
- Gain IV access; start continuous ECG monitoring.
- Correct contributing factors (e.g. acidosis, hypovolaemia).
- Give one or more of the following in the dosages outlined above:
  - Dextrose and insulin IV
  - Salbutamol nebulised or IV
  - Sodium bicarbonate ($NaHCO_3^-$) IV if acidotic
  - Calcium resonium exchange resin PO or PR
  - Frusemide IV.
- Monitor the serum K^+ concentration every 1–2 hours until it is <6 mmol/L.

Mild hyperkalaemia

- Serum K^+ >5.5 mmol/L.
- ECG shows minor peaked T waves only.
- Cause is not progressive.
- Correct contributing factors as above.
- Give one or more of the following in the dosages outlined above:
  - Calcium resonium exchange resin PO or PR
  - Frusemide IV.
- Re-measure the serum K^+ concentration 4–6 hours later, depending on the cause.

Hypokalaemia

Hypokalaemia is defined as a serum potassium (K^+) below 3.5 mmol/L.

Causes

- **Inadequate intake** (over 1–2 weeks)
  - Associated with alcoholism, eating disorders and starvation
- **Extrarenal losses** (urine K^+ <20 mmol/day)
  - Diarrhoea
  - Intestinal fistula
  - Laxative misuse

- **Abnormal renal losses** (urine K$^+$ >20 mmol/day)
  - Vomiting or NG suction (hydrogen ions are lost with vomiting or NG suction, inducing a metabolic alkalosis that results in renal K$^+$ wasting)
  - Hyperaldosteronism and glucocorticoid excess
  - Conn's and Cushing's syndromes
  - Bartter's syndrome (rare inherited defects usually affecting thick ascending limb of loop of Henle leading to hypokalaemia and a metabolic alkalosis)
  - Fanconi's syndrome
  - RTA (classic type I)
  - Medications
    - Loop and thiazide diuretics, acetazolamide, steroids
    - Salbutamol, adrenaline
    - Penicillins, amphotericin B, aminoglycosides, cisplatin
  - Magnesium deficiency
  - Chronic metabolic alkalosis
- **Shift from extracellular to intracellular space**
  - Acute metabolic alkalosis
  - Insulin therapy
  - Drugs (vitamin B12 therapy, salbutamol, lithium, aminophylline)
  - Hypokalaemic periodic paralysis
  - Hypothermia

Clinical features
Cardiac
Hypokalaemia is associated with an increased incidence of cardiac arrhythmias, especially in patients with pre-existing heart disease or on digoxin.
- Premature atrial contractions (PACs)
- Premature ventricular contractions (PVCs)
- Ventricular arrhythmias, including torsades de pointes (polymorphic VT)
- Other ECG changes (see Figure 43.2) are usually non-specific, but may include:

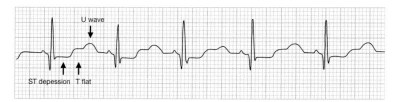

Figure 43.2 ECG manifestations of hypokalaemia. Copyright Tor Ercleve.

- T wave flattening or inversion
- Enlarging U waves
- Prolongation of PR interval
- ST-segment depression.

Neuromuscular
- Ileus, constipation
- Weakness, fatigue
- Paraesthesiae, leg cramps
- Depressed deep tendon reflexes
- Ascending paralysis and respiratory failure

Miscellaneous
- Nephrogenic diabetes insipidus
- Metabolic alkalosis
- Worsening of hepatic encephalopathy
- Chronic digoxin toxicity

Management
- Correct the underlying cause.
- Assess the severity based on the serum K^+ concentration, the ECG findings and the clinical setting in which hypokalaemia has occurred (see below).

Severe hypokalaemia
- Serum K^+ <2.5 mmol/L.
  - Or serum K^+ <3.0 mmol/L associated with cardiac arrhythmias, chronic heart failure, in the setting of myocardial ischaemia or with chronic digoxin toxicity.
- Call your senior and start continuous ECG monitoring.
- Give K^+ replacement therapy with 10 mmol KCl in 100 mL normal saline IV over 1 hour using a fluid infusion device, ideally under ECG control. Repeat once or twice as necessary. *Never* exceed a K^+ replacement rate >40 mmol K^+ in 1 hour.
  - KCl in small volumes should preferably be given through a CVL if available, as it is painful and high concentrations of K^+ are sclerosing to peripheral veins. Achieve further replacement with maintenance therapy of up to 40 mmol KCl/L of IV fluid at a maximum rate of 20 mmol KCl/h. K^+ may also be given PO, but check how many mmoL are in each tablet as their strength varies (see *Formulary*).
- In intractable severe hypokalaemia give 10 mmol or 2.5 g magnesium sulfate in 100 mL normal saline over 30–45 minutes in addition, as magnesium enhances potassium uptake and helps maintain intracellular potassium levels.

- Recheck serum K$^+$ level after each 20–30 mmol dose of KCl has been given IV.

Moderate hypokalaemia

- Serum K$^+$ <3.0 mmol/L.
- PACs but no (or infrequent) PVCs plus no evidence of ischaemia or digoxin toxicity.
- Inform your senior. Give oral K$^+$ supplementation.
- IV replacement therapy is reserved for patients who are unable to take oral supplements (see recommendations above).
- Recheck serum K$^+$ level in the morning, or sooner if clinically indicated.

Mild hypokalaemia

- Serum K$^+$ between 3.1 and 3.5 mmol/L.
- No (or infrequent) PACs and patient asymptomatic.
- Oral supplementation is usually adequate (see previous recommendations).
- Recheck serum K$^+$ level in the morning, or sooner if clinically indicated.

Handy hints

- Serious hyperkalaemia may occur with K$^+$ supplementation, so watch serum K$^+$ levels closely during IV treatment, which *must* be given through an infusion device if >20 mmoL/h. Be particularly cautious with patients with renal impairment.
- In hyperkalaemia, an abnormal ECG is a more important determinant of severity than the serum potassium level.
- Hypokalaemia and hypomagnesaemia may coexist. Correction of hypokalaemia may be unsuccessful unless hypomagnesaemia is corrected simultaneously (see above).
- Hypokalaemia and hypocalcaemia may coexist. Correction of hypokalaemia without accompanying correction of hypocalcaemia may increase the risk of ventricular arrhythmias, particularly torsades de pointes.

SECTION D – Investigations

44

Calcium disorders

Calcium (Ca^{2+}) is the most abundant mineral in the body and is essential for bone strength, neuromuscular function and a myriad of intracellular processes. It accounts for 1.5% of total body weight, with 99% stored as hydroxyapatite in the bone matrix.

Less than 1% is found in the ECF, where half of the calcium is in an active ionised form and freely diffusible, and the other half is bound to albumin and inactive.

Hypercalcaemia

Hypercalcaemia is defined as a serum Ca^{2+} level of >2.6 mmol/L after correction for albumin. The main causes are hyperparathyroidism and malignancy.

Causes

- **Increased intake**
  - Excessive calcium supplementation (with chronic renal failure)
  - Milk-alkali syndrome (from excessive calcium-containing antacid ingestion)
- **Increased GI absorption**
  - Hyperparathyroidism (usually primary, or tertiary)
  - Sarcoidosis, tuberculosis and other granulomatous diseases
  - Vitamin D intoxication
  - Acromegaly
  - Chronic lithium use
- **Increased production or resorption from bone**
  - Malignancy—four mechanisms result in hypercalcaemia associated with malignancy:
    - Bony metastases—breast, lung, thyroid, kidney and prostate primary
    - Parathyroid hormone-like substance produced by tumour cells—lung, kidney, ovary and colon
    - Prostaglandin E2 (increases bony resorption)—multiple myeloma, breast
    - Osteoclast-activating factor—multiple myeloma, lymphoproliferative disorders

- Addison's disease
- Thyrotoxicosis
- Vitamin A excess
- Immobilisation (e.g. following spinal cord injury, stroke)
- Paget's disease (particularly with bed rest)
- **Decreased excretion (increased renal resorption)**
  - Thiazide diuretics
  - Familial hypocalciuric hypercalcaemia
- **Other**
  - Prolonged tourniquet effect
  - Hyperalbuminaemia, dehydration

Clinical features

The classic aphorism 'stones, bones, abdominal groans and psychic moans' originally referred to hypercalcaemia from primary hyperparathyroidism, but it is still a useful aid to remembering the clinical manifestations of hypercalcaemia. These features are numerous and non-specific:

- Excessive thirst (polydipsia), polyuria
- Anorexia, nausea, vomiting
- Lethargy, weakness, hyporeflexia
- Nephrolithiasis ('stones')
- Bone pain, fractures ('bones')
- Abdominal pain, constipation, pancreatitis ('abdominal groans')
- Depression, confusion, delirium and coma ('psychic moans').

The ECG findings are also non-specific and include:

- Prolonged P–R interval
- Widened QRS
- Short QT interval
- Bradycardia, AV block and cardiac arrest.

Management

- The severity is determined by a combination of the:
  - Clinical manifestations
  - Serum calcium concentration
  - Rate of progression of symptoms
  - Degree of dehydration.
- The definition of hypercalcaemia severity based on the total serum calcium concentration includes:
  - **Normal:**   2.2–2.6 mmol/L
  - **Mild:**   2.6–2.9 mmol/L
  - **Moderate:** 2.9–3.2 mmol/L
  - **Severe:**   >3.2 mmol/L.

If the patient is hypoalbuminaemic, use a correction factor to estimate the total calcium concentration. Add 0.2 mmol/L to the serum calcium value for each 10 g/L of measured hypoalbuminaemia.

> *Example:* if the measured serum calcium level is 2.6 mmol/L (upper limit of normal), but the serum albumin value is low at 30 g/L (anticipated normal concentration of 40 g/L), the corrected serum calcium value is 0.2 + 2.6 = 2.8 mmol/L (i.e. mildly elevated).

Most laboratories measure the total serum calcium, which includes ionised plus albumin-bound, although the primary determinant of the physiological effects is the ionised component.

- The percentage of Ca^{2+} in ionised form is affected by the pH:
  - Acidosis increases the amount of Ca^{2+} available in ionised form (increases its effect)
  - Alkalosis increases the amount of calcium bound to albumin (decreases its effect).

A symptomatic patient with hypercalcaemia and progressive clinical manifestations requires urgent evaluation and treatment.

Severe hypercalcaemia

Severe hypercalcaemia (>3.2 mmol/L) requires immediate treatment because of the danger of a fatal cardiac arrhythmia.

- **Correct the volume depletion and expand the extracellular volume.**
  - Commence rehydration with normal saline at 500 mL/h, then titrate the normal saline maintenance rate to keep the patient slightly volume-expanded, with a urine output of at least 1.5–2 mL/kg/h.
  - This replaces free water and helps reduce the Ca^{2+} level by haemodilution, plus enhances the urinary excretion of Na^+ and Ca^{2+} ions.
    - *Caution:* potassium and magnesium will also be lost with enhanced urinary excretion, so their levels must be monitored carefully during this volume-expansion process.
  - If the patient has a history of CCF, undertake the volume expansion in a monitored ICU/high-dependency area to allow close monitoring of the volume status.
- **Establish diuresis >2500 mL/day.**
  - Administer frusemide 40 mg IV to initiate a diuresis if there is volume overload, but otherwise its regular use is not recommended.
  - *Note:* **do not** use a thiazide diuretic agent to establish the diuresis, as thiazides increase the renal tubular reabsorption of calcium, therefore increasing its level.
- **Consider dialysis.**
  - Haemodialysis or peritoneal dialysis is indicated in a patient with:
    - Serum Ca^{2+} level >4.5 mmol/L
    - Cardiovascular instability

— Significant renal impairment, unable to tolerate forced saline diuresis.

Drugs used to treat hypercalcaemia

One of the following medications may be of value in addition to administering the normal saline as above:

- **Corticosteroids**–prednisone 40–100 mg PO daily, or hydrocortisone 200–500 mg IV daily in divided doses
  - Steroids antagonise the peripheral action of vitamin D (decrease Ca^{2+} absorption, decrease mobilisation from bone and decrease renal tubular reabsorption).
  - Most useful when hypercalcaemia is secondary to malignancy (and sarcoidosis or vitamin D intoxication).
- **Bisphosphonates**–disodium pamidronate 60–90 mg in 1000 mL normal saline IV over 2–4 hours
  - Bisphosphonates have revolutionised the management of hypercalcaemia associated with malignancy, including bone metastases secondary to breast carcinoma, and in Paget's disease.
  - They work by inhibiting osteoclast activity and reducing bone turnover. Normocalcaemia is restored in >90%, with a maximal effect within 5–7 days that lasts 3–4 weeks.
  - *Note:* bisphosphonates are an effective treatment for hypercalcaemia due to bone resorption from any cause (not just malignancy).
- **Calcitonin**
  - Calcitonin 5–10 units/kg/day by slow IV infusion may be used in the emergency treatment of hypercalcaemia, in conjunction with a bisphosphonate.
  - Calcitonin inhibits osteoclast activity and the renal reabsorption of Ca^{2+} to rapidly lower Ca^{2+} within 2–3 hours, but its effect only lasts 2–3 days.
- **Indomethacin**
  - Indomethacin 50 mg PO 8-hourly inhibits the synthesis of prostaglandin E2, which is produced by some solid tumours (e.g. breast) and stimulates bone resorption.

Moderate hypercalcaemia or symptomatic mild hypercalcaemia

- Correct volume depletion and expand ECF volume with 1000 mL normal saline IV over 1–2 hours. Give further normal saline at a rate to keep the patient slightly volume-expanded, with a urine output of at least 1.5–2 mL/kg/h.
- Address any other aggravating factors such as thiazide diuretic or lithium use, prolonged bed rest and excessive dietary calcium.
- Phosphate supplementation with 0.5–3 g/day PO may be given to patients with low or normal serum phosphate levels in the face of hypercalcaemia to lower serum calcium.
  - GI intolerance (diarrhoea, flatulence) may limit its use.

SECTION D – Investigations

Asymptomatic mild hypercalcaemia

Asymptomatic mild hypercalcaemia (2.6–2.9 mmol/L) does not require immediate treatment, but will need investigating, which can be arranged for the morning.

Hypocalcaemia

Hypocalcaemia is defined as a serum Ca^{2+} level <2.1 mmol/L after correction for albumin. It is most commonly associated with respiratory alkalosis associated with hyperventilation or hypoalbuminaemia.

Causes

- **Artefact** (need to correct calcium level)
  - Hypoalbuminaemia
- **Metabolic**
  - Primary respiratory alkalosis (hyperventilation)
  - Metabolic alkalosis (vomiting, fistula)
- **Decreased intake of calcium** (usually taken in dairy products)
  - Decreased GI absorption
  - Vitamin D deficiency
  - Malabsorption
  - Chronic pancreatic disease
  - Intestinal bypass surgery
  - Short bowel syndrome
- **Decreased production or mobilisation from bone**
  - Acute hyperphosphataemia (precipitates calcium in serum)
    - Tumour lysis syndrome
    - Chronic renal failure
    - Rhabdomyolysis
- **Malignancy**
  - Paradoxical hypocalcaemia associated with osteoblastic metastases (breast, lung, prostate)
  - Medullary carcinoma of the thyroid (calcitonin-producing tumour)
- **Parathyroid hormone (PTH) deficiency or resistance**
  - Hypoparathyroidism (decreased PTH level)—autoimmune or postoperative
  - Pseudohypoparathyroidism (resistance to PTH whose level is actually high)
  - Hypomagnesaemia
- **Medications**
  - Anti-infectives (e.g. aminoglycosides, ketaconazole, foscarnet)
  - Frusemide, especially in patients with hypoparathyroidism
  - Anticonvulsants (e.g. phenytoin)
  - Chemotherapeutic agents, denosumab

- **Other**
  - Sepsis and toxic shock syndrome
  - Massive blood transfusion (citrate toxicity, particularly with hepatic or renal failure)
  - Plasmapheresis

Clinical features

The earliest symptoms are paraesthesiae of the lips, fingers, toes and face.
- Additional features include:
  - Carpopedal spasm, muscle cramps, tetany
  - Laryngeal spasm with stridor
  - Hyperreflexia
  - Generalised tonic–clonic seizures
  - Confusion, irritability, depression
  - Papilloedema, diplopia
  - Cardiac failure.

Specific signs

- ECG findings:
  - T wave inversion
  - QT prolongation (see Figure 21A)
  - Torsades de pointes (polymorphic VT) related to QT prolongation (see Figure 21B)
  - Cardiac arrest, including from torsades de pointes.
- **Chvostek's sign**—facial muscle spasm is elicited by tapping the facial nerve immediately anterior to the earlobe and below the zygomatic arch (normal finding in 10% of the population).
- **Trousseau's sign**—carpal spasm elicited by occluding the arterial blood flow to the forearm for 3–5 minutes using a sphygmomanometer cuff.

Management

- Assess the severity. This is based on:
  - Clinical manifestations, particularly cardiac arrhythmias, seizures, stridor, tetany
  - Serum calcium level
  - Serum albumin level
  - Serum phosphate level.
- Total serum Ca^{2+} concentration in hypocalcaemia:
  - **Normal:**   2.2–2.6 mmol/L
  - **Mild:**   1.9–2.2 mmol/L
  - **Moderate:**   1.5–1.9 mmol/L
  - **Severe:**   <1.5 mmol/L.

SECTION D – Investigations

If the serum albumin is not within the normal range, use a correction factor (see earlier) to estimate the total serum calcium (ionised plus albumin-bound).

Severe symptomatic hypocalcaemia

Severe symptomatic hypocalcaemia (<1.5 mmol/L) requires immediate treatment with parenteral Ca^{2+} to prevent respiratory failure from laryngospasm and tetany.

- Give 10–20 mL of 10% calcium gluconate (2.2–4.4 mmol elemental calcium) in 50–100 mL of 5% dextrose IV over 5–10 minutes.
- Commence an infusion containing 10 mL of 10% calcium gluconate in 500 mL of 5% dextrose over 6 hours.
- Administer a further infusion containing 15 mL of 10% calcium gluconate in 500 mL 5% dextrose if the serum Ca^{2+} level is <1.9 mmol/L after 6 hours.
  - *Note:* patients may require up to 3 mmol of elemental calcium *per hour* following a parathyroidectomy.
- Measure serum Ca^{2+} every 4–6 hours to maintain serum level >2.0 mmol/L.
- Commence oral replacement therapy with 0.5–2 g elemental Ca^{2+} TDS, once a satisfactory response has been achieved with parenteral calcium gluconate.
- *Note:* calcium chloride 10% solution (6.8 mmol elemental calcium/10 mL, i.e. 3-fold the amount present in the gluconate salt) is an alternative means of giving parenteral calcium.
- Calcium chloride delivers a much higher amount of elemental Ca^{2+} and is useful when rapid correction is needed. However, as it can cause significant venous irritation when administered peripherally, it should preferably be given by central venous administration.
- *Remember:* patients with cardiac arrhythmias or patients on digoxin therapy need continuous ECG monitoring during Ca^{2+} replacement. Calcium potentiates digitalis toxicity and may promote fatal arrhythmias. A pacing system may be needed.

Mild and moderate asymptomatic hypocalcaemia

- Hypocalcaemic patients who are asymptomatic do not require urgent correction with parenteral calcium.
- Start oral replacement with elemental calcium 1000–1500 mg/day to achieve a corrected serum level between 2.2 and 2.6 mmol/L.
- Longer-term treatment with oral Ca^{2+} or vitamin D depends on the cause, which can be evaluated in the morning.

45

Anaemia

Serum haemoglobin (Hb) measurement is a common laboratory test in hospitalised patients. Laboratory-recorded Hb is a *concentration* whose value will be modified by both a change in its content and a change in its *diluent* (plasma).

Thus, a patient's Hb may not be reduced (i.e. remain in the 'normal' range) despite a sudden loss of intravascular volume, as is seen with acute haemorrhage.

Remember to treat the patient, not the laboratory value. Avoid the reflex administration of RBC transfusion to correct a low Hb level, because of the potential complications with blood transfusions, which include the possibility of transfusion-related illness, haemolytic or anaphylactic reactions, volume overload or acute lung injury (see Chapter 34).

Low haemoglobin (anaemia)

Anaemia is defined as Hb <125 g/L in adults or 110 g/L in children. It is important to take an accurate history and perform a systematic examination, including vital signs and postural blood pressure. Then review the mean corpuscular volume (MCV) and mean corpuscular haemoglobin (MCH), and determine the presence of additional cells such as reticulocytes to define the underlying cause(s) of anaemia.

Causes
- **Physiological**
  - Pregnancy (iron and folate deficient)
- **Reduced RBC production**
  - **Microcytic (↓MCV), hypochromic (↓MCH)**
    - **Iron deficiency:** menorrhagia; colon cancer or polyps often with occult bleeding; dietary lack; NSAID use; malabsorption
    - Thalassaemia minor; HbE trait (e.g. Vietnamese)
    - Lead poisoning (+ basophilic stippling of RBCs)
  - **Normocytic (normal MCV), normochromic (normal MCH)**
    - Primary marrow failure: myelofibrosis, aplastic anaemia

- Secondary marrow failure: anaemia of chronic disease (e.g. chronic inflammation, endocrine failure, liver disease); uraemia, alcohol excess
- **Macrocytic (↑MCV), normochromic (normal MCH)**
  - **Folate deficiency:** pregnancy; dietary including the elderly; chronic alcohol use; malabsorption including coeliac disease; medications (e.g. trimethoprim, methotrexate, phenytoin); prolonged haemolysis
  - **Vitamin B12 deficiency:** intrinsic factor deficiency (e.g. pernicious anaemia, post-gastrectomy); terminal ileitis in Crohn's disease; malabsorption including coeliac disease; chronic alcohol use; dietary e.g. vegan diet; rarely medications (e.g. omeprazole, metformin)
- **Increased RBC loss (usually normal MCH and MCV)**
  - GI haemorrhage
  - Vaginal bleeding (uterine or cervical)
  - Trauma (external or concealed)
  - Internal (concealed) haemorrhage— postoperative bleeding, retroperitoneal haematoma, ruptured aortic aneurysm, ruptured ectopic pregnancy
- **Haemolysis (haemolytic anaemias)**
  - **Genetic**
    - Membrane protein defect (hereditary spherocytosis)
    - Enzyme defect (G6PD deficiency, pyruvate kinase deficiency)
    - Haemoglobinopathy (thalassaemia, sickle-cell disease)
  - **Acquired immune** (associated with spherocyte formation)
    - Iso-immune (Rhesus disease of the newborn, blood transfusion)
    - Autoimmune (warm haemaglutinin, cold haemaglutinin, drug related e.g. quinine)
  - **Acquired non-immune** (associated with schistocytes/fragmented RBCs)
    - Microangiopathic (DIC, TTP, HUS, pre-eclampsia, HELLP)
    - Infection (e.g. malaria, septicaemia, mycoplasma)
    - Mechanical cardiac valve, hypersplenism, metastatic carcinoma
    - Hyperthermia

Clinical manifestations

The manifestations of anaemia depend on its severity (absolute Hb level), rapidity of onset and any comorbid medical conditions, such as angina.

The body's reaction to an acute reduction in RBC mass usually includes compensatory changes in the cardiovascular and respiratory systems. Thus, anaemia secondary to acute haemorrhage is associated with the symptoms and signs of intravascular volume depletion with their autonomic sympathetic system compensation.

Symptoms of anaemia
- Fatigue, lethargy
- Dyspnoea
- Palpitations
- Worsening of prior conditions such as angina pectoris, peripheral vascular disease with intermittent claudication, and cerebrovascular disease with TIA
- GI disturbance with anorexia, nausea, bowel irregularity (because of shunting of blood from the splanchnic bed)
- Irregular menstrual pattern

Signs of anaemia
- Pallor
- Tachypnoea
- Tachycardia, wide pulse pressure
- Jaundice, hepatomegaly or splenomegaly (e.g. in some haemolytic anaemias)

Management
Assess the severity
Severity is determined by the Hb level, the patient's volume status, the rapidity with which the anaemia developed and whether the underlying disease process is continuing.

General treatment
- The treatment of anaemia from blood loss includes the investigation and correction of the underlying cause, and oral administration of ferrous sulfate to reverse the anaemia and to replenish the body's stores of iron.
- Few indications exist for the use of parenteral iron therapy, which has been associated with anaphylaxis when given IV.
- Reserve blood transfusion for the treatment of hypoxia, shock, ongoing active bleeding or significant organ dysfunction such as angina or TIA (but get senior advice about the rate and amount of blood to be transfused).

Treatment of the bleeding patient who is volume-depleted
Anaemia secondary to acute blood loss is associated with intravascular volume depletion and results in a compensatory tachycardia and tachypnoea. Hypotension or shock will result if the body's

haemodynamic compensation is incomplete or inadequate (see Chapters 11 and 18):

- Notify your senior immediately.
- Ensure that at least one and preferably two large-bore (14–16G) cannulae are in place.
- Organise urgent cross-matching of 2–6 units of packed RBCs, depending on the estimated blood loss.
- **Restore intravascular volume:** temporarily restore haemodynamic stability by giving IV fluid such as normal saline or Hartmann's solution 10–20 mL/kg IV rapidly.
- **Transfusion of packed RBCs:** reserve for patients who are actively bleeding, and for patients with acute end-organ dysfunction such as tachypnoea, chest pain, oliguria or confusion.
  - Give O-negative blood in an emergency only, usually reserved for acute trauma victims.
- **Determine the aetiology of acute blood loss:**
  - Look for obvious signs of external bleeding—haematemesis, melaena, menstrual bleeding, gross haematuria, IV sites, skin lesions.
  - Examine for signs of occult (concealed) blood loss such as abdominal pain (AAA or ectopic pregnancy) and, in particular, perform a PR examination to look for melaena or fresh rectal blood.
  - Occult blood loss should also be suspected if there is swelling at biopsy or surgical sites (e.g. flank swelling after renal biopsy, abdominal swelling after liver biopsy); or if there is bruising in the flank (Grey Turner's sign indicating retroperitoneal bleeding) or periumbilical bruising (Cullen's sign indicating a possible haemoperitoneum).
  - Suspect a ruptured ectopic pregnancy in *every* female patient of childbearing age, perform an immediate beta-hCG pregnancy test and arrange an urgent pelvic USS. Alert the O&G team, theatre and the duty anaesthetist.
  - Suspect a ruptured AAA in a man over 45 years or a postmenopausal woman who presents with any features of abdominal or back pain, shock or unexplained tachycardia, and a tender abdomen with or without a pulsatile mass. Arrange an urgent abdominal USS and alert the surgeons, theatre and the duty anaesthetist.
- Review the chart for exacerbating factors that may be contributing to ongoing haemorrhage, such as administration of aspirin, clopidogrel, heparin, warfarin or a NOAC, or a recent thrombolytic agent.
  - Look for pertinent laboratory values indicating a coagulopathy, such as a prolonged aPTT or PT, and low platelets.

Treatment of the patient who is normovolaemic

Mild chronic anaemia (Hb 100–120 g/L) with a normal intravascular volume does not tend to alter the patient's vital signs. Patients may even tolerate a severe anaemia (Hb <70 g/L) if it develops slowly.

Transfusion therapy is seldom warranted on an urgent basis if the patient is normovolaemic.

Once the presence of active haemorrhage has been excluded (see above), the anaemia will have been caused by chronic blood loss, inadequate production of RBCs or a haemolytic process.

- **What is the patient's usual Hb?** Look at the current or old chart to determine whether the anaemia is new. If the current Hb is more than 10–20 g/L lower than previous values, assume that the underlying cause of anaemia has worsened or a second factor has developed (e.g. a patient with a chronic disease, such as SLE, may normally have an Hb of 90 g/L; a new value of 75 g/L may represent further marrow suppression, haemolysis or new onset of bleeding).
- Reconfirm an unexpectedly low Hb result <100 g/L with a repeat sample to exclude a laboratory error while other assessments are taking place.
  - An asymptomatic patient with mild anaemia (Hb 100–120 g/L) and normal vital signs can usually wait if other problems of higher priority exist. However, always keep in mind that if active bleeding is responsible for the anaemia, a stable patient may rapidly become unstable.
  - Further investigations can be done in the morning if the patient is comfortable, has a normal cardiovascular examination and physical examination reveals no suspicion of active bleeding.
- Baseline studies to help diagnose the cause of the anaemia include:
  - MCV to classify the anaemia secondary to decreased RBC production (microcytic, normocytic or macrocytic).
  - Reticulocyte count to provide a measure of marrow erythropoiesis.
    - Elevated reticulocyte count suggests haemolysis, recent haemorrhage or a recently treated chronic anaemia (e.g. vitamin B12 deficiency).
    - Inappropriately low reticulocyte count suggests failure to produce RBCs (e.g. untreated iron, vitamin B12 or folate deficiency, or anaemia of chronic disease).
  - Examination of a blood film and differential may provide additional evidence of the underlying aetiology (e.g. spherocytes, schistocytes, poikilocytes, basophilic stippling,

Howell–Jolly bodies, red cell agglutinates, and immature or atypical white cells suggesting bone marrow failure or infiltration).

- Iron, ferritin, iron-binding capacity and transferrin; folate and vitamin B12 level according to the suspected aetiology.
- A bone marrow aspiration arranged by the usual medical team to further evaluate for a haematological disorder.

46

Coagulation disorders

While on call, you may be confronted with abnormal results of coagulation tests, which must be interpreted in the clinical context in which the measurements were made. Bleeding is the most common clinical manifestation of a coagulation disorder:

- Bleeding associated with vessel or platelet abnormalities causes non-blanching skin bleeding seen as small petechiae ('flea bites'), larger purpura (bruises) or generalised 'easy bruising'. The bleeding is characteristically superficial (e.g. oozing from mucous membranes or IV site).
- Bleeding related to a coagulation factor deficiency (or warfarin or NOAC use) may occur spontaneously and in deeper organ sites (e.g. visceral haemorrhage, retroperitoneal bleeding, a haemarthrosis or intracerebral bleeding). It tends to be slow, delayed and/or prolonged.
- Bleeding associated with a thrombolytic agent usually manifests as a continuous ooze from an IV site, but also as a sudden acute intracerebral haemorrhage or GI bleed.

Assessment of haemostasis

Various laboratory parameters that measure specific functions of the coagulation system are available:

- Prothrombin time (PT)
- International normalised ratio (INR)
- Activated partial thromboplastin time (aPTT)
- Platelet count.

The aPTT and PT/INR results provided in the coagulation profile should be reviewed together to determine the probable cause of the clotting derangement (see Table 46.1).

Prothrombin time and international normalised ratio

The PT evaluates the extrinsic and common pathways of the coagulation system, and their contribution to a patient's bleeding and/or clotting tendencies. Thromboplastin (tissue factor or coagulation factor III)

Table 46.1 Combination of prothrombin time (PT) and activated partial thromboplastin time (aPTT) in the coagulation profile		
aPTT	PT normal	PT elevated
Normal	A	B
Elevated	C	D

A: Normal result (factor levels at least 35% of normal)

B: Isolated factor VII deficiency
- Congenital deficiency
- Acquired
- Warfarin therapy
- Vitamin K deficiency
- Early liver disease

C: Intrinsic pathway abnormality
- Heparin treatment
- Factor VIII deficiency
- Typical pattern in haemophilia and von Willebrand's disease
- Low levels of factors VIII, IX, XI and XII
- Antiphospholipid antibody
- Black snake (*Pseudechis* spp) bite

D: Common pathway abnormality
- Low levels of factors I, II, V and X
- Venom-induced consumptive coagulopathy (VICC)

Combined intrinsic and extrinsic pathway defects
- DIC
- Full warfarin and high-dose heparin treatment
- Vitamin K deficiency
- Advanced liver disease

Note: LMWH does not prolong the PT or aPTT. It exerts its anticoagulant effect by binding to antithrombin III, resulting in anti-factor Xa and IIa activities.

and calcium are added to plasma in the laboratory to assess any potential deficit or antagonism of the clotting factors II, V, VII and X.

The PT test is most sensitive to a decrease in factor VII, which is one of the vitamin K-dependent factors.

However, as each laboratory uses different reagents and types of animal thromboplastin to measure the PT, analysis of PT across different institutions is potentially confusing.

Thus, the INR was introduced to standardise the reporting of PT from different laboratories. The international sensitivity index (ISI) is supplied with every batch of thrompoplastin reagent, and is used by the haematology laboratory to calculate the INR:

$$INR = (\text{patient's PT}/\text{laboratory's control PT})^{ISI}.$$

A normal INR is between 0.9 and 1.2, and is the best means of standardising PT, for instance to monitor oral anticoagulant therapy.

Causes of an elevated prothrombin time/international normalised ratio

- **Deficiency of clotting factors**
  - Fibrinogen
  - Factors II, V, VII, X
- **Vitamin K deficiency** (leading to a deficiency of vitamin K-dependent factors II, VII, IX, X)
  - Infants
  - Chronic liver disease
  - Biliary disease with cholestasis
  - Malabsorption, including coeliac disease, inflammatory bowel disease
  - Post-abdominal surgery
- **Medications and other substances**
  - Warfarin anticoagulation (used to monitor this)
  - Unfractionated heparin (UFH)—only at high dose
  - Indomethacin, mefanamic acid, aspirin (>1 g/day)
  - Phenytoin, thyroxine, anabolic steroids
- **Other**
  - Nephrotic syndrome
  - Massive blood transfusion
  - DIC

Factors that disturb the interpretation of prothrombin time/international normalised ratio

- External contamination:
  - EDTA cross-contamination if coagulation profile tube is not filled *first*, as interferes with the activation process
- Alteration of whole blood to citrated anticoagulant ratio (normal 9:1):
  - Underfilled sample
  - Polycythaemia
  - Blood withdrawn from a line if not properly flushed e.g. heparin in CVL
- Factors leading to laboratory error:
  - Haemolysis, hyperbilirubinaemia
  - Lipaemia, hyperproteinaemia

Activated partial thromboplastin time

The aPTT is a test of the intrinsic coagulation system. The aPTT is most sensitive to deficiencies and abnormalities that occur before factor X activation in the coagulation cascade.

It is the time taken for plasma to form a fibrin clot and is measured in seconds (normal aPTT is 25–35 sec). It is used to monitor UFH IV therapy.

Causes of a prolonged activated partial thromboplastin time

- **Deficiency of clotting factors**
  - Factor VIII deficiency (haemophilia A)
  - Factor IX deficiency (haemophilia B or 'Christmas disease')
  - von Willebrand's disease (variable effect, related to reduced levels of factor VIII)
  - High-molecular-weight kininogen, prekallikrein (contact factor deficiency)
- **Anticoagulant therapy**
  - UFH therapy (used to monitor this)
  - Warfarin therapy (aPTT rise relatively insensitive, so is *not* used as a monitor)
- **Other**
  - Antiphospholipid antibody syndrome (primary or secondary to SLE etc)
  - Increased FDPs (abruptio placentae, septicaemia, DIC, transfusion reaction)
  - Black snake (*Pseudechis* spp) envenomation
  - Severe vitamin K deficiency
  - Severe liver disease

Factors that disturb the interpretation of activated partial thromboplastin time

- External contamination:
  - Lithium–heparin cross-contamination if coagulation profile tube is not filled *first*, as it interferes with the activation process
- Alteration in whole blood to citrated anticoagulant ratio (normal 9:1):
  - Underfilled sample

Platelet count

Disorders of haemostasis can occur due to platelet abnormalities that include:
- Reduction in total platelet count (thrombocytopenia):
  - Reduced production
  - Increased destruction

- Impaired platelet function
- Vessel abnormalities.

Disorders associated with a low platelet count (thrombocytopenia)

Decreased marrow production
- Primary marrow disease (leukaemia, lymphoma, myeloma)
- Marrow replacement
  - Metastatic neoplasm, TB, sarcoid, storage disease such as Gaucher's disease
- Defective marrow maturation from vitamin B12 or folate deficiency
- Infections such as viral hepatitis, CMV, leptospirosis, brucellosis, malaria, TB, severe sepsis
- Medications and other substances
  - Chemotherapeutic agents, thiazides, interferon
  - Ethanol, chloramphenicol

Increased peripheral destruction
- **Immune-mediated**
  - Idiopathic (immune-mediated) thrombocytopenic purpura (ITP)—note HIV or SLE may underlie or be associated with this
  - Medications
    - Quinine/quinidine, sulfonamides, rifampicin, vancomycin, thiazides, NSAIDs
    - Heparin (HITS: unfractionated > low-molecular-weight), gold, penicillamine, cimetidine/ranitidine
  - Connective tissue disorders (SLE)
  - Lymphoproliferative disorders (CLL)
  - HIV infection
  - Post-transfusion purpura
  - Neonatal
- **Non-immune-mediated**
  - Increased consumption (DIC, prosthetic valves, TTP, HUS)
  - Dilutional (e.g. massive transfusion)
- **Sequestration**
  - Hypersplenism including chronic liver disease with portal hypertension

Factitious thrombocytopenia
  - Platelet clumping giving a falsely low platelet count when the blood sample is exposed to EDTA, a preservative used in full blood collection tubes (maroon-topped). This is verified by direct examination of the blood smear.

- An accurate platelet count may be obtained in these patients by collecting a blood sample in a sodium citrate (blue-topped) tube.

Platelet function or vessel abnormalities

Bleeding may still occur even if the patient has a normal PT/INR, aPTT and platelet count, and is not receiving LMWH.

This will be a result of either impaired platelet function or vessel abnormalities.

Impaired platelet function
- **Hereditary disorders**
  - von Willebrand's disease
  - Bernard–Soulier's disease
  - Glanzmann's disease (thrombasthenia)
- **Acquired disorders**
  - Medications
    - NSAIDs, aspirin, clopidogrel, glycoprotein IIb/IIIa receptor blockers
    - High-dose penicillin, cephalosporins, nitrofurantoin
  - Uraemia
  - Paraproteins
    - Multiple myeloma, amyloidosis
    - Waldenström's macroglobulinemia
  - Myeloproliferative disorder
    - Chronic myelocytic leukaemia, essential thrombocytosis
    - Post-cardiopulmonary bypass

Vessel abnormalities
- **Hereditary disorders**
  - Hereditary haemorrhagic telangiectasia (Osler–Weber–Rendu syndrome)
  - Marfan's syndrome, Ehlers–Danlos syndrome
  - Pseudoxanthoma elasticum
  - Osteogenesis imperfecta
- **Acquired disorders**
  - Vasculitis
    - Meningococcal, pneumococcal, gonococcal or Rickettsial infection
    - Henoch–Schönlein purpura
    - SLE, polyarteritis nodosa, rheumatoid arthritis
    - Cryoglobulinaemia
  - Increased vascular fragility
    - Senile purpura
    - Cushing's syndrome
    - Trauma
    - Scurvy

Management of bleeding in coagulation disorders

Bleeding in a patient with a coagulation disorder is of concern for two reasons:
- Progressive loss of intravascular volume may lead to hypovolaemia and/or anaemia if uncorrected with inadequate perfusion of vital organs.
- Haemorrhage into specific organ sites may produce critical local tissue or organ injury (e.g. intracerebral haemorrhage, epidural haemorrhage with spinal cord compression or a haemarthrosis).

Bleeding due to anticoagulant therapy

Bleeding caused by anticoagulant therapy can be reversed slowly or rapidly, depending on the patient's clinical status, the site of bleeding and the underlying medical condition for which the anticoagulation was given.

Unfractionated heparin

- Minor bleeding secondary to heparin-induced coagulopathy:
  - Discontinue the heparin infusion.
- Significant haemorrhage:
  - More rapid and specific reversal of UFH is achieved by giving 1 mg protamine sulfate IV slowly for each 100 units of unfractionated heparin recently delivered.
  - Determine protamine dose by estimating the amount of circulating heparin (see Table 46.2).
  - Discontinue the heparin infusion.
  - *Example:* a patient who bleeds when on a maintenance infusion of UFH 1000 units/h IV must have the heparin infusion stopped and be given sufficient protamine to neutralise approximately half of the preceding hour's dose. In this case, a total of 5 mg protamine.
  - *Caution:* do not give more than 50 mg protamine per single dose in a 10-minute period. Significant side effects such as hypotension, bradycardia or flushing may occur.

Table 46.2 Calculation of protamine dose for reversal of unfractionated heparin

Time since cessation of heparin infusion (min)	Dose of protamine to neutralise 100 U of heparin (mg)
<30	1
30–60	0.5
60–120	0.375
>120	0.25

SECTION D – Investigations

Low-molecular-weight heparin

- LMWH has a longer half-life than UFH. The aPTT has no value for monitoring the degree of anticoagulation, but anti-factor Xa levels may be useful if they can be measured.
- Protamine sulfate only partially reverses the anticoagulant effect of LMWH.
- Administer approximately 1 mg protamine for every 1 mg or 100 units (anti-factor Xa activity) of LMWH. Give lower doses of protamine if there is a delay in protamine administration, just as with UFH (see Table 46.3).
- A second infusion of 0.5 mg protamine sulfate for each 100 units anti-factor Xa activity may be given after 2–4 hours if the patient has not responded.

Table 46.3 **Calculation of protamine dose for reversal with low-molecular-weight heparin (partial effect only)**

Time since last dose of LMWH (hours)	Dose of protamine to neutralise 100 U of heparin (mg)
<8	1
8–12	0.5
>12	Protamine usually not required

Warfarin

- When considering changes to warfarin anticoagulation therapy, always review the medical notes for the clinical indication, target INR (see Table 46.4) and predicted duration of therapy.
- The decision to commence or cease warfarin should be made (or approved) by a senior doctor, who *must* be consulted. Clearly document any changes to the warfarin regimen in the medical notes.

Table 46.4 **Recommended ranges for the international normalised ratio (INR) according to clinical indication**

Recommended INR range	Condition
2.0–3.0	Preventing DVT (high-risk patients) Therapy for DVT or PE Preventing systemic embolisation in AF, valvular heart disease, post AMI, bioprosthetic heart valves (first 3 months)
2.5–3.5	Bileaflet mechanical heart valve (aortic)
3.0–4.5	Mechanical prosthetic valve (high risk) Thrombosis in antiphospholipid syndrome

- Major bleeding is a common and potentially hazardous complication associated with warfarin. There is a close relationship between the INR and the risk of bleeding, especially with INR >4.
- Management of a highly elevated INR with haemorrhage includes cessation of the warfarin therapy and administration of vitamin K, fresh frozen plasma (FFP), a prothrombin complex concentrate or recombinant factor VIIa (see Table 46.5).
- Vitamin K may be used to partially or completely reverse the effects of warfarin anticoagulation. However, warfarin reversal with vitamin K takes up to 24 hours for maximal effect.
- Low-dose vitamin K (0.5–1.0 mg) is used to partially reverse warfarin anticoagulation. Larger doses (5–10 mg) are used in cases of life-threatening haemorrhage, or when full reversal of anticoagulation is required (and is not contraindicated, as in a patient with a mechanical prosthetic heart valve who will *not* tolerate loss of the normal anticoagulation state).

Table 46.5 **Reversal of warfarin anticoagulation according to international normalised ratio (INR)**

INR	Clinical situation	Action
3.0–5.0	No bleeding	Reduce dose of warfarin and consider omitting next dose Monitor INR daily Restart warfarin at a reduced dose when INR is in normal therapeutic range
5.0–9.0	No bleeding	Stop warfarin Re-measure INR in 6–12 hours Recommence warfarin at lower dose when INR <5.0
5.0–9.0	Minor bleed *and* increased risk of bleeding	Stop warfarin Consider vitamin K 1–2 mg oral *or* 0.5–1mg slow IV bolus over 2 min Re-measure INR in 6–12 hours Recommence warfarin at lower dose when INR <5.0
>9.0	No bleeding *and* low risk of bleeding *or* minor bleeding	Stop warfarin Give 2–5 mg vitamin K oral *or* 1 mg slow IV bolus Re-measure INR in 6–12 hours **Discuss with haematologist before restarting**
>9.0 Or whenever warfarin use is considered contributory	Serious bleeding	Stop warfarin **Seek senior advice** Give 5–10 mg vitamin K (slow IV bolus) +Prothrombinex-VF 50 IU/kg +fresh frozen plasma 150–300 mL Repeat INR in 6–12 hours

- Vitamin K is administered PO or IV.
- *Remember:* larger doses of vitamin K produce resistance to re-anticoagulation and should be discussed with your senior or the haematologist on call.
- When immediate reversal of anticoagulation is required, the combination of prothrombin complex concentrate and FFP will cover the interim period before vitamin K reaches its full effect.

New oral anticoagulants

- New oral anticoagulants (NOACs) are non-warfarin oral anticoagulants, also known as *novel* oral anticoagulants or *direct* oral anticoagulants (DOAC).
- They include dabigatran, a competitive inhibitor of thrombin, and apixaban and rivaroxaban, which are direct competitive antagonists of factor Xa.
- Patients with renal impairment including advanced age are at increased risk of bleeding, although drug and food interactions are much less than with warfarin.
- Routine coagulation monitoring is not required; however, determining the presence and degree of NOAC-related anticoagulation in a bleeding patient or one needing urgent surgery is complex.
  - A normal thrombin time (TT) excludes clinically relevant dabigatran effect.
  - A normal specific chromogenic anti-Xa assay result excludes clinically relevant apixaban or rivaroxaban effect, but this test may not be immediately available.
  - Discussion with a haematologist is essential.
- Dabigatran is fully reversed by giving idarucizumab 5 g IV bolus. There is currently no reversal agent for the factor Xa antagonists.
- Contact your senior, and discuss with a haematologist the management of any patient on a NOAC who is bleeding or needs urgent surgery.

Bleeding secondary to coagulation factor abnormalities
Clinical features

- The clinical features of a coagulation factor abnormality are many and various, and tend to manifest at deeper organ sites (e.g. visceral haemorrhage, retroperitoneal bleeding or a haemarthrosis). Bleeding may be slow, delayed and/or prolonged.
- Thrombotic thrombocytopenic purpura (TTP) presents with a constellation of features that include haemolytic anaemia, thrombocytopenia, fever, neurological disorders and renal dysfunction.

- Haemolytic–uraemic syndrome (HUS) presents similarly to TTP, but *without* the neurological manifestations.
- These two syndromes must be distinguished from DIC, in which a prolonged aPTT and PT, reduced fibrinogen level and elevated fibrin degradation products are seen (see Table 46.6). DIC most often occurs with infection (e.g. Gram-negative sepsis), an obstetric catastrophe such as septic abortion or amniotic fluid embolus (if the patient survives), malignancy (e.g. prostate cancer) and traumatic tissue damage or shock.

Treatment

Treatment of coagulation factor abnormalities is dependent on the specific factor deficiency or deficiencies. All specific factor deficiencies should always be treated in consultation with a haematologist.

- Factor VIII deficiency (haemophilia A) is best treated with factor VIII concentrate. However, it may also be treated with FFP, cryoprecipitate and non-blood products such as DDAVP or EACA.
- Factor IX deficiency (haemophilia B) is treated with factor IX concentrate, but may be treated with FFP.
- Liver disease with active bleeding in patients with an elevated PT, aPTT or INR is managed with FFP. Many patients with liver disease are also vitamin K-deficient, so administer vitamin K 10 mg PO daily for 3 days as well.
  - However, factor IX concentrate carries a risk of thrombosis and is contraindicated in liver disease.
- Vitamin K deficiency—identify and treat the underlying cause of the vitamin K deficiency.
- DIC treatment is complicated and controversial, and should be discussed with the haematologist on call. Essentially, management involves treating the underlying cause. Additionally, a patient with DIC may require coagulation factor and platelet support with FFP, cryoprecipitate and platelet transfusions. The use of heparin in the treatment of DIC is possible.
- Thrombolytic agent bleeding may be localised oozing at sites of invasive procedures and is managed by local pressure dressings, and avoidance of other invasive procedures (especially a central line). Discontinue the thrombolytic agent if more serious haemorrhage occurs and seek urgent senior advice.
  - FFP may be required to replace fibrinogen as many fibrinolytic agents are not fibrin-specific and cause systemic fibrinogenolysis.
  - Cryoprecipitate may be used to replace fibrinogen and factor VIII levels.
  - EACA, which is an inhibitor of plasminogen activator, can also be used (20–30 g/day), but should not be initiated without consulting a haematologist.

SECTION D – Investigations

Table 46.6 Laboratory features of common coagulation disorders

Disorder	Diagnostic laboratory test				
	aPTT	PT/INR	Platelets	Bleeding time	Other
Vessel abnormalities					
Vasculitis	N	N	N	N or ↑	
Increased vascular fragility	N	N	N	↑	
Hereditary connective tissue disorders	N	N	N	↑	
Paraproteinaemias	N	N	N	↑	
Coagulation factor abnormalities					
Unfractionated heparin	↑	↑ or N	N or ↓	N or ↑	
LMWH	N	N	N	N or ↑	
Warfarin	N or ↑	↑	N	N	
Vitamin K deficiency	↑	↑	N	N	
DIC	↑	↑	↓	N or ↑*	↑ FDP↓ Fibrinogen
Factor VIII deficiency	↑	N	N	N	↓ Factor VIII assay
Factor IX deficiency	↑	N	N	N	N factor IX assay
von Willebrand's disease	N or ↑	N	N	N or ↑	↓ Factor VIII antigen / N or ↓ Factor VIII assay
Liver disease	↑	↑	N or ↓	N or ↑	
Platelet disorders					
Thrombocytopenia	N	N	↓	N or ↑*	
Impaired platelet function	N	N	N	↑	

N, normal.
*Depends on degree of thrombocytopenia.

Management of bleeding in platelet or vessel disorders

Management of a patient with bleeding due to a platelet or vessel disorder will depend on whether the underlying cause is related to a platelet abnormality or vessel abnormality.

Platelet abnormalities

The treatment of bleeding in a patient with thrombocytopenia varies according to the presence of either an abnormality in platelet production or an increase in platelet destruction:

- Decreased marrow production of platelets is treated by identifying and, if possible, correcting the underlying cause (e.g. chemotherapy for tumour, removal of marrow toxins, vitamin B12 or folate supplementation).
- In the short term, treat any serious bleeding complication by a platelet transfusion with a minimum of five units of platelets at a time. One unit of platelets should increase the platelet count by 1000 in a patient with inadequate marrow production of platelets, although the biological half-life is short (1–2 days).
- Increased peripheral destruction of platelets is best managed by identifying and correcting the underlying problem (e.g. systemic corticosteroids or other immunosuppressive agents). Patients tend to have less serious bleeding manifestations than those with inadequate marrow production of platelets, but platelet transfusion may be required for a life-threatening bleeding episode.
- Significant bleeding in patients with ITP responds to immune globulin IV (quicker response) or steroids, or both, followed by platelet transfusion if needed.
- However, platelet transfusion therapy should *not* be used to treat thrombocytopenia in a patient with TTP, as it may actually worsen the condition ('adding fuel to the fire'). Platelet abnormality in TTP is treated urgently with plasma exchange.
- Dilutional thrombocytopenia from massive RBC transfusion and IV fluid therapy is treated with platelet transfusion as necessary.
  - This dilutional thrombocytopenia may be prevented by transfusing 5 units of platelets for every 5 units of RBCs transfused (i.e. 1:1). In addition, as massive transfusion results in consumption and dilution of coagulation factors, also administer FFP if there is evidence of bleeding or a significantly elevated PT, aPTT or INR.
- von Willebrand's disease is treated with factor VIII concentrates or cryoprecipitate. DDAVP injection is useful for long-term therapy of type 1 von Willebrand's disease, but may exacerbate thrombocytopenia in type 2 disease.

SECTION D – Investigations

- Bleeding disorders resulting from acquired platelet dysfunction are managed by identifying and correcting the underlying problem. Temporary treatment of bleeding disorders caused by these conditions may involve platelet transfusion or other more specialised measures (e.g. cryoprecipitate, DDAVP injection, plasmapheresis, conjugated oestrogens and haemodialysis in uraemia). Seek senior advice and involve a haematologist.

Vessel abnormalities

Treatment of bleeding caused by vessel abnormalities consists of dealing with the underlying disorder:

- Serious bleeding due to hereditary disorders of connective tissue or hereditary haemorrhagic telangiectasia requires local mechanical or surgical measures at the site of haemorrhage to control blood loss, such as cautery of a persistent epistaxis. Some patients with hereditary haemorrhagic telangiectasia may benefit from aminocaproic acid.
- Control of bleeding is best achieved by the use of corticosteroids, other immunosuppressive agents, or both, in vasculitis such as SLE.
- Purpura in Cushing's syndrome is preventable with normalisation of plasma cortisol levels, although in a patient receiving therapeutic corticosteroids, the underlying indication for therapy may prevent any significant reduction in dose. Haemorrhages associated with scurvy do not recur after adequate dietary supplementation of ascorbic acid (vitamin C).
- There is no good treatment for the increased vascular fragility that results from senile purpura of old age.
- Treat septicaemia with vasculitis from meningococcal, pneumococcal or gonococcal infection aggressively with antibiotics and supportive measures. Make certain your senior is involved immediately.

Practical procedures

47

General preparation for a practical procedure

Prepare yourself

- Familiarise yourself with the procedure, including the indications, contraindications, technique, anatomical landmarks and potential complications.
- *Never* perform a procedure unless you have first observed that procedure being performed, and then performed the procedure at least once under supervision. Never be afraid to ask for help. Do not bluff your way at the patient's expense.
- Inform nursing staff that a procedure is to be performed.
- Adhere to aseptic practices for all procedures such as the aseptic non-touch technique (ANTT).

Prepare the patient

- Ensure that you have the correct patient for the correct procedure. Ask the patient's name and date of birth and double-check this with the patient's name band. Then check and confirm you have the correct side and mark it if necessary.
- Introduce yourself: be polite, courteous and empathic. Gaining the confidence and trust of the patient is invaluable, especially when faced with a painful or lengthy procedure, or should complications arise.
- Use simple language to explain what you are doing and why, and obtain verbal consent from the patient.
- Examine the patient, confirm anatomical landmarks and look for potential complicating factors such as local sepsis, deformities or scarring.
- Place the patient in the most appropriate position for the procedure and ensure that the patient is as comfortable as possible. Do not perform any potentially painful procedure with the patient standing up in case he or she faints.

- Review requirements for premedication, sedation, analgesia and monitoring.

Prepare the equipment

Try to visualise the procedure and any potential complications in your mind. Locate all equipment required for the procedure and place on the lower shelf of a trolley. Commonly required equipment includes:

- **Absorbent blue plastic-and-paper pad ('bluey')**—essential for all procedures. When placed correctly before commencing a procedure, the absorbent pad will protect the bed linen and the patient's clothes from cleaning solution or spilled blood.
- **Dressing pack**—contents are sterile and usually contain:
  - Folded plastic sheet (unfold and place sterile equipment onto it)
  - Plastic tray to hold cleaning solution
  - Gauze or cotton swabs
  - Disposable forceps
  - Simple sterile drape (green or blue paper).
- **Skin cleaning solutions**
  - Chlorhexidine 1% or 2%—chemical antiseptic agent effective against Gram-positive and -negative microbes, facultative aerobes, anaerobes and yeasts. Use for general skin cleansing and wound irrigation, often in combination with cetrimide, another antiseptic agent. Both agents bind strongly to skin, mucosa and other tissues, but are poorly absorbed. Their activity is reduced by the presence of blood or body fluids. May also be combined with 75% ethanol or 70% isopropyl alcohol.
  - Povidone–iodine solution (Betadine)—provides its antiseptic effect by slowly releasing iodine (iodophor). The preferred skin cleanser for major and minor surgical procedures. Its action persists while the colour remains when in the presence of blood, serum, purulent exudate and necrotic (dead) tissue. Avoid in patients who have an allergy to iodine, so ask first.
  - Alcohol swab—gamma-irradiated, individual, sterile swab impregnated with 70% isopropyl alcohol. Only use as an antiseptic skin cleanser prior to an injection.
- **Syringes**—these vary in size from 1 mL to 60 mL. Common sizes needed for a procedure include 5, 10, 20 and 50 mL. The nozzle of the syringe may be a Luer-lock (locks the needle onto the tip of the syringe), a slip tip (secures the needle by compressing the slightly tapered needle hub onto the nozzle) or a catheter tip (fitted to 50 mL syringes to access drains [e.g. NGT], sometimes using a spigot).

Table 47.1	Needle sizes and uses	
Gauge	**Hub colour**	**Use**
18G	Pink	Drawing-up needle
21G	Green	Joint aspiration, deep anaesthetic infiltration, most phlebotomies
22G	Blue	Deep IM injections
23G	Black	Deeper infiltration of local anaesthetic
25G	Orange	Superficial dermal local anaesthetic administration, ring block

- **Needles**—the translucent hub to visualise fluid/blood flashback is colour-coded according to the gauge of the needle (see Table 47.1). However, these colours are *not* standard across all manufacturers. The **smaller** the gauge, the **larger** the diameter of the needle. Needle length varies from 1.25 cm (e.g. for SC injections) to 4 cm (e.g. for deep IM injection or joint aspiration).
- **Sharps bin**—it is *essential* to have easy access to a sharps bin before performing any procedure as it reduces the risk of needlestick injury to you or other members of staff. Use a kidney dish as a temporary store for unwanted sharps only if a sharps bin is not readily accessible.
  - **Sharps safety:** *never* **recap a used needle or re-sheath a disposable blade. Do not fill a sharps bin above the full line or use your fingers to push overflowing contents inside.**

Prepare for the procedure

- Gather all the equipment required for the procedure. Place it on the lower shelf of the trolley and put the dressing pack on the top of the trolley.
- Open the dressing pack onto the upper shelf of the trolley to create your sterile field. Remove the outer package or tape and open the dressing pack with the tips of your fingers, only touching the corners.
- Peel and open all needles and syringes required and drop them onto the dressing pack without touching them, so they remain sterile.
- Wash your hands thoroughly, dry with sterile paper towel and put on sterile gloves.
- Use an aseptic technique at all times.

Post-procedural care

- Evaluate the effectiveness of the procedure and for any signs of a complication.

- Dispose of all contaminated material. This is your responsibility as the proceduralist:
  - Place all sharps in a sharps bin
  - Place contaminated rubbish in a yellow plastic bag
  - Place contaminated linen in a clear bag, then in a linen bin.
- Remove gloves and wash hands.
- Record details of the procedure in the patient's medical notes:
  - Date, time and type of procedure performed
  - Equipment used, size of catheter/cannulae/drain placed
  - Report any complications or adverse side effects encountered.
- Write appropriate aftercare management.
- Chart any medication given and prescribe further analgesia or fluids as required.

48

Infection control and standard precautions

Previously known by various names including 'universal precautions', standard precautions are designed to reduce the risk of microorganism transfer from recognised and unrecognised sources to a susceptible host.

Hospital infection is the result of a combination of factors:

microbial source + transmission + susceptible host

= nosocomial infection

Standard precautions include:
- Handwashing
- Aseptic practice
- Personal protective equipment (PPE)
- Safe handling and disposal of infectious material, particularly sharps
- Reprocessing of reusable equipment and instruments
- Environmental control.

Handwashing

This practice is the single most effective form of infection control. It is essential and central to reducing the spread of infection within hospitals, yet it is also the most commonly breached precaution. Human hands carry a plethora of resident and transient flora.
- **Resident microbes** are always present on the skin, where they are generally non-pathogenic. However, these microorganisms are of concern when performing invasive procedures or dealing with immunosuppressed patients. They may be reduced or inhibited by washing with an antimicrobial solution.
- **Transient microbes** include potentially pathogenic organisms, usually from another patient or the hospital environment. They contaminate the hands of hospital staff during daily activities. These microbes can be readily passed from one person to another via hand contact, and can survive on the skin for up to 24 hours. Routine handwashing will remove transient microbial flora.

> **BOX 48.1 The 5 moments for hand hygiene**
> 1. Before touching a patient
> 2. Before a procedure
> 3. After a procedure or body fluid exposure risk
> 4. After touching a patient
> 5. After touching a patient's surroundings
> © World Health Organization 2016, www.who.int/gpsc/5may/background/5moments/en

- In many hospitals, alcohol gel has been introduced to complement handwashing. Alcohol gel can substitute for a handwash prior to contact with a clean, external patient body surface if the hands are already clean.
- Examination gloves are an important component of hand hygiene procedures when in contact with patient body fluids or blood products.

Hands should always be washed:
- **Before** every significant patient contact, interventional procedure or eating and drinking. Significant contact includes the examination of a patient or wound, and any form of contact with invasive devices such as catheters, cannulae or drains.
- **After** performing an activity likely to cause significant contamination, such as direct contact with bodily secretions or excretions, wounds, mucous membranes or drain sites.
- **Between** examining patients (even if you are on a busy ward round). See Box 48.1.

Remember: disinfect your stethoscope periodically as a matter of routine, and especially after examining a patient with a surgical wound, chronic skin condition or long-term IV line or other medical device, and known epidemiologically important organisms such as methicillin-resistant *Staphylococcus aureus* (MRSA) or vancomycin-resistant enterococci (VRE) (in addition to any designated local infection control practice 'contact precautions' for that patient).

Handwashing procedure
- Wet the hands thoroughly and lather with soap or skin cleanser (antiseptic preparations are not required).
- Rub the hands vigorously together for at least 15 seconds, paying attention to the fingertips, interdigital areas, thumbs and wrists.
- Rinse and dry thoroughly with a paper towel.

Aseptic practice

Asepsis is the state of being free from disease-causing contaminants (such as bacteria, viruses, fungi and parasites). When performing an invasive procedure it is essential to promote or induce asepsis to prevent contamination of a person, object or area by microorganisms and thereby avoid infection.

Personal protective equipment

PPE provides a barrier between the microbial source and the operator or patient. PPE includes gloves, plastic aprons, gowns, protective eyewear, masks and adequate footwear and should be worn when splashing or spillage from any source is likely.

Determine the requirement for PPE before performing a procedure.

As well as other standard precautions, PPE reduces the potential for microbial transmission, but does not negate the need for safe work practices or handwashing.

- Gloves are worn whenever contact with blood, body fluid, mucous membranes, broken skin or contaminated equipment is anticipated. Choose the type of gloves most appropriate to the task. Avoid latex gloves if the patient or operator is allergic.
  - General-purpose utility gloves are used for manual decontamination and cleaning of spills, used instruments and equipment.
  - Sterile gloves are used when performing invasive procedures on normally clean areas of the body or into sterile body cavities.
  - Non-sterile examination gloves are used for all other patient contact.
- Gowns and aprons are worn to protect clothing and skin from contamination with blood and body fluids, and in the care of patients infected or colonised with epidemiologically important microorganisms such as MRSA or VRE.
- Protective eyewear includes goggles, glasses and face shields with visors. They are worn during procedures likely to be associated with splashing, spraying or splattering of blood or body fluids.
- Masks protect the mucous membranes of the mouth and nose from blood or body-fluid splashes. Special high-filtration masks are required when nursing or examining patients known or suspected to be infected with pathogens spread by the airborne route (e.g. TB).

Disposal of infectious material

Determine what is 'dirty', what is 'clean' and what is 'sterile', and know what these terms actually mean. Keep these environments separate and immediately remedy any contamination:

- Contaminated skin surfaces or mucous membranes should be washed immediately. If heavy contamination occurs, showering

and change of clothes are recommended. In all instances, wash hands as soon as gloves are removed.
- Any body fluid spillage must be cleaned up immediately with a disposable towel, which is then placed in a designated contaminated waste bin. The floor should be washed with soap and water.
- Put soiled linen in a clear or blue plastic bag before placing in a laundry bag.

Additional precautions

Special precautions are required in certain situations, *in addition* to standard precautions. These are based on the risk of disease transmission and are situation-specific. They mainly relate to:
- Patients colonised with epidemiologically important microorganisms
- Patients colonised with highly transmissible pathogens that can cause infection by potential:
  - Airborne transmission (e.g. TB, measles)
  - Droplet transmission (e.g. pertussis, influenza, rubella, mumps)
  - Contact transmission (e.g. MRSA)
- Immunocompromised patients
- Patients with large areas of infected skin or large, open, purulent wounds.

Additional special precautions include (but are not limited to):
- Handwashing with antiseptic cleansers
- Isolating the patient in a normal single room
- Using suitable easily visible signs warning other patients and staff of the potential infection risk
- Cohorting patients infected with the same microorganism (e.g. respiratory syncytial virus)
- Treating the patient in a purpose-designed isolation room, ideally with negative-pressure ventilatory capability
- Standard use of gowns, gloves, masks, protective eyewear and impervious dressings for all contact
- Double-sterilising all equipment used.

SECTION E – Practical procedures

49

Venepuncture

You are responsible for checking that the correct patient is being bled, that all the specimens for laboratory analysis are correctly labelled and signed as per hospital policy and that enough blood is drawn on the first attempt.

Indication

- Draw blood for laboratory analysis.

Contraindications and cautions

- Never draw blood from the AV fistula arm of a patient on renal dialysis.
- Never place a tourniquet on the arm of a patient with lymphoedema.
- Do not draw blood from an arm with a distally sited IV drip with running line.
- Avoid skin sites that are infected, or bruised from multiple previous venepuncture attempts.
- Ask your senior to perform, if you are unable to find any suitable vein even by palpation, if you fail once on a 'difficult' patient, or after two attempts on an 'easy' patient.

Equipment

- Non-sterile gloves
- Tourniquet
- Alcohol swabs × 2
- Syringe: 10 mL or 20 mL
- Needles: 18G or 20G or evacuated-tube aspiration system, such as Vacutainer®, with 20G butterfly needle and paper tape
- Blood tubes: select the correct blood tubes prior to performing the procedure and have them within reach, particularly when using the Vacutainer® system
- Sharps container
- Absorbent pad or 'bluey'
- Sticking plaster

Procedural technique

- Explain the procedure to the patient, who is reclining on a bed or seated in a comfortable chair, but *never* standing up.
- Ask the patient which is the preferred arm. An alert, conscious patient will usually inform you of the best arm to use, generally the non-dominant one.
- Enquire about any fistulae or lymphoedema, and look for evidence of a running IV line and avoid these (see *Contraindications and cautions*).
- Apply the tourniquet 10–15 cm above the proposed venepuncture site. Check distal pulses are still palpable as this ensures the highest venous pressure.
- Put on non-sterile gloves and palpate the antecubital fossa (or sometimes forearm or hand) for a suitable vein.
- Prepare the area with an alcohol swab and attach the needle to the syringe.
- Hold the skin taut to anchor the vein and gently, but firmly, advance the needle, bevel up, at 15–30 degrees to the horizontal, directly over and in line with the vein.
  - You will see a small flashback within the proximal portion of the needle when successful if using a needle and syringe. Hold the syringe and needle steady in the vein and slowly draw back the syringe and collect the blood. Do not aspirate too vigorously as this may collapse the vein and stop blood flow.
  - When using the Vacutainer® system, push the first tube onto the multi-sample needle. Allow the tube to fill fully and then remove the tube by pulling gently. Additional tubes may be filled by repeating this procedure.
- Undo the tourniquet, withdraw the needle and apply firm pressure with a dry cotton-wool ball or gauze swab to the site.
- Dispose of any used sharps immediately in the sharps container.
- Gently transfer the blood from the syringe into an uncapped blood tube and then replace the cap. Never inject into a blood tube held in the hand (high risk of needlestick injury). Be careful not to cause haemolysis of the blood by overly vigorous injection.
- Invert all blood tubes several times following collection, regardless of the method, to ensure blood is thoroughly mixed and does not clot.
- Ensure there is no further bleeding from the site and that the patient remains comfortable and is not feeling faint.

Complications

- Needlestick injury or blood splash to a mucous membrane.
  - Most likely when evacuated tubes or blood tubes are held in the hand and directly injected with blood. *Never* do this.

SECTION E – Practical procedures

- Promptly wash away the blood or body fluid and encourage bleeding. Use soap, except for the eyes and mouth, and rinse well with water.
- Report the incident to your supervisor as soon as possible.
- Haemolysis producing unreliable automated laboratory results.
  - Can be caused by incorrect venepuncture technique such as pulling the tourniquet too tight or leaving it on for too long, using needles that are too small (>20G), insufficient amount of blood, incorrect filling of the blood collection tubes or too vigorous shaking of the tubes.

Handy hints

- Check that you are taking blood at the required time, as some tests are time-specific (e.g. serum digoxin level, which is assessed 6 hours after a digoxin dose, or a fasting blood for a lipid profile).
- Try hanging the patient's arm over the edge of the bed and gently tap the antecubital fossa, forearm and back of the hand veins if you can not easily find a vein. Inflate the cuff to just above DBP, and/or apply a warmed pack to the patient's arm, to enhance venous filling.
- Ultrasound is useful for finding a vein and guiding venepuncture or cannulation in patients with difficult venous access.
- Do not use excessive suction to extract blood, as this may cause haemolysis and makes the vein collapse and stops the blood flow. Using a small 2 or 5 mL syringe to withdraw blood allows better control of evacuation pressure and is less likely to collapse veins than the 10 or 20 mL size. This is especially important in children, or venesection from a small vein.
- Never, ever recap a needle.
- Always invert filled blood tubes gently, especially those containing anticoagulant.
- Never underfill anticoagulant tubes (citrate/blue top).
- Never overfill heparinised tubes (green top), as this will cause the sample to clot.
- Remember to double-check that all samples have been labelled and that the correct patient's details, the date and time are entered prior to sending samples to the laboratory.

50

Blood cultures

Blood culture is not a routine procedure and is not performed just because a patient has a fever (see *Indication*).

Best results are obtained when blood is withdrawn and inoculated carefully, following the procedure outlined below, and *two* sets of cultures are taken on *every* occasion, from two different venepuncture sites.

Indications

- Blood cultures are requested for patients with fever, rigors and/or other features of systemic infection, such as raised or very low white cell count or suspected severe sepsis or septic shock.
- Where possible, they should be collected at, or shortly after, a temperature 'spike' and prior to starting antibiotic treatment.

Contraindications and cautions

- Never choose the AV fistula arm of a patient on renal dialysis.
- Never place a tourniquet on the arm of a patient with lymphoedema.
- Do not draw blood from an arm with a distally sited IV drip with running line.

Equipment

- Non-sterile gloves
- Tourniquet
- Alcohol swabs × 8
- Syringes: 10 mL × 4
- Butterfly × 2, or alternative IV cannulae × 2
- Needles: 18G × 4
- Correct blood culture bottles × 2 sets (one anaerobic and one aerobic per set)
- Sharps container
- Absorbent pad or 'bluey'
- Sticking plasters

Procedural technique

- Identify the patient and explain the procedure.
- Prepare and position the patient for venepuncture, either in a comfortable chair or reclining on a bed.
- An alert, conscious patient will usually inform you of the best arm to use.
- Wash your hands and put on non-sterile gloves.
- Remove the plastic shield from the top of each blood culture bottle without touching the rubber septum.
- Wipe the top of each bottle with an alcohol swab or 1% chlorhexidine with 75% ethanol swab and allow to dry.
- Select an appropriate vein and apply the tourniquet 10–15 cm proximal to the chosen site. Palpate the vein and identify its position carefully. Prepare the skin surface with an alcohol-based swab, moving from the centre outwards.
  - Repeat the process with a second alcohol swab or 1% chlorhexidine with 75% ethanol swab and allow to air dry for at least 1 minute.
- Without retouching the vein, cannulate and use the 10 mL syringes to withdraw blood samples, using one syringe for each bottle, or preferably use a Vacutainer® system with closed leash transfer attachment.
- Undo the tourniquet, withdraw the needle and apply firm pressure with a dry swab to the venepuncture site.
- Insert the needle into the sterile septum of the blood culture bottle and inject a minimum of 5 mL of blood. Start with the anaerobic bottle if using a syringe, to avoid any air entering from the top (last part) of the syringe. Withdraw the needle and repeat for the aerobic culture bottle.
  - When using a Vacutainer® system, or a butterfly, fill the aerobic bottle first, as there will be air in the leash tubing, before filling the anaerobic bottle second.
- Dispose of all used sharps immediately in the sharps container.
- Label blood culture bottles with the patient's name, ward, date, time *and* site of venepuncture.
- Repeat the whole procedure on the other arm, or at a different skin site, as two paired sets of cultures are required at a time to most reliably differentiate a skin contaminant (present in one set of blood cultures only) from a pathogen (present in both sets of blood cultures), particularly for suspected infective endocarditis or indwelling line sepsis.

Handy hints

- Do not touch or palpate the vein after swabbing, unless there is difficult venous access, in which case adopt full aseptic technique with sterile gloves and field.

- It is *not* necessary to replace the needle after withdrawing blood and prior to inserting it in the culture bottles. This increases the risk of needlestick injury and contamination.

- Avoid placing a label over the barcode of the blood culture bottles.

- Inoculate blood culture bottles first if part of a series of blood tests, to avoid a low rate of genuine positive results and a high false-positive rate due to skin contaminants.

- Avoid inoculating blood culture bottles with 20 mL syringes. They are more likely to contaminate the cultures and are prone to overfilling if allowed to discharge passively.

- Neutropenic haematology and oncology patients often have CVL-associated bacteraemia. If trained, collect one blood culture set via the CVL and one from a peripheral vein to distinguish line-associated infection from other sources of systemic infection.

- Suspected infective endocarditis—carefully collect three sets of blood cultures from perpheral veins at regularly spaced intervals. Remember to accurately document the time of venesection on the blood culture bottles, request and continuation notes.

- If there is a very small quantity available (e.g. 5 mL total), inoculate all into one aerobic bottle and note 'difficult venesection' on the lab request.

- If less than 3 mL (shocked patient, paediatric patient), inoculate all into a paediatric blood culture bottle.

SECTION E – Practical procedures

51

Peripheral venous cannulation

Indications

- Administration of maintenance or replacement IV fluids, including blood.
- Administration of IV medication.

Contraindications and cautions

- Never draw blood from the AV fistula in a patient on renal dialysis.
- Avoid using an arm with lymphoedema secondary to axillary node clearance.
- Avoid skin sites that are infected, or bruised from multiple previous venepuncture or cannulation attempts.
- Ask your senior to perform, if you are unable to find any suitable vein even by palpation, if you fail once on a 'difficult' patient, or after two attempts on an 'easy' patient.

Equipment

- Non-sterile gloves
- Tourniquet
- Alcohol swab
- Absorbent pad or 'bluey'
- Cannulae × 2 and with choice of sizes
- Sterile gauze swabs
- Sharps container
- 3 mL syringe
- Local anaesthetic agent (1% lignocaine)
- Needle: 25G
- 10 mL syringe
- 10 mL normal saline (flush)
- IV bung, or primed three-way tap with extension tubing (according to local practice)

- Non-allergenic tape
- Transparent semi-permeable, adhesive dressing or suitable tape

Procedural technique

- Explain the procedure to the patient.
- **Choose the best vein.**
  - **Site:** ask the patient which is the preferred arm (usually the non-dominant arm) and carefully examine both arms for the most appropriate vessels.
  - When a high flow rate is required or an irritant drug is to be administered, look for a large proximal vein with good blood flow.
    - Review the metacarpal, cephalic and basillic veins.
    - The antecubital fossa usually has the largest palpable vein and is the preferred site in an emergency. Otherwise *avoid*, as this site is uncomfortable and awkward when an extended elbow is essential to maintain fluid flow.
    - Use foot veins only as a last resort, as they thrombose more readily and are prone to infection.
  - **Character of vein:** Look for veins that are large, straight, visibly or palpably prominent (rather than just 'look blue'), bouncy and refill when depressed.
    - Avoid veins that are small, tortuous, cord-like or hard, with poor refill and a lack of resilience (as may be thrombosed, sclerosed, inflamed or in spasm).
    - Avoid using veins in areas with broken skin, infection, inflammation or oedema.
- **Choose the correct gauge of cannula (see Table 51.1).**
  - Determine the type of fluid therapy to be infused (e.g. blood or blood products, or an irritant solution such as sodium bicarbonate or calcium chloride), the rate of infusion flow required, the duration of time the cannula will remain in place and the patient's activity level and age.
  - Choose the shortest length and largest diameter for the task required, carefully differentiating maintenance or slow fluid use (smaller cannula) from resuscitation or rapid fluid use (larger cannula).
  - Large cannulae are associated with insertion trauma to the vein, insertion-site pain and mechanical phlebitis secondary to friction exerted by the cannula on the intima of the vein.
  - Smaller cannulae allow better flow of blood around the cannula, allowing haemodilution of solutions, and minimise insertion trauma but they restrict overall flow rate.

SECTION E – Practical procedures

SECTION E – Practical procedures

Table 51.1		Peripheral cannula gauge selection		
Colour	**Gauge**	**Flow rate (mL/min)**	**Application**	**Considerations**
Brown Grey	14G 16G	300–330 200–220	Urgent fluid resuscitation including blood or rapid crystalloid infusion in haemorrhagic shock, volume depletion, trauma, high-risk surgical procedure (such as prior to AAA or ectopic repair)	Increased pain on insertion (consider administering local anaesthetic) Requires a larger vein to accommodate the cannula May create increased mechanical irritation to vein wall, depending on location
Green	18G	90–105	Major surgery, fluid replacement, most emergency situations *excluding* those above Minimum gauge for viscous solutions and whole blood/ RBC transfusion	Requires a vein large enough to accommodate the cannula Commonly selected gauge size

Table 51.1 Peripheral cannula gauge selection—*Continued*

Colour	Gauge	Flow rate (mL/min)	Application	Considerations
Pink	20G	55–60	Suitable for maintenance infusions only Minor surgical procedures, routine outpatient or radiological procedures requiring IV access. IV medication	Versatile Commonly selected gauge size Red cell components (blood) will *not* flow freely, so avoid when blood is needed
Blue	22G	33–35	Suitable for most infusions in children Routine administration of antibiotics and hydration therapies at slow flow rates Recommended for small and/ or fragile veins, and general use in children	Easier to insert into small, thin, fragile veins Red cell components (blood) will *not* flow freely, so avoid when blood is needed May be difficult to insert through tough skin Easy to kink or pull out
Yellow	24G	20	Suitable only for infusions or IV drugs in children at slowest flow rates	Neonatal, paediatric and elderly patients Extremely small veins when larger veins are not accessible Difficult to insert through tough skin Easy to kink or pull out

SECTION E – Practical procedures

- Use standard infection control procedures such as ANTT. Prepare equipment, select cannulae and apply a tourniquet to the preferred arm, above the elbow.
- Having identified a suitable vein, wipe the selected site thoroughly with an alcohol swab, or 1% chlorhexidine with alcohol swab, and allow site to dry for 1 minute.
- Anchor the vein and hold the skin taut with the non-dominant hand, without touching swabbed area again.
- Warn patient of a sharp, stinging sensation as the needle is inserted.
- Insert the needle firmly through the skin directly over the vein, bevel up, at a flat angle of approach of no more than 15–30 degrees to the horizontal.
  - *Note:* most 'misses' are caused by entering the skin too steeply (vertically) and going straight through the back of the vein, which then 'blows' or 'tissues' and is unusable.
- As the needle enters the vein you will feel a 'give' or 'pop' sensation and see 'flashback' of blood up the cannula.
- Reduce the angle of the cannula until it is almost parallel to the skin and advance the tip a further 3–5 mm up the vein.
  - *Note:* the larger the cannula, the further it must be advanced, to avoid it remaining outside the vein lumen.
- Withdraw the needle slowly 1–2 mm without moving the cannula and confirm that the blood flows up the cannula tubing.
- Slide the cannula smoothly down off the needle into the vein as far as its hub and withdraw the needle from the cannula.
- Occlude the vein proximally at the end of the cannula tip with external pressure by your non-dominant hand.
- Dispose of any sharps immediately in a sharps bin and cap the cannula hub with the IV bung with a Luer connection, or three-way tap and extension tubing.
- Secure the cannula in place with a suitable transparent dressing and tape.
- Flush with 5 mL normal saline to confirm patency and fluid flow.
- Record and date the time of cannula insertion in an obvious location near the insertion site.

Complications

- **Local**
  - Local tissue sequestration ('tissuing') following through-and-through vein perforation or cannula dislodgement

- Haematoma, usually from vein perforation
- Line occlusion secondary to kinking of tubing or backflow of blood
- Vein irritation and chemical thrombophlebitis
- Local infection with bacterial thrombophlebitis
  - IV cannulae should ideally be replaced every 48–72 hours to minimise the risk of infection
- Nerve, tendon or ligament damage, particularly when inserting into the antecubital fossa
- **Systemic**
  - Vasovagal reaction on insertion—always have patient reclining comfortably
  - Systemic infection
  - Air embolism, usually with a large-bore cannula sited in a central vein

---

Handy hints

- Venous distension may be enhanced by using a BP cuff as a tourniquet, applying a heat pack, lowering the arm below the level of the heart, opening and closing the fist, and light tapping over the vein.
- If you cannot feel a vein in the first site, stop and review the other sites.
- Ultrasound is helpful for finding a vein and guiding venepuncture or cannulation in a patient with difficult venous access.
- Subcutaneous infiltration with local anaesthetic (0.3 mL 1% lignocaine) significantly reduces the pain of cannulation and reduces persistent discomfort at the site of cannulation (see Chapter 54). Use for large cannulae such as 16G or 14G.

SECTION E – Practical procedures

52

Arterial puncture

Indications

- Evaluate the adequacy of oxygenation, ventilation and acid–base status (diagnostic evaluation).
- Evaluate the patient's initial response to therapy (therapeutic evaluation).
- Monitor ongoing progression and severity of a known disease process (prognostic evaluation).
- Remember a VBG (with pulse oximetry) is usually sufficient in most clinical situations, and is much simpler and safer.

Contraindications and cautions

- Modified Allen test gives a negative result—that is, it indicates an inadequate collateral circulation to the hand when radial artery is occluded (see below).
- Local cellulitis or infection.
- Uncontrolled bleeding diathesis.
- Peripheral vascular disease involving the selected limb.
- Do not perform distal to a surgical shunt (e.g. AV fistula).

Equipment

- Non-surgical gloves
- Arterial blood gas (ABG) syringe (pre-heparinised)
- Alcohol swab
- Gauze, cotton wool or plaster
- Adhesive tape
- Needles: 25G orange × 2 or 23G blue (radial artery); 21G green (femoral artery)
- 3 mL syringe
- Local anaesthetic agent (1% lignocaine)
- Towel
- Sharps container

Procedural technique

- Identify the patient and carefully explain the procedure.
- **Choose the appropriate artery.**
  - **Radial artery:** readily accessible, easy to palpate, less commonly associated with venous sample or nerve damage (than femoral or brachial), and easy to control haemorrhage.
    - First check the ulnar artery collateral circulation using the modified Allen test. Ask the patient to make a tight fist, then occlude the radial artery manually at the wrist with direct pressure. Still maintaining pressure over the radial artery, ask the patient to next relax the fist. If the hand remains white after 10–15 seconds, do *not* use the radial site for arterial puncture. The ulnar collateral circulation is inadequate and an alternative site to the radial artery should be sought, as inadvertent radial artery damage can lead to hand ischaemia.
  - **Femoral artery:** large artery with good anatomical landmarks. However, direct pressure must be applied for at least 3–5 minutes following the procedure, and the artery lies in close proximity to the femoral vein, which may be punctured instead.
  - **Brachial artery:** 'last resort' as it is technically more difficult and associated with significant risk of local injury (e.g. median nerve).
- Arterial puncture is considerably more painful than venepuncture and the unprepared patient may move abruptly on needle insertion. Therefore, always administer local anaesthetic first, particularly if the patient requests it. This does not increase the likelihood of failure.
- Make sure the patient is in a comfortable position, preferably lying on a bed.
- Use bedside ultrasound guidance to locate the artery if hard to find.
- Put on non-sterile gloves and prepare the ABG syringe. Have a gauze swab or a cotton-wool ball and tape ready for pressure over the site after completion.
- Cleanse the skin with an alcohol swab and allow to dry.

Radial artery

- Position the patient's limb in a supinated position, ideally with the dorsal aspect of the wrist resting comfortably on a bag of saline or a rolled-up towel.
- Palpate the artery with the index and middle fingers of your non-dominant hand to identify the course of the artery.
- Administer local anaesthetic.
- Attach a 25G needle to the ABG syringe. Hold the syringe with a pencil grip and, keeping the skin taut, insert the needle through

the skin, bevel up, at an angle of approximately 30–45 degrees to the skin, directly over the pulse.

- *Note:* some operators prefer a 23G needle as the success rate may be better, especially in arteriosclerotic or low-flow situations.
- Advance slowly over the line of the artery until a flashback of bright-red arterial blood is observed. Hold the needle steady and allow the syringe to fill. A minimum of 0.5 mL is required.
- Withdraw the needle and apply firm pressure to the puncture site with a gauze swab or cotton wool for 2–3 minutes (or at least 5 minutes if the patient is on warfarin or a NOAC, or has a bleeding tendency).
- Dispose of the needle immediately in the sharps bin.
- Hold the syringe upright and expel any excess air by tapping the syringe gently.
- Cap the syringe and invert 3–4 times to ensure adequate mixing of anticoagulant.

Femoral artery

- Lay the patient supine with the hip in extension and external rotation. Locate the femoral pulse at the mid-inguinal point, halfway between the anterior superior iliac spine and the pubic tubercle (see Figure 52.1). Or use bedside ultrasound guidance.
- Cleanse the groin with an alcohol swab. Attach a 21G needle to the ABG syringe and insert perpendicular to the skin directly over the artery.
- Advance until there is a flashback and allow the syringe to fill. Withdraw the needle slowly and apply firm pressure to the puncture site with a gauze swab or cotton wool for at least 3–5 minutes.
- Dispose of the needle immediately in the sharps bin.
- Hold the syringe upright and expel any excess air by tapping the syringe gently.
- Cap the syringe and invert 3–4 times to ensure adequate mixing of anticoagulant.

Complications

- Pain over puncture site (use local anaesthetic)
- Vasovagal response
- Failure (arteriospasm or simple miss)
- Haematoma or overt haemorrhage from trauma to the vessel
- Arterial occlusion
- Air or distal clotted-blood emboli
- Pseudoaneurysm (late complication)

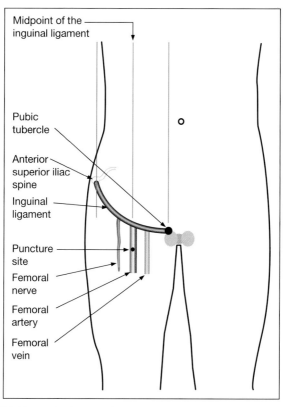

Midpoint of the inguinal ligament

Pubic tubercle

Anterior superior iliac spine

Inguinal ligament

Puncture site

Femoral nerve

Femoral artery

Femoral vein

Figure 52.1 Femoral artery: anatomy.

Handy hints

- If you fail to enter the artery on the first pass, withdraw the needle slightly (without removing from the skin), re-palpate the artery and advance the needle slowly once more, this time at a shallower angle.
- Transport the sample to the ABG machine or laboratory on ice if there will be a delay to specimen testing. This curtails the ongoing cellular use of oxygen for up to 1 hour.

SECTION E – Practical procedures

53

Administering an injection

Equipment

- Non-sterile gloves
- 25G (orange) needle (SC) *or* 21 (blue)–23G (green) needle (IM)
- Vial or ampoule of medication
- Syringe—1 mL or 5 mL
- Alcohol swabs
- Sticking plaster
- Cotton swab
- Sharps container

Subcutaneous (SC) injection

Route of administration for small volumes (0.5–1.0 mL) of water-soluble medication into the loose connective tissue underneath the dermis. Absorption is slow, but usually complete in patients without circulatory compromise, although the onset of action can be delayed (up to 30–45 minutes).

Contraindications

- Known allergy
- Circulatory shock
- Reduced local tissue perfusion
- Thin or emaciated patients (may have inadequate adipose tissue for SC injection)

Anatomical sites

- Central abdomen, below costal margins
- Posterolateral aspect of upper arms
- Anterior thigh
- Scapular region of back

Procedural technique

- Identify the correct patient.
- Confirm medication and dose, and that it has been checked by someone else.

- Review contraindications, including known allergies.
- Gain verbal consent from the patient and explain the procedure.
- Warn the patient that the injection may cause a slight burning or stinging sensation.
- **Select a suitable site.**
  - Choose a site with high adipose content (see Figure 53.1).
  - Avoid areas with broken skin, bruising, infection, inflammation or oedema, and areas in proximity to bony prominences.
  - Palpate the site to ensure no tenderness or masses.
  - Rotate the site for injection regularly if injections are given frequently, such as insulin.
- **Check the correct needle size and angle of insertion.**
  - The depth of the SC layer is determined by body weight.
  - Needle length should be half the height of a skinfold grasped between the forefinger and thumb (see Figure 53.2).

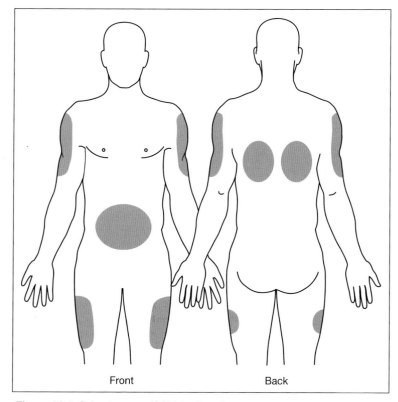

Front   Back

Figure 53.1 Subcutaneous (SC) injection sites.

SECTION E – Practical procedures

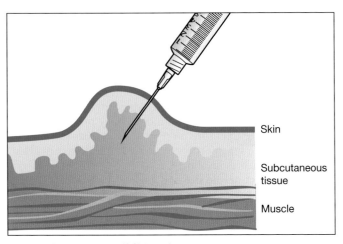

Skin

Subcutaneous tissue

Muscle

Figure 53.2 Subcutaneous (SC) injection.

- Ensure that the patient is in a comfortable position, either reclining on a bed or seated on a comfortable chair. Do not administer to a patient who is standing up, as there is a risk of fainting.
- Put on gloves, cleanse the site with an alcohol swab and allow to dry.
- Pinch up the skin at the site between the thumb and forefinger of your non-dominant hand.
- Insert the needle with your dominant hand quickly at 45–60-degree angle, or vertically at a right angle if using a short needle such as on an insulin syringe or heparin syringe, and release the skin.
- Grasp the lower end of the syringe barrel with your non-dominant hand and move your dominant hand to the end of the plunger, being careful not to dislodge the needle in the skin.
- Draw back on the plunger to ensure not injecting directly into a blood vessel (blood is aspirated). This is not indicated in heparin administration as it increases local haematoma risk.
- Slowly depress the plunger to administer medication (too rapid injection will increase pain).
- Withdraw the needle and apply alcohol swab or cotton swab gently over site. Stabilising the tissue around the injection site minimises discomfort during needle withdrawal.
- Dispose of any sharps immediately in the sharps bin, including needle and glass ampoule plus top.

Complications

- Local tissue pain or irritation, haematoma (particularly with heparin), erythema or inflammation
- Sterile abscess (collection of medication within the skin that appears as a hard, painful lump)
- Lipodystrophy (delayed, possibly immunological complication) following insulin injection

Intramuscular (IM) injection

The IM route has certain advantages compared with SC administration, which include:
- Faster rate of absorption (from 5 to 15 minutes) related to the greater vascularity of muscle
- Viscous solutions and substances irritant to subcutaneous tissues may be administered safely
- Larger volumes up to 3–5 mL can be given.

Contraindications

- Known allergy
- Circulatory shock
- Reduced local tissue perfusion due to peripheral vascular disease
- Bleeding disorder
- Muscle atrophy

Anatomical sites

- **Upper outer buttock (ventrogluteal)**
  - This is a safe site for all patients and is the preferred site for adults and children over 7 months of age (see Figure 53.3).
  - Locate the injection site by placing the heel of your hand over the greater trochanter of the hip, with the thumb directed towards the patient's groin and fingers towards the patient's head.
  - Place your index finger over the anterior superior iliac spine and extend the middle finger back over the iliac crest towards the buttock. This delineates a triangular area, the centre of which is the injection site.
  - Slight flexion of the hips and knee in the recumbent patient will relax the muscles.
- **Upper outer thigh (vastus lateralis)**
  - Commonly used for IM injections in adults as it is thick, usually well-developed and easily accessible, even through clothing in an emergency such as for adrenaline in anaphylaxis.

SECTION E – Practical procedures

- Middle third of the muscle is the best site for administration and is located over the anterolateral aspect of the mid thigh.
- Injections are best administered with the patient lying flat with the knee slightly flexed to relax the muscle.
- **Upper outer arm (deltoid)**
  - Deltoid muscle is easily accessible, but may not be well developed and should only be used for small volumes of medication.
  - Fully expose the patient's upper arm (do not roll up a tight-fitting sleeve). Relax the patient's arm by flexing at the elbow and palpate the acromion process.
  - Inject 3–5 cm below the acromion process, in the midline of the lateral aspect of the upper arm.

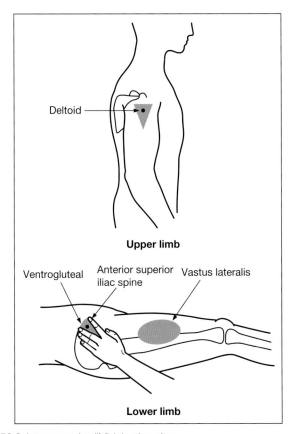

Figure 53.3 Intramuscular (IM) injection sites.

Procedural technique

- Identify the correct patient.
- Confirm medication and dose, and that it has been checked.
- Review contraindications and known allergies.
- Gain verbal consent from the patient and explain the procedure.
- Warn the patient that the injection can be painful and may cause a slight burning or stinging sensation.
- **Choose the correct site.**
  - Choose a site with adequate muscle bulk (see Figure 53.3).
  - Avoid areas with broken skin, bruising, infection, inflammation or oedema.
  - Palpate the site to ensure no tenderness or masses.
  - Rotate the site for injection regularly if injections are given frequently.
- **Choose the correct needle size and angle of insertion.**
  - A longer, heavier needle is used compared with SC injections (at least a 21–23G needle, not 25G).
- Ensure that the patient is in a comfortable position, either reclining on a bed or seated on a comfortable chair.
- Put on gloves, clean the site with an alcohol swab and allow to dry.
- Position your non-dominant hand at the injection site and hold the skin taut (to prevent leakage of the injected medication on needle withdrawal).
- Insert the needle quickly and firmly with your dominant hand while retaining tension on the skin at 90 degrees to the surface of the skin (see Figure 53.4).
- Draw back on the plunger to ensure not injecting directly into a blood vessel (blood is aspirated).

SECTION E – Practical procedures

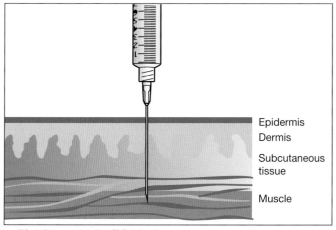

Figure 53.4 Intramuscular (IM) injection.

Epidermis
Dermis
Subcutaneous tissue
Muscle

- Inject medication slowly. Withdraw the needle steadily and release the skin.
- Dispose of sharps immediately in the sharps bin, including any glass ampoules, and apply a sticking plaster.
- Do *not* massage the injection site.

Complications

- Direct injection into blood vessel (always pull back on the plunger to reduce this risk)
- Sciatic nerve injury with incorrect approach (*note:* dorsogluteal approach is no longer used)
- Brachial artery or radial nerve injury with deltoid injection

Handy hints

- Do not give adrenaline SC in anaphylaxis, but IM into the upper outer thigh for optimal absorption.
- Be particularly careful when disposing of sharps to avoid inadvertent needlestick injury to self or others.

54

Local anaesthetic infiltration

Indication

- Local anaesthesia for painful procedure such as suturing, wound debridement, foreign body retrieval, reduction of a dislocated small joint such as in a finger or toe, and arterial puncture.

Contraindications and cautions

- Local anaesthetic allergy (true allergy is rare and usually associated with the esters such as benzocaine, amethocaine/tetracaine or procaine).
- Avoid using lignocaine with adrenaline to infiltrate areas with an end-arterial supply such as fingers, toes, penis, the pinna or nose (even though there is little evidence for ischaemic complications following lignocaine with adrenaline use in digital blocks of the finger or toe).
- Make sure to test sensory function before injecting any local anaesthetic, especially with a digital injury.

Equipment

- Alcohol swab
- Skin cleansing solution (e.g. 1% chlorhexidine)
- Local anaesthetic agent (e.g. lignocaine)
- Syringe: 5 mL or 10 mL
- Needle: 25G and 21G

Choose the local anaesthetic agent

- Lignocaine is a short-acting, amide-type local anaesthetic agent. It is supplied in 0.5%, 1% and 2% concentrations without (plain) or with adrenaline. Onset of action is within 1–2 minutes and duration is 0.5–1 hours (plain) or 2–5 hours (with adrenaline) (see Table 54.1).

Table 54.1   Maximum recommended safe dose and duration of action of common local anaesthetics

Medication	Dose (mg/kg)*	Duration (h)
Lignocaine	3	0.5–1
Lignocaine with adrenaline	7	2–5
Prilocaine	6	0.5–1.5
Bupivacaine	2	2–4
Ropivacaine	1–3[+]	2–8[+]

*A 1% solution contains 10 mg/mL.
[+]Depending on site.

- Small volumes of a more concentrated solution (i.e. 2%) are used for anatomically restricted areas of infiltration, such as a ring block for interphalangeal joint relocation.
- Use a larger volume of a less concentrated solution (e.g. 1%) around larger joints, such as for knee joint aspiration.
- Select lignocaine with adrenaline for vascular sites or for sites where the skin is incised, as adrenaline causes vasoconstriction and so will reduce systemic absorption, maintain a higher anaesthetic concentration near nerve fibres and prolong local anaesthetic conduction blockade. Avoid its use around end arteries in the nose, the pinna of the ear or the penis, and in digital nerve blocks (but see note under *Contraindications and cautions*).
- Bupivacaine and ropivacaine are longer-acting, amide-type local anaesthetic agents. Onset of action is slightly slower than lignocaine, but the duration of action is much longer (see Table 54.1). These agents are typically used for nerve blocks (e.g. femoral nerve block) or epidural anaesthesia, and may also be used instead of lignocaine to provide a longer anaesthetic effect (but *never* use bupivacaine for a Bier block, only ever lignocaine or prilocaine).

Calculate the maximum safe dose of a local anaesthetic agent

Local anaesthetics are toxic if absorbed systemically, with adverse effects ranging from perioral tingling at a low plasma toxic level, to convulsions, apnoea and cardiovascular collapse at the highest plasma toxic levels (see Box 54.1). Thus, it is essential to know their maximum safe doses per kg:

- Maximum safe dose of lignocaine **without** adrenaline is 3 mg/kg.
- Maximum safe dose of lignocaine **with** adrenaline is 7 mg/kg.

BOX 54.1 Features of systemic local anaesthetic toxicity (in order of increasing plasma level)

- Circumoral tingling
- Dizziness
- Tinnitus
- Visual disturbance
- Muscular twitching
- Confusion
- Convulsions
- Coma
- Apnoea
- Cardiovascular collapse (highest plasma levels)

- Local anaesthetic concentration in various solutions:
  - 0.5% = 0.5 g/100 mL or 5 mg/mL
  - 1% = 1 g/100 mL or 10 mg/mL
  - 2% = 2 g/100 mL or 20 mg/mL.
- Thus, in a 70 kg patient do *not* use more than:
  - 20 mL 1% plain lignocaine
  - 10 mL 2% plain lignocaine
  - 48 mL 1% lignocaine with adrenaline
  - 24 mL 2% lignocaine with adrenaline.

Procedural technique

- Attach a 25G needle to a syringe filled with local anaesthetic, after re-checking the dilution, dose and safety related to body weight.
- Enter the dermis of the skin at 45 degrees and aspirate to ensure that the needle is not in a blood vessel. Infiltrate 1–2 mL local anaesthetic to raise a subdermal 'bleb' on the skin.
- Exchange the 25G needle for a 21G needle and enter the skin through the previously anaesthetised skin site.
- Advance the needle into the deeper tissues. Again, aspirate for blood before injecting any tissue. If you draw blood, withdraw a little and try again.
- Infiltrate the area to be anaesthetised and remove the needle.
- When an incision is to be made in the skin, direct the 25G needle along the line of the incision at the level of the dermis, to extend the area of superficial anaesthesia.
- Wait at least 2 minutes for the local anaesthetic to take effect, and longer for a ring block or femoral nerve block.

SECTION E – Practical procedures

55

Nasogastric tube insertion

Nasogastric tube (NGT) insertion is one of the more uncomfortable procedures in medicine. Nurses are highly experienced in placing NGTs, so if you are called to place one it is usually because they have failed, and/or the patient is uncooperative with the procedure.

Indications

- Aspiration of stomach contents to decompress the stomach of fluid or air.
- Reducing the risk of vomiting or aspiration, such as in bowel obstruction.
- Introducing liquids to the stomach such as charcoal, enteral feeds or oral contrast media.

Contraindications

- Base of skull fracture or severe mid-face trauma (risk of cribriform plate disruption, with the NGT inadvertently entering the brain)
- Caustic ingestion or known oesophageal stricture (risk of perforation)

Equipment

- Gloves (non-sterile)
- Apron
- NG tube (size 12–16F)
- Kidney dish
- Lubricating jelly
- Litmus paper
- 50 mL syringe (catheter tip)
- Catheter drainage bag
- Glass of water
- Non-allergenic tape
- Stethoscope

Procedural technique

- Explain to the patient exactly what you are about to do and why.
- Assess the patient's ability to swallow and the patency of either nostril.
- Prepare a trolley with all the equipment.
- Sit the patient upright with the neck slightly flexed.
- Measure the required length of tube (from nose to earlobe, then earlobe to xiphoid process and add 15 cm).
- Cover the tip of the NGT with lubricating jelly and insert into the largest patent nostril horizontally and backwards, at a right angle to the face (under the inferior turbinate) and not upwards toward the nasal bridge.
- Gently advance the tube into the pharynx. Ask the patient to swallow when the tube is felt at the back of the mouth and, as the patient swallows, carefully push the tube down further. A sip of water may help the patient to swallow.
- Insert the tube down to the pre-selected distance.
- Assess that it is positioned correctly:
  - Aspirate slowly on the tube using the 50 mL syringe. Check syringe contents with blue litmus paper (gastric contents are acid and will turn blue litmus paper red).
  - Rapidly inject 20 mL of air into the tube while auscultating over the left hypochondrium. Listen for 'bubbling' over the stomach (correct position).
  - Perform a CXR. Look for the path of the tube and trace its course below the diaphragm, deviating to the left into the gastric area (not entering the chest or coiled in the oesophagus).
- Attach the drainage bag.
- Secure the NGT to the tip of the nose with non-allergenic tape, taking care to avoid pressure on the medial or lateral nostril.

Complications

- Epistaxis (turbinate trauma)
- Misplacement, such as inadvertent tracheal placement (you may have noticed coughing when NGT inserted) or curled back on itself in the oesophagus or pharynx

Handy hints

- Do not attempt to re-use an NGT that has already been used in a failed insertion. Use a fresh tube from the fridge (the colder, the better), as these are more rigid and less pliable, and are therefore easier to pass.

SECTION E – Practical procedures

Continued

Handy hints—Continued

- If the tube continually curls up in the pharynx, flex the patient's neck as much as possible, which may change the angle sufficiently to pass an obstruction, and re-insert the tube.
- Nebulised lignocaine (4 mL of 10%) or lignocaine lubricating gel 2% can be administered prior to insertion of the tube to reduce discomfort and increase patient compliance.
- **Do not** use the NGT for any fluid administration until CXR confirmation of position.

Urinary catheterisation

Indications

- **Continuous**
  - Acute or chronic urinary retention.
  - Measurement of urine output to monitor fluid balance (e.g. volume resuscitation, shock therapy).
  - Short term (e.g. postoperatively).
  - Long term (e.g. when TURP is medically contraindicated or awaited).
- **Intermittent**
  - Obtaining uncontaminated urine for microscopy and culture (especially in females or young children).
  - Measurement of bladder residual volume.
  - Facilitating adequate bladder emptying (e.g. in conditions associated with atonic bladder).
  - Intravesical installation of contrast or medications (e.g. in suspected bladder trauma, for a micturating cysto-urethrogram or instillation of local cytotoxic agent).
  - Urodynamic assessment.

Contraindications

- Urethral disruption in the setting of pelvic trauma suggested by penile, scrotal or perineal haematoma, blood at the urethral meatus and a high-riding prostate on rectal examination.
- Postoperative urological patients. Always consult the urologist first if the patient has had bladder neck or prostate surgery.
- Known stricture or 'impossible insertion last time'.

Equipment

- Catheter dressing pack (kidney bowl, small 'wash pots' ×2, gauze swabs, sterile fenestrated drape)
- Catheter (appropriate size ×2)
- 10 mL syringe with 10 mL sterile water

- Skin cleansing solution (e.g. saline)
- Lignocaine gel 2%
- Sterile gloves
- Sterile urine drainage bag and bedside holder
- Woven adhesive tape
- Specimen jar for laboratory urine analysis

Choose the correct catheter
Lumen
- Single lumen—these catheters have no balloon and are used for in–out catheterisations only.
- Double lumen—two-way catheters have a draining lumen and a balloon inflation lumen and are used for continuous catheterisation.
- Triple lumen—three-way catheters have a draining lumen, a balloon inflation lumen and an irrigation lumen. Inserted when blood, clots or debris are to be washed out of the bladder (e.g. post TURP).

Size
- Catheter size refers to the circumference of the catheter, not the luminal diameter and is recorded in French sizes (1 French [F] = 1 Charrière = 0.33 mm).
- Choose the optimal catheter that facilitates insertion and allows adequate urinary drainage. Sizes 16–18F are suitable for adult men and women. Use up to 20F if the patient has urine with blood clots or gross haematuria, mucus or debris that may occlude a smaller lumen.
- A 22F triple lumen is the standard size for bladder irrigation and 'washout'.
- Smaller sizes (6–10F) are available for children.

Procedural technique

Male catheterisation
- Explain the procedure to the patient.
- Open all necessary equipment onto a clean trolley.
- Wash your hands thoroughly, perform thorough antiseptic hand-wash and put on sterile gloves.
- Draw up sterile water for balloon inflation.
- Place fenestrated drape over the patient's perineum.
- Gently retract the patient's foreskin and swab the urethral opening and glans with sterile gauze soaked in saline.
- Hold the penis firmly and in an upright position and retract the foreskin with sterile gauze using your middle and ring fingers,

leaving the thumb and index finger free to manipulate the catheter.
- Instil lignocaine gel 2% into the urethra. Approximately 20 mL (two syringes) of gel is required to reach the proximal end of the urethra in a male. Gently squeeze the tip of the glans to close off the urethra so that lubricant gel is retained and does not ooze straight back out.
- Hold the penis in this position for 90 seconds to allow the anaesthetic gel time to work.
- Open the catheter wrapping at the distal (tip) end only and insert the catheter gently and slowly into the urethra, withdrawing the plastic covering in stages, avoiding unnecessary touching of the sterile outside surface.
- Advance the catheter to the hilt and wait for urine to flow. If no urine flows, consider blockage with gel (see *Handy hints*) or malposition within urethra, which requires gentle re-insertion. Only proceed when urine flow is seen.
- Inflate the balloon with 10 mL sterile water (or as indicated on the hilt of the catheter). Stop immediately if the patient experiences pain, as it may have become malpositioned.
- Once the balloon is inflated, gently retract the catheter until resistance is felt.
- *Always* reposition the foreskin to prevent a paraphimosis developing later.
- Connect the bag aseptically to the catheter.
- Attach the catheter to the patient's inner upper thigh using non-allergenic tape, allowing a gentle curve from the external urethral meatus to the skin, without tension.

Reasons for failure
- Urethral or penile stricture: be careful, never use force and if in doubt, call a urologist.
- Enlarged prostate: generally the larger the prostate, the larger the catheter required.
- Malposition with catheter coiled within urethra: usually no urine will flow.

Female catheterisation
- Explain the procedure to the patient.
- Open all necessary equipment onto a clean trolley.
- Wash your hands thoroughly, perform thorough antiseptic hand-wash and put on sterile gloves.
- Draw up sterile water for balloon inflation.
- Open the catheter wrapping at the distal (tip) end and, holding the proximal portion (still in the wrapping), lubricate the catheter tip with lignocaine gel 2%.

- Position the patient as for a vaginal examination, flat on her back with knees and hips flexed and ankles together. Allow the legs to rest gently in full abduction.
- Drape the perineum using the fenestrated sheet.
- Use your non-dominant gloved hand to gently separate the labia minora and cleanse the area with saline.
    - *Note:* the hand holding the labia must be kept in place until the catheter is successfully inserted and urine flows.
- Locate the urethral opening (inferior to the clitoris, but may still be difficult to define), and swab anterior to posterior with cleansing solution.
- Instil a small amount of lignocaine gel into the tip of the urethral meatus and introduce well-lubricated catheter along the urethra until urine flows.
- Inflate the balloon with 10 mL of sterile water.
- Connect the bag aseptically to the catheter.
- Attach the catheter to the patient's upper thigh using non-allergenic tape, allowing a gentle curve from the external urethral meatus to the skin, without tension.

Complications
- Unable to pass catheter
    - Do not persist with multiple attempts at catheterisation, as this will only result in urethral trauma. Consult urology early for consideration of suprapubic catheterisation.
- Urethral trauma (e.g. creation of a false passage).
- Paraphimosis from failure to replace foreskin.
- Introduction of infection, bacteraemia (was the catheterisation definitely necessary?).

Documentation
Always document the procedure fully in the notes for both male and female catheterisation:
- Date, time and reason for catheter insertion.
- Catheter make, size (F), material, balloon size and amount of fluid used in balloon.
- Any problems encountered during or following catheter placement, such as traumatic catheterisation or, in particular, failure to pass.

Handy hints

- Urine must flow from an inserted catheter *before* the balloon is inflated. Urine may not flow initially because of obstruction by lubricating gel. You may be able to expedite flow by gently suctioning the catheter with a syringe or applying suprapubic pressure.

Handy hints—Continued

- Do not over- or underfill the catheter balloon, as this will lead to balloon distortion, causing the catheter tip to deviate within the bladder, and can potentially result in bladder wall necrosis.
- If the patient is immunosuppressed, or has a prosthetic heart valve, catheter insertion may cause serious bacteraemia with bacterial seeding. Seek senior advice as regards prophylactic antibiotics prior to catheter insertion and/or whether the catheter is really necessary.

57

Paracentesis

Indications

- **Diagnostic**
  - Determine cause of new-onset ascites, ascites of unknown origin or suspected malignant ascites.
  - Suspicion of bacterial peritonitis in a patient with known ascites associated with any one of a pyrexia, hypotension, tachycardia or encephalopathy.
- **Therapeutic**
  - Remove excess intraperitoneal fluid.

Contraindications

- Problems at proposed puncture site
  - Local skin infection/cellulitis
  - Hernia
  - Caput medusae or superficial veins
- Uncooperative patient
- Uncorrected bleeding diathesis (in particular, platelet count $<50 \times 10^9$/L or INR >1.5)
- Suspected abdominal adhesions or loculated fluid collection (e.g. seen on ultrasound)
- Bowel distension

Equipment

- Sterile occlusive dressing
- Gauze swabs
- Sticking plaster
- Local anaesthetic (10 mL 2% lignocaine)
- Syringes: 10 mL, 20 mL, 50 mL Luer-lock
- Needles: 21G × 2, 25G × 1

- Cannula: 16G and long, or a peritoneal dialysis catheter, suprapubic catheter or ascitic drain
- Skin preparation fluid (chlorhexidine)
- Sterile gloves
- Drape
- Three-way tap
- Scalpel with blade
- Sterile specimen containers
- Assistant

Procedural technique

- Explain the procedure to the patient and ensure that there is a patent IV line with normal saline attached.
- Record baseline observations of HR, BP, RR and oxygen saturation. Record pre-drainage weight if performing a therapeutic procedure.
- Ask the patient to empty the bladder immediately before commencing the procedure to reduce the risk of inadvertent puncture.
- Ask the patient to lie on the bed and expose the whole abdomen. Percuss the abdomen to demonstrate shifting dullness and the extent of the ascites.
- Identify the landmarks for proposed puncture site, confirm dullness to percussion and mark with a pen. Preferably use bedside ultrasound to find the optimal insertion site (see below).
- The preferred and safest sites are located in the right and left lower quadrants two finger-breadths medial, and two finger-breadths superior (cephalad) to the anterior superior iliac spine.
  - Note: if the ascites is poorly defined clinically, do not proceed; make sure an USS is used to mark the best puncture site.
- Using aseptic technique, put on gloves and cleanse and drape the proposed entry site.
- Draw up 10 mL lignocaine 2%.
  - Use the 25G needle to raise a subcutaneous bleb on the surface of the skin at the proposed entry site.
  - Infiltrate local anaesthetic with the 21G needle beneath the skin and working towards the peritoneum.
  - Take care to draw back on the syringe before infiltrating and stop when fluid is aspirated, which confirms correct intraperitoneal placement.

SECTION E – Practical procedures

Diagnostic tap

- Attach a new 21G needle to a 20 mL syringe and insert along the anaesthetised track, bevel up, at 90 degrees to the skin.
- Maintain constant negative pressure on the syringe by drawing back on the plunger as the needle is advanced.
- When fluid is aspirated, withdraw 20 mL of fluid.
- Remove the needle and press firmly over the site with a gauze swab.
- Send fluid for biochemistry (protein, glucose, LDH), microbiology (MCS and Gram stain) and cytology.
- Apply a sterile occlusive dressing.

Therapeutic tap

- Cannula:
    - Insert a 16G cannula along the anaesthetised track at 90 degrees to the surface of the skin. When flashback is seen, hold the stylet steady and advance the plastic cannula fully into the peritoneal cavity.
    - Remove the stylet and place a gloved thumb over the cannula. Attach the three-way tap and 50 mL syringe, and secure the cannula with tape.
    - Withdraw fluid into the syringe and switch the three-way tap settings to empty the syringe contents into an appropriately sized container.
- Suprapubic catheter, peritoneal dialysis catheter or ascitic drain:
    - All these devices are specially manufactured with their own blunt introducer that is less likely to cause bowel perforation, or use a Seldinger technique with guidewire and dilator.
    - Nick the skin over the anaesthetised track with a scalpel blade. Enter the skin at 90 degrees and gently push the device through the peritoneum into the peritoneal cavity.
    - Aspirate the catheter with a 20 mL syringe to ensure ascitic fluid flows, withdraw the introducer and advance the plastic sheath as far into the peritoneum as it will go.
    - Attach to the drain and secure the catheter to the skin with tape or a single suture. Temporarily clamp the drain once 1000 mL of fluid has been removed.
    - *Note:* large-volume therapeutic aspiration (5000 mL) should be accompanied by IV albumin replacement (500 mL of 4% albumin if dehydrated, or 100 mL of 20% albumin if hypervolaemic).
    - Do not drain more than 5000 mL during a single therapeutic procedure (risk of profound hypotension).

Complications

- Shock
- Hypovolaemia
- Renal failure
- Perforation of viscera (bowel, bladder)
- Peritonitis
- Haemorrhage (e.g. from an abdominal wall vessel laceration)
- Persistent fluid leak

Handy hints

- Ultrasound-guided paracentesis should be performed whenever possible, certainly in patients who are pregnant, have multiple abdominal scars or a history of bowel adhesions.
- **No aspiration**
  - Re-percuss the abdomen and try again. If still unsuccessful, request USS to confirm ascitic fluid volume.
- **No drainage**
  - Kinked or blocked tube: untwist and flush with sterile saline.
- Drain not secured properly and no longer in peritoneum: remove drain and re-insert, as a new procedure (do *not* just push back in).

58

Pleural tap

Indications

- **Diagnostic**
  - Determine the cause of pleural effusion.
- **Therapeutic**
  - Remove excess pleural fluid to assist respiration and provide symptomatic relief.

Contraindications and cautions

- Local skin infection
- Uncooperative patient
- Uncorrected bleeding diathesis (in particular, platelet count $<50 \times 10^9$/L or INR >1.5).
- Take special care with:
  - Small effusion
  - Bullous lung disease
  - Single functioning lung

Equipment

- Sterile dressing pack
- Gauze swabs
- Adhesive tape
- Local anaesthetic (10 mL 2% plain lignocaine)
- Syringes: 10 mL × 1, 20 mL × 1
- 50 mL Luer-lock syringe attached to three-way tap
- Needles: 21G × 2, 25G × 1
- Cannula: 16G
- Sterile gloves
- Drape
- Skin cleansing solution (e.g. chlorhexidine)
- Sterile specimen containers
- Occlusive dressing

- Assistant
- Pulse oximeter

Procedural technique

- Explain the procedure to the patient.
- Record baseline observations of HR, BP, RR and oxygen saturation, and attach a pulse oximeter to the patient.
- Sit the patient on the edge of the bed, arms folded in front of the body and leaning forwards over a bedside tray table. Expose the whole of the patient's back.
- Re-confirm the site and size of the pleural effusion:
  - Review the most recent CXR.
  - Percuss down the patient's chest to confirm the upper border of the effusion (stony dull percussion), then auscultate (decreased breath sounds and decreased vocal resonance).
  - Mark the site for aspiration—posterolateral aspect of the chest wall (midscapular or posterior axillary line), 1–2 intercostal spaces below the percussed upper border of the effusion.
  - Ideally use bedside ultrasound to confirm the optimal site for aspirating, particularly when the effusion is poorly defined clinically.
  - Ensure that the proposed aspiration site is directly over a palpable intercostal space, and above the level of the diaphragm (that is, no lower than the 8th intercostal space).
- Using aseptic technique, put on gloves, then cleanse and drape the proposed entry site.
- Draw up 10 mL lignocaine 2%.
  - Use the 25G needle to raise a subcutaneous bleb on the surface of the skin at the proposed entry site.
  - Infiltrate local anaesthetic with the 21G needle, working towards the upper border of the inferior rib to avoid hitting the neurovascular bundle (i.e. work 'just above the rib below').
- The most pain-sensitive structures are skin, periosteum and pleura, so ensure that these are all well anaesthetised.
- Take care to draw back on the syringe before infiltrating and stop when fluid is aspirated from the pleural cavity.

Diagnostic tap

- Attach a new 21G needle to a 20 mL syringe and insert along the anaesthetised track, bevel up, at 90 degrees to the surface of the skin, working 'just above the rib below'.

- Maintain constant negative pressure on the syringe by drawing back on the plunger as the needle is advanced.
- When fluid is aspirated, withdraw a 20 mL sample.
- Remove the needle and press firmly over the site with a gauze swab.
- Send fluid for biochemistry (protein or albumin, glucose, LDH, pH, triglycerides [chylothorax] and amylase), microbiology (MCS and Gram stain) and for tumour markers and cytology.
- Apply an occlusive dressing.
- Document the procedure, the appearance of the fluid, the volume aspirated and vital signs in the patient's notes and order a CXR (even after a failed tap).

Therapeutic tap

- Insert a 16G cannula along the anaesthetised track, bevel up, at 90 degrees to the surface of the skin, working 'just above the rib below'.
- When flashback is seen, hold the stylet steady and advance the plastic cannula as far into the thorax as it will go.
- Remove the stylet while the patient holds a breath in expiration and place your gloved thumb over the cannula.
- Secure the cannula with tape and attach the three-way tap and 50 mL syringe, again with the patient holding a breath in expiration (this reduces the risk of causing a pneumothorax).
- Withdraw 50 mL of fluid into the syringe and switch the three-way tap settings to empty the syringe contents into an appropriately sized container.
- Once 1000–1500 mL of fluid has been drained, remove the cannula and press firmly over the site with a gauze swab.
- Apply an occlusive dressing.
- Document the procedure, the appearance of the fluid, the volume aspirated and vital signs in the patient's notes and order a CXR (even after a failed tap).

Complications

- Pneumothorax
- Haemopneumothorax
- Hypotension due to a vasovagal response
- Re-expansion pulmonary oedema (large volume aspirated)
- Infection, either skin site or with empyema developing
- Spleen or liver puncture
- Air embolism

Handy hints

- A dry tap may indicate a loculated effusion or empyema. Ultrasound will help define the problem.

- When requesting USS, if not done at the bedside, accompany the patient to observe the marking and positioning of the patient. Ensure that the mark is in an optimal position and ask the radiologist to quantify the likely amount of fluid for removal during a therapeutic tap.

- Do not withdraw fluid too rapidly when performing a therapeutic tap, or remove more than 1500 mL, as this will increase the risk of re-expansion pulmonary oedema.

- Risk of haemothorax is decreased by avoiding the superior portion of the intercostal space (neurovascular bundle runs under the rib above) and never puncturing medial to the midclavicular line (internal mammary vessels).

SECTION E – Practical procedures

59

Chest drain insertion and removal

Chest drain insertion

Indications
- Drainage of a symptomatic pneumothorax, haemothorax, empyema or large pleural effusion.
- Prophylactic insertion, prior to positive-pressure ventilation or aeromedical transport, in a patient with a chest injury and rib fractures or flail chest, or even a small pneumothorax.

Contraindications
- Infection over insertion site
- Uncorrected bleeding diathesis (in particular, platelet count $<50 \times 10^9$/L or INR >1.5)

Equipment
- Appropriate-sized chest tubes
- Sterile tray, gown, gloves and drapes
- Suture material: 00 or 0 nylon (*not* 2/0 as it is not strong enough)
- Chest-drain insertion kit (including sponge-holding forceps, scalpel handle, artery forceps, toothed forceps, needle holder, scissors)
- Scalpel blades
- Gauze swabs
- Skin cleansing solution (e.g. chlorhexidine)
- Local anaesthetic (20 mL 1–2% plain lignocaine)
- Syringes: 10 mL $\times 2$
- Needles: 21G $\times 2$, 25G $\times 1$
- Underwater sealed chest drain unit prepared with sterile saline
- Dressing: drain swabs and occlusive dressing
- Absorbent pad or 'bluey'

Procedural technique

- Explain the procedure to the patient.
- Record baseline observations of HR, BP, RR and oxygen saturation. Attach a cardiac monitor and pulse oximeter to the patient and administer oxygen.
- Re-confirm the side, position and size of the pneumothorax or fluid:
  - Review recent CXR
  - Percuss down the patient's chest to confirm the upper border of the haemothorax/effusion (stony dull percussion) or pneumothorax (resonant percussion), then auscultate the chest (reduced breath sounds).
- Give analgesia or procedural sedation in the haemodynamically stable patient, as this procedure is painful and distressing:
  - Analgesia—0.05–0.1 mg/kg morphine IV, titrated to effect
  - Procedural sedation—0.05 mg/kg midazolam IV, titrated to effect (reduce doses of both if given together).
- Select size of chest tube:
  - Adult   20–24F for pneumothorax
                    28–36F for effusion, haemothorax or empyema
  - Child   18–22F
  - Newborn   12–14F.
- Select site for chest tube insertion: just anterior to the mid-axillary line, in the 4th or 5th intercostal space on a line lateral to the nipple.
- Position the patient lying comfortably on a bed with upper end raised at 30–45 degrees, and with the ipsilateral arm placed above the head.
- Using full sterile technique put on a mask, gown and gloves, then cleanse and drape the site.
- Draw up 20 mL lignocaine 1% and anaesthetise the insertion site:
  - Use the 25G needle to infiltrate at least 4–5 cm of the surface skin over the desired intercostal space (you will be taking a scalpel through this area, so ensure it is well anaesthetised!).
  - Change to the 21G needle and infiltrate local anaesthetic deeper towards the pleura. Aim for the upper border of the rib below, to avoid hitting the neurovascular bundle.
  - Use liberal doses of local anaesthetic, particularly at the pleural entry site (further lignocaine may be required after initial dissection).
  - Take care to draw back on the syringe before infiltrating and stop if air or fluid is aspirated from the pleural cavity.
- Make a 2–4 cm incision through the anaesthetised skin, parallel to the line of the ribs, at the level of the upper border of the rib.

- Using artery forceps, blunt dissect through the intercostal space just above the upper border of the rib below, until the pleura is reached. Infiltrate more local anaesthetic.
- Use the index finger of your dominant hand, or a Kelly clamp/ large needle holder, to push through the pleura between the ribs. Once through, sweep in a 360-degree plane with the finger flexed within the pleural cavity to ensure that the cavity has indeed been breached and no adherent lung is present.
- Leave your finger or the needle holder/forceps in the pleural space, particularly in an obese patient, to maintain a tract.
- Remove the trocar (introducer) from the chest tube and pass the tube into the pleural cavity to a distance of 10–14 cm. Ensure that the side hole of the tube is well inside the pleural cavity.
- *Never, ever use the trocar to force a tube into the chest, as serious internal damage will occur.*
- Connect the chest tube to an underwater sealed drain and ask the patient to cough to check the drain is swinging, bubbling and/or draining freely.
- Secure the chest tube in place:
  - Insert 00 or 0 nylon sutures to either side of the chest drain, keeping the ends of the suture material long (5–10 cm). Tie the outer sutures as normal, pulling the skin taut around the chest tube, and use the additional length of the remaining suture material to wrap around and lock onto the tube tightly to secure it in position.
  - Do *not* leave a purse-string suture for 'later' skin closure, as it will become colonised and increase the risk of infection if tied on drain removal (insert a fresh suture at time of drain removal).
  - Place cut gauze swabs around the chest tube and secure with a small occlusive dressing (do not cover the chest wall in sticky tape, especially in males!).
- Check the position of the chest tube with a post-procedure CXR.

Complications
- Malposition, either extrathoracic (obvious on CXR, as the drain runs up external to the chest wall) or intrathoracic but extrapleural (not obvious on CXR, but exceedingly painful). In neither case will the drain swing, bubble and/or drain freely.
- Subcutaneous emphysema
- Trauma with haemorrhage (e.g. haemothorax from intercostal vessel injury)
- Local nerve injury (eg. long thoracic nerve)
- Infection, either skin site or with empyema developing
- Re-expansion pulmonary oedema
- Trauma to heart, liver, lung or spleen (e.g. use of trocar, or re-insertion through a recent drain site—*never* do either of these)

Handy hints

- Keep the underwater sealed chest drain below the level of the heart at all times.
- Regularly check that the fluid in the drain is swinging with normal respiration. If the fluid level fails to swing at all, look to see if the chest tube is kinked, blocked or in the wrong place.

Chest drain removal

Indication

- Resolution of pneumothorax or haemothorax with re-expansion of collapsed lung and no chest drain bubbling or air leak for 24 hours.

Equipment

- Dressing pack and suture pack
- 3/0 nylon suture
- Sterile scissors
- Sterile gauze swabs
- Skin cleansing solution (e.g. chlorhexidine)
- Clamping forceps
- Occlusive dressing
- Assistant

Procedural technique

- Explain the procedure to the patient and position the patient upright in bed.
- Remove the dressings from around the chest tube.
- Clamp the tube with forceps.
- Cleanse the skin and surrounding area thoroughly with chlorhexidine.
- Cut the ends of the suture material securing the chest tube in place, taking care not to remove the actual sutures holding the skin incision closed.
- Insert a *new* purse-string suture around the tube insertion site.
- Ask the patient to take a deep breath in, expire fully, then hold a breath.
- As your assistant removes the chest tube in a single movement, pull on the free ends of the new purse-string suture to bring the skin edges together and secure with a knot.
- Cleanse and dress the area with an occlusive dressing.
- Observe the patient and repeat the CXR 2–6 hours after removal.
- Remove the sutures after 1 week.

SECTION E – Practical procedures

60

Lumbar puncture

Lumbar puncture (LP) is an uncomfortable, often frightening, procedure for any patient. It is essential to position the patient correctly and take your time.

Indications

- **Diagnostic**
  - Analyse CSF in suspected meningitis or encephalitis, SAH, carcinomatosis, multiple sclerosis and syndromes such as Guillain–Barré syndrome.
  - Measure CSF pressure.
- **Therapeutic**
  - Intrathecal administration of medications.
  - Removal of CSF in benign intracranial hypertension.

Indications for a CT head scan *prior* to lumbar puncture
- Objective evidence of raised ICP (see below), including altered level of consciousness (ALOC) or focal neurological deficits
- Suspected SAH
- Known CNS lesion (e.g. stroke, mass lesion, focal CNS infection)
- Seizure activity in preceding week
- Immunocompromise
- Age >60 years

Contraindications

- Signs of increased ICP with or without mass effect, such as focal neurological signs, papilloedema, ALOC, bradycardia and hypertension, or abnormal respiratory pattern (irrespective of what the CT head scan shows)
- Space-occupying lesion on CT
- Intracranial masses, particularly in the posterior fossa, which may cause brain herniation and compress the brainstem

- Uncontrolled bleeding diathesis
  - Patients with coagulopathy including INR >1.5, platelet count <50×10^9/L or taking anticoagulant medication are at increased risk of epidural haematoma
- Local skin infection of the lower back

Equipment

- Sterile gloves and gown
- Dressing pack
- Local anaesthetic (10 mL of 2% lignocaine)
- 10 mL syringe
- Needles (21G and 25G)
- Spinal needles (20G [black], 18G [yellow])
- Skin cleansing antiseptic solution (e.g. chlorhexidine)
- Gauze swabs
- Manometer with three-way tap
- Three sterile collection bottles (check which type of containers the laboratory needs before commencing procedure and confirm correct specimens to send)
- Assistant to reassure patient and to help with CSF collection
- Absorbent pad or 'bluey'
- Sticking plaster

Procedural technique

- Identify the correct patient and explain the procedure and gain verbal consent, warning about the risks of post-LP headache, which occurs in 10–30% cases.
- If the patient is anxious or unable to lie still for 15–30 minutes, sedate with 0.05 mg/kg midazolam IV, titrated to effect.
- **Spend time positioning the patient correctly** (see Figure 60.1):
  - Lie the patient on their left-hand side on the bed with the back as close as possible to the right edge of the bed.
  - Place one hand on the patient's right shoulder and one on the right anterior superior iliac spine and ask the patient to flex the hips, knees and neck as much as possible (i.e. fetal position).
  - Ensure that the patient's back remains straight, the vertebral column parallel to the edge of the bed and the shoulders square to the hips, both at a right angle to the bed.
- **Determine the site of needle insertion:**
  - Palpate the iliac crests and locate the vertebra lying on an imaginary line between them (L4 vertebra).
  - Feel the space above this vertebra (L3–4 space) and the space above that (L2–3 space). Mark each with a pen cap or fingernail indent.

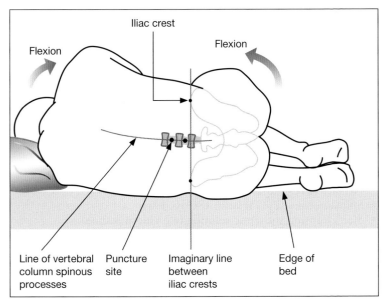

Iliac crest

Flexion

Flexion

Line of vertebral
column spinous
processes

Puncture
site

Imaginary line
between
iliac crests

Edge of
bed

Figure 60.1 Patient positioning for lumbar puncture.

- Wash your hands and put on sterile gown and gloves.
- Ensure that you are in a comfortable position, seated by the side of the bed with the patient's spine at the level of your sternum.
- Use an aseptic non-touch technique to prepare and drape the site.
- Anaesthetise the skin using the 25G needle and SC infiltration. Use the 21G needle for deeper infiltration down to the interspinous ligament. Wait 2–3 minutes for full effect of local anaesthetic.
- Confirm that the stylet releases freely from within the LP needle and check the manometer tap. Examine the needle bevel for orientation.
- Locate the L3 and L4 vertebrae with the index and middle fingers of your non-dominant hand, and use as physical landmarks. The anaesthetised area should be in the midline directly between these fingers.
- Place the LP needle, bevel up and at 90 degrees to the skin in all planes, or 5–10 degrees caudad (i.e. needle tip pointing up to the head) over the intervertebral space (see Figure 60.2).
- Advance the needle through the skin, between the spinous processes, aiming cranially towards the patient's umbilicus.
- Stop if bone is contacted, withdraw and re-advance the needle.
- Feel for increased resistance (interspinous ligament) and then a 'give' as the needle passes through the ligamentum flavum.

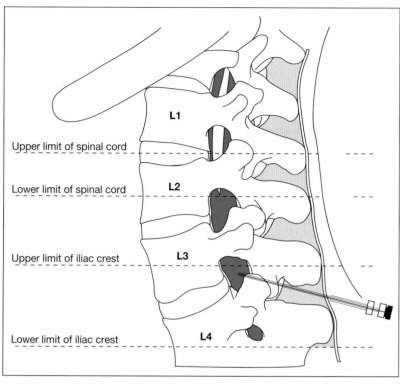

Figure 60.2 Needle insertion for lumbar puncture. Copyright Tor Ercleve.

- Withdraw the stylet and look for a flashback of CSF. If there is none, replace the stylet and advance the needle another few millimetres, checking for evidence of CSF return each time.
- Once the subarachnoid space has been reached, and CSF is draining, remove the stylet fully and attach the manometer.
- Measure the CSF pressure (normal opening pressure is 6–18 cm H_2O).
- Disconnect the manometer and collect CSF drops from the open end of the spinal needle. Collect 10–20 drops into three specimen containers and label them 1, 2 and 3.
- Send to laboratory for cell count with differential, Gram stain plus culture for bacteriology, cytology, PCR testing (meningitis/encephalitis), India ink staining for fungi (*Cryptococcus neoformans*) and xanthochromia (subarachnoid haemorrhage). Depending on the pathology service requirements, a further tube with preservative may be required to analyse biochemistry and glucose.
- Re-insert the stylet (reduces post-LP headache risk) and slowly remove the entire spinal needle.

- Cleanse the patient's back and place a small dressing or plaster over the puncture site.
- Move the patient gently into a prone position if possible (stomach down, back uppermost) to reduce CSF leak by gravity.
- Recommend bed rest for 1–2 hours (depending on local hospital policy), although it does not influence the likelihood of post-LP headache.

Complications

- Failure—ask a senior doctor for help
- Post-LP headache—more likely with larger-bore needle, multiple attempts, excessive CSF removal, dehydration and in females
  - Can reduce risk by using an atraumatic needle (e.g. Sprotte or Whitacre) rather than a cutting needle (e.g. Quincke) to separate rather than cut dural fibres, and by orienting the bevel of the needle parallel to the long axis of the spine
- Local skin haemorrhage
- Epidural haematoma, with signs of acute spinal cord compression
- Infection (rare)—meningitis, epidural abscess
- Brainstem compression secondary to brain herniation (controversial but devastating)

Handy hints

- **If you do not enter the epidural space:**
  - Reposition the patient correctly.
  - Ensure the needle remains at 90 degrees to the skin in all planes, in the midline between the two vertebrae.
  - Ask the patient if the needle feels like it is dead centre. People can usually tell if it feels like the needle is off to one side.
  - If you think you are in the correct place, slowly rotate the needle through 90–180 degrees to release the needle bevel.
- **If you still cannot drain CSF:**
  - Give yourself and the patient a short break. Call your senior for help.
  - Try repositioning the patient in a sitting position, with hips flexed (increases the interspinous width) and the head and shoulders draped forwards over a table. Re-determine landmarks and repeat procedure.
  - In the sitting position the midline is easier to determine and CSF flows are higher, especially in a dehydrated patient; however, manometer readings are unreliable.
- Do not remove too much CSF; usually 10–20 drops (1–2 mL) only are required per specimen container. Excessive removal (>20 mL) leads to an increased risk of post-LP headache.
- **Never** apply suction to the spinal needle.

Joint aspiration

Common joints requiring fluid aspiration and/or steroid injection include the knee, elbow and shoulder.

The anatomical landmarks for the site of injection will vary, but the principles of anaesthetic administration and use of an aseptic technique are similar for all joints.

Indications

- **Diagnostic**
  - Remove joint fluid for biochemical testing, including polarising light microscopy, microbiology and cytology.
  - Unexplained joint effusion to differentiate a septic arthritis from an inflammatory (gouty) or bloody (haemarthrosis) effusion.
- **Therapeutic**
  - Remove excess fluid or blood from the joint to provide symptomatic relief, increase mobility and decrease pain in a large effusion, crystal-induced arthropathy or haemarthrosis.
  - Intra-articular steroid injection (must first discuss with orthopaedics or rheumatology consultant).

Contraindications

- Local skin cellulitis/infection
- Uncooperative patient
- Acute fracture (may introduce infection)
- Joint prosthesis (may introduce infection)
- Uncorrected bleeding diathesis (in particular, platelet count $<50 \times 10^9$/L or INR>1.5)

Equipment

- Sterile dressing pack
- Syringes: 10 mL, 20 mL, 50 mL
- Needles: 25G and 21G ×2
- Cannula: 16G or 14G

- Local anaesthetic (plain lignocaine 1% or 2%)
- Sterile gloves and gown
- Skin cleansing solution (e.g. chlorhexidine or povidone–iodine solution)
- Sterile specimen containers ×3
- Sterile fenestrated drape
- Alcohol swab
- Absorbent pad or 'bluey'
- Sticking plaster

Procedural technique

- Explain the procedure to the patient.
- Position the patient comfortably on the bed, with the affected joint fully exposed.
- Examine the joint fully to ascertain the site where maximal fluid is felt, and to define the anatomical landmarks.
- Identify the proposed puncture site with a skin marker pen.
- Wash hands thoroughly and put on sterile gown and gloves.
- Cleanse the skin over the joint with povidone–iodine or chlorhexidine solution using a circular motion, commencing at the puncture site and working from the inside out (i.e. do not return to a previously swabbed area). Place a fenestrated drape over the area and allow the skin to air dry.
- Wipe over the proposed puncture site with an alcohol swab prior to infiltrating anaesthetic if using povidone–iodine solution (a small amount of contamination may inhibit bacterial culture growth).
- Draw up 10 mL lignocaine and infiltrate the surface of the skin over the entry site using the 25G needle. Wait 45–60 seconds.
- Switch to the 21G needle and infiltrate the subcutaneous tissue with local anaesthetic. Avoid injecting lignocaine directly into the joint, as it can have a bactericidal effect. Wait for 45–60 seconds for anaesthesia to take effect.
- Attach the second 21G needle to a 20 mL syringe. Stabilise the joint by holding the skin taut over the joint effusion with your non-dominant hand and 'milk' the effusion fluid towards the point of the needle.
- Advance the needle slowly along the anaesthetised track, maintaining a slight negative pressure.
- Observe for flashback of joint fluid as the joint capsule is breached and slowly aspirate the fluid from the joint. Keep the needle as steady as possible, without touching the bone or cartilage surfaces (painful!).
- If joint contents are too thick or viscid to aspirate, change to a 16G or 14G cannula with syringe attached.

- Do not apply too great a negative pressure on the syringe, as it will cause the local tissues to collapse into and occlude the needle bevel.
- Massage the area surrounding the needle insertion site over the joint to increase the local accumulation of effusion.

Diagnostic tap

- Aspirate 15–20 mL fluid from the joint, then withdraw the syringe and needle. Apply firm pressure over the puncture site and apply a sticking plaster.
- Transfer 5 mL of fluid to each of the three sterile containers and label for biochemical testing, including polarising light microscopy, microbiology and cytology.

Therapeutic tap

- Aspirate the first 15–20 mL of fluid from the joint and disconnect the syringe, leaving the needle or cannula in place.
- Attach a second syringe (20 mL or 50 mL) and continue this procedure until sufficient fluid has been drained.
- Alternatively, attach a three-way tap first to avoid the need to change aspirating syringe, which can then be emptied when full.
- Apply a firm crepe bandage around the joint if a large volume of fluid has been removed.

Complications

- Joint infection—introduction of skin organisms from poor aseptic technique may result in septic arthritis
- Local haematoma
- Haemarthrosis
- Synovial fistula

SECTION E – Practical procedures

62

Cardiac monitoring and the electrocardiograph

The ECG is one of the most useful investigations in medicine. Electrodes provide the physical contact between the monitoring equipment and the patient, and the leads are the different viewpoints of the heart's electrical activity.

Ten electrodes attached to the chest and/or limbs (six praecordial and four limb electrodes) record small voltage changes as potential differences, which are transposed into a visual tracing.

* The 12-lead ECG collects information from all 10 electrodes to provide 12 different views (leads) of the heart's electrical activity.
* Single-lead monitoring is used for continuous bedside cardiac monitoring and telemetry. It focuses on one lead and requires two, three or five electrodes placed on the praecordium to provide the trace.

Indications

* Diagnose specific cardiac disorders (e.g. acute MI).
* Identify cardiac rhythm disturbances (e.g. SVT, VT, AF, heart block).
* Identify certain systemic disorders (e.g. electrolyte disturbance, drug toxicity).
* As part of non-invasive vital signs monitoring in critical patients.

Equipment

* ECG machine or cardiac monitor
* Adhesive electrodes
* Razor

Procedural technique

* Explain to the patient what you are about to do and why. Reassure the patient that the procedure is completely painless and harmless.

- Expose the patient's chest and limbs.
- Shave areas covered with hair with a razor to ensure good electrical contact.
- Attach the electrodes to the patient's skin. Electrode leads are usually colour-coded or labelled to allow correct identification and placement (see Table 62.1).
  - **12-lead ECG:**
    - Place upper limb electrodes on the inner aspect of each forearm just above the wrist.
    - Place lower limb electrodes on the lateral aspect of each leg, just above the ankle.
    - Place the electrodes as distal as possible on the affected limb in the patient with an amputation or with limbs immobilised in non-conducting material such as a plaster cast, and mirror this position on the unaffected side, being careful to ensure that the electrodes remain equidistant from the heart.
  - **Single-lead monitoring:**
    - All leads should be placed on the praecordium equidistant from the heart.

Table 62.1	**Electrocardiogram electrode systems**		
Electrode	**Colour**	**Position**	**System**
RA	White ('snow')	Right arm	3-electrode 5-electrode 12-lead ECG
RL	Green ('grass')	Right leg	5-electrode 12-lead ECG
LA	Black ('smoke')	Left arm	3-electrode 5-electrode 12-lead ECG
LL	Red ('fire')	Left leg	3-electrode 5-electrode 12-lead ECG
C	Brown	Central chest, over sternum	5-electrode
V1	Red	Right 4th ICS, sternal edge	12-lead ECG
V2	Yellow	Left 4th ICS, sternal edge	12-lead ECG
V3	Green	Between V2 and V4	12-lead ECG
V4	Blue	Left 5th ICS, mid-clavicular line	12-lead ECG
V5	Orange	Between V4–V5 in left 5th ICS	12-lead ECG
V6	Purple	Left 5th ICS, mid-axillary line	12-lead ECG

RA, right arm; RL, right leg; LA, left arm; LL, left leg; ICS, intercostal space.

SECTION E – Practical procedures

- Check the leads are in the correct position.
- Ensure that no cables (e.g. a monitor mains lead) are in contact with or cross over the electrode leads.
- Switch on the ECG machine or the monitor.
- Enter the patient details if required and switch on the filter button.

Electrocardiogram recording systems
3-electrode system (see Figure 62.1)

- Uses three electrodes (right arm [RA], left arm [LA] and left leg [LL]).
- Monitor will display the bipolar leads (I, II and III).
- *Note:* electrodes are usually placed on the chest wall rather than the specific limb, and should remain equidistant from the heart to get the best result.

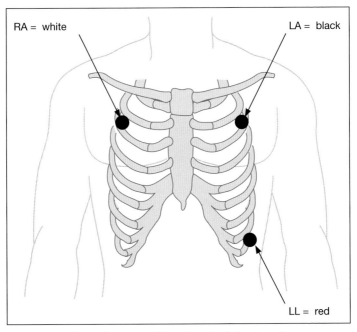

RA = white

LA = black

LL = red

Figure 62.1 3-electrode system. Generates single-lead continuous monitoring. Common for cardiac monitoring in hospitals and for transport monitors.

5-electrode system (see Figure 62.2)

- Uses five electrodes (RA, right leg [RL], LA, LL and chest).
- Monitor will display the bipolar leads (I, II and III) and a single unipolar lead, which depends on the position of the brown chest lead (positions V1–6).

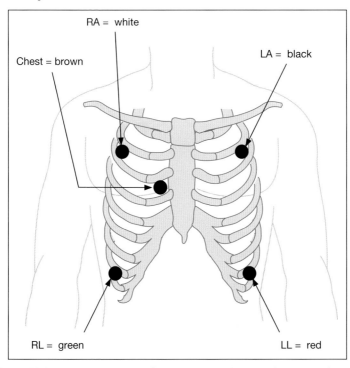

Figure 62.2 5-electrode system. Generates single-lead continuous monitoring.

12-lead electrocardiogram (see Figure 62.3)

- Electrodes on all four limbs (RA, LA, LL, RL).
- Electrodes on praecordium (V1–6).
- Monitors 12 leads (V1–6), (I, II, III) and (aVR, aVF, aVL).
- Allows interpretation of specific 'anatomical' areas of the heart:
  - 'Inferior'   II, III, aVF
  - 'Lateral'   I, aVL, V5, V6
  - 'Anterior'   V1–4
  - 'Right ventricular'   V4R (V4 placed on the right side of the chest, same level)
  - 'Posterior'   V7–9 (V7 level with V6 in left posterior axillary line, V8 midway between V7 and V9, and V9 level with V7 at left spinal border).

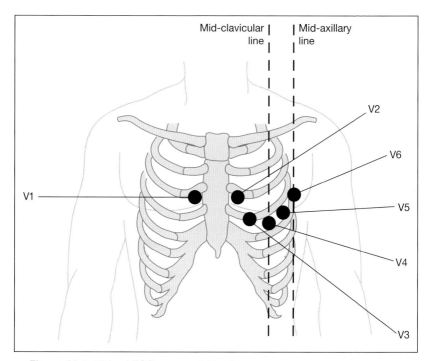

Figure 62.3 12-lead ECG praecordial leads.

V_1 = R 4th ICS by sternum
V_2 = L 4th ICS on sternal border
V_3 = midway between V_2 and V_4
V_4 = L 5th ICS in mid-clavicular line
V_5 = L 5th ICS between V_4 and V_6
V_6 = L 5th ICS in mid-axillary line

Handy hints

- An easy way to remember the placement of the limb electrodes for single-lead continuous ECG monitoring is:
  - *White is always right*, and
  - *Smoke over Fire* and *Snow over Grass* (see Table 62.1).
- Reduce tremor artefact or a wandering baseline on the 12-lead ECG by:
  - Ensuring the patient is completely relaxed. Ask the patient not to talk, and to take shallow breaths if possible, until the ECG is acquired.
  - Reducing shivering by covering the patient with clothing, gown or a light blanket prior to recording.
  - Re-locating the limb leads proximally (e.g. on hips and shoulders) to reduce the interference form peripheral muscle groups (skeletal muscle electrical signals).
    - This also minimises the distal tremor of Parkinson's disease.
- If a bizarre axis is encountered, check the limb electrodes, as they are often the culprit.

63

Defibrillation

Defibrillation is the passage of an electrical current across the myocardium to depolarise a critical mass of myocardium, and is the *only* treatment proven to be effective for terminating ventricular fibrillation (VF) or pulseless ventricular tachycardia (pVT).

Depolarisation allows the restoration of coordinated myocardial electrical activity following recapture by a single pacemaker. Success depends on the ability of the depolarised myocardium to begin synchronous excitation and contraction.

Defibrillation must be initiated as soon as possible and *never* be delayed for any other interventions, as the likelihood of successful defibrillation decreases rapidly with time.

Indications

- VF
- pVT
- Asystole (*only* when fine VF cannot confidently be excluded)

Equipment

Defibrillator models
- Manual defibrillator: all modern defibrillators are biphasic.
- Semi-automated external defibrillator (SAED): often found in hospitals, where there is some degree of medical expertise available for its use.
- Automated external defibrillator (AED) or 'shock-advisory defibrillator': usually biphasic and may be found in public places where expertise is limited.

Self-adhesive pads or paddles
- Disposable self-adhesive gel pads with electrode wires that connect directly to the defibrillator have now largely replaced paddles.

- Defibrillator paddles are attached to the defibrillator by insulated leads. Electrical contact is made with the patient's skin over a gel pad or electrode jelly placed on the chest wall.
  - *Note:* self-adhesive defibrillation pads and paddles are both safe and effective, with similar transthoracic impedance and efficacy. Self-adhesive pads also allow the operator to defibrillate at a safe distance from the patient, enable quicker delivery of the first shock and can be used for longer-term monitoring in the peri-arrest situation.

Procedural technique

- **Ensure safe operating practice:**
  - Check that the chest is dry and that the operator is not standing in a pool of body fluid, blood or water.
  - Ensure that no metal object, ECG electrode or GTN patch is underneath a pad or paddle and that an internal pacemaker is at least 5 cm away from any contact points.
  - Move any free oxygen source (oxygen mask, nasal prongs or disconnected ventilation tubing) at least 1 m away from the patient to reduce the risk of fire or burns.
  - All personnel should be clear of any contact with the patient or bed prior to administration of a shock.
  - Paddles should either remain held on the patient's chest or be placed back in the machine in between shocks, and should never be moved while charging or charged.

Reduce the transthoracic impedance to a minimum to increase the amount of electrical energy reaching the heart.

- **Choose the correct paddle size:**
  - Optimum size for adults is 10–13 cm in diameter (smaller in children).
  - If too small, focal myocardial damage may occur.
  - If too large, contact with the chest wall becomes difficult and impedance is increased with the charge delivered decreased.
- **Choose the correct pad/paddle site:**
  - Do not place over female breast (increased impedance).
  - **Standard placement:**
    - Right chest: 2nd intercostal space, mid-clavicular line
    - Left chest: 5–6th intercostal space, mid-axillary line
  - **Anteroposterior placement:**
    - Anterior chest: 5–6th intercostal space, anterior or mid-axillary line
    - Posterior chest: over left or right infrascapular region.

- **Shave the chest** (if time allows): prevents air being trapped beneath the electrode and increases electrical conduction.
- **Use conductive pads:** if paddles are used, always place gel pad or electrode jelly on the skin to reduce the transthoracic impedance and apply firm pressure with paddles (5–8 kg on each paddle).
- **Watch the respiratory phase delivery:** defibrillation should ideally occur in end expiration (ventilation) when transthoracic impedance is least.
- *Note:* patients with COPD or significant asthma with lung hyper-expansion (gas trapping) often require higher than normal energy levels for successful defibrillation.
- **Choose the correct energy:**
  - Biphasic (modern) defibrillators—use 150–200 J for each shock.

Defibrillation technique

Manual defibrillation with self-adhesive pads (*preferred* to paddles)
- Place self-adhesive pads on chest (as above).
- Turn defibrillator on, observe ECG trace and identify rhythm.
- Select energy level.
- Charge. Once the defibrillator is charged, state loudly: '*Stop CPR and move away.*' Visually confirm the shockable rhythm is still present.
- Check that no personnel are in physical contact with the patient or bed and state loudly: '*Delivering shock.*'
- Press 'Shock' on the defibrillator. Immediately state loudly '*Recommence CPR*' without checking the rhythm or pulse.

Manual defibrillation with paddles
- Review ECG trace on monitor and identify rhythm.
- Attach gel pads or electrode jelly to chest wall.
- Turn on defibrillator and select required energy level.
- Put paddles on patient's chest.
- Charge using 'Charge' button on right-hand (apex) paddle. Once the defibrillator is charged, state loudly: '*Stop CPR and move away.*'
- Check that no personnel are in physical contact with the patient or bed and state loudly: '*Delivering shock.*'
- Discharge pads with 'Shock' button on paddles. Immediately state loudly '*Recommence CPR*' without checking the rhythm or pulse.

Complications

- Burns to skin
- Myocardial injury to epicardial and subepicardial tissue
- Post-defibrillation arrhythmias
- Pacemaker malfunction (avoid area)
- Electrical injury to bystanders
- Failure (check correct charge was set, correct pressure applied if using paddles, charge was actually delivered i.e. tonic patient muscle contraction)
  - Consider anteroposterior pad or paddle placement

64

Electrical cardioversion (DC reversion)

Indications

- Emergency treatment of a haemodynamically unstable patient (hypotension, SOB, chest pain) with tachyarrhythmia.
- Elective treatment of a stable patient with a tachyarrhythmia such as new-onset atrial fibrillation within previous 24–48 hours (do *not* revert if onset is longer or unknown).
- In both cases, an electrical current is applied across the chest and is synchronised with the R wave of the ECG to reduce the risk of precipitating VF, if the shock was delivered in the relative refractory period of the cardiac cycle (i.e. with the T wave).

Contraindications

- Sinus tachycardia
- Multifocal atrial tachycardia

Procedural technique

- Explain the procedure to the patient.
- Enquire about fasting status (relative contraindication to elective treatment only).
- Use procedural sedation such as low-dose propofol 0.5–1.0 mg/kg or fentanyl 0.5 microgram/kg plus midazolam 0.05 mg/kg titrated to effect for conscious patients undergoing elective cardioversion (less if shocked).
- Technique is similar to that for defibrillation, except that the defibrillator is set to 'Synchronised' mode so that the shock is delivered with the R wave.
- Energy requirements are less than those required when defibrillating to terminate VF.
  - Atrial fibrillation (AF)
    - Biphasic waveform: 120–150 J.

- Atrial flutter and paroxysmal SVT other than AF
  — Biphasic: 70–120 J.
- Stable monomorphic VT
  — Biphasic: 120–150 J for the initial shock.

Complications

These are essentially the same as for defibrillation:
- Pain if inadequately sedated
- Burns to skin
- Myocardial injury to epicardial and subepicardial tissue if shocks repeated
- Pacemaker malfunction (avoid area)
- Electrical injury to bystanders
- Failure (check correct charge was set, correct pressure applied if using paddles, charge was actually delivered i.e. tonic patient muscle contraction).
    - Consider anteroposterior pad or paddle placement.
- *Note:* remember to switch off the 'Synchronised' mode if the arrhythmia deteriorates into VF and immediate defibrillation is needed.

65

Transthoracic cardiac pacing

Indications

- Symptomatic bradycardia with a palpable pulse in a patient who has not responded to pharmacological therapy.
- High-grade AV block.
- Cardiac arrest with ventricular standstill, but atrial activity present.

Contraindication

- Asystolic cardiac arrest

Procedural technique

- Explain to the patient what you are about to do and why. Provide supplemental oxygen and gain IV access.
- Ensure that the skin is clean, dry and shaven to allow electrical contact.
- Some patients require sedation to tolerate the discomfort associated with pacing, especially if higher currents are needed. Use fentanyl 0.5 microgram/kg plus midazolam 0.05 mg/kg titrated to effect.
- Sandwich the heart between an anterior electrode (placed over the praecordium to the left of the sternum) and a posterior electrode (placed between the left scapula and the vertebral column). Ventricular pacing may also be done using standard anterior pad placement as per defibrillation.
- Set the defibrillator to 'Pacing' mode—once the pacing option is activated, ensure that the monitor is sensing any intrinsic QRS complexes, signalled by a marker on the monitor.
- Select the pacing rate: usually 60–80 beats/min.
- Select the pacing current: start at 5 mA and increase in increments of 5 mA until electrical capture is visible on the ECG monitor. Capture generally occurs at 50–80 mA.

- As the current rises and electrical capture with a ventricular contraction occurs, the monitor will start to show QRS–T complexes after each pacing spike.
- Check that mechanical capture is also occurring by palpating the patient's pulse.
- Set the current at least 5 mA above the minimum current at which capture occurs.

Complications

- Failure to capture.
- Patient discomfort, so ensure adequate analgesia and sedation.
- Failure to recognise fine VF because of the size of the pacing artefact on the ECG screen. Palpate the pulse and/or look for absence of signs of life.
- Occurrence of another arrhythmia.

Central venous cannulation

This procedure can be associated with significant complications and must always be performed under supervision until competence is attained. In addition, the use of ultrasound guidance is now the 'standard of care' at the bedside.

Commonly used sites are the femoral vein, internal jugular vein (IJV) and subclavian vein. All are all located close to arteries and nerves that may be damaged by a misplaced needle. In addition, the subclavian vein lies near the pleura of the lung, so there is a risk of pneumothorax.

The same basic principles, techniques and equipment are required for all sites. The specific anatomical considerations and complications for each site are considered individually.

Indications

- IV administration of specific drugs (e.g. noradrenaline or adrenaline).
- Inability to obtain timely, adequate peripheral IV access in the critically unwell patient.
- Central venous pressure monitoring.
- Haemodialysis or plasmapharesis.
- Hyperalimentation such as TPN administration.
- Long-term chemotherapy, antibiotic therapy or administration of other medications (Hickman line or portacath, which are inserted operatively in a fully sterile environment).
- Cardiopulmonary resuscitation, usually to deliver post-resuscitation care.

Contraindications

- Uncooperative patient
- Inexperienced, unsupervised proceduralist
- Less invasive forms of IV access are possible and adequate

- Overlying cellulitis or skin burn
- Uncorrected bleeding diathesis (especially for a subclavian line, as it cannot be easily compressed)

Equipment

- Tilting trolley or bed
- Comprehensive non-invasive monitoring equipment
- Portable ultrasound machine with vascular probe
- Sterile drape and dressing pack, including gown
- Surgical facemask
- Appropriate central venous cannula (CVC) complete with preprepared insertion pack chosen for a particular patient, duration and purpose. Almost all types use the Seldinger insertion technique (see below).
- Needles: 25G×1, 21G×1
- Syringes: 5 mL×2, 10 mL×2, 20 mL×1
- Lignocaine 1% or 2%
- 10 mL sodium chloride 0.9% for injection
- Skin-cleansing solution (e.g. chlorhexidine)
- Swabs
- Forceps
- Tape
- Disposable scalpel
- Suture set
- Suture material (e.g. 4/0 nylon)
- Sterile occlusive, transparent dressing (e.g. Opsite)
- IV bungs ×3
- Primed IV fluid line with 500 mL normal saline

Procedural technique (Seldinger)

- Confirm with a senior doctor that central venous access is definitely needed, select the most appropriate route, explain the procedure to the patient and obtain verbal consent.
- Have a trolley ready with all sterile contents laid out. Position the patient for the specific route chosen and identify the anatomical landmarks and then use ultrasound guidance.
- Wash your hands well and put on sterile gown and gloves. Use a strict aseptic technique to prepare and check central line equipment, in particular that the guidewire passes through the large-bore needle.
- Use the 10 mL syringe to draw up 10 mL normal saline and prime all the central venous cannula ports and tubing with saline.
- Use the 5 mL syringe to prepare the 1% lignocaine local anaesthetic, and cap with a sheathed 25G needle.

- Cleanse a wide area of skin around the insertion site with chlorhexidine on a swab held with a pair of forceps. Use a circular motion, commencing at the insertion site and working from the inside out (i.e. do not return to a previously swabbed area).
- Dispose of swab away from sterile area and repeat. Cover the sterile area with a large fenestrated drape.
- Infiltrate the skin and deeper tissues with local anaesthetic. Work around the site and towards the vein. Remember to draw back on the plunger before injecting each time to ensure that the vein has not been penetrated.
- Attach a syringe to the large-bore insertion needle and insert through the needle into the skin. Aspirate gently while advancing the needle until the central vein is entered.
- Once in the vein, ensure that you can easily aspirate blood. Remove the syringe and thread the guidewire down through the needle and into the vein. The wire should advance easily and need no force. Insert 10–15 cm of guidewire into the vein (the mean distance from skin to right atrium is 18 cm in adults). Do not over-insert the wire, as it may cause cardiac arrhythmias, kink or even perforate the vessel wall.
- Use one hand to secure the guidewire at all times, and remove the needle. Make a 2–3 mm skin incision where the wire penetrates the skin.
- Thread the dilator over the wire and into the vein with a light twisting motion. Push it firmly through the skin as far as it will go.
- Remove the dilator, being careful not to dislodge the guidewire.
- Now thread the CVC over the guidewire towards the skin. Hold the catheter steady when the tip is 2 cm above the surface of the skin and slowly reverse the guidewire up the catheter tube away from the patient, until the wire tip appears from the line port (i.e. the central brown port).
- Holding the proximal portion of the wire protruding from the catheter port, advance the catheter through the skin down the guidewire and into the vein. Do not allow the wire to be pushed further into the vein while advancing the catheter.
- Withdraw the wire and close off the insertion port. Check that blood can be aspirated freely from all lumens of the catheter and then flush each with saline.
- Secure the catheter in place with sutures and cover with a sterile dressing. Tape any redundant tubing, carefully avoiding kinking or loops that may snag and pull the catheter out.
- With IJV and subclavian lines, order a CXR to confirm the position of the catheter tip and to exclude a pneumo-, hydro- or haemothorax. The tip of the CVP line should lie in the superior vena cava just above its junction with the right atrium, around the level of the carina.

SECTION E – Practical procedures

Femoral vein

Advantages
- Rapid, easy access with a high success rate, even in inexperienced hands.
- Does not interfere with airway management or other resuscitation processes.
- No risk of pneumothorax.
- Easy to control haemorrhage with direct pressure.

Disadvantages
- Infection and thrombosis are the most common problems, so is not recommended for long-term use >24 hours.
- Reduces patient's mobility.
- Easily dislodged.

Contraindications
- Vascular insufficiency or trauma on the same side as the line is to be inserted.
- If CVP monitoring is required.
- Pelvic trauma or significant intra-abdominal injury.

Anatomy
- The femoral vein lies approximately 1 cm medial to the femoral artery within the femoral triangle of the upper thigh. The femoral artery is usually found midway along the inguinal ligament, and should be easily palpable in the groin.
- Access the vein below the level of the inguinal ligament, which runs between the anterior superior iliac spine and the pubic tubercle, to avoid inadvertently entering the peritoneal cavity.
- The femoral nerve lies lateral to the femoral artery (VAN = vein, artery, nerve from medial to lateral) (see Figure 52.1).

Procedural technique
- Lie the patient supine, with the leg slightly abducted and externally rotated.
- Palpate the femoral artery 2 fingerbreadths below the inguinal ligament using your non-dominant hand. Ideally use ultrasound guidance, although this site is the safest on which to use the landmark technique alone, when time critical.
- Insert the needle, bevel up, a fingerbreadth **medial** to the femoral pulsation and aim towards the umbilicus at an angle of 20–30 degrees to the skin. In adults, the vein is normally found 2–4 cm beneath the skin.

- Reduce the elevation on the needle to 10–15 degrees in small children as the vein lies more superficially.
- *Note:* keep a finger over the artery during the procedure to reduce the risk of arterial puncture. The right leg is therefore easier to use for the right-handed operator.

Internal jugular vein

Advantages

- Pneumothorax is rare.
- Easy to control haemorrhage with direct pressure.
- Lower incidence of complications compared with the subclavian approach.

Disadvantages

- Carotid artery puncture relatively frequent as the IJV may overlie the carotid artery to some extent in 50% of cases.
- Landmarks are difficult to palpate in obese or oedematous patients.
- Protracted periods of Trendelenburg (head-down) tilt may not be tolerated.
- Access to the IJV may be difficult in patients with a tracheostomy, and is contraindicated in suspected cervical spine trauma.

Anatomy

- The IJV passes vertically down the neck within the carotid sheath, initially lying posterior to the internal carotid artery, before running lateral and then anterolateral to the artery.
- It is most superficial between the heads of the sternocleidomastoid (SCM), then runs deep to join the subclavian vein behind the sternal end of the clavicle.

Procedural technique

- Lie the patient supine with the table tilted head down to enhance central venous distension and reduce the risk of air embolism.
- Turn the patient's head 30–60 degrees to the contralateral side to allow better access to the IJV.
  - *Note:* turning the head too far laterally increases the risk of arterial puncture.
- Stand at the head of the patient and palpate the carotid artery at the level of the cricoid cartilage, at the apex of the triangle formed by the heads of SCM.
- Using ultrasound guidance, insert the needle, bevel up, at an angle of 30–40 degrees 1 fingerbreadth lateral to the artery. Aim for the

vessel seen on the ultrasound screen, which anatomically is towards the ipsilateral nipple in men and the ipsilateral anterior superior iliac spine in women.
- Always direct the needle **away** from the artery.
- The vein is usually only 2–3 cm under the skin, so if the vein is not entered, re-direct the needle tip more laterally.

Subclavian vein

Advantages
- Wide-calibre vein (1–2 cm) in haemodynamically stable patients.
- Not affected by head movement in conscious patients.
- Useful in a trauma patient with suspected cervical spine injury.
- Easy to secure with reduced rate of dislodgement.
- Low infection rate.

Disadvantages
- Increased risk of complications, such as pneumothorax and arterial puncture.
- Haemorrhage from accidental arterial puncture is difficult to control.
- Technically a more difficult ultrasound skill than ultrasound-guided IJV access.

Anatomy
- The subclavian vein is a continuation of the axillary vein, commencing at the lower border of the first rib and draining blood from the arm.
- It is bounded medially by the posterior border of the SCM muscle, caudally by the middle third of the clavicle and laterally by the anterior border of the trapezius muscle.

Procedural technique
- Lie the patient supine with both arms by the sides and the table tilted head down to distend the central veins and prevent air embolism.
- Turn the head away from the side to be cannulated. Normally, the right subclavian is cannulated. The thoracic duct is on the left and may occasionally be damaged during cannulation, resulting in a chylothorax.
- Access to the vein may be facilitated by caudal traction on the ipsilateral arm, or by placing a roll under the ipsilateral shoulder.
- Stand beside the patient on the side to be cannulated. Identify the mid-clavicular point and the sternal notch. Insert the needle

through the skin 1 cm below and lateral to the mid-clavicular point. Watch its progress on the ultrasound screen.
* Keeping the needle horizontal, advance just under the clavicle, aiming for the sternal notch. If the needle hits the clavicle, 'walk off the bone', moving inferiorly, and direct slightly deeper to pass beneath it, again watching its progress at all times on the ultrasound screen.
* Do not pass the needle further than the sternal head of the clavicle.

Complications

* **Early (immediate):**
    * Arterial puncture
        – Less likely with subclavian route than with IJV or femoral
        – However, haemorrhage from the femoral or carotid artery is much easier to control with direct pressure than haemorrhage from the subclavian artery
    * Arterial dissection, laceration and false aneurysm formation
    * Pneumothorax (particularly subclavian route), haemothorax
    * Cardiac arrhythmia (usually disappears on pulling guidewire back)
    * Malposition of the tip of a subclavian line, which may ascend up into the IJV or horizontally across the midline
    * Injury to surrounding nerves
    * Air embolism
    * Loss of the guidewire (requires radiologically guided removal)
* **Late:**
    * Local infection—more common with femoral access than with IJV or subclavian
    * Systemic infection, bacteraemia and endocarditis—more common with femoral than with IJV, which in turn is more likely than subclavian
    * Venous thrombosis: incidence of proximal venous thrombosis is as high as 10–25% for femoral catheters left in-situ for more than 24 hours
    * Cardiac tamponade
    * Hydrothorax

Treatment

* **Arterial puncture:**
    * Usually obvious, but may be missed in the severely hypotensive or hypoxic patient.
    * Withdraw the needle and apply firm direct pressure to the site for at least 10 minutes, or longer if there is continuing bleeding.

Seek senior assistance, then retry if there is minimal swelling, or change to a different route.

- **Suspected pneumothorax:**
  - Suspect if air is easily aspirated from the syringe or the patient becomes acutely breathless.
  - Stop the procedure and obtain an urgent CXR.
  - If central access is absolutely necessary, try another route *on the same side*, or one or other femoral veins. *Never* attempt either the subclavian or the jugular route on the *other* side, as bilateral pneumothorax may occur.
- **Cardiac arrhythmia:**
  - Usually occurs when the wire or catheter is inserted too far. Withdraw the wire or catheter.

Aftercare (all routes)

Care and use of a central line

- The central line should be connected to a closed infusion system, and accessed as infrequently as possible to minimise the risk of infection.
- Each time the line is accessed, the injection port must be thoroughly swabbed with antiseptic solution, such as chlorhexidine or an alcohol swab.
- When injecting through a central line, it is important to avoid inadvertent introduction of air bubbles.
- Any central line inserted in an emergency situation should be replaced as soon as practically possible, due to the increased risk of infection.

Measuring central venous pressure

- Ensure that the infusion line is patent and that the CVP line is connected to the distal port of the CVC and the infusion solution is a crystalloid.
- Place the patient supine or with bed head up to 45 degrees.
- Measurements may be made using the right atrium as the reference point. Locate the 4th intercostal space at the right mid-axillary line. Place the zero mark at this point.
- Use an electronic invasive monitoring channel if available, and zero the device before displaying CVP trace on the monitor.
- Alter the infusion rate or medications to the prescribed order.

Removing a central venous catheter

- Ensure that the patient's coagulation and platelet profile is within satisfactory limits.

- If sepsis is suspected, obtain the following:
  - Peripheral and CVC blood cultures
  - Swab from entry site if discharge present for culture
  - Catheter tip when removed, to send for culture.
- Turn off and disconnect all infusions.
- Wash hands, put on sterile gloves, remove old dressing and cleanse around the site with chlorhexidine. Remove sutures.
- Instruct the patient to hold a deep breath while the catheter is removed in a slow constant motion for IJV and subclavian lines. This increases intrathoracic pressure and prevents air embolism.
- Apply firm pressure over the exit site with a sterile gauze swab for at least 5 minutes.
- Inspect the catheter for completeness.
- Apply an occlusive dressing over the exit site for 48 hours.

Handy hints

- Do not shave hair at the insertion site unless it interferes with dressing adhesive, as it increases the risk of infection from disruption of the epidermal barrier by microscopic skin lacerations.
- Draw up normal saline in a 10 mL syringe and lignocaine in a 5 mL syringe to ensure that these two agents are not mistaken during the procedure.
- Always use ultrasound guidance and ECG monitoring during insertion of IJV and subclavian lines.

SECTION E – Practical procedures

Formulary

On-call formulary

This formulary is a quick reference for information on medications commonly used by inpatients, or prescribed by the doctor on call. It is not a comprehensive list, but provides information on the common indications, contraindications, actions and adverse reactions of most of the prescribed medications. Short monographs are included for uncommonly used drugs.

The formulary does *not* include drugs usually prescribed in specialist units including general anaesthetic agents, some blood products, vitamins and minerals, vaccines and antivenoms, obstetric and gynaecological medications, antimycobacterials, antiretrovirals, antineoplastics and immunomodulators.

All doses are for adult patients with normal renal and hepatic function, unless otherwise stated. Always check appropriateness in children, potential pregnancy, pregnancy and lactation. Pregnancy risk category is noted in brackets following the drug name, which includes the following notations:

Pregnancy risk categories:
A: Taken by a large number of pregnant or potentially pregnant women with no harm being observed.
B1: Taken by a limited number of pregnant women without evidence of harm. Animal studies have shown no evidence of increased incidence of harm.
B2: Taken by a limited number of pregnant women without evidence of harm. Inadequate animal studies but no evidence of increased incidence of harm.
B3: Taken by a limited number of pregnant women without evidence of harm, but animal studies have shown an increased incidence of harm.
C: Suspected to cause harmful pharmacological effects on the fetus without malformations.
D: Suspected to cause an increased incidence of damage or adverse pharmacological effects to the fetus.
X: High risk of permanent damage to the fetus.

Cardiovascular

- Cardiac arrest
- Antiarrhythmics
- Inotropes, chronotropes and vasopressors
- Hypertension, heart failure, angina
- Drugs affecting blood clotting
- Lipid-modifying drugs

Respiratory and allergy

- Bronchodilators
- Cough medicines
- Antihistamines

Gastrointestinal

- Antiemetics
- Antiulcer drugs
- Antidiarrhoeals, antispasmodics, inflammatory bowel disease
- Laxatives

Neuromuscular

- Analgesics and musculoskeletal drugs
- Antimigraine drugs
- Anticonvulsants
- Neurodegenerative and movement disorders
- Local anaesthetics

Psychotropics

- Sedatives, anxiolytics and drugs for sleep disorders
- Mood disorders
- Antipsychotics
- Drugs for attention-deficit hyperactivity disorder
- Drug-dependence syndromes

Antimicrobials

- Antibacterials
- Antifungals
- Anthelminthics
- Antiprotozoals
- Antivirals

Endocrine

- Diabetes
- Thyroid
- Bone disease
- Other endocrine disorders

Genitourinary

- Drugs affecting bladder function
- Erectile dysfunction

Antidotes

Cardiovascular

Cardiac arrest
Adrenaline (epinephrine)

Indication: Cardiac arrest—give immediately if bradyasystolic rhythm or after the second shock if VF/pVT.

Actions: Non-selective adrenergic agonist causing peripheral vasoconstriction improving efficacy of CPR. Positive inotrope and chronotrope (beta-1 receptors); and bronchodilator plus mast cell stabiliser (beta-2 receptors).

Adverse effects: Not relevant during cardiac arrest, but will cause dilated pupils.

Cautions: Ensure reliable IV access; do not use cardiac arrest dose in a patient with a pulse.

Comments: Can be given via intraosseous route if IV access not available.

Dose: Available in 1 mg ampoules or rapid-access syringes (1:1000 (equivalent 1 mg/mL) and 1:10,000 ampoules (equivalent 0.1 mg/mL) concentrations). *Cardiac arrest:* 1 mg rapid IV (using 1 mL of 1:1000 solution or 10 mL of 1:10,000 solution). This is repeated every 3–5 min followed by a 20 mL normal saline flush to ensure central delivery of the drug.

Amiodarone (see also *Antiarrhythmics*)

Indication: Cardiac arrest—give following 3rd shock in refractory VF/pVT.

Actions: Membrane-stabilising antiarrhythmic.

Adverse effects: Proarrhythmic—may worsen bradyarrhythmias.

Cautions: Thrombophlebitis when injected into a peripheral vein. Not compatible with normal saline.

Comments: Can be given via intraosseous route if IV access not available.
Dose: Available in 150 mg ampoules. *Cardiac arrest:* Give 300 mg IV by bolus injection over 1–2 min if VF/pVT persists after the 3rd shock. Repeat 150 mg dose in 3–5 min if VF/pVT persists.

Calcium

Indication: Cardiac arrest associated with hyperkalaemia (not due to digoxin toxicity), hypocalcaemia, calcium-channel blocker toxicity.
Actions: Stabilises myocardial membrane.
Adverse effects: Not relevant during cardiac arrest.
Cautions: Thrombophlebitis when injected into a peripheral vein. Not compatible with sodium bicarbonate.
Comments: Can be given via intraosseous route if IV access not available.
Dose: Available as 10% calcium chloride (6.8 mmol in 10 mL) and 10% calcium gluconate (2.2 mmol in 10 mL) ampoules. *Cardiac arrest:* 10 mL of Ca chloride or 30 mL of Ca gluconate as rapid IV bolus. Repeat in 3–5 min if no response.

Lignocaine

Indication: Cardiac arrest—give following 3rd shock in refractory VF/pVT if amiodarone unavailable.
Actions: Membrane-stabilising antiarrhythmic.
Adverse effects: Proarrhythmic—may worsen bradyarrhythmias.
Cautions: Nil.
Comments: Can be given via intraosseous route if IV access not available.
Dose: Available in 100 mg ampoules or rapid-access syringes. *Cardiac arrest:* 100 mg rapid IV bolus. Repeat in 3–5 min if no response.

Magnesium

Indication: Cardiac arrest associated with hypomagnesaemia, torsades de pointes or digoxin toxicity. Third-line agent in refractory VF/pVT.
Actions: Stabilises myocardial membrane.
Adverse effects: Not relevant during cardiac arrest.
Cautions: Nil.
Comments: Can be given via intraosseous route if IV access not available.
Dose: Available as 50% magnesium sulfate ampoules (2.5 g/10 mmol in 5 mL). *Cardiac arrest:* 10 mmol rapid IV bolus. Repeat in 3–5 min if no response.

Sodium bicarbonate

Indication: Cardiac arrest associated with hyperkalaemia, sodium-channel blocker toxicity or severe metabolic acidosis.

Actions: Causes intracellular shift of potassium; antidote to sodium-channel toxicity; buffers acidosis.

Adverse effects: May worsen intracellular acidosis.

Cautions: Not compatible with calcium.

Comments: Can be given via intraosseous route if IV access not available.

Dose: Available in 100 mL of 8.4% (100 mmol) ampoules or 50 mL of 8.4% (50 mmol) rapid-access syringes. *Cardiac arrest:* 50 mmol rapid IV bolus. Repeat in 3–5 min if no response.

Antiarrhythmics
Adenosine (B2)

Indication: Narrow-complex paroxysmal supraventricular (re-entry) tachycardia.

Actions: Inhibits AV nodal conduction and increases the AV nodal refractory period.

Adverse effects: Short-lived facial flushing, chest pain, dyspnoea, bronchospasm, choking sensation, nausea, light-headedness; brief periods of asystole or bradycardia. At the time of conversion, a variety of new rhythms may briefly appear on the ECG.

Caution: Contraindicated in patients taking dipyridamole (increases the half-life of adenosine), those with asthma, second- or third-degree AV block and sick sinus syndrome (unless paced). May induce torsades de pointes in patients with a prolonged QT interval and is less effective in patients taking theophylline.

Comments: Must administer with full cardiac monitoring. Verapamil may be preferable in patients with asthma or those who have previously experienced severe adverse effects.

Dose: Available as 6 mg/2 mL ampoules. *PSVT:* 6 mg rapid IV over 2 seconds into a central or large peripheral vein followed immediately with a 20 mL normal saline flush. If necessary give a further 12 mg after 1–2 min, and then 18 mg after a further 1–2 min.

Amiodarone (see also *Cardiac arrest*) (C)

Indications: Rate control of atrial fibrillation/flutter. Haemodynamically stable broad-complex tachycardias. PSVT not reverted with other drugs. Atrial tachycardias.

Actions: Membrane-stabilising antiarrhythmic. Increases the duration of the action potential and refractory period in the atria and ventricles.

Adverse effects: Hypotension, prolongation of QT interval, bradycardia because of excess AV block, cardiac arrest, cardiogenic shock. IV administration may produce vasodilation and hypotension. Multiple adverse effects with chronic use.

Cautions: Thrombophlebitis when injected into a peripheral vein. Use with extreme caution in patients predisposed to bradycardia or AV block. Contraindicated if iodine allergy.

Comments: Monitor the ECG throughout initial administration.

Dose: Available in 150 mg ampoules and 100 mg and 200 mg tablets. *Stable arrhythmias:* Loading dose 150–300 mg diluted in 100 mL 5% dextrose IV over 30–60 min. Maintenance infusion: 900–1200 mg diluted in 500 mL 5% dextrose over 24 h. Commence PO treatment as soon as possible and aim to overlap IV treatment by 2 days. Maximum cumulative dose is 2.2 g/24 h (IV). *Chronic treatment of tachyarrhythmia:* Oral dose is 200 mg TDS for 1 week, followed by 200 mg BD for 1 week. Maintenance dose is 100–400 mg once daily; monitor for adverse effects.

Atropine (A)

Indications: Symptomatic bradycardia; also used in organophosphate poisoning.

Actions: Antimuscarinic; blocks vagal stimuli to heart improving cardiac electrical contraction, particularly of atria.

Adverse effects: Dilated pupils and blurred vision, dry mouth, flushing, urinary retention, constipation. Large doses may cause anticholinergic delirium, tachycardia.

Cautions: Contraindicated in glaucoma, urinary or gastrointestinal obstruction, myasthenia gravis.

Comments: Maximum dose 3 mg (complete vagolytic dose), but most patients who improve will respond to 1.2–1.8 mg.

Dose: Commonly available in 600 microgram, 1.2 mg ampoules or 1 mg rapid-access syringes. *Bradyarrhythmias:* 1.2 mg IV bolus followed by 600 microgram IV boluses until acceptable improvement in heart rate.

Beta-adrenergic blockers

See *Antihypertensives.*

Calcium-channel blockers

See *Antihypertensives.*

Digoxin (A)

Indications: Rate control in AF or atrial flutter. Heart failure, especially if associated with chronic AF.

Actions: Mildly increases force of myocardial contraction and decreases AV nodal conduction, predominantly by vagotonic effect.

Adverse effects: Serious adverse effects, including worsening of the arrhythmia (proarrhythmic effect). Common—anorexia, nausea, vomiting, diarrhoea, blurred vision, visual disturbances with yellow vision (chromatopsia), confusion, drowsiness, dizziness, nightmares, agitation, depression.

Cautions: Do not give in: second- or third-degree heart block without pacemaker; SVT mediated by a bypass tract (WPW syndrome); ventricular tachycardia; HCM. Caution in renal failure. Halve the loading and maintenance dose in the elderly and those with renal impairment.

Comments: Narrow therapeutic margin. Adverse effects are related to the plasma concentration, and are rare if <0.8 microgram/L. Onset of effect occurs 4–6 h after initial oral dose. Characteristic changes to the ECG, such as a prolonged PR interval, ST depression or T wave inversion ('reverse tick' T waves).

Dose: Available in 500 microgram ampoules, and 62.5 microgram and 250 microgram tablets. Loading: 250–500 microgram PO or IV 4–6-hourly, to a maximum of 1.5 mg. Only necessary if acute rate control required. IV administration offers little therapeutic advantage over oral dosing, but increases risk of adverse effects. Maintenance: 125–250 microgram PO once daily. Tailor dose according to renal function, clinical response and therapeutic drug monitoring.

Lignocaine (see also *Cardiac arrest*) (A)

Indication: Ventricular arrhythmias, if amiodarone unavailable or ineffective.

Actions: Lengthens the effective refractory period in the ventricular conducting system, decreases ventricular automaticity and stablises potentially excitable membranes, preventing initiation and transmission of nerve impulses.

Adverse effects: Nausea, vomiting, dizziness, paraesthesia or drowsiness, particularly if too rapid injection. Other CNS effects with toxicity include confusion, respiratory depression, convulsions and hypotension with bradycardia leading to cardiac arrest.

Cautions: Proarrhythmic. Contraindicated in bradyarrhythmias and known lignocaine or amide local anaesthetic hypersensitivity.

Comments: Lower maintenance dose in the elderly. Avoid in patients with CCF, liver disease or hypotension.

Dose: Available in 100 mg ampoules or rapid-access syringes. *Ventricular tachyarrhythmia without shock:* 100 mg IV bolus over a few minutes followed by IV infusion of 4 mg/min for 30 min, 2 mg/min for 2 h, then 1 mg/min. Reduce concentration further if infusion continued beyond 24 h. ECG monitoring is essential.

Magnesium sulfate (see also *Cardiac arrest*) (A)

Indications: Arrhythmias associated with hypomagnesaemia, hypokalaemia; digitalis-induced arrhythmias; torsades de pointes (polymorphic VT), third-line agent in rate control in AF/atrial flutter or rhythm control in PSVT. Also used in severe asthma, and pre-eclampsia.

Actions: Influences Na^+/K^+ ATPase, sodium channels, certain potassium and calcium channels. It is effectively a 'physiological calcium antagonist'.

Adverse effects: Hypotension, flushing and headache with too-rapid IV infusion.

Cautions: May exacerbate heart block. Excessive administration results in hypermagnesaemia, causing predictable nausea, vomiting, flushing, hypotension, muscle weakness, muscle paralysis, blurred or double vision, CNS and respiratory depression and loss of reflexes as the serum level increases. Use with caution in renal failure, because of accumulation.

Comments: Hypokalaemia is often associated with hypomagnesaemia and requires magnesium replacement to help retain supplemental potassium. *Note:* The total adult dose should not exceed 30–40 g of magnesium sulfate per day.

Dose: Available as 50% magnesium sulfate ampoules (2.5 g/10 mmol in 5 mL).

Give 1.25–2.5 g IV diluted in 5% dextrose over 20 min. In emergency situations such as polymorphic VT, this dose can be given over 1–2 min. If an infusion is required, the usual dose is 1 g per hour.

- **Disopyramide:** Sodium-channel blocking agent used for rate or rhythm control of atrial or ventricular tachyarrhythmias.
- **Flecainide:** Sodium-channel blocking agent used for rate or rhythm control of atrial tachyarrhythmias; used under specialist supervision only.

Inotropes, chronotropes and vasopressors
Adrenaline (see also *Cardiac arrest*) (A)

Indications: Chronotropic support for symptomatic bradycardia (after trial of atropine). Inotropic and vasopressor support in acute heart failure, cardiogenic shock, anaphylactic shock and septic shock; severe bronchospasm; anaphylaxis.

Actions: Non-selective adrenergic agonist. Positive inotrope and chronotrope (beta-1 receptors). Vasodilator at low dose (beta-2 receptors); vasoconstrictor at high dose (alpha receptors). Bronchodilation (beta-2 receptors). Mast cell stabiliser.

Adverse effects: Anxiety, headache, palpitations, tachycardia, restlessness, tremor, dizziness, dyspnoea, weakness, sweating, pallor, hypertension, hyperglycaemia. **Overdose or too-rapid IV administration:** arrhythmias (ventricular and supraventricular), severe hypertension, cerebral haemorrhage and pulmonary oedema. Extravasation causes necrosis of surrounding tissue, so preferably given via CVC.

Cautions: Correct hypovolaemia before use in circulatory shock. Contraindicated in uncontrolled hypertension, phaeochromocytoma, tachyarrhythmias, thyrotoxicosis. Do not give a full cardiac arrest dose to a patient with a pulse, but use small boluses only.

Comments: IV adrenaline in conscious patients should only be administered by experienced physicians when continuous cardiac and BP monitoring are available. Different hospitals and departments will have their own administration protocols.

Dose: Available in 1 mg ampoules or rapid-access syringes (1:1000 [equivalent 1 mg/mL]) and 1:10,000 ampoules (equivalent 0.1 mg/mL). *Circulatory shock, symptomatic bradycardias, severe bronchospasm, anaphylaxis:* Place 2 mg (1 mL of 1:1000) of adrenaline in 500 mL of normal saline and administer IV infusion at an initial rate of 30 mL/h (approx 2 microgram/min). Titrate this every 5–10 min according to clinical response. Alternatively, dilute 1 mg (1 mL) of 1:1000 solution in 20 mL normal saline and carefully give 0.5–1 mL (25–50 micrograms) IV boluses every 2–3 min.

Dobutamine (B2)

Indications: Inotropic support in acute heart failure, cardiogenic shock.

Actions: Catecholamine with beta-adrenergic effects (predominantly beta-1) causing increased myocardial contractility with peripheral vasodilation.

Adverse effects: Headache, dizziness, tachycardia, tremor, flushing.

Cautions: Ensure hypovolaemia corrected prior to use, because the beta effects cause vasodilation and may worsen hypotension.

Comments: Should only be used as a titrated infusion and administered by experienced physicians when continuous cardiac and BP monitoring are available. Different hospitals and departments will have their own administration protocols.

Dose: Available in 250 mg ampoules. *Cardiogenic shock:* Place 250 mg in 500 mL of normal saline and administer IV infusion at an initial rate of 25 mL/h (approx 3 microgram/kg/min). Titrate this every 5–10 min according to clinical response.

Dopamine (B3)

Indications: Chronotropic support for symptomatic bradycardia (in place of adrenaline). Inotropic and vasopressor support in acute heart failure, cardiogenic shock, septic chock.

Actions: Catecholamine with dopaminergic, beta-1-adrenergic and alpha-adrenergic effects. Positive inotrope and chronotrope from rates of 2 microgram/kg/min; vasoconstrictor from rates of 5 microgram/kg/min.

Adverse effects: Common—ectopic beats, nausea, vomiting, tachycardia, angina, palpitations, dyspnoea, headache, hypotension if volume depleted and at low doses, or hypertension.

Cautions: As per adrenaline.

Comments: Should only be used as a titrated infusion and administered by experienced physicians when continuous cardiac and BP monitoring is available. Different hospitals and departments will have their own administration protocols.

Dose: Available in 200 mg ampoules. *Circulatory shock; symptomatic bradycardias:* Place 200 mg in 500 mL of normal saline and administer IV infusion at an initial rate of 20 mL/h (approx 2 microgram/kg/min). Titrate this every 5–10 min according to clinical response.

Isoprenaline (A)

Indications: Chronotropic support for transient episodes of heart block not requiring pacemaker. May be used to initially overdrive pace torsades de pointes.

Actions: Predominant beta-2-adrenergic agonist with marked chronotropic effects.

Adverse effects: Headache, dizziness, tachycardia, tremor, flushing.

Cautions: Ensure hypovolaemia corrected prior to use, because the beta effects cause vasodilation and may worsen hypotension. Avoid in digitalis toxicity and recent MI or angina (increases myocardial oxygen demand). ECG monitoring is essential.

Comments: Should only be used as a titrated infusion and administered by experienced physicians when continuous cardiac and BP monitoring are available. Different hospitals and departments will have their own administration protocols.

Dose: Available in 200 microgram and 1 mg ampoules. *Symptomatic bradycardias:* Place 2 mg in 500 mL of normal saline and administer IV infusion at an initial rate of 30 mL/h (approx 2 microgram/min). Titrate this every 5–10 min according to clinical response.

Noradrenaline (A)

Indications: Vasopressor support in distributive shock, particularly septic shock.

Actions: Catecholamine with predominant alpha-adrenergic effects. Potent peripheral vasoconstrictor.

Adverse effects: Common—anxiety, palpitations, headache. Infrequent—hypertension, bradycardia (reflex consequence of increased BP); extravasation may cause tissue necrosis.

Cautions: As per adrenaline.

Comments: Although vasopressors raise the BP, they do so at the expense of perfusion of vital organs such as the kidney and gut mucosa. May be combined with an inotropic vasodilator such as dobutamine. Should only be used as a titrated infusion and administered by experienced physicians when continuous cardiac and BP monitoring are available. Different hospitals and departments will have their own dilution protocols.

Dose: Available in 2 mg ampoules. *Circulatory shock:* Place 2 mg in 500 mL of normal saline and administer IV infusion at an initial rate of 15 mL/h (approx 1 microgram/min). Titrate this every 5–10 min according to clinical response.

- **Ephedrine:** Non-selective catecholamine with similar effects to adrenaline, but less potent and more long-lasting. Usually used as a vasopressor for transient, drug-induced hypotension.
- **Metaraminol:** Catecholamine selective for alpha receptors with similar effects to noradrenaline, but less potent and more longlasting. Commonly used as a vasopressor for transient, drug-induced hypotension. Usually given in 0.5–1 mg titrated IV boluses.
- **Milrinone:** Phosphodiesterase inhibitor with moderate cardiac inotropic effects usually used as an IV infusion for severe chronic heart failure.
- **Phenylephrine:** Catecholamine selective for alpha receptors with similar effects to noradrenaline, but less potent and more long-lasting. Uncommonly used as a vasopressor for transient, drug-induced hypotension.
- **Vasopressin:** Potent peripheral and splanchnic vasoconstrictor used for refractory vasodilatory shock. Available in 20 IU ampoules. Usually given as a continuous IV infusion titrated to cardiovascular parameters in shock refractory to other vasopressors.

Hypertension, heart failure, angina
Angiotensin-converting enzyme (ACE) inhibitors (D)

Indications: One of the first-choice agents for uncomplicated hypertension. Improve LV dysfunction in post-AMI patients. Prevent adverse LV remodelling, delay progression of heart failure, and decrease sudden death and recurrent MI. Also used in asymptomatic LV dysfunction (especially if ejection fraction <40%), CCF, renal disease such as diabetic nephropathy with clinical hypertension, and the prevention of progressive renal failure in patients with persistent proteinuria (>1 g/day).

Actions: Inhibit conversion of angiotensin I to angiotensin II and degradation of bradykinins; decrease levels of aldosterone; and increase levels of bradykinin and vasodilator prostaglandins. Results in reduced vasoconstriction, reduced sodium retention and vasodilation in many vascular beds.

Adverse effects: Hypotension (esp. first dose), cough, hyperkalaemia, headache, dizziness, fatigue, nausea, renal impairment. Cough is probably caused by accumulation of prostaglandins, kinins or substance P, and is often expressed as continuous clearing of the throat. There is no apparent difference in the frequency of cough among the various ACE inhibitors.

Cautions: Cease potassium supplements and potassium-sparing diuretics and check renal function before starting therapy. Significant hypotension occurs in patients with dehydration, hypovolaemia, aortic or mitral valve stenosis, or cardiac outflow tract obstruction, particularly with the first dose. Hyperkalaemia occurs in patients with renal impairment, hypovolaemia, renal artery stenosis, or if taking NSAIDs, potassium supplements or potassium-sparing diuretics. Onset of ACE-inhibitor-associated angio-oedema (can be oral, facial, abdominal etc) usually occurs in the first weeks of use, but may be delayed up to 1–2 years after commencing.

Comments: Claimed advantages for specific ACE inhibitors are based on pharmacokinetic, metabolic or tissue ACE-binding characteristics; however, these do not translate into significant clinical differences. Start with low-dose oral administration, especially in the elderly, who are more predisposed to first-dose hypotension and hyperkalaemia. Halve initial dose if: patient already taking diuretics; ACE inhibitor is in a combination medicine with a diuretic; patient is hyponatraemic, has renal impairment or is elderly (>65 years). ACE inhibitor/calcium-channel blocker combination tablets are not used to initiate therapy.

Drug	Usual initial adult dose	Maximum adult dose
Captopril	6.25 mg TDS	50 mg TDS
Enalapril	2.5 mg BD	40 mg once daily or 20 mg BD
Fosinopril	10 mg once daily	40 mg once daily
Lisinopril	5 mg once daily	40 mg once daily
Perindopril	4 or 5 mg once daily	8 or 10 mg once daily
Quinapril	5 mg once daily	40 mg once daily or 20 mg BD
Ramipril	2.5 mg once daily	10 mg once daily
Trandolapril	0.5 mg once daily	4 mg once daily

Angiotensin II receptor blockers (ARBs, sartans) (D)

Indications: As per ACE inhibitors.

Actions: Block angiotensin receptor and have similar actions to ACE inhibitors but are less likely to inhibit degradation of bradykinins. Can be tried in patients with ACE inhibitor-induced cough, or in addition to ACE inhibitors for intractable heart failure, although adding an aldosterone antagonist is preferred.

Adverse effects: As per ACE inhibitors, but less likely to cause angio-oedema or cough.

Cautions: As per ACE inhibitors.

Comments: As per ACE inhibitors.

Drug	Usual initial adult dose	Maximum adult dose
Candesartan	4 mg once daily	32 mg once daily
Eprosartan	400 mg once daily	800 mg once daily
Irbesartan	150 mg once daily	300 mg once daily
Losartan	50 mg once daily or 25 mg BD	100 mg once daily
Olmesartan	20 mg once daily	40 mg once daily
Telmisartan	40 mg once daily	80 mg once daily
Valsartan	80 mg once daily or 40 mg BD	160 mg BD

Beta-adrenergic blockers (C)

Indications: Reduce cardiovascular morbidity and mortality in hypertension and ACS (acute and long-term treatment). Also used for rate control in tachyarrhythmias. Used as adjunct in controlled heart failure, phaeochromocytoma with concurrent alpha-blocker treatment, and diastolic heart dysfunction. Propranolol used for migraine prophylaxis (or atenolol), essential tremor, tetralogy of Fallot, thyrotoxicosis, HCM.

Actions: Antihypertensive effect of reducing cardiac output by reducing contractility of the myocardium and the heart rate, without increasing peripheral vascular resistance. Antianginal effect because of reduction in left ventricular work and oxygen use. Antiarrhythmic effect because of depressed sinus node function and AVN conduction, and prolonged atrial refractory periods.

Adverse effects: Hypotension, bradycardia, bronchospasm, nausea, fatigue, nightmares; alteration in glucose metabolism, blunts sympathetic symptoms in diabetic hypoglycaemia; cool peripheries. Adverse-effect profile depends on relative cardioselectivity and lipid solubility.

SECTION F – Formulary

Cautions: Contraindicated in asthma and COPD; bradyarrhythmias, shock, uncontrolled heart failure. Cardioselective agents are useful in patients with peripheral vascular disease. Withdraw treatment slowly when ceasing.

Comments: Start with a small dose and increase as required. Use predominantly renal-excreted beta-blockers in hepatic failure, and vice versa, or adjust doses accordingly.

Drug	Usual initial adult dose	Maximum adult dose	Comments
Atenolol	25 mg daily	200 mg once daily or 100 mg BD	Renal elimination; cardioselective, used for hypertension, IHD, AF rate control.
Bisoprolol	1.25 mg once daily	10 mg once daily	Hepatic and renal elimination; highly cardioselective; useful adjunct in heart failure.
Carvedilol	3.125 mg BD	25 mg BD	Hepatic elimination; non-selective with some alpha-receptor blockade; useful adjunct in heart failure.
Esmolol	500 microgram IV bolus over 1 min, followed by 40 microgram/min infusion.	Complex IV dose titration	Cardioselective; extremely short half-life. IV administration under specialist supervision only.
Labetalol	100 mg BD	600 mg QID	Hepatic elimination; non-selective with alpha-receptor blockade, used for hypertension.
Metoprolol	25 mg BD PO Available in 5 mg ampoules: give slow 2.5 mg IV boluses every 5–10 min up to 10 mg	150 mg BD PO	Hepatic elimination; cardioselective, used for hypertension, IHD, AF rate control. Extended-release preparation useful adjunct in heart failure. IV administration for tachyarrhythmia rate control (including in acute thyrotoxicosis) requires ECG and BP monitoring under specialist supervision.

Drug	Usual initial adult dose	Maximum adult dose	Comments
Nebivolol	1.25 mg daily	10 mg daily	Renal and hepatic clearance. Used for heart failure but less evidence of benefit than other beta-blockers
Oxprenolol	20 mg BD or TDS	160 mg BD	Hepatic elimination; non-selective, used for hypertension.
Pindolol	5 mg once daily	10 mg TDS	Hepatic and renal elimination; non-selective, used for hypertension.
Propranolol	20 mg BD or TDS	80 mg QID	Hepatic elimination; non-selective; readily crosses blood–brain barrier.
Sotalol	80 mg BD PO Available in 40 mg ampoules.	320 mg BD	Renal elimination; non-selective; proarrhythmic; potassium-channel blocking effects, so used predominantly for rate or rhythm control of atrial tachyarrhythmias under specialist supervision only.

Calcium-channel blockers (C)

Indications: Hypertension, angina, some supraventricular arrhythmias.

Actions: Inhibit calcium influx into cells in vascular smooth muscle, myocardium and cardiac conduction system. Dihydropyridines act predominantly as peripheral vasodilators; verapamil acts predominantly on cardiac muscle and conducting system; diltiazem acts on both.

Adverse effects: Adverse-effect profile varies according to the relative effects on vascular, myocardial and conducting tissue. Common— hypotension, flushing, dizziness, GI upset, headache, peripheral oedema, constipation (verapamil).

Cautions: Cardiogenic shock, sick sinus syndrome, bradyarrhythmias, hepatic impairment, elderly.

Comments: Absorption is highly variable. The absorption of dihydropyridines is significantly enhanced by grapefruit juice.

Drug	Usual initial adult dose	Maximum adult dose	Comments
Amlodipine	2.5 mg once daily	10 mg once daily	Dihydropyridine
Diltiazem	180 mg once daily for extended-release capsules	360 mg once daily for extended-release capsules	Useful for hypertension. Can also be used for chronic rate control of AF, or for ACS in patients unable to tolerate beta-blockers.
Felodipine	2.5 mg once daily for extended-release tablets	20 mg once daily for extended-release tablets	Dihydropyridine
Lercanidipine	10 mg once daily	20 mg once daily	Dihydropyridine
Nifedipine	10 mg BD or 30 mg once daily for controlled-release tablets	40 mg BD or 120 mg once daily for controlled-release tablets	Dihydropyridine
Nimodipine	30–60 mg 4-hourly PO. May follow an initial IV infusion. Treatment duration 10–14 days		Dihydropyridine used to prevent vasospasm post-SAH. Use under specialist supervision only.
Verapamil	40 mg BD or TDS or 120 mg once daily for sustained-release tablets. Available in 5 mg ampoules: give slow 2.5 mg IV boluses every 5–10 min up to 15 mg.	160 mg TDS or 240 mg BD for sustained-release tablets	Useful for hypertension. Can also be used for chronic rate control of AF, or for ACS in patients unable to tolerate beta-blockers. IV preparation useful for rhythm control of PSVT in patients unable to tolerate adenosine, or in acute rate control of AF in patients unable to tolerate beta-blockers; requires ECG and BP monitoring.

Clonidine (B3)

Indications: Acute and chronic hypertension, opioid withdrawal, perioperative sedation, migraine prophylaxis. May be useful in amphetamine intoxication, neuropathic pain, insomnia, ADHD.

Actions: Central alpha-2 adrenergic agonist, stimulating the presynaptic receptors of the vasomotor centre in the brainstem to decrease sympathetic tone.

Adverse effects: Common—drowsiness, dry mouth, constipation, fatigue.

Cautions: Bradyarrhythmias, sick sinus syndrome; do not cease abruptly.

Comments: Potentiates other antihypertensives and sedatives.

Dose: Available in 100 microgram and 150 microgram tablets, 150 microgram ampoules. *Migraine prophylaxis:* Commence at 25 micrograms BD PO and titrate to maximum 75 micrograms BD PO. *Chronic hypertension:* Commence at 75 micrograms BD PO and titrate up to maximum 300 micrograms TDS PO. Acute IV administration: Slow IV bolus over 5 min of 100–300 micrograms every 3 h until effect achieved.

Diuretics—loop (C)

Indications: Oedema associated with heart failure, hepatic cirrhosis, renal impairment and nephrotic syndrome. Severe hypercalcaemia, in combination with IV rehydration.

Actions: Inhibit reabsorption of sodium and chloride in the ascending limb of the loop of Henle. Intense diuresis with a short duration of action of 4–6 h.

Adverse effects: Electrolyte disturbances, dehydration, hyperuricaemia, gout, dizziness, orthostatic hypotension, syncope, renal impairment or anuria, ototoxicity.

Cautions: Severe sodium and fluid depletion from excessive or prolonged use, or if used together with thiazide diuretics (synergistic effect). Caution if patient is allergic to sulfonamides because frusemide and many other diuretics contain a sulfa moiety. Monitor weight and electrolytes. IV administration has a greater risk of electrolyte disturbance, hearing loss, renal impairment. Ethacrynic acid more ototoxic.

Comments: 1 mg bumetanide, or 50 mg ethacrynic acid, or 20 mg IV frusemide are equivalent to 40 mg oral frusemide.

Drug	Usual initial adult dose	Maximum adult dose
Frusemide	20 mg once daily PO	500 mg BD PO
Bumetanide	0.5 mg once daily	5 mg BD
Ethacrynic acid	50 mg once daily	200 mg BD

SECTION F – Formulary

Diuretics—potassium-sparing and aldosterone antagonists (B3; amiloride C)

Indications: See table below.

Actions: Inhibit sodium absorption in the distal tubule either by blocking sodium channels (amiloride, triamterene) or antagonising aldosterone (spironolactone, eplerenone). Interfere with sodium/potassium exchange and reduce urinary potassium excretion. Useful in severe heart or hepatic failure, hypertension.

Adverse effects: Gynaecomastia, breast pain, menstrual abnormalities, sexual dysfunction (aldosterone antagonists); drowsiness, headache, blood dyscrasias, hyperkalaemia, renal impairment, muscle cramps, nausea, vomiting, weakness, hypotension.

Cautions: Severe renal impairment and anuria. Monitor electrolytes. Avoid aldosterone antagonsists in Addison's disease.

Drug	Usual initial adult dose	Maximum adult dose	Comments
Amiloride	5 mg once daily	10 mg BD	Usually combined with a hydrochlorothiazide diuretic. Used for diuretic-associated hypokalaemia, oedema associated with heart or hepatic failure, hypertension.
Triamterene	50 mg once daily	100 mg BD	Used as combination medicine with hydrochlorothiazide to prevent diuretic-associated hypokalaemia.
Spironolactone	25 mg once daily	200 mg once daily or 100 mg BD	Used for oedema in heart failure, hepatic failure, renal failure; hypertension; hyperaldosteronism; prevent diuretic-associated hypokalaemia; female hirsutism.
Eplerenone	25 mg once daily	50 mg once daily	Used for cardiovascular death risk reduction post-MI.

Diuretics—thiazide type (C)

Indications: Mild-to-moderate hypertension. Oedema associated with heart or hepatic failure.

Actions: Inhibit reabsorption of sodium and chloride in the distal convoluted tubule. Also have a mild vasodilator effect.

Adverse effects: Common—dizziness, weakness, muscle cramps, polyuria, orthostatic hypotension, electrolyte disturbances.

Cautions: Addison's disease, severe renal impairment and anuria, gout.

Comments: Use the lowest dose to reduce metabolic adverse effects. Higher doses increase this risk without additional antihypertensive effect. Synergistic with loop diuretics short term in patients with severe heart failure to augment the diuresis.

Drug	Usual initial adult dose	Maximum adult dose
Indapamide	1.25 mg once daily	2.5 mg once daily
Hydrochlorothiazide	12.5 mg once daily	50 mg once daily
Chlorthalidone	12.5 mg once daily	50 mg once daily

Glyceryl trinitrate (GTN) (B2; isosorbide dinitrate B1; isosorbide mononitrate B2)

Indications: Acute relief of angina (short-acting preparations); adjunct for treatment of IHD or chronic LVF (long-acting preparations); acute LVF (IV preparation); malignant hypertension (IV preparation).

Actions: Provides exogenous source of nitric oxide, causing venodilation. Reduces venous return and thus cardiac preload, reducing myocardial oxygen requirement.

Adverse effects: Common—headache, flushing, palpitations, orthostatic hypotension, syncope, peripheral oedema.

Cautions: Hypotension (do not give if SBP <90 mmHg), hypovolaemia, HCM, cardiac tamponade, aortic or mitral stenosis, cor pulmonale, marked anaemia, raised ICP.

Comments: Nitrate tolerance may develop with prolonged, continuous administration; attempt a daily period free of drug if possible. Avoid use with other potent vasodilators such as sildenafil (Viagra).

Drug	Usual initial adult dose	Maximum adult dose
GTN tablets	300–600 microgram SL to relieve angina	Can repeat dose every 5 min to max. of 1800 microgram SL if tolerated by BP
GTN spray	400 microgram SL to relieve angina	Can repeat dose every 5 min up to max. of 1600 microgram SL if tolerated by BP
GTN patch	5 mg or 24 h patch once daily	15 mg or 24 h patch once daily

Continued

SECTION F – Formulary

Drug	Usual initial adult dose	Maximum adult dose
Glyceryl trinitrate (GTN) injection	Available in 50 mg ampoules: Dilute 50 mg in 100 mL of 5% dextrose and commence infusion at 1 mL/h (500 microgram/h)	Increase dose by 1–2 mL/h every 5 min to max. of 20 mL/h (10 mg/h)
Isosorbide dinitrate	5 mg SL to relieve angina	Can repeat dose every 10 min up to max. of 10 mg SL if tolerated by BP
Isosorbide mononitrate	30 mg once daily	180 mg once daily

Hydralazine (C)

Indications: Moderate to severe hypertension; hypertensive crisis, including preeclampsia.

Actions: Arteriolar vasodilator by directly relaxing smooth muscle tissue in vascular resistance vessels.

Adverse effects: Tachycardia, SLE reaction in chronic use, palpitations, flushing, hypotension, fluid retention, GI disturbances, headache, dizziness.

Cautions: Hepatic impairment, renal impairment; coronary artery disease, as may provoke angina. Avoid after MI. Cerebrovascular disease. Not to be used if idiopathic SLE, high-output heart failure, cor pulmonale, myocardial insufficiency due to mechanical obstruction such as severe aortic stenosis.

Comments: Limited effect on veins and preload, so postural hypotension unusual.

Dose: Available in 25 mg and 50 mg tablets; 20 mg ampoules. *Chronic hypertension:* 25 mg PO BD initially, can be gradually increased up to 200 mg daily in two divided doses. *Hypertensive crisis:* 5 mg slowly IV, repeat doses every 20–30 min if necessary.

Methyldopa (A)

Indications: Moderate-to-severe hypertension; hypertensive crisis, including preeclampsia.

Actions: Centrally acting alpha-2 agonist, decreases sympathetic tone.

Adverse effects: Drowsiness, dry mouth, haemolytic anaemia, drug-induced fever, hepatic abnormalities, blood dyscrasias, hypotension, dizziness, oedema.

Cautions: Hepatic impairment, renal impairment; coronary artery disease, as may provoke angina; comcomitant use of MAOIs.

Dose: Available in 250 mg tablets. *Chronic hypertension:* 250 mg PO BD initially; can be gradually increased up 750 mg QID if necessary.

Phentolamine (B1)

Indications: Hypertensive episodes due to phaeochromocytoma. Local vasodilation after inadvertent soft-tissue injection of adrenaline. Erectile dysfunction adjunct.

Actions: Competitively blocks the effects of adrenaline and noradrenaline at alpha-1- and alpha-2-adrenergic receptors, to cause arteriolar and slight venular vasodilation, with a compensatory increase in heart rate and contractility.

Adverse effects: Hypotension, tachycardia, angina, cerebral ischaemia, GI symptoms.

Cautions: Conditions where sudden hypotension is undesirable (e.g. stroke or coronary artery disease).

Comments: Used mainly during surgery for phaeochromocytoma. Limited availability in Australia.

Dose: Available in 10 mg ampoules. *Emergency control of hypertension:* Slow 2–5 mg IV bolus; best given by infusion at a rate of 5–10 microgram/kg/min. *Local infiltration:* Doses of 1 mg locally infiltrated at site of adrenaline injection.

Prazosin (B2)

Indications: Hypertension, benign prostatic hypertrophy, Raynaud's syndrome, severe chronic heart failure.

Actions: Competitively blocks the effects of adrenaline and noradrenaline at alpha-1-adrenergic receptors, to cause arteriolar and slight venular vasodilation.

Adverse effects: Hypotension (first-dose effects common and severe), tachycardia, oedema, dry mouth, weakness, headache, drowsiness, nasal congestion, blurred vision, angina, cerebral ischaemia, GI symptoms.

Cautions: Conditions where sudden hypotension is undesirable (e.g. stroke or coronary artery disease); severe aortic or mitral stenosis

Dose: Available in 1 mg, 2 mg and 5 mg tablets. *Chronic hypertension, severe CCF:* First dose 0.25 mg at night, then 0.5 mg BD, gradually increased up to 10 mg BD if necessary. *Benign prostatic hypertrophy:* Commence as above, gradually increase to 2 mg BD.

- **Diazoxide:** Direct peripheral vasodilator available as IV use, only for acute hypertensive crises.
- **Ivabradine:** Blocks Na^+–K^+ channel at the sinoatrial node, thus decreasing heart rate. May be used to treat chronic stable angina in patients unable to tolerate beta-blockers; used under specialist supervision only.
- **Minoxidil:** Direct potent peripheral vasodilator used for severe refractory hypertension; used under specialist supervision only.

SECTION F – Formulary

- **Moxonidine:** Centrally acting imidazoline and alpha receptor agonist with similar effects to clonidine; used for hypertension not responding to usual agents.
- **Nicorandil:** Potassium-channel opener also with nitrate effects, used for control of angina. Can cause GI ulceration.
- **Perhexiline:** Non-selective calcium-channel blocker used for control of intractable angina. Adverse effects limit use.
- **Phenoxybenzamine:** Peripheral alpha-blocker; used for hypertension associated with phaeochromocytoma.
- **Sodium nitroprusside:** Non-selective arteriolar and venous dilator; used in critical care for hypertensive emergencies. Requires careful titration and invasive monitoring.
- **Terazosin:** Alpha blocker similar to prazosin used for hypertension.

Drugs affecting blood clotting
Aspirin (acetylsalicylic acid) (C)

Indications: Secondary prophylaxis and treatment of thromboembolic arterial occlusions including TIA, stroke, ACS, IHD, peripheral vascular occlusion, including DVT. Benefit of primary prevention for patients without symptomatic vascular disease is not proven.

Actions: Irreversibly inhibits cyclooxygenase, reducing platelet synthesis of thromboxane A2 (an inducer of platelet aggregation) for the life of the platelet (7–10 days).

Adverse effects: Bleeding, gastritis.

Cautions: GI haemorrhage, renal impairment, severe hepatic disease, gout, children.

Comments: Can also use half of a 300 mg tablet if preferred. No definite benefit of enteric-coated preparations.

Dose: Low-dose aspirin available in 100 mg tablets. Usual dose 100 mg once daily.

Clopidogrel (B1)

Indications: Prevention of vascular events in patients with symptomatic vascular disease, ACS, prevention of restenosis following coronary stent insertion.

Actions: Irreversibly inhibits platelet ADP receptor with inhibition of platelet aggregation and cross-linking of fibrin.

Adverse effects: Bleeding, diarrhoea, rash.

Cautions: Hepatic impairment, pregnancy, children. Clopidogrel effect decreased by proton-pump inhibitors (less with pantoprazole).

Comments: Usually used if aspirin is not tolerated, poses too high a risk of GI bleeding or has not been effective. Used together with aspirin for high-risk ACS or post-stent insertion.

Dose: Available in 75 mg tablets. Usual dose 75 mg once daily. For high-risk ACS prior to percutaneous coronary interventions give 300 mg loading dose.

Coagulation factors

Indications: Prophylaxis and treatment of bleeding due to specific factor deficiencies; reversal of warfarin anticoagulation in patients with bleeding (prothrombin complex concentrate); treatment of life-threatening bleeding with associated coagulopathy (prothrombin complex concentrate, eptacog alpha).

Actions: Replacement of coagulation factor deficits.

Adverse effects: Fever, rash, clotting with thrombosis, dizziness, flushing, risk of DIC.

Cautions: **Pregnancy, children.**

Comments: Monitor coagulation.

Drug	Indications	Usual adult dose	Comments
Cryoprecipitate	Hypofibrinogenaemia esp. when associated with DIC; factor VIII or von Willebrand's disease when specific factors not available	Hypofibrinogenaemia: 1 unit of cryoprecipitate IV for each 10 kg body weight	Each 15 mL unit typically contains 100 IU of factor VIII, and 250 mg of fibrinogen. It also contains von Willebrand factor, fibronectin and factor XIII.
Eptacog alfa (factor VIIa)	Life-threatening bleeding not responding to other blood product replacement	35–120 microgram/kg IV every 2–3 h	Use under specialist supervision only.
Factor VIII (including octocog alfa, moroctocog alfa)	Treatment or prophylaxis of bleeding secondary to factor VIII deficiency	*Prophylaxis:* 10–50 IU/kg IV twice weekly *Treatment:* minor bleeding 10–20 IU/kg; major bleeding 40–50 IU/kg IV, which may need to be repeated 12 hourly	Pooled human donor factor VIII also contains therapeutic amounts of von Willebrand factor for use if bleeding is unresponsive to desmopressin.

Continued

Drug	Indications	Usual adult dose	Comments
Factor IX (including nonacog alfa and nonacog gamma as rDNA products)	Treatment or prophylaxis of bleeding secondary to factor IX deficiency	*Prophylaxis:* 25–40 IU/kg IV twice weekly *Treatment:* 20–100 IU/kg IV depending on severity of bleeding	
Prothrombin complex concentrate	Treatment of bleeding secondary to deficiencies of factor II, IX or X when specific factors not available; warfarin toxicity	*Treatment of warfarin toxicity with bleeding:* 50 IU/kg IV	When reconstituted, contains factor IX 500 IU, factors II and X approximately 500 IU each, low levels of factors V and VII, antithrombin III 25 IU, heparin sodium 192 IU.

Direct oral anticoagulants/new oral anticoagulants (C)

Indications: Equivalent benefits to warfarin for thromboprophylaxis in non-valvular atrial fibrillation and postoperative lower limb arthroplasty; treatment of venous thromboembolic disease and prevention of subsequent VTE.

Actions: Dabigatran is a competitive inhibitor of thrombin. Apixaban and rivaroxaban are direct competitive antagonists of factor Xa, thus preventing conversion of prothrombin to thrombin. All prevent conversion of fibrinogen to fibrin, clot formation and platelet aggregation.

Adverse effects: GI disturbance, bleeding.

Cautions: Contraindicated in pregnancy, lactation, high risk of bleeding, severe renal impairment, cirrhosis. Renal impairment can lead to accumulation and excessive anticoagulation and requires dose adjustment.

Comments: Low potential for interactions with diet or alcohol, but can be affected by liver enzyme inducers/inhibitors or protease inhibitors. Absorption of dabigatran reduced if patient taking proton pump inhibitors. No routine monitoring required. Dabigatran is fully reversed by giving monoclonal antibody fragment (Fab) idarucizumab 5 g IV bolus. Otherwise, prothrombin complex concentrates or recombinant factor VIIa may be tried to reverse bleeding with apixaban and rivaroxaban.

Dose: Dabigatran available in 75 mg, 110 mg and 150 mg tablets. Apixaban available in 2.5 mg and 5 mg tablets. Rivaroxaban available in 10 mg, 15 mg and 20 mg tablets.

Drug	Usual adult dose	Comments
Apixaban	2.5 mg BD for postop prophylaxis or prevention of subsequent VTE, 5 mg BD for AF, 10 mg BD for 7 days for VTE treatment then 5 mg BD	Not indicated in surgery of hip fracture. Consider decreasing dose if age >80 years, weight <60 kg or renal impairment.
Dabigatran	220 mg daily for postop prophylaxis. 150 mg BD for AF or 110 mg BD if >75 years. Same doses (150 or 110 mg) for treatment of VTE, but after at least 5 days of parenteral anticoagulant.	Reduce to 110 mg dosage in patients aged >75 years, or with renal impairment. Avoid if creatinine clearance <30mL/min. Full immediate reversal with idarucizumab 5 g IV monoclonal antibody fragment.
Rivaroxaban	10 mg daily for postop prophylaxis, 15 mg BD for acute treatment of VTE for first 3 weeks then 20 mg once daily. 20 mg daily for AF or prevention of subsequent VTE	Not indicated in surgery of hip fracture. Decrease dose if renal impairment. Avoid if creatinine clearance <30mL/min.

Fibrinolytics (C)

Indications: Acute STEMI or new LBBB with pain; acute massive venous thromboembolism in patients who are haemodynamically unstable; peripheral arterial thromboembolism; thrombosed IV cannulae, central venous catheters, haemodialysis shunts or blocked chest drains; acute ischaemic stroke on CT scan within 4.5 h of onset of symptoms (alteplase under specialist supervision only).

Actions: Converts plasminogen to plasmin, which catalyses the breakdown of fibrin.

Adverse effects: Common—bleeding, including bleeding at injection sites, intracerebral bleeding, internal bleeding (e.g. GI, genitourinary). Infrequent—allergic reactions, including fever, chills, rash, nausea, headache, bronchospasm, anaphylaxis (particularly streptokinase), vasculitis, nephritis, hypotension.

Cautions: Contraindications include active internal bleeding; recent (<0.5 year) thrombotic CVA; recent (<1 month) major surgery or trauma; intracranial neoplasm; prior intracranial haemorrhage; bleeding disorder; non-compressible vascular puncture (including

LP); severe uncontrolled hypertension (SBP >200 mmHg or DBP >110 mmHg); bacterial endocarditis, pericarditis; haemorrhagic retinopathy; suspicion of left heart thrombus (e.g. mitral stenosis with AF); recent (<10 days) prolonged or traumatic CPR.

Comments: Avoid IM injections and other invasive procedures during thrombolytic treatment. In case of severe bleeding not controlled by local pressure, stop infusion of thrombolytic. Give fibrinogen, platelets, coagulation factors, tranexamic acid (and protamine if heparin has been used).

Drug	Indications	Usual adult dose	Comments
Alteplase	STEMI, PE (haemo-dynamically unstable), stroke, arterial occlusion, chest drain blockage	15 mg bolus, then infusion of 0.75 mg/kg in 30 min (max. 50 mg), then 0.5 mg/kg in 60 min (max. dose 35 mg); give with weight-adjusted heparin. *PE, stroke, chest drain blockage:* consult hospital guidelines.	Plasminogen activators produced by recombinant DNA technology; more fibrin-specific than streptokinase. Thrombolytic agents of choice in Aboriginal people because of their frequent high levels of anti-streptococcal antibodies.
Tenecteplase	STEMI	Weight-dependent as a single bolus; give with weight-adjusted heparin: <60 kg: 30 mg IV (6000 units); >90 kg: 50 mg IV (10,000 units).	
Reteplase	STEMI	2 injections of 10 units, 30 min apart; give each bolus injection slowly IV over <2 min. Give with weight-adjusted heparin.	

Heparins and injectable antithrombins (C)

Indications: Prophylaxis and treatment of DVT, PE, embolic stroke; adjunct in the treatment of high-risk ACS; management of acute peripheral arterial occlusion; prevention of clotting in haemodialysis circuits.

Actions: Enhances the activity of antithrombin III by forming complexes that inactivate several coagulation enzymes, particularly thrombin and factor Xa. Highly protein-bound. LMWHs catalyse antithrombin to neutralise several procoagulant enzymes,

including thrombin, factor IIa and factor Xa. Fondaparinux is a
direct Xa inhibitor.

Adverse effects: Haemorrhage, thrombocytopenia, local irritation,
pain and bruising.

Comments: UFH has a rapid initiation of anticoagulation, but a
shorter duration of action than LMWH. More suitable than
LMWH for patients at high risk of bleeding, as can be terminated
rapidly by stopping the infusion or giving protamine. For UFH,
monitor the aPTT within 4–6 h of initiating or changing IV doses.
LMWH are given SC, are less plasma protein binding than UFH
and almost completely excreted by the renal route. Therapeutic
dosing is more predictable and the kinetics are not dose-
dependent. The aPTT does not need to be measured.

Cautions: Elderly; hypersensitivity; hepatic and renal impairment and
pregnancy. Prior heparin-induced thrombocytopenia syndrome
(HITS), bleeding diathesis, acute GI or PV bleeding, epidural
anaesthesia, severe hypertension.

Drug	Usual adult dose	Comments
Heparin	*DVT prophylaxis:* 5000 U SC BD or TDS. *DVT/PE/ACS treatment:* 5000 U IV bolus followed by IV infusion of 1000 U/h.	Adjust IV loading and infusion doses based on patient weight and monitor with aPTT.
Enoxaparin	*DVT prophylaxis:* 40 mg SC once daily. *DVT/PE treatment:* 1.5 mg/kg SC once daily. *ACS:* 1 mg/kg SC BD.	Reduce dose in renal impairment.
Dalteparin	*DVT prophylaxis:* 2500–5000 U SC once daily. *DVT/PE treatment:* 100 U/kg SC BD. *ACS:* 120 U/kg SC BD. Max. dose 10,000 U in 12 h.	Does not accumulate in renal impairment.
Danaparoid	*DVT prophylaxis:* 750 units SC BD. *DVT/PE treatment:* 2500 U IV, then 400 U/h for 2 h, then 300 U/h for 2 h and then 200 U/h for 5 days.	Mixture of non-heparin glycosaminoglycans derived from porcine mucosa, with an action similar to LMWH in inhibiting factor Xa. Indicated in those with thromboembolic disease and heparin-induced thrombocytopenia.

Continued

SECTION F – Formulary

Drug	Usual adult dose	Comments
Fondaparinux	*DVT prophylaxis:* 2.5 mg SC once daily. *DVT/PE treatment:* 5–10 mg SC once daily (adjust dose according to weight). *Treatment of high-risk NSTEACS:* 2.5 mg daily.	Factor Xa inhibitor and the intrinsic limb of the coagulation system. More specific than heparin for antithrombin III and less risk of thrombocytopenia.

Phytomenadione (vitamin K)

Indications: Vitamin K deficiency, reversal of warfarin effect.

Actions: Essential for hepatic synthesis of factors II, VII, IX and X, and proteins C and S.

Adverse effects: Pain, tenderness and erythema and haematoma formation with SC or IM administration. Allergic reactions, including anaphylaxis (especially with rapid IV injection).

Comments: Patients with fat malabsorption, especially in biliary obstruction or hepatic disease, may become deficient because vitamin K is fat-soluble. Therefore, to prevent vitamin K deficiency in malabsorption syndromes, a water-soluble preparation, menadiol sodium phosphate, must be used. The usual dose is 10 mg PO daily.

Cautions: IV vitamin K occasionally causes an anaphylactic reaction, so should be given cautiously. Vitamin K1 is administered PO or IV, but should not be given SC or IM, especially in patients with active bleeding. Larger doses of vitamin K1 produce resistance to re-anticoagulation and should be given under specialist supervision.

Dose: Available in 10 mg tablets, 2 mg and 10 mg ampoules. Dose of 0.5–10 mg PO or slowly IV, depending on INR and presence of minor or major bleeding (see Chapter 46). Low-dose vitamin K1 (0.5–1.0 mg) is used to partially reverse warfarin anticoagulation. Larger doses (5–10 mg) are used in cases of life-threatening haemorrhage or when full reversal of anticoagulation is required. Maximum IV dose 40 mg/day.

Protamine (B2)

Indications: Counteracts anticoagulant effect of heparin and, to some extent, LMWH in cases of severe haemorrhage or after cardiopulmonary bypass.

Actions: Combines with heparin to form a stable inactive complex, reversing the anticoagulant effect of heparin.

Adverse effects: Common—sensation of warmth, flushing, nausea, vomiting, lassitude. Infrequent—hypotension, bradycardia, dyspnoea (especially if given too rapidly), allergic reaction, rebound bleeding with excessive doses.

Cautions: Overdosage may paradoxically result in worsening haemorrhage, as protamine possesses anticoagulant activity.

Comments: Protamine neutralises the antithrombin activity of LMWH but only partially neutralises the anti-factor Xa effect.

Dose: Available in 50 mg ampoules. 1 mg slow IV injection over 10 min neutralises 100 units of heparin when given within 15 min of heparin. If time since heparin is >5 min, less protamine is required as heparin is rapidly bound to protein. Maximum single dose 50 mg.

Tranexamic acid (B1)

Indications: Prevention and treatment of bleeding due to excessive fibrinolysis (e.g. prevention of haemorrhage in patients with mild-to-moderate coagulopathies undergoing minor surgery, major trauma with bleeding, menorrhagia, prevention of hereditary angio-oedema, hyphaema). Can also be used topically (IV preparation) for difficult to control dental, ENT or skin bleeding.

Actions: Competitively inhibits the activation of plasminogen and (at high doses) non-competitively inhibits plasmin, preventing the breakdown of clots.

Adverse effects: Common—nausea, vomiting, diarrhoea. Infrequent—thrombosis, hypotension.

Cautions: Contraindications include history or risk of thrombosis, active thromboembolic disease (DVT, PE, cerebral thrombosis); disturbances of colour vision; SAH (may increase cerebral ischaemic complications). Use with caution in patients with haematuria because of renal parenchymal disease and renal haemorrhage, as thrombosis may lead to renal obstruction. Establish the cause of menorrhagia prior to use, and avoid in females <15 years old.

Comments: Reduce dose in renal impairment.

Dose: Available in 500 mg tablets, and 500 mg, 1 g and 2 g ampoules. Usual dose 1–1.5 g 2–4 times daily for varying duration according to indication. *Trauma (start within 3 hours of injury):* 1 g over 10 minutes followed by 1 g over 8 hours.

Warfarin (D)

Indications: Prophylaxis and treatment of DVT and PE; prevention of thromboembolism in patients with prosthetic heart valves; prevention of cardioembolism in patients with AF, including before and after cardioversion.

Actions: Inhibits synthesis of the vitamin-K-dependent clotting factors II, VII, IX and X, and the antithrombotic factors protein C and protein S, thus inhibiting the extrinsic clotting cascade.

Adverse effects: Common—bleeding. Infrequent—allergy and idiosyncratic reactions.

Cautions: Contraindications—bleeding disorders, previous GI bleeding, haemorrhagic retinopathy, intracerebral aneurysm or haemorrhage, severe hypertension, bacterial endocarditis, alcoholism, unsupervised dementia and/or frequent falls. Caution in renal and hepatic failure, as increased risk of bleeding. Caution performing invasive procedures such as central venous catheter. LP contraindicated.

Comments: Warfarin interacts with many drugs, making dosing more complicated. Regular monitoring of the INR is essential, particularly when starting warfarin. Check thyroid function if the patient is extremely sensitive or resistant to warfarin doses. For more information regarding monitoring of warfarin levels and management in the event of raised INR, see Chapter 46.

Dose: Available in 1 mg, 2 mg, 3 mg and 5 mg tablets. Usually 5 mg PO daily for 2 days, then adjust according to INR. *Usual maintenance dose:* 1–10 mg PO daily, taken at the same time each day, with a target INR of 2–3 for most indications except heart valves (3.5–4.5).

- **Abciximab:** Platelet glycoprotein IIb/IIIa inhibitor given IV as adjunctive therapy in patients undergoing PCI to decrease risk of acute reocclusion and need for revascularisation in the short term.
- **Antithrombin III:** Antithrombotic used IV for prevention of thromboembolic disease in hereditary antithrombin III deficiency.
- **Bivalirudin:** Short-acting direct thrombin inhibitor used IV for patients undergoing PCI.
- **Dipyrimadole:** Inhibits phosphodiesterase, which increases platelet cAMP and prevents aggregation.
- **Eptifibatide:** Platelet glycoprotein IIb/IIIa inhibitor used IV in high-risk ACS, in particular for patients undergoing PCI.
- **Prasugrel:** Similar to clopidogrel but used preferentially in ACS when managed with PCI (together with aspirin) in patients aged <75 years. Loading dose 60 mg with maintenance dose 10 mg daily.
- **Ticagrelor:** Reversible platelet ADP antagonist used preferentially in ACS (together with aspirin) unless patient is bradycardic, or has chronic dyspnoea or hepatic impairment. Usual loading dose 180 mg.
- **Tirofiban:** Glycoprotein IIb/IIIa inhibitor preventing platelet aggregation. Used IV in high-risk ACS as adjunct to usual antiplatelet therapy and heparin.

Lipid-modifying drugs
Cholestyramine (B2)

Indications: Adjuvant therapy in hypercholesterolaemia not responsive to diet therapy; relief of cholestatic pruritis; relief of diarrhoea from ileal disease.

Actions: Binds bile acids in the GI tract, which are then excreted in faeces. Plasma cholesterol is then converted to bile acids to compensate, thus decreasing circulating cholesterol levels.

Adverse effects: GI disturbance, especially constipation; may decrease fat and vitamin absorption in prolonged use; increased risk of gallstones, tooth erosion.

Cautions: Complete biliary obstruction. Renal and hepatic disease.

Comments: Advised to separate the ingestion of cholestyramine from that of other drugs by several hours.

Dose: Available in 4 g powder sachets. Commence at 4 g BD. Maximum dose 24 g daily.

Gemfibrozil (B3)

Indications: Hypertriglyceridaemia, hypercholesterolaemia not responding to dietary therapy or if more potent agents not tolerated.

Actions: Fibric acid derivative increasing the activity of lipoprotein lipase, altering the hepatic synthesis of lipids. Useful for type III and type IV hyperlipidaemia.

Adverse effects: GI disturbance, myopathy, rhabdomyolysis, rash, photosensitivity, gallstones, abnormal LFTs, pancreatitis.

Cautions: Not to be used with statins or other fibrates, as increased risk of myalgias and myopathy; hepatic and renal dysfunction.

Comments: Monitor LFTs.

Dose: Available in 600 mg tablets. Usual dose 600 mg BD PO.

HMG CoA reductase inhibitors (statins) (D)

Indications: Treatment of hypercholesterolaemia not responding to dietary therapy. Can be used initially in high-risk patients: symptomatic cardiovascular, cerebrovascular, peripheral vascular disease; strong family history; high-risk diabetes.

Actions: Blocks hepatic synthesis of cholesterol with an increased blood clearance of LDL and VLDL with slight rises in HDL.

Adverse effects: GI disturbances, myopathy with raised muscle enzymes and myalgias, headache, fatigue.

Cautions: Abnormal LFTs, liver disease, renal impairment. Monitor LFTs.

Comments: Beneficial outcomes seem unrelated to changes in lipid profile and may be related to an as yet undefined anti-inflammatory effect. Atorvastatin and rosuvastatin appear to have greatest efficacy at maximum doses.

SECTION F – Formulary

Drug	Usual initial adult dose	Maximum adult dose
Atorvastatin	10 mg once daily	80 mg once daily
Fluvastatin	20 mg once daily	40 mg BD
Pravastatin	10 mg once daily	80 mg once daily
Rosuvastatin	5 mg once daily	40 mg once daily
Simvastatin	10 mg once daily	80 mg once daily

- **Colestipol:** Bile acid sequestrant similar to cholestyramine.
- **Ezetimibe:** Inhibits intestinal cholesterol absorption. Used as adjunct to diet and statin use for hypercholesterolaemia or familial phytosterolaemia.
- **Fenofibrate:** Fibric acid derivative similar to gemfibrozil.
- **Fish oil:** Reduce plasma triglyceride levels with daily doses of 2 g of omega-3 fatty acids. Other lipid and haemostatic effects.
- **Nicotinic acid (niacin):** Blocks fat breakdown thus decreasing circulating levels of free fatty acids and VLDL. Used as adjunctive therapy for hyperlipoproteinaemia and hyperlipidaemia; pellagra (niacin deficiency).

Respiratory and allergy

Bronchodilators
Aminophylline (A)

Indications: Reversible bronchospasm in chronic bronchitis, emphysema and asthma, and paroxysmal dyspnoea in left heart failure. Rarely used because of narrow therapeutic margin (i.e. toxic adverse effects are common) with minimal benefits as adjuvant to other bronchodilator therapy.

Actions: Phosphodiesterase inhibitor. Direct bronchial smooth muscle dilator. Directly stimulates the respiratory centre.

Adverse effects: Arrhythmias, nausea, vomiting, headaches, insomnia, nightmares. Seizures occur if given too rapidly by IV infusion.

Cautions: Precautions include hypertension, hyperthyroidism, peptic ulcer, epilepsy, fever, hepatic impairment, pregnancy and breastfeeding. Determine theophylline level prior to initiating therapy in patients already on theophylline, and omit the loading dose.

Dose: Available in 250 mg ampoules. *Loading dose:* 6 mg/kg IV over 30 min, to a maximum of 500 mg. *Maintenance infusion:* 0.5–0.7 mg/kg/h to provide a peak serum theophylline concentration of approximately 10 microgram/mL (55 micromol/L). Reduce maintenance dose (0.3 mg/kg/h) in patients with CCF or liver disease, and in the elderly.

Beta-2 agonists (see also *Adrenaline* under *Cardiac arrest*) (A; eformoterol/salmeterol B3)

Indications: Treatment and prophylaxis of bronchospasm associated with asthma, COPD; treatment of bronchospasm of other causes, including heart failure, aspiration syndromes. Salbutamol also used as adjunct in treatment of hyperkalaemia and for treatment of premature labour.

Actions: Selective beta-2 adrenergic receptor agonists with bronchodilator effect, and potential mast-cell-stabilising effects with inhibition of inflammatory mediator release.

Adverse effects: Tachycardia, arrhythmias, tremor, agitation, anxiety, headache, GI disturbance, hypotension, hypokalaemia, muscle cramps. Adverse effects more common with IV, oral or high-dose nebulised administration. Inhaled preparations may cause sore throat, hoarseness, dry mouth.

Cautions: Cardiovascular disease, hypertension, hyperthyroidism. Long-acting beta-agonists should be used together with preventer medications in asthma.

Comments: Long-acting agents (salmeterol, eformoterol, indacaterol) predominantly used for prevention. Short-acting preparations (salbutamol, terbutaline) used for acute exacerbations. Inhalers more efficacious when used with a spacer device. Use of nebulisers may not provide additional benefit to inhalers with spacers in most patients. IV preparations only for use in critically ill patients under specialist supervision.

Drug	Usual initial adult dose	Maximum adult dose	Comments
Eformoterol inhaler	12 microgram BD	24 microgram BD	For prophylactic use; can also be used acutely in patients already receiving long-term eformoterol and steroid therapy.
Indacaterol	150 microgram daily	300 microgram daily	For prophylactic use. Also available as combination with glycopyrronium.
Salbutamol inhaler	100–200 microgram PRN	Can repeat dose every 4 h	If more frequent use required for asthma control, requires medical review.
Salbutamol syrup	4 mg QID	8 mg QID	Generally used as prophylaxis only in patients unable to tolerate inhaler.

Continued

Drug	Usual initial adult dose	Maximum adult dose	Comments
Salbutamol injection	5 microgram/ kg slow IV bolus over 3–5 min followed by infusion	Titrate infusion according to response and adverse effects	Use only in critical patients under specialist supervision and with local administration guidelines. Alternative administration is 250 microgram SC 4-hourly.
Salbutamol nebuliser solution	2.5–5 mg diluted up to 4 mL with saline	Can use continuously as 5–10 mg doses	Use continuously in acute severe asthma.
Salmeterol	50 microgram BD by inhaler	100 microgram BD by inhaler	For prophylactic use only.
Terbutaline inhaler	500 microgram QID	1 mg QID	
Terbutaline elixir	3 mg TDS	4.5 mg TDS	Generally used as prophylaxis only in patients unable to tolerate inhaler.
Terbutaline injection	250 microgram every 6 h		Salbutamol injection more commonly used.
Terbutaline nebuliser solution	2.5–5 mg every 6 h	20 mg every 6 h	
Vilanterol	25 microgram daily	25 microgram daily	For prophylactic use. Only available as combination with umeclidinium or with fluticasone.

Corticosteroid inhalations (B3; budesonide A) (see also *Corticosteroids* under *Antidiarrhoeals, antispasmodics, inflammatory bowel disease* and *Analgesics and musculoskeletal drugs*)

Indications: Prophylaxis and treatment of bronchospasm associated with asthma, exercise or allergens.

Actions: Reduce bronchial inflammation, oedema and hyperreactivity.

Adverse effects: Dry mouth, throat irritation, dysphonia, oropharyngeal candidiasis. High-dose use may lead to systemic adverse effects.

Cautions: Trial of other preventers prior to use of corticosteroids in children. Use in acute asthma probably beneficial but may offer

no benefits over oral corticosteroids. Not for use if possible pulmonary TB or severe pulmonary infection.
Comments: Local adverse effects minimised by use of spacer and rinsing mouth after use.

Drug	Usual initial adult dose	Maximum adult dose	Comments
Beclomethasone	50 microgram BD by inhaler	400 microgram BD by inhaler	
Budesonide	200 microgram BD by inhaler; 1 mg BD by nebuliser	600 microgram QID by inhaler; 2 mg BD by nebuliser	Combined with eformoterol as inhaler. Can also be used for croup in children as single 2 mg dose by nebuliser.
Ciclesonide	80–160 microgram once daily by inhaler	320 microgram once daily by inhaler	
Fluticasone	100 microgram BD by inhaler; 2 mg BD by nebuliser	1000 microgram BD by inhaler; 2 mg BD by nebuliser	Combined with long-acting beta-agonists as inhaler.

Cromoglycate (B1)

Indications: Prophylaxis of bronchospasm associated with asthma, exercise or allergens.
Actions: Direct mast-cell-stabilising agent.
Adverse effects: Dry mouth, throat irritation, cough, nasal congestion, GI upset, headache, bronchospasm.
Cautions: Pregnancy, lactation.
Comments: Not for use in acute management.
Dose: Available as sodium cromoglycate in 20 mg nebuliser solution, 1 mg and 5 mg inhalers, 20 mg spincaps. Usual dose 20 mg QID–4-hourly by nebuliser, 2–20 mg QID by inhaler. Also available as nedocromil 2 mg inhaler, usual dose 4 mg BD or QID.

Ipratropium (B1)

Indications: Treatment and prophylaxis of bronchospasm associated with asthma, COPD.
Actions: Topical muscarinic receptor antagonist with bronchodilator effect.
Adverse effects: Dry mouth, throat irritation, headache, tachycardia, urinary retention, constipation, blurred vision.

Cautions: Narrow-angle glaucoma, urinary retention risk such as prostatic hypertrophy, bladder neck obstruction.

Comments: Has minor additional benefits to beta-2 agonists in acute exacerbations of COPD.

Dose: Available in 250 microgram/mL and 500 microgram/mL nebuliser solutions, 21 microgram inhaler. *Acute bronchospasm:* 42–84 microgram QID as inhaler; 500 microgram QID as nebuliser. In severe episodes, can give 500 microgram nebulisers every 20 minutes for 3 doses, followed by 500 microgram 4-hourly. Can mix with salbutamol nebuliser solution if required.

- **Aclidinium:** Long-acting inhaled anticholinergic used in chronic management of COPD. Usual dose 322 microgram BD.
- **Glycopyrronium:** Long-acting inhaled anticholinergic used in chronic management of COPD. Usual dose 50 microgram daily. Available as combination with indacaterol.
- **Montelukast:** Leukotriene receptor antagonist used for prophylaxis of asthma, especially in children. Usual dose 4–20 mg once daily PO.
- **Nedocromil:** Similar action and use to cromoglycate.
- **Omalizumab:** IgE selective monoclonal antibody for prophylaxis of moderate to severe chronic allergic asthma, given as SC injection every 2–4 weeks.
- **Theophylline:** Oral preparation of aminophylline with similar indications and adverse-effect profile. Available in syrup, tablets and modified-release tablets. Initial adult dose 200 mg BD (modified-release tablets) adjusted to serum levels. Also available as choline theophyllinate syrup.
- **Tiotropium:** Long-acting preparation of ipratropium for use as prophylaxis for COPD. Usual dose 18 microgram once daily as dry powder inhaler, or 5 microgram daily as MDI.
- **Umeclidinium:** Long-acting inhaled anticholinergic used in prophylaxis of COPD. Usual dose 62.5 microgram daily. Also available as combination with vilanterol (ultra-long-acting beta-agonist).
- **Zafirlukast:** Leukotriene receptor antagonist used for prophylaxis of asthma. Usual dose 20–40 mg BD PO.

Cough medicines
Cough suppressants (A)

Indications: Treatment of dry, irritating cough associated with upper respiratory tract infection, malignancy.

Actions: Opioid-receptor agonists causing CNS depression.

Adverse effects: Drowsiness, confusion, constipation, withdrawal syndromes after prolonged use.

Cautions: Lower respiratory tract infection with mucus production; bronchiectasis, acute or chronic bronchitis: may cause sputum retention. Elderly patients may have more neurological adverse effects. Not recommended for children <6 years.

Comments: Require high doses to produce an antitussive effect, usually limited by adverse effects. Can lead to dependency. For malignant cough, potent opioids such as morphine, hydrocodone or oxycodone are preferred.

Drug	Usual adult dose
Codeine	30 mg TDS to QID PO
Dextromethorphan	30 mg TDS to QID PO
Dihydrocodeine	10–20 mg TDS to QID PO
Pholcodine	15 mg TDS to QID PO

Expectorants and mucolytics (A; dornase alfa B1; acetylcysteine B2)

Indications: Treatment of chest congestion and cough associated with upper respiratory tract infection. Acetylcysteine inhalation and dornase alfa inhalation are used as mucolytics in bronchopulmonary disease, especially cystic fibrosis.

Actions: Usually have soothing effect on swallowing; unknown effectiveness on decreasing mucus viscosity.

Adverse effects: GI upset, dizziness, headache, rash.

Comments: Little evidence of any effect on expectoration. Warm honey and lemon drink may be as effective.

Drug	Usual adult dose
Acetylcysteine	200 mg QID nebuliser
Bromhexine	8–16 mg TDS PO
Dornase alfa	2.5 mg daily nebuliser
Guaifenesin	200 mg TDS to QID PO
Senega and ammonia mixture	250 mg/ 250 mg PO 4-hourly in warm water

Antihistamines
Promethazine (C)

Indications: Allergic conditions, itch, nausea and vomiting (drug of choice for motion sickness), sedation.

Actions: Phenothiazine acting as antagonist at H1 receptors, reducing histamine-induced vasodilation and permeability. Also has anticholinergic and alpha-adrenergic antagonistic effects.

Adverse effects: Sedation, dry mouth, blurred vision, dizziness, anxiety, sleep disturbance, constipation, urinary retention, abdominal discomfort, hypotension, delirium.

SECTION F – Formulary

Cautions: Avoid in patients at risk of urinary retention, with glaucoma, in elderly due to risk of delirium and other adverse effects. Can lead to thrombophlebitis if IV administration. Has been used extensively in pregnancy without evidence of adverse fetal effects. Dose: Available in 10 mg and 25 mg tablets, oral liquid and 50 mg ampoules. Usual dose 10–25 mg PO BD or TDS, or 25–50 mg IM/ IV as a single dose.

- **Brompheniramine:** Moderate sedating effects, available only as combination with decongestants/analgesics.
- **Cetirizine:** Less-sedating antihistamine used for allergic rhinitis, conjunctivitis and chronic urticaria. Can be sedating in some individuals. Decrease dose in renal impairment.
- **Chlorpheniramine:** Moderate sedating effects, available only as combination with decongestants/analgesics.
- **Cyclizine:** Slight sedating effects, used as antiemetic—see antiemetics.
- **Cyproheptadine:** Used for allergic conditions, sedating and has some antiserotoninergic effects. Can be used to shorten duration of mild serotonin syndrome.
- **Desloratidine:** Less-sedating antihistamine used for allergic rhinitis, conjunctivitis and chronic urticaria.
- **Dexchlorpheniramine:** Sedating antihistamine. Used for allergic reactions.
- **Dimenhydrinate:** Significant anticholinergic and sedating effects. Available as combination with hyoscine hydrobromide as treatment for motion sickness.
- **Fexofenadine:** Less-sedating antihistamine used for allergic rhinitis, conjunctivitis and chronic urticaria.
- **Levocetirizine:** Less-sedating antihistamine used for allergic rhinitis, conjunctivitis and chronic urticaria. Can be sedating in some individuals. Decrease dose or increase dosing interval in renal impairment.
- **Loratidine:** Less-sedating antihistamine used for allergic rhinitis, conjunctivitis and chronic urticaria.
- **Pheniramine:** Sedating antihistamine. Used for allergic conditions, motion sickness, Ménière's disease.
- **Trimeprazine:** Sedating antihistamine. Used for allergic reactions. Has been used for sedation in children.

Gastrointestinal

Antiemetics
Metoclopramide (A)

Indications: Nausea, vomiting, migraines, enhancement of gastric emptying in gastroparesis.

Actions: Central dopamine antagonist and GI tract cholinergic effects, both having an antiemetic action.

Adverse effects: Dystonic reactions including oculogyric crises, akathisia (esp. with rapid IV injection), drowsiness, dry mouth, rarely neuroleptic malignant syndrome.

Cautions: GI bleeding, perforation or bowel obstruction where increased gastric emptying may worsen symptoms; young adults and children are more likely to suffer dystonic reactions, so need dose carefully calculated and only used if severe vomiting.

Comments: Not effective in motion sickness or nausea related to vestibulopathies.

Dose: Available in 10 mg tablets, 10 mg ampoules. Usual adult dose 10–20 mg PO, IM or IV QID.

Prochlorperazine (C)

Indications: Nausea, vomiting, migraines, vertigo.

Actions: Phenothiazine with central dopaminergic effects on the chemoreceptor trigger zone and peripheral antiemetic properties.

Adverse effects: Anticholinergic effects including dry mouth, blurred vision, urinary retention, constipation; dystonic reactions including oculogyric crises, akathisia; drowsiness, hypotension, rarely neuroleptic malignant syndrome, QT interval prolongation.

Cautions: Narrow-angle glaucoma, children.

Comments: Lower dose in elderly. Careful dose titration in children as can cause severe dystonic reactions.

Dose: Available in 5 mg tablets, 25 mg suppositories, 12.5 mg ampoules. Usual adult dose 5–10 mg QID PO, 25 mg QID PR, 12.5 mg IM or IV QID.

Serotonin-3 antagonists (setrons) (B1; tropisetron B3)

Indications: Nausea, vomiting not responsive to usual antiemetics, particularly chemotherapy or radiotherapy induced.

Actions: Central and peripheral serotonin receptor antagonist.

Adverse effects: Diarrhoea, dizziness, taste disturbance, abdominal pain, headache, extrapyramidal effects.

Cautions: Give IV preparations slowly.

Comments: All have similar effectiveness.

Drug	Usual adult dose
Granisetron	1–3 mg IV daily or 2 mg PO daily
Ondansetron	4–12 mg IV/IM/PO/SL 8–12-hourly or 16 mg 8–12 hourly PR
Palonosetron	250 microgram IV before chemotherapy
Tropisetron	2–5 mg IV daily or 5 mg PO daily

- **Aprepitant:** Substance P neurokinin-1 receptor antagonist used PO as adjuvant with other antiemetics for prevention and treatment of cytotoxic chemotherapy-associated nausea and vomiting.
- **Cyclizine:** Antihistamine used primarily for postoperative, motion-induced or radiotherapy-induced nausea and vomiting. Dose 25–50 mg TDS IV or PO.
- **Dexamethasone:** Potent antiemetic for postoperative or chemotherapy-associated nausea and vomiting, or if unreponsive to other agents.
- **Dimenhydrinate:** Anticholinergic antihistamine with similar uses as promethazine.
- **Domperidone:** Dopamine antagonist that does not cross the blood–brain barrier, used for treatment of diabetic gastroparesis, intractable nausea and vomiting of any cause. Usual dose 10–20 mg PO QID.
- **Doxylamine:** Sedating antihistamine used for nausea and vomiting in pregnancy. Usual dose 12.5–25 mg PO.
- **Droperidol:** Anticholinergic and central antidopaminergic effects useful for postoperative nausea and vomiting, or if not reponsive to other therapies. Small doses of 0.5 mg IV are usually sufficient.
- **Fosaprepitant:** Substance P neurokinin-1 receptor antagonist used IV as adjuvant with other antiemetics for prevention and treatment of cytotoxic chemotherapy-associated nausea and vomiting.
- **Hyoscine hydrobromide (scopolamine):** Anticholinergic used for prophylaxis or treatment of motion sickness. Usual dose 300–600 microgram QID with maximum of 1.2 mg in 24 h.
- **Lorazepam:** Benzodiazepine with sedating and anxiolytic effects useful for anticipatory nausea associated with cancer treatment. Can also be beneficial as a vestibular suppressant in vertigo-associated nausea and vomiting. Other benzodiazepines have similar effects.
- **Promethazine:** Phenothiazine antihistamine with central antiemetic effects, used for postoperative or vestibular-associated nausea and vomiting, or if unresponsive to other antiemetics. Drug of choice for motion sickness. Usual doses 10 mg PO QID or 12.5 mg IM/slow IV QID.

Antiulcer drugs
Antacids (A)
Indications: Symptomatic relief of dyspepsia, gastro-oesophageal reflux, peptic ulcer disease.
Actions: Neutralise stomach acid.

Adverse effects: Diarrhoea (magnesium-based preparations), constipation (calcium- or aluminium-based preparations), prolonged or excessive use can cause milk-alkali syndrome.

Cautions: Calcium-based antacids in hypercalcaemia or nephrolithiasis. Renal impairment for aluminium- or magnesium-based preparations. Some preparations contain sodium, avoid in heart and renal failure.

Comments: Aluminium hydroxide, calcium carbonate, magnesium carbonate, magnesium hydroxide and sodium bicarbonate are the commonly used active ingredients, often in combination with each other or with simethicone or alginic acid or local anaesthetic, which may reduce symptoms. Best taken 1–3 h after meals. Liquid preparations more effective.

Dose: Varies with preparations. Usually 1 or 2 tablets or 20–40 mL of liquid PO as required.

H2 receptor antagonists (B1; nizatadine B3)

Indications: Symptomatic relief and treatment of dyspepsia, gastro-oesophageal reflux, peptic ulcer disease. Stress ulcer prophylaxis. May also help itch in allergic skin conditions.

Actions: Reduce gastric acid secretion by blocking H2 receptors on stomach parietal cells.

Adverse effects: Uncommon. Cimetidine can cause changes in libido or gynaecomastia. Ranitidine IV preparations need to be given slowly due to risk of arrhythmias.

Cautions: Cimetidine has high rate of drug interactions.

Comments: Similar efficacy of all preparations. Halve initial doses for maintenance therapy.

Drug	Usual adult dose
Cimetidine	400–800 mg PO daily
Famotidine	40 mg PO daily
Nizatadine	300 mg PO daily
Ranitidine	300 mg PO daily or 50 mg IV 6–8 hourly

Proton-pump inhibitors (PPIs) (B3)

Indications: Symptomatic relief and treatment of dyspepsia, gastro-oesophageal reflux, peptic ulcer disease, scleroderma oesophagus. Adjunct in *Helicobacter pylori* eradication. Stress or NSAID ulcer prophylaxis. Acute upper GI bleed to prevent rebleeding following endoscopic interventions.

Actions: Inactivates the H^+/K^+ ATPase pump, suppressing stomach acid secretion.

Adverse effects: Headache, GI disturbance, abdominal pain.

Cautions: Exclude upper GI malignancy. Associated with increased risk of community-acquired pneumonia and some enteric infections. PPIs (except pantoprazole) interfere with clopidogrel function. Use pantoprazole if required following ACS or coronary stent insertions.

Comments: Similar efficacy for all preparations. Halve initial doses for maintenance therapy. Higher doses are required for Zollinger–Ellison syndrome. Dose for acute GI bleeding is 80 mg slow IV bolus (esomeprazole, omeprazole or pantoprazole) followed by 80 mg IV infusion over 10 h.

Drug	Usual adult dose
Esomeprazole	20–40 mg PO daily
Lansoprazole	15–30 mg PO daily or BD
Omeprazole	20–40 mg PO daily
Pantoprazole	40–80 mg PO or IV daily
Rabeprazole	20–40 mg PO daily or BD

- **Misoprostol:** Prostaglandin E1 analogue increases stomach mucus secretion and duodenal bicarbonate secretion. Used for symptomatic relief and treatment of peptic ulcer disease.
- **Sucralfate:** Forms cytoprotective barrier on stomach mucosa, used to prevent stress-induced ulcers.

Antidiarrhoeals, antispasmodics, inflammatory bowel disease
Opioids (A; diphenoxylate C; loperamide B3)

Indications: Short-term treatment of diarrhoea. Reduce bowel frequency and fluid in short-bowel syndromes.

Actions: Reduce bowel motility by activating bowel wall opioid receptors.

Adverse effects: Abdominal pain and bloating, nausea, vomiting, drowsiness, dizziness.

Cautions: Contraindicated in dysentery or invasive enterocolitis as may prolong illness or worsen systemic infection. Contraindicated in bowel obstruction or exacerbations of ulcerative colitis—may precipitate toxic megacolon. Codeine has addictive potential.

Comments: Most diarrhoeal illnesses are self-limiting and do not require drug treatment. Opioids are most effective generic antidiarrhoeals. Loperamide preferred.

Drug	Usual adult dose
Codeine	30–60 mg PO QID
Diphenoxylate	5 mg QID
Loperamide	*Acute diarrhoea:* 4 mg initially PO followed by 2 mg after each loose bowel motion *Chronic diarrhoea:* 2–4 mg PO BD or TDS titrated to effect

Corticosteroids (see also *Corticosteroids* under *Bronchodilators* and *Analgesics and musculoskeletal drugs*)

Oral, IV or rectal steroids are used for acute inflammatory bowel disease. Budesonide tablets may have a better topical to systemic effect but are more expensive—usual dose 9 mg PO daily. Hydrocortisone rectal foam, prednisolone suppositories or enemas can also be used daily or BD for rectosigmoid disease. Severe exacerbations may require oral prednisolone 50 mg daily PO or hydrocortisone 100–200 mg IV QID.

Salicylates (C; sulfasalazine A—use with folate supplementation)

Indications: Inducing or maintaining remission in inflammatory bowel disease.

Actions: Local anti-inflammatory effects in bowel wall.

Adverse effects: Nausea, rash, diarrhoea, nephritis, blood dyscrasias.

Cautions: Sulfasalazine has additional adverse effects due to the sulfa moiety, including severe allergic reactions, oligospermia, haemolysis, orange skin or urine discolouration. Monitor urinalysis, LFTs and FBC regularly.

Drug	Usual adult dose	Comments
Balsalazide	*Acute ulcerative colitis:* 2.25 g PO TDS until remission. *Maintenance dose:* 1.5 g PO BD titrated to effect	Pro-drug of mesalazine.
Mesalazine	*Ulcerative colitis:* 1 g suppository PR daily or 2–4 g enema PR daily *Acute ulcerative colitis or Crohn's disease:* 500 mg TDS PO up to 1 g QID PO *Ulcerative colitis or Crohn's disease maintenance:* 250–500 mg BD or TDS PO	Different preparations have different formulations and doses.
Olsalazine	*Acute ulcerative colitis:* 1 g PO BD or TDS *Ulcerative colitis maintenance:* 500 mg BD PO	
Sulfasalazine	*Acute ulcerative colitis or mild colonic Crohn's disease:* 1–2 g QID PO *Ulcerative colitis maintenance:* 500 mg QID	

- **Adalimumab, golimumab, infliximab:** TNF-alpha antagonists used as immunosuppressants for refractory moderate or severe ulcerative colitis or Crohn's disease.
- **Hyoscine N-butylbromide:** Anticholinergic with smooth muscle relaxant properties. Used for abdominal cramps, biliary spasm, ureteric colic, irritable bowel syndrome. Efficacy unclear.
- **Mebeverine:** Anticholinergic with smooth muscle relaxant properties. Used for abdominal cramps, irritable bowel syndrome. Minor effects in reducing symptoms of irritable bowel syndrome.
- **Peppermint oil:** Direct smooth muscle relaxant. Minor effects in reducing symptoms of irritable bowel syndrome.
- **Vedolizumab:** Recombinant antibody against leucocyte integrin resulting in inhibition of GIT inflammation. Used for Crohn's disease or ulcerative colitis refractory to TNF-alpha antagonists.

Laxatives (A)

Drug	Usual adult dose	Comments
Bisacodyl	5–15 mg PO nocte or 10 mg suppository PR or 5 mg enema PR as required	Direct stimulant of bowel to increase motility. Can be used chronically in chronic constipation due to opioid use or neurological dysfunction.
Bulking agents	Various, usually titrated to effect	Absorb water in faeces; increase bulk and stimulate bowel motility. Avoid in opioid-associated constipation as may lead to faecal impaction or obstruction.
Docusate/ poloxamer	100–150 mg BD PO or 50 mg enema PR	Stool softener, helps mix water with stool and increase intestinal fluid secretion. Onset of action 1–3 days following oral doses, 10–30 minutes following enema. Often combined with senna. Poloxamer used in children.
Glycerin	1 suppository PR as required	Non-absorbable sugar causing osmotic laxative effect, and direct stimulant of bowel wall.
Lactulose	Initially 15 mL PO BD and titrate to effect. Use 30 mL PO hourly until laxative effect achieved in hepatic encephalopathy	Osmotic laxative, onset of action is 1–3 days with normal dosing. Used in higher doses to treat hepatic encephalopathy by decreasing ammonia absorption, as well as laxative effect decreasing protein absorption.

Drug	Usual adult dose	Comments
Paraffin	20–40 mL PO daily titrated to effect	Lubricates faeces to assist passage and may stimulate bowel activity. Emulsified liquid preparations are more viscous and decrease risk of aspiration pneumonitis.
Phosphate, citrate, magnesium salts	Various	Poorly absorbed salts with osmotic laxative effect. Usually used as bowel preparations or enemas for faecal impaction. Avoid in dehydration, heart failure, renal impairment. Onset of action 1–3 hours after oral administration and 10–30 minutes after rectal administration.
Polyethylene glycol	Various. Usually sachet powder is mixed with water and 1–2 L is given over 1–2 hours	Osmotic laxative. Used as bowel preparation or for intractable constipation or faecal impaction. Also used for whole bowel irrigation for selected poisonings.
Senna	7.5–30 mg PO nocte	Direct stimulant of bowel to increase motility.
Sodium picosulfate	2.5–10 mg PO nocte	Usually used as a bowel preparation combined with magnesium salts.
Sorbitol	20 mL PO daily to TDS titrated to response	Non-absorbable sugar with osmotic laxative effect.

Drugs for obesity

Orlistat: Inhibits GIT lipases preventing some dietary fat absorption. Can cause oily stools or increased flatus. Contraindicated if pancreatic deficiency states, malabsorption syndromes.

Phentermine: Central CNS stimulant increases activity and energy expenditure. Common adverse effects related to CNS stimulation. Multiple contraindications and drug interactions, subject to misuse.

Neuromuscular

Analgesics and musculoskeletal drugs
Allopurinol (B2)

Indications: Gout, uric acid nephropathy and tumour lysis syndrome (from urate/uric acid deposition).

Actions: Inhibits xanthine oxidase, reducing the oxidation of hypoxanthine and xanthine in the formation of uric acid.

SECTION F – Formulary

Cautions: May prolong acute manifestations of gout—*not* indicated in an acute attack (commence 2–3 weeks after acute attack has settled).

Adverse effects: Rash, fever, GI upset, hepatotoxicity.

Comments: Attacks of acute gout may occur shortly after starting allopurinol. Reduce the dose in renal or hepatic failure.

Dose: Available in 100 mg and 300 mg tablets. Usual dose 300 mg PO daily after meals. Up to 800 mg/day can be used for maintenance therapy in severe cases. If the daily dose exceeds 300 mg, it should be taken in divided doses.

Aspirin (acetylsalicylic acid) (C) (see also *Drugs affecting blood clotting*)

Indications: Mild-to-moderate pain, fever. Anti-inflammatory effects in rheumatic fever, rheumatoid arthritis, Kawasaki disease.

Actions: Non-selective NSAID, irreversibly inhibits cyclooxygenases 1 and 2.

Adverse effects: Nausea, gastritis and peptic ulceration, bleeding (can be asymptomatic), renal impairment with sodium and fluid retention. High doses can cause tinnitus and dizziness.

Cautions: GI haemorrhage, renal impairment, severe hepatic disease, heart failure, gout, children (associated with Reye's syndrome). Allergic cross-reactivity with other NSAIDs.

Comments: Often combined with codeine. Enteric-coated preparations do not decrease risk of GI adverse effects.

Dose: Available in 300 mg tablets. Usual dose 600–900 mg QID PO. Higher doses of 20 mg/kg PO QID used as anti-inflammatory dose for specific conditions.

Colchicine (B2)

Indications: Treatment or prevention of acute gout.

Actions: Inhibits neutrophil function, reducing inflammatory response to uric acid crystals.

Adverse effects: Diarrhoea, nausea, abdominal pain, GI bleeding, rash.

Cautions: Patients with renal or hepatic impairment, or taking liver enzyme-inducing medications (including digoxin, some antifungals, macrolide antibiotics, some antiretrovirals, fibrates, statins and grapefruit juice) are more susceptible to toxicity.

Dose: Available in 500 microgram tablets. For acute gout give 1 mg initially, followed by 500 microgram 1 hour later and do not repeat within 3 days. For gout prevention give 500 microgram daily or BD.

Corticosteroids (A) (see also *Corticosteroids* under *Bronchodilators* and *Antidiarrhoeals, antispasmodics, inflammatory bowel disease*)

Indications: Adrenal insufficiency. Immunosuppression in transplantation and autoimmune diseases. Anti-inflammatory in inflammatory bowel disease, asthma, croup, rheumatological and autoimmune disorders, giant cell arteritis, allergy and skin conditions. Adjunctive treatment for chemotherapy- or malignancy-induced nausea and vomiting or pain.

Actions: Regulate gene expression that results in glucocorticoid effects (e.g. raising blood fats and blood glucose, suppression of immune responses) and mineralocorticoid effects (e.g. sodium and water retention, hypertension, potassium loss).

Adverse effects: Usually occur when corticosteroids are used for other than adrenal insufficiency. Can occur even with topical or local therapy. Short courses of high-dose systemic corticosteroids cause fewer adverse effects than prolonged courses at lower doses. Common—dyspepsia, candidiasis, sleep disturbance, dysphoria, bloating. *Chronic therapy*—increased susceptibility to infection, masking of signs of infection; acne, oedema, hypertension, hypokalaemia, hyperglycaemia, adrenal suppression, osteoporosis, spontaneous fractures, increased appetite, delayed wound healing, bruising, skin atrophy, proximal myopathy, fat redistribution (producing Cushingoid appearance with central obesity, 'buffalo hump'), amenorrhoea, psychosis, euphoria, depression.

Comments: Altered glucose tolerance—may increase insulin requirement or precipitate the need for insulin. Hypertension, heart failure—may be worsened by sodium and water retention (mineralocorticoid effect) and enhanced vascular reactivity; more likely to occur with cortisone or hydrocortisone (consider using alternative corticosteroid). Psychiatric disorders—may exacerbate psychosis and mood swings.

Drug*	Indications	Usual adult dose	Comments
Betamethasone	Intra-articular or soft-tissue anti-inflammatory injections; topical skin conditions.	*Joint injection:* 1–2 mL/injection (1 mL = 5.7 mg) *Skin:* apply thin layer TDS (0.2 mg/g in 100 mg tube)	

Continued

Drug*	Indications	Usual adult dose	Comments
Dexamethasone	Cerebral oedema, chemotherapy- or malignancy-induced nausea and vomiting or pain; croup, asthma; adjuvant to antibiotic treatment of meningitis.	0.5–10 mg PO daily. *Cerebral oedema:* 10 mg IV initially, then 4 mg IV QDS *Bacterial meningitis:* 10 mg IV QDS, started with first dose of antibiotic	No mineralo-corticoid effects.
Hydrocortisone	Acute asthma, anaphylaxis, angio-oedema, acute transplant rejection, adrenocortical insufficiency; topical skin conditions.	*Acute severe asthma:* 100–250 mg IV 6-hourly *Acute transplant rejection:* 0.5–1 g IV 8-hourly	Relatively high mineralocorticoid activity, so unsuitable for disease suppression on a long-term basis.
Methylprednisolone	*Acetate:* Intra-articular or soft-tissue anti-inflammatory injections. *Sodium succinate:* Used IV for exacerbations of multiple sclerosis.	*Joint injection:* 1–2 mL/injection (1 mL = 40 mg) *Skin:* apply thin layer once daily (1 mg/g in 15 g tube)	Similar to predisolone but used as injection, has slightly less mineralocorticoid effects.
Prednisolone	Suppression of allergic and inflammatory disorders.	Variable. *Acute severe asthma:* 50 mg PO once daily for 5–7 days. *Initial autoimmune or inflammatory disease:* 1–2 mg/kg once daily and taper according to response	Commonly used for long-term disease suppression.
Triamcinolone	Intra-articular or soft-tissue anti-inflammatory injections; topical skin conditions.	40–80 mg local injection (IM, SC, intra-/peri-articular)	

*Relative anti-inflammatory equivalence: dexamethasone 0.75 mg = hydrocortisone 20 mg = methylprednisolone 4 mg = prednisolone 5 mg.

Ketamine (A)

Indications: Adjunct in severe or intractable pain.

Actions: NMDA receptor antagonist causing dissociation, analgesia and CNS depression.

Adverse effects: Increased muscle tone and jerking, nausea and vomiting, emergence delirium, lacrimation, hypersalivation, diplopia, nystagmus.

Cautions: Use by experienced personnel only.

Dose: Available in 200 mg ampoules. Careful titration of 5–10 mg IV boluses for acute pain, or 2–3 mg/kg for procedural sedation with analgesia.

Methoxyflurane (A)

Indications: Short-term analgesia in acute trauma or for painful procedures.

Actions: Inhaled volatile anaesthetic.

Adverse effects: Nephrotoxic at anaesthetic doses or in chronic use. Can cause confusion or sedation.

Cautions: Do not use in patients with renal impairment, or with altered mental status or haemodynamic instability. Do not use in very young children or patients unable to self-administer. Do not use more than 6 mL per day or 15 mL per week.

Comments: Available on PBS Doctor's Bag list due to rapid action, portability and ease of administration.

Dose: Available in 3 mL bottles together with a single-use inhaler. Pour 3 mL of methoxyflurane into the inhaler and instruct the patient to inhale and exhale into the mouthpiece. An additional 3 mL can be used after 25–30 min if ongoing analgesia is required, up to 60 min.

NSAIDs (C)

Indications: Mild-to-moderate pain, fever, especially due to inflammation including dysmenorrhoea, metastatic bone pain, renal colic, migraine, pericarditis. Inflammatory arthritides including acute gout.

Actions: Cyclooxygenase (COX) 1 and 2 inhibition, producing anti-inflammatory and analgesic effects.

Adverse effects: Nausea, gastritis and peptic ulceration, bleeding (can be asymptomatic), diarrhoea, headache, dizziness, renal impairment with sodium and fluid retention and worsening hypertension.

SECTION F – Formulary

Cautions: GI haemorrhage, renal impairment, severe hepatic
disease, heart failure. Allergic cross-reactivity across NSAIDs
and aspirin. Associated with increased risk of cardiovascular
events. Elderly have an increased risk of serious adverse
effects.

Comments: Enteric-coated preparations do not decrease risk
of GI adverse effects. Similar rates of serious GI events between
selective and non-selective agents. Topical administration
may slightly reduce systemic adverse effects. Take medication
with food.

Drug	Usual adult dose	Comments
Celecoxib	100 mg PO BD	Selective COX-2 inhibitor.
Diclofenac	25–50 mg PO TDS, or topical gel applied to affected area QID	Can be used for dysfunctional uterine bleeding.
Etoricoxib	30–60 mg PO daily. Can give 120 mg daily short term for acute exacerbations of gout	Selective COX-2 inhibitor. Contraindicated in severe heart, hepatic or renal dysfunction, or in poorly controlled hypertension, or coronary, cerebral or peripheral vascular disease.
Ibuprofen	200–400 mg PO QID, or topical gel applied to affected area QID	Can decrease antiplatelet effect of aspirin, so choose an alternative NSAID if prolonged use is expected. Combination with codeine not recommended due to lack of benefit.
Indomethacin	25–50 mg PO BD or QID, or 100 mg suppository PR BD	Vertigo is common adverse reaction.
Ketoprofen	200 mg PO daily, or 100 mg suppository PR daily, or topical gel applied to affected area QID	
Ketorolac	15–30 mg IV/IM QID to max 60 mg daily dose, or 10 mg PO QID	Contraindicated in renal impairment or dehydration. Give IV injection slowly.

Drug	Usual adult dose	Comments
Mefenamic acid	500 mg PO TDS	
Meloxicam	7.5–15 mg PO daily	Dose-dependent COX-2 selectivity, so use lowest effective dose.
Naproxen	250–500 mg PO BD, or 750–1000 mg PO daily for controlled-release preparation	Can decrease antiplatelet effect of aspirin, so choose an alternative NSAID if prolonged use is expected.
Parecoxib	20–40 mg IV/IM	Selective COX-2 inhibitor. Used IV or IM as single dose for postoperative pain.
Piroxicam	10–20 mg PO daily	Higher risk of serious skin reactions.
Sulindac	200 mg PO daily or BD	

Opioids (C; codeine A)

Indications: Moderate to severe acute or chronic pain.

Actions: Activate opioid receptors in peripheral and central nervous systems.

Adverse effects: Common—nausea, vomiting, anorexia, drowsiness, itch, dizziness, constipation, headache. Uncommon—bronchospasm, altered mental status including dysphoria, confusion, agitation, urticaria, paralytic ileus, local or generalised flushing due to histamine release (except fentanyl-type opioids).

Cautions: Respiratory depression and coma are the most serious adverse effects. More common in elderly, hepatic disease (reduce dose), renal impairment, severe respiratory disease. Hypotension and shock can occur with large doses. All opioids can cause spasm of the sphincter of Oddi and biliary pain. Physical dependence and tolerance are common. Tolerance to constipation does not occur, so a stimulant laxative is recommended.

Comments: Dosages are a guide and individual variation is common, so titrated doses are required. Older or opioid-naïve patients generally require lower doses. Morphine is the preferred opioid analgesic due to cost, familiarity and availability but others can be used if unacceptable adverse effects or allergy. Most longer-acting opioids can also be used as cough suppressants.

SECTION F – Formulary

Drug	Usual adult dose	Approximate comparison doses	Comments
Buprenorphine	*Acute pain:* 300–600 microgram IM/IV QID or 200–400 microgram SL QID. *Chronic pain:* Commence with 5 microgram/h topical patch and titrate dose every 3 days.	5 microgram/h patch equivalent to 10 mg total daily dose of PO morphine.	Partial agonist, so less efficacious than full agonists and may precipitate withdrawal if dependence on other opioids. Usually used for chronic pain management. Steady-state effects take at least 3 days with a patch.
Codeine	30–60 mg PO/SC/IM 4-hourly	100 mg SC/IM or 200 mg PO equivalent to 10 mg SC/IM morphine.	Also used for diarrhoea and cough suppression. Do not use in renal impairment. Analgesic effect limited by adverse effects (esp nausea and vomiting). Morphine is active metabolite—approx 8% of Caucasians, 1% Asians do not obtain analgesia from codeine due to lack of metabolism to morphine. Approx 10% of Caucasians, 1% Asians, 29% Ethiopians are rapid metabolisers and obtain higher morphine concentrations. No evidence that lower-dose codeine adds analgesic efficacy to paracetamol or NSAIDs alone.
Dextropopoxyphene	Usually used in combination with paracetamol. Various preparations		Not recommended for use. No added analgesic effect compared to paracetamol alone in single dose. Toxic in overdosage and accumulation if regular use.

Drug	Usual adult dose	Approximate comparison doses	Comments
Fentanyl	*Acute pain:* Careful titration of 25 microgram IV boluses with cardiorespiratory monitoring. Also used via intranasal route for acute pain or palliative care breakthrough pain in dose of 1–1.5 microgram/kg. *Breakthrough pain:* 200 microgram lozenge PO or careful IV titration as above. *Chronic pain:* Not used for opioid-naïve patients. Use patch once patient stabilised on other opioid.	100 microgram IV equivalent to 10 mg morphine IV.	No histamine release and more cardiovascularly stable than other opioids. More likely to cause respiratory depression. Contributes to serotonin syndrome if combined with other serotinergic drugs. Preferred in renal impairment.
Hydromorphone	*Acute pain:* 2–4 mg PO 4-hourly of standard release preparation or 0.1 mg IV titrated to response. *Chronic pain:* Individual dosing dependent on previous opioid use.	1 mg equivalent to 5–8 mg morphine (either PO or parenteral).	IV preparations uncommonly used for acute pain but can be used for breakthrough pain.
Methadone	Not suitable for acute pain. *Chronic pain:* Individual dosing dependent on previous opioid use.	10 mg IM/SC equivalent to 10 mg morphine SC/IM; 20 mg PO equivalent to 30 mg PO morphine acutely but 200 mg with chronic administration.	Do not use if risk of prolonged QT syndromes. Also used for chronic management of opioid dependence.

Continued

SECTION F – Formulary

Drug	Usual adult dose	Approximate comparison doses	Comments
Morphine	*Acute or breakthrough pain:* Titrated IV boluses of 1–2.5 mg every 3–5 minutes, or 5–10 mg SC Q2H. Use lower doses in elderly or with multiple comorbid conditions. *Chronic pain:* Convert the 24-h opioid requirement into an equivalent dose of controlled-release preparation and give half-dose every 12 h. *Breakthrough pain:* Use one-sixth of usual total morphine dose as oral liquid, or use IV or SC titration as above. *Intractable cough:* 5–10 mg via nebuliser 4-hourly.	10 mg IV morphine equivalent to 30 mg PO morphine.	Active metabolites may accumulate in renal impairment. Peak analgesia occurs within 10 minutes with IV, 30 minutes SC, 60 minutes PO. Do not use controlled-release preparations for acute pain management.
Oxycodone	*Acute pain:* 5–10 mg PO 4-hourly titrated to response. *Chronic pain:* Individual dosing dependent on previous opioid use.	15 mg PO equivalent to 30 mg PO morphine.	IV preparations uncommonly used. Can be used as an alternative to morphine for acute or chronic pain. Preferred if renal impairment or in elderly (less sedation). Available in standard and controlled-release preparations. Also as controlled-release combination with naloxone to decrease risk of adverse effects.

Drug	Usual adult dose	Approximate comparison doses	Comments
Pethidine	*Acute or breakthrough pain*: Titrated IV boluses of 10–25 mg every 3–5 min, or 50–100 mg IM Q2H. Use lower doses in elderly or with multiple comorbid conditions.	100 mg IV equivalent to 10 mg IV morphine.	Avoid in renal impairment. Contributes to serotonin syndrome if combined with other serotinergic drugs.
Tapentadol	50 mg BD PO	100 mg PO equivalent to 40 mg PO morphine.	Mu receptor agonist and inhibits noradrenaline reupake. Used for chronic pain. Dose titrated to maximum 250 mg BD. Benefit compared to placebo is questionable. Avoid or reduce dose in renal or hepatic impairment.
Tramadol	*Acute pain*: 50–100 mg IV/IM/PO 4-hourly. Max 400 mg/day. Reduce dose in elderly. *Chronic pain*: 50–200 mg BD using 12-h controlled-release product, or 100–400 mg daily using 24-h controlled-release product. Titrate dose to effect.	100 mg IV equivalent to 10 mg morphine IV. 50 mg PO equivalent to 10 mg morphine PO.	Weak affinity for opioid receptors so effective for moderate pain and less constipating effect. Also prevents reuptake of noradrenaline and serotonin, so may have additional effects in neuropathic pain. Approx 8% of Caucasians, 1% Asians do not obtain analgesia from tramadol due to lack of metabolism to active metabolite. Contributes to serotonin syndrome if combined with other serotinergic drugs. Avoid or reduce dose in renal or hepatic impairment.

SECTION F – Formulary

Paracetamol (A)

Indications: Mild-to-moderate pain, fever. Adjunct in severe pain.
Actions: Unclear, probably central inhibition of prostaglandin
synthesis. No anti-inflammatory effect.
Adverse effects: Abnormal LFTs common, allergic reactions rare.
Cautions: Abnormal liver function.
Comments: Often combined with codeine as analgesic preparation,
metoclopramide for migraine treatment. Contained in many
cough and cold products. Evidence of additional analgesic effect of
NSAID over paracetamol alone for undifferentiated (non-
inflammatory) pain is lacking. IV preparation has more rapid onset
but no other benefits and is more expensive. Rectal absorption is
erratic.
Dose: Most commonly used preparations are 500 mg tablets or
665 mg slow-release tablets; multiple children's liquid
preparations; suppositories; 500 mg and 1000 mg ampoules. Usual
dose 1 g QID PO (15 mg/kg QID PO for children).

- **Febuxostat:** Xanthine oxidase inhibitor second-line treatment for
  gout prophylaxis or hyperuricaemia from tumour lysis syndrome.
- **Hylans:** Visco supplements containing hyaluronic acid used to
  treat osteoarthritis. Efficacy is unclear.
- **Nitrous oxide:** Inhaled gaseous analgesic and anaesthetic
  adjunct. Used as premixed 50:50 mixture with oxygen for
  undifferentiated acute pain. Can cause distension of gas-filled
  cavities, so contraindicated in bowel obstruction, pneumothorax,
  air embolism, middle ear occlusion, pneumocranium.
- **Probenecid:** Increases renal excretion of uric acid, so used for gout
  prophylaxis if intolerant of allopurinol (usual dose 500–1000 mg
  PO BD). Also used to increase plasma concentrations of penicillin
  antibiotics (usual dose 500 mg PO QID).

Antimigraine drugs
Metoclopramide (see also *Antiemetics*)

Used orally as single agent or in combination with paracetamol or
NSAIDs as first-line agent in aborting or treating acute migraine. Usual
dose 10 mg PO/IV/IM.

Phenothiazines (see also *Antiemetics* and *Antipsychotics*)

Used parenterally are effective treatments for acute migraine if no
response to initial simple analgesics (paracetamol or NSAIDs) or abortive therapy (triptan or ergotamine/caffeine or metoclopramide). Usual
dose is prochlorperazine 12.5 mg IV/IM or chlorpromazine 12.5–
25 mg IV together with IV fluids.

Triptans (B3)

Indications: Acute treatment or prophylaxis of migraine.

Actions: Constricts cranial vessels by acting selectively at $5HT_{1B/1D}$ receptors, particularly of the dilated carotid arterial circulation in migraine. Also thought to inhibit the abnormal activation of trigeminal nociceptors.

Adverse effects: Sensations of tingling, heat, pain, heaviness or tightness in any part of the body, including chest and throat, flushing, dizziness, feeling of weakness, drowsiness, fatigue, nausea, vomiting, dry mouth, transient increase in BP.

Cautions: Can cause coronary artery spasm, so contraindicated in history of MI, IHD, coronary vasospasm (e.g. Prinzmetal's angina); uncontrolled hypertension; history of CVA or TIA; peripheral vascular disease.

Comments: Dependence may occur with overuse, resulting in recurrent and/or rebound migraine headaches and withdrawal syndrome. Do not use IV (increased risk of coronary vasospasm). Avoid if ergot compounds used within 24 hours as increases risk of vasospasm. Give first SC injection under medical supervision. Use as soon as possible after onset of headache.

Drug	Usual adult dose
Eletriptan	40 mg with repeat after 2 h if required.
Naratriptan	2.5 mg PO with repeat after 4 h if required.
Rizatriptan	10 mg with repeat after at least 2 hours if required.
Sumatriptan	50–100 mg PO with repeat after 2 h if required or 6 mg SC with repeat dose after 1 h if required or 10–20 mg intranasal spray repeated after 2 h if required.
Zolmitriptan	2.5 mg PO with repeat after 2 h if required.

- **Caffeine:** Used for relief of migraine headache, usually in combination with paracetamol. The benefit of adding caffeine to paracetamol is uncertain.
- **Droperidol:** Used parenterally is most effective treatment for acute migraine if no response to initial simple analgesics (paracetamol or NSAIDs) or abortive therapy (triptan or ergotamine/caffeine or metoclopramide). Usual dose is 0.625–1.25 mg IV together with IV fluids.
- **Methysergide:** Ergot alkaloid serotonin antagonist causing vasoconstriction. Used to prevent migraine when other treatments ineffective. Multiple adverse events and contraindications.
- **Pizotifen:** Serotonin antagonist with antihistamine and anticholinergic effects. Used for prevention of migraine and cluster headache, but high rate of adverse effects.

SECTION F – Formulary

Anticonvulsants
Benzodiazepines (C)
Indications: First-line management in acute treatment of seizures, and used as adjuncts for treatment of epilepsy.

Actions: Potentiate GABA effects in the CNS, resulting in sedative and anticonvulsive effects. Also provide antiemetic effects and provide effective labyrinthine suppression for vertigo.

Adverse effects: Drowsiness, sedation, ataxia and falls, slurred speech, confusion, euphoria, hypotension and dizziness. IV–hypotension, arrhythmias from too-rapid delivery, thrombophlebitis, skin necrosis.

Cautions: Generally not suitable for long-term management due to sedation and development of tolerance and dependence.

Comments: Diazepam not suitable for IM administration (use midazolam or clonazepam). Marked individual dose variation can occur depending on age and tolerance. Decrease dose in elderly.

Drug	Usual adult dose	Comments
Clobazam	5–10 mg PO nocte, increased if required.	Used for absence and myoclonic seizures refractory to other agents.
Clonazepam	0.5–1 mg PO nocte, increased if required. *Status epilepticus:* 1 mg IV, repeated as necessary. *Ongoing seizure control:* 2–8 mg IV infusion over 24 h.	Used for absence and myoclonic seizures refractory to other agents. Also used IV/IM for status epilepticus or other seizures requiring ongoing acute management.
Diazepam	*Status epilepticus:* 5–10 mg slow IV boluses repeated every 5 minutes, or 10–20 mg PR. *Prevention of withdrawal seizures:* 10–20 mg PO hourly titrated to withdrawal features.	Acute seizure control, including status epilepticus, or prevention of drug-withdrawal seizures.
Midazolam	5–10 mg IV/IM/ buccal/ intranasal repeated every 5 minutes.	Used for status epilepticus.

Carbamazepine (D)
Indications: First-line management in partial seizures. Also used for trigeminal and glossopharyngeal neuralgias and as a mood stabiliser in bipolar disorder.

Actions: Prevents repetitive neuronal discharge by sodium-channel blockade.

Adverse effects: Drowsiness, ataxia, dizziness, blurred or double vision, headache, rash, GI upset, blood dyscrasias, hyponatraemia. Severe skin reactions including life-threatening toxic epidermal necrolysis or Stevens–Johnson syndrome (more likely if Asian ancestry due to HLA type). Use of controlled-release agents may decrease concentration-dependent adverse effects (dizziness, blurred vision).

Cautions: Hypersensitivity cross-reactivity occurs across most anticonvulsants. Check blood counts regularly. Consider prophylaxis for osteoporosis if chronic use.

Comments: Contraindicated in patients with cardiac AV conduction abnormalities, history of bone marrow depression.

Dose: Available in 100 mg and 200 mg standard tablets and 200 mg and 400 mg controlled-release tablets. Usual initial dose 100 mg PO BD, increase every 2–4 weeks according to response. Usual range 200–600 mg PO BD. Halve initial dose in elderly.

Phenytoin (D)

Indications: Simple and complex partial seizures, and generalised tonic–clonic seizures, particularly in status epilepticus.

Actions: Prevents repetitive neuronal discharge in the cerebral cortex by blocking sodium channels.

Adverse effects: Nausea, vomiting, insomnia, sedation, confusion, ataxia, nystagmus and vertigo, diplopia, blurred vision, agitation and behavioural disturbances, impaired learning (dose-related). Long-term use can cause gingival hypertrophy, skin eruption, coarse facies, hirsutism, loss of bone density. IV—hypotension, arrhythmias from too-rapid delivery, thrombophlebitis, skin necrosis.

Cautions: Phenytoin interacts with many drugs and must be given dissolved in normal saline *slowly* IV under ECG control with an in-line filter. Reduce the dose in hepatic impairment. Do not use IM.

Comments: Therapeutic range is 10–20 mg/L (40–80 micromol/L). A small change in dosage may result in a disproportionately large change in serum phenytoin concentration because of the saturation of its hepatic metabolism. If a decision is made to withdraw treatment, preferably do so over 6 months at a rate not greater than 25 mg/week or 100 mg/month.

Dose: Available in 30 mg, 50 mg and 100 mg tablets, 6 mg/mL syrup, and 100 mg and 250 mg ampoules. *Epilepsy:* Initially 5 mg/kg PO daily in 1 or 2 doses; increase by 30 mg daily once every 2 weeks according to clinical response and plasma concentration. Usual range: 200–500 mg PO daily. *Status epilepticus:* 15 mg/kg IV by slow infusion at no greater than 50 mg/min. An additional dose of 5 mg/kg IV may be given after 12 hours if necessary.

Valproate (D)

Indications: First-line treatment for generalised tonic–clonic or absence seizures. Can also be used for other primary epileptic generalised seizures and for partial seizures. May have benefit in bipolar disorder resistant to other therapies and for migraine prevention.

Actions: Prevents repetitive neuronal discharge in the cerebral cortex by blocking sodium channels.

Adverse effects: Nausea, vomiting, increased appetite and weight gain, tremor, drowsiness, ataxia, hair loss.

Cautions: Contraindicated if pancreatic dysfunction, porphyria, severe hepatic impairment (can induce hepatic failure, especially if other anticonvulsants used).

Comments: Injectable form used in patients unable to tolerate oral preparation. Efficacy in status epilepticus unknown.

Dose: Available in 100 mg, 200 mg and 500 mg tablets, 40 mg/mL syrup and 400 mg injectable preparation. Usual starting dose 600 mg PO BD increasing by 200 mg every 3 days until adequate response.

- **Acetazolamide:** Used for menstrual-related seizures.
- **Ethosuximide:** Can be considered as first-line agent for absence seizures.
- **Gabapentin:** Adjunctive therapy for partial seizures not controlled by other drugs. Also used for neuropathic pain with initial dose of 100 mg at night.
- **Lacosamide:** Adjunctive therapy for partial seizures. Also available as IV formulation.
- **Lamotrigine:** Adjunctive or monotherapy for partial or generalised seizures. Also used in bipolar disorder to prevent depressive episodes.
- **Levetiracetam:** Monotherapy or adjunctive therapy of partial seizures, or adjunctive therapy of generalised seizures or juvenile myoclonic epilepsy. IV preparation can be use in patients unable to take oral therapy. Its role in acute management of seizures or non-convulsive status epilepticus is unclear.
- **Oxcarbazepine:** Adjunctive or monotherapy of partial or generalised tonic–clonic seizures.
- **Perampanel:** Adjunctive treatment for partial seizures.
- **Phenobarbitone:** Second-line agent for epilepsy including partial seizures, generalised tonic–clonic seizures, neonatal seizures. Can be used for status epilepticus not responding to benzodiazepines and phenytoin (usual dose 15 mg/kg IV infusion over 30 minutes).
- **Pregabalin:** Adjunctive treatment of partial seizures. Also used for neuropathic pain with initial dose of 75 mg BD.

- **Primidone:** Prodrug of phenobarbitone. Used orally for similar indications.
- **Tiagabine:** Adjunctive treatment of partial seizures.
- **Topiramate:** Monotherapy or adjunctive therapy for partial seizures, generalised tonic–clonic seizures or Lennox–Gastaut syndrome.
- **Vigabactrin:** Adjunctive therapy for complex partial seizures not responding to other agents; 20–40% of patients may develop permanent visual field defects, so uncommonly used.
- **Zonisamide:** Adjunctive treatment or monotherapy for partial seizures.

Neurodegenerative and movement disorders
Benztropine mesylate (B2)

Indications: Drug-induced extrapyramidal reactions (except tardive dyskinesia). Drug of choice for terminating acute dystonic reactions. Useful for symptomatic treatment of Parkinson's disease.

Actions: Anticholinergic (antimuscarinic) agent with antihistamine and local anaesthetic properties.

Adverse effects: Tachycardia, dizziness, mydriasis and cycloplegia, dry mouth, urinary hesitancy/retention.

Cautions: Contraindicated in closed-angle glaucoma, GI obstruction, urinary obstruction (may exacerbate symptoms of prostatic hypertrophy), myasthenia gravis. Avoid combination with other drugs with anticholinergic effects. Use with caution in the elderly and in children.

Comments: Onset of effect is 2–3 minutes after IM or IV injection or 1–2 hours after oral dose (effects may persist for 24 hours or longer). May increase effects of alcohol (avoid driving/operating machinery).

Dose: Available in 2 mg tablets and ampoules. 1–2 mg PO, IM or IV for acute dystonic reactions. If symptoms return, dose can be repeated. *Parkinson's disease:* 0.5–1 mg PO daily, increased gradually to 6 mg daily.

Levodopa–carbidopa/benserazide (B3)

Indications: Parkinson's disease.

Actions: Levodopa is converted to dopamine in the basal ganglia. The carbidopa or benserazide inhibits the peripheral production of levodopa, decreasing adverse effects.

Adverse effects: Common—anorexia, nausea, vomiting, abdominal pain, dysrhythmias, behavioural changes, orthostatic hypotension, involuntary movements.

Cautions: Contraindicated in closed-angle glaucoma. Breastfeeding— may inhibit lactation. May develop sudden changes in efficacy

(i.e. 'on/off' phenomenon). Do not use with non-selective MAOIs or conventional antipsychotics. Do not stop suddenly.
Comments: Dosage is expressed as levodopa.
Dose: Available in multiple tablet dosages and combinations, and an intestinal gel for gastrostomy use. Dosing schedule is complex. Initiate therapy with one 100/25 mg tablet TDS, then increase according to response up to eight 100/25 mg tablets daily; if more levodopa is needed, substitute the 250/25 mg tablets.

- **Amantadine:** Increases dopamine release, NMDA antagonist, anticholinergic. May be used as monotherapy for early Parkinson's disease or as adjunct for drug-induced dyskinesias.
- **Apomorpine:** Stimulates central dopamine receptors. Used in Parkinson's disease for frequent motor fluctuations (on/off periods) refractory to other drugs. Can cause hypotension, respiratory depression. Highly emetogenic, so requires pretreatment with domperidone in initial phase of use. Also used for acromegaly, hyperprolactinaemia, suppression of lactation.
- **Baclofen:** GABA agonist used for muscle spasms and spasticity related to CNS disorders.
- **Benzhexol:** Similar to benztropine. Used for drug-induced movement disorders and Parkinson's disease.
- **Biperiden:** Similar to benztropine. Used for drug-induced movement disorders and Parkinson's disease.
- **Bromocriptine:** Stimulates central dopamine receptors. Can be used in early Parkinson's disease as monotherapy or as adjunct to levodopa. Not as effective as levodopa and has risk of tissue fibrosis (ergot derivative). May require domperidone treatment due to nausea. Dopamine agonists can also cause problems with impulse control such as pathological gambling, hypersexuality, overspending. Also used as treatment for acromegaly and hyperprolactinaemia.
- **Cabergoline:** Central dopamine agonist with similar uses, effects and adverse reactions (esp cardiac fibrosis) to bromocriptine.
- **Dantrolene:** Direct-acting muscle relaxant, interferes with calcium release from sarcoplasmic reticulum. Used for chronic spasticity related to CNS pathology and for malignant hyperthermia.
- **Dimethyl fumarate:** Antioxidant and immunomodulatory effects. Decreases risk of relapses in relapsing-remitting multiple sclerosis.
- **Donepazil:** Anticholinesterase used to prevent deterioration of cognition in Alzheimer's disease.
- **Entacapone:** Used as adjunct to levodopa for motor fluctuations in Parkinson's disease. Increases duration of motor improvement but increased risk of dyskinesias.

- **Fampridine:** Potassium channel blocker used to increase walking speed in multiple sclerosis. Exact mechanism of action unknown.
- **Fingolimod:** Sphingosine receptor modulator reduces lymphocyte infiltration of the CNS reducing demyelination. Used for relapsing-remitting or secondary progressive multiple sclerosis.
- **Galantamine:** Anticholinesterase used to prevent deterioration of cognition in Alzheimer's disease.
- **Glatiramer:** Synthetic polypeptide with unknown mechanism of action. Used to decrease risk of relapses in multiple sclerosis.
- **Interferon beta:** Immunomodulatory actions used to decrease risk of relapse in multiple sclerosis.
- **Memantine:** NMDA antagonist used to prevent deterioration of cognition in Alzheimer's disease.
- **Natalizumab:** Integrin antibody decreasing CNS inflammation used to decrease risk of relapses in multiple sclerosis.
- **Neostigmine:** Anticholinesterase used SC or IM for treatment of myasthenia gravis when oral route is inappropriate, and to reverse neuromuscular blockade in anaesthesia.
- **Orphenadrine:** Similar to benztropine but used mainly for treatment of muscle spasm. Efficacy is unclear.
- **Pergolide:** Dopamine agonist used as adjunct to levodopa for Parkinson's disease. Similar to cabergoline.
- **Pramipexole:** Non-ergot-derived dopamine agonist. Used as adjunct for treatment of Parkinson's disease with levodopa when ergot derivatives are contraindicated or not tolerated. Has also been used for restless leg syndrome.
- **Pyridostigmine:** Anticholinesterase used as first-line for long-term therapy of myasthenia gravis.
- **Rasagiline:** MAO-B inhibitor reduces breakdown of dopamine. Used for Parkinson's disease generally as an adjunct to levodopa.
- **Riluzole:** Inhibits glutamate neurotransmission, slightly prolongs survival in amyotrophic lateral sclerosis.
- **Rivastigmine:** Anticholinesterase used to prevent deterioration of cognition in Alzheimer's disease.
- **Ropinirole:** Dopamine agonist used for restless leg syndrome.
- **Rotigotine:** Similar to pramipexole but available as patch, so used if patient unable to tolerate or swallow oral medication.
- **Selegiline:** Reduces dopamine destruction and reuptake. Can be used as monotherapy in early Parkinson's disease or as adjunct to levodopa for motor fluctuations.
- **Teriflunomide:** Inhibits leucocyte activation in the CNS, used to decrease risk of relapse and disease progression in multiple sclerosis.
- **Tetrabenazine:** Depletes dopamine in CNS, used for choreiform, dystonic and other movement disorders (not Parkinson's disease).

SECTION F – Formulary

Local anaesthetics
Lignocaine (A)
Indications: Local anaesthesia including topical, infiltration, nerve or plexus block, ophthalmic, intra-articular. Adjunctive to other analgesics for epidural or intrathecal anaesthesia. Can be used for IV regional anaesthesia, but not first-line agent. Swallowed lignocaine gel also used for intractable hiccups.

Actions: Reversibly blocks sodium channels in peripheral nerves and other excitable membranes, inhibiting depolarisation.

Adverse effects: Usually well tolerated. Adverse reactions usually occur from exceeding the recommended dose or due to the effects of the anaesthesia rather than the medication.

Cautions: Contraindications are usually related to the procedure (local infection, anticoagulation) rather than the agent. Caution when used in patients with haemodynamic instability, seizure disorder, cardiac conduction defects, renal (bupivicaine, ropivicaine, procaine) or hepatic dysfunction (lignocaine and prilocaine).

Comments: There is no allergic cross-reaction between amides and esters.

Dose: Available in 2% liquid gel for topical oral and upper GI anaesthesia; 4% liquid, 5% ointment, 10% spray for topical use; 0.5%, 1% and 2% ampoules; 2% gel for urethral catheterisation; 5% nasal spray (together with 0.5% phenylephrine). Combined with adrenaline as various preparations. Maximum dose 3 mg/kg (7 mg/kg if used in combination with adrenaline). Patch (5%) also available for post-herpetic neuralgia.

- **Amethocaine (tetracaine):** Slow-onset, long-acting amide anaesthetic, used topically for wounds or corneal anaesthesia. Maximum dose 1 mg/kg.
- **Bupivicaine:** Long-acting amide anaesthetic used for infiltration, nerve or plexus block, epidural and intrathecal anaesthesia. Duration: 3–4 h after infiltration or 6–12 h after nerve block. Maximum dose 2 mg/kg.
- **Cocaine:** Short-acting ester anaesthetic, used for topical anaesthesia for ENT or upper GI procedures. Vasoconstrictive so can be used in epistaxis. Maximum dose 1.5 mg/kg.
- **Levobupivicaine:** S-isomer of bupivicaine.
- **Prilocaine:** Amide anaesthetic, less toxic than other amides. Used predominantly for IV regional anaesthesia, epidural anaesthesia, or mixed with lignocaine as cream for topical use. Causes dose-related methaemoglobinaemia. Maximum dose 6 mg/kg.
- **Procaine:** Short-acting ester anaesthetic, used for infiltration and nerve block anaesthesia. Maximum dose 8 mg/kg.

- **Ropivicaine:** Long-acting amide anaesthetic similar to bupivicaine. Maximum dose 3 mg/kg.

Psychotropics

Sedatives, anxiolytics and drugs for sleep disorders

Benzodiazepines (C) (see also *Anticonvulsants*)

Indications: Anxiety, panic disorder, insomnia, behavioural sedation, drug intoxication and withdrawal syndromes, procedural sedation or premedication.

Actions: Potentiate the inhibitory effects of GABA within the CNS.

Adverse effects: Drowsiness and oversedation, dizziness, poor concentration and memory, slurred speech, confusion.

Cautions: May worsen respiratory failure. Will worsen muscle weakness in myasthenia gravis. Avoid long-acting agents in hepatic impairment. Addictive potential with physical tolerance and withdrawal symptoms. Reduce dose in elderly.

Comments: Short-term use preferred. Large variation in dose and tolerance.

Drug	Usual adult dose	Comments
Alprazolam	0.25–0.5 mg PO TDS for anxiety. *Panic disorder:* increase dose to max 10 mg per day.	Used for anxiety and panic disorder. Short duration of action (6–12 h).
Bromazepam	3–6 mg PO BD to TDS	Medium duration of action (12–24 h).
Clobazam	10–30 mg daily	Long duration of action (>24 h).
Diazepam	1–10 mg PO up to TDS; 5–10 mg IV for sedation, repeated as necessary	Used for drug withdrawal, anxiety, premedication, IV sedation. Ensure reliable IV access as extravasation can lead to tissue necrosis. Not for IM administration. Rapid onset of action but long-acting due to active metabolites.
Flunitrazepam	0.5–2 mg nocte PO	Long-acting but rapid onset of action. Controlled drug.
Lorazepam	1–2.5 mg daily PO or SL	Also used as antiemetic for anticipatory nausea and vomiting from chemotherapy. Medium duration of action.

SECTION F – Formulary

Continued

Drug	Usual adult dose	Comments
Midazolam	2.5–5 mg IV boluses for sedation	Very short-acting. Used for acute behavioural sedation or control of withdrawal symptoms, procedural sedation, to abort seizures.
Nitrazepam	20 mg nocte	Used for insomnia as single evening dose. Long-acting.
Oxazepam	7.5–15 mg TDS for anxiety, increased to 30 mg PO QID as maximal dose. *Insomnia:* 7.5–30 mg nocte.	Short-acting (6–12 h).
Temazepam	5–20 mg nocte	Used for insomnia as single evening dose. Short-acting (6–12 h) with rapid onset.
Triazolam	0.125–0.25 mg nocte	Used for insomnia as single evening dose. Very short-acting (<6 h) with rapid onset. High dependence potential.

- **Buspirone:** Partial serotonin agonist used for anxiety syndromes. May be preferred in patients at risk of benzodiazepine dependence.
- **Melatonin:** Pineal gland hormone used for short-term treatment of insomnia, particularly in patients aged over 55 years, who may have increased adverse effects from alternative medications.
- **Modafinil:** Non-amphetamine CNS stimulant used for narcolepsy, severe shift-work sleep disorder. Risk of abuse, increased risk of psychiatric adverse effects. Avoid in cardiovascular disease.
- **Zolpidem:** Non-benzodiazepine that potentiates effects of GABA, used for short-term treatment of insomnia.
- **Zopiclone:** Non-benzodiazepine that potentiates effects of GABA, used for short-term treatment of insomnia.

Mood disorders
Lithium (D)
Indications: Bipolar disorder, acute mania, schizoaffective disorder, adjunct for depression not responding to other agents.
Actions: Mechanism of action unknown, but inhibits dopamine release and enhances serotonin release.
Adverse effects: Metallic taste, GI disturbance, dyspepsia, weight gain, fatigue, vertigo, tremor. Can cause nephrogenic diabetes insipidus with polyuria and polydipsia.

Cautions: Can worsen psoriasis. Toxicity more likely in hyponatraemia, renal impairment. Can contribute to serotonin syndrome.

Comments: Onset of action delayed by 6–10 days. Monitor renal and thyroid function. Withdraw slowly to prevent relapse.

Dose: Available in 250 mg standard-release and 450 mg controlled-release tablets. Usual dose for acute mania is 250 mg PO TDS, increasing dose by 250 mg daily until symptoms resolve, to maximum of 2500 mg daily. Chronic therapy requires titration according to clinical effect and serum concentration (0.4–1.0 mmol/L).

Selective serotonin reuptake inhibitors (SSRIs) (C)

Indications: Major depression, some anxiety disorders including obsessive–compulsive disorder, some eating disorders.

Actions: Increase synaptic serotonin levels by inhibiting presynaptic uptake.

Adverse effects: Nausea, agitation, sleep disturbance, drowsiness, dry mouth, GI disturbance, weight changes, sexual dysfunction. Increased suicidality can occur in the early stage of treatment. May provoke mania in patients with bipolar disorder.

Cautions: In the elderly, use a lower starting dose and a more gradual dose increase because of the greater risk of adverse effects. Taper dose prior to cessation. Serotonin syndrome can occur with coadministration of other antidepressants (TCAs, SSRIs, MAOIs), some opioids (fentanyl, pethidine, tramadol), stimulants (amphetamines), lithium and others.

Comments: All SSRIs are equally efficacious in the management of depression. Efficacy in posttraumatic stress disorder, premenstrual dysphoric syndrome is unclear. Doses for obsessive–compulsive disorder or panic disorder are usually higher, although higher doses can also increase anxiety. Take in morning to minimise insomnia.

Drug	Usual adult dose	Comments
Citalopram	20 mg daily. Slowly increase to 60 mg daily if used for obsessive–compulsive or eating disorders. Doses >20 mg usually not required for depression.	Use lower dose in elderly.
Escitalopram	10 mg daily, slowly increased to 20 mg daily if required. Doses >10 mg usually not required.	Use lower dose in elderly.

Continued

Drug	Usual adult dose	Comments
Fluoxetine	20 mg daily, slowly increased to max of 60 mg daily if required. 10–20 mg daily for panic disorder.	Used for major depression, obsessive–compulsive disorder, premenstrual dysphoric disorder, bulimia, panic disorder, posttraumatic stress disorder.
Fluvoxamine	50 mg daily, slowly increased to 150 mg daily to BD. Doses >100 mg usually not required.	Used for major depression, obsessive–compulsive disorder, panic disorder.
Paroxetine	20 mg daily, slowly increased to max of 50 mg daily. Doses >20 mg usually not required. Use 10–20 mg in posttraumatic stress disorder.	Most likely to cause withdrawal if stopped suddenly due to shorter half-life and no active metabolites.
Sertraline	50 mg daily, slowly increased to max of 200 mg daily if required. Doses >50 mg usually not required.	Used for major depression, obsessive–compulsive disorder, panic disorder, social phobia, premenstrual dysphoric syndrome.

Tricyclic antidepressants (TCAs) (C)

Indications: Major depression, adjunct in analgesia, particularly chronic and neuropathic pain, attention-deficit hyperactivity disorder, urge incontinence, migraine prophylaxis.

Actions: Increase synaptic serotonin and noradrenaline levels by inhibiting presynaptic uptake. They also block cholinergic, histaminergic, serotonergic, alpha-1 adrenergic receptors and sodium channels.

Adverse effects: Sedation, dry mouth, blurred vision, constipation, weight gain, dizziness from orthostatic hypotension, palpitations, sexual dysfunction, anxiety. May provoke mania in patients with bipolar disorder.

Cautions: Anticholinergic adverse effects may precipitate urinary retention, acute glaucoma, arrhythmias. Can lower seizure threshold. Highly toxic in overdose. Can precipitate serotonin syndrome (see SSRIs above). Suicidality may increase during early treatment. Taper slowly to avoid withdrawal symptoms. Use lower doses in elderly who have a higher rate of confusion and other adverse effects.

Comments: Take in evening to minimise daytime drowsiness, unless daytime sedation required.

Drug	Usual adult dose	Comments
Amitriptyline	25–75 mg nocte initially, increased every 3–4 days up to a max of 300 mg daily (150 mg if used as pain adjuvant). *Urinary urge incontinence:* use 10–25 mg up to TDS.	Used for major depression, analgesic adjuvant, urinary urge incontinence. Sedating, strong anticholinergic and orthostatic effects.
Clomipramine	As per amitriptyline for depression	Treatment of choice for obsessive–compulsive disorder and narcolepsy.
Dothiepin	As per amitriptyline for depression	Used for major depression. Less sedating, anticholinergic and orthostatic effects than most other agents.
Doxepin	As per amitriptyline for depression	Used for major depression. Most sedating agent.
Imipramine	As per amitriptyline	Used for major depression, panic disorder, urinary urge incontinence, ADHD. Similar adverse effects to dothiepin.
Notriptyline	25–75 mg nocte initially, increased every 3–4 days up to a max of 150 mg daily. As per amitriptyline for urge incontinence.	Used for major depression, urinary urge incontinence. Least sedating, anticholinergic and orthostatic adverse effects.

Venlafaxine (B2)

Indications: Major depression, anxiety disorders including generalised anxiety, social phobia and panic disorder.

Actions: Serotonin and noradrenaline reuptake inhibition (SNRI).

Adverse effects: Rash, GI disturbance, sweating, weakness, sexual dysfunction, sleep disturbance, anorexia.

Cautions: Reduce dose in hepatic or renal impairment. May provoke mania in patients with bipolar disorder. May lower seizure threshold. Inhibits platelet aggregation. Can cause hyponatraemia. Avoid combinations which could provoke serotonin syndrome. Potentially fatal cardiotoxicity and delayed seizures in overdose.

Dose: Available in 37.5 mg, 75 mg and 150 mg controlled-release capsules. Usual starting dose 75 mg once daily, increased to 150 mg once daily.

SECTION F – Formulary

- **Desvenlafaxine:** Major active metabolite of venlafaxine.
- **Duloxetine:** Serotonin and noradrenaline reuptake inhibitor. Used for major depression, generalised anxiety and painful peripheral neuropathy. High rate of adverse effects necessitating change to another agent.
- **Mianserin:** Tetracyclic antidepressant with similar effects to the tricyclic antidepressants. More sedating, but less anticholinergic and cardiovascular adverse effects.
- **Mirtazepine:** Postsynaptic serotonin receptor blocker, and presynaptic central alpha-2 blocker. Used for major depression. Can cause increased appetite and weight gain, sedation.
- **Moclobemide:** Selective MAO-A inhibitor used for major depression, social phobia and panic disorder. Less likely to cause sexual dysfunction than non-selective MAOIs and SSRIs.
- **Phenelzine:** Non-selective MAOI used for major depression and panic disorder. Infrequently used due to multiple drug and food interactions.
- **Reboxetine:** Noradrenaline reuptake inhibitor with weak serotonin reuptake inhibition. Used for major depression.
- **Tranylcypromine:** Similar to phenelzine.
- **Vortioxetine:** Serotonin transporter inhibitor increases CNS serotonin activity. Used for major depression.

Antipsychotics
Indications: Primarily treatment of psychotic disorders. If used for non-psychotic illnesses, prescribe the lowest dose for the shortest possible time period. Other indications include second-line to benzodiazepines for behavioural sedation, and for acute treatment of migraine and intractable hiccups.

Actions: All antipsychotics block cental dopaminergic (D2) receptors. Variable ability to block D1 dopamine receptors, serotonin, alpha-adrenergic receptors, H1 histamine and cholinergic receptors. Relative blockade of different receptors determines predominant adverse effects.

Adverse effects: Dopamine receptor blockade causes sedation and impaired performance, extrapyramidal effects including drug-induced parkinsonism, acute dystonic reactions, akathisia and tardive dyskinesia, and endocrinological adverse effects such as hyperprolactinaemia. Autonomic blockade at muscarinic and adrenoreceptors causes anticholinergic effects and postural hypotension. *Neuroleptic malignant syndrome:* fevers, muscle rigidity, altered consciousness and autonomic instability may be caused by antipsychotics—potentially fatal.

Cautions: In the elderly, use a lower starting dose and a more gradual dose increase because of the greater risk of adverse effects, including stroke, diabetes and dyslipidaemia.

Drug	Usual adult dose	Cautions	Comments
Amisulpride	*Acute psychosis:* 200–400 mg BD, 50–300 mg daily for maintenance.	Relatively higher risk of hyperprolactinaemia.	
Aripiprazole	10–15 mg daily, slow increase to max 30 mg daily.	Cautious use if history of IHD.	
Asenapine	5–10 mg BD as sublingual wafers	Higher dose may not provide additional benefit but increases risk of adverse effects.	Prevents short-term relapse in bipolar disorder, also used for schizophrenia.
Chlorpromazine	*Disturbed behaviour:* 12.5–25 mg IV/IM. Repeat after 1 h if required, or 25–50 mg PO (max QDS). 25–100 mg QID for chronic psychoses.	Avoid use in moderate to severe hepatic impairment. Significant hypotensive effect. Photosensitivity and phototoxicity reactions can occur. Relatively higher risk of sedation and anticholinergic effects with some risk of metabolic effects (weight gain and hyperglycaemia).	Acute and chronic psychoses. Short-term management of anxiety/ agitation or disturbed behaviour in non-psychotic disorders. Intractable hiccups if non-drug treatment fails. Headache. Useful in behavioural disturbance associated with amphetamine use (also lowers elevated BP in such patients).
Clozapine	12.5 mg PO initial dose, increase by daily increments to 300 mg daily.	Can cause bone marrow depression and agranulocytosis, cardiomyopathy, interstitial nephritis. First dose may precipitate severe hypotension or cardiorespiratory failure. Hyperpyrexia can occur in 5% of patients.	Used only in schizophrenia resistant to other agents, due to high risk of serious adverse reactions.

Continued

Drug	Usual adult dose	Cautions	Comments
Droperidol	1 mg IV boluses titrated to effect.	Similar to haloperidol.	Used for acute behavioural sedation, adjunct to anaesthesia, antiemetic.
Flupenthixol	20–40 mg IM every 2–4 weeks.	Maximum dose 100 mg IM every 2 weeks.	Depot antipsychotic.
Fluphenazine	12.5–50 mg IM every 2–6 weeks.	Maximum dose 100 mg IM every 2 weeks.	Depot antipsychotic.
Haloperidol	*Disturbed behaviour:* PO 1–5 mg BD to TDS or 2–10 mg IM/IV repeated every 2–6 h PRN. Reduce dose in elderly (0.5–5 mg daily).	May prolong QT interval and increase risk of arrhythmias such as torsades de pointes—check ECG. Lower incidence of hypotension and anticholinergic effects, but relatively higher incidence of extrapyramidal effects.	Acute and chronic psychoses, acute mania, chorea. Adjunct in treatment of alcoholic hallucinosis. Intractable nausea and vomiting. Intractable hiccups. Short-term management of acute agitation/ disturbed behaviour in non-psychotic disorders.
Lurasidone	40 mg once daily.	Higher dose may not provide additional benefit but increases risk of adverse effects.	
Olanzepine	Initial dose 10 mg PO daily, increasing by 2.5 mg/day to total dose of 20 mg daily. *Acute mania or psychosis:* 5–10 mg IM/SL.	Increased likelihood of metabolic effects compared to conventional antipsychotics. Extrapyramidal adverse effects uncommon.	Used for schizophrenia and related psychoses; adjunct for bipolar disorder. Can be used for acute behavioural control of psychosis. Wafer can be used for acute treatment of psychosis.

Drug	Usual adult dose	Cautions	Comments
Paliperidone	6 mg PO daily with slow increase to max 12 mg daily.	Extrapyramidal adverse effects, hyperprolactinaemia, sexual problems, orthostatic hypotension common.	
Pericyazine	10–40 mg PO BD		
Quetiapine	25 mg PO BD with gradual increase up to a max daily dose of 800 mg.	Moderate relative risk of orthostatic hypotension and metabolic effects.	Used for schizophrenia and related psychoses; adjunct for bipolar disorder or treatment-resistant depression.
Risperidone	1 mg PO BD, gradual increase to 4–6 mg PO daily. *Acute behavioural disturbance:* can be given as 0.5–1.0 mg SL.	Use half recommended doses in elderly patients.	Used for psychotic illnesses, acute mania, behavioural disturbance in dementia, autism or mental retardation.
Trifluoperazine	2–15 mg PO BD		Used for psychotic illnesses and for short-term management of anxiety and agitation.
Ziprasidone	Initially 40 mg PO BD titrated to max 80 mg PO BD. Decrease dose for maintenance.	Cautious use if history of IHD.	Used for psychotic illnesses, acute mania.
Zuclopenthixol	10–50 mg PO daily		Usually used as depot antipsychotic. Intermediate-acting preparation can be used for acute psychosis.

SECTION F – Formulary

Drugs for attention-deficit hyperactivity disorder

- **Atomoxetine:** Inhibits CNS noradrenaline uptake. Used if no response or in patients intolerant of psychostimulants. Has cardiovascular sympathomimetic activity so avoid in patients with cardiovascular or cerebrovascular disease.
- **Dexamphetamine:** Amphetamine causing enhanced central dopaminergic and noradrenergic neurotransmission. Avoid in cardiovascular disease or other psychiatric conditions.
- **Lisdexamfetamine:** Metabolised to dexamphetamine as the active metabolite.
- **Methylphenidate:** Non-amphetamine CNS stimulant with similar effects to amphetamines.

Drug-dependence syndromes

- **Acamprosate:** GABA analogue used to maintain abstinence in alcohol dependence.
- **Buprenorphine:** Partial opioid receptor agonist used for maintenance of opioid abstinence by reducing opioid withdrawal symptoms and reduced effects of opioids.
- **Buproprion:** Inhibits neuronal uptake of dopamine and noradrenaline. Used as adjunct to stop smoking. May worsen psychiatric conditions.
- **Disulfiram:** Irreversibly inhibits aldehyde dehydrogenase preventing aldehyde metabolism following alcohol ingestion. Accumulation of aldehyde produces unpleasant effects. Used to maintain abstinence in alcohol dependence.
- **Methadone:** Long-acting opioid used for maintenance of opioid abstinence.
- **Naltrexone:** Long-acting opioid antagonist, reduces craving for alcohol by blocking endogenous opioid effects. Used also for maintenance of opioid abstinence by preventing pleasurable effects of opioids.
- **Nicotine:** Replacement therapy reduces severity of nicotine withdrawal symptoms to assist with smoking cessation. Available as patches, chewing gum, lozenges, inhalers, sublingual tablets.
- **Varenicline:** Partial agonist at neuronal nicotinic receptors blocking binding of nicotine and reducing pleasurable effects of smoking. Partial agonist activity reduces nicotine withdrawal symptoms. May cause severe behavioural changes.

Antimicrobials

Antibacterials
Aminoglycosides (D)

Indications: Moderate-to-severe Gram-negative systemic infections, usually in combination with another antibiotic. Antibacterial sensitivities should always be performed.

Actions: Interfere with the initiation of bacterial protein synthesis in susceptible organisms. Active against aerobic Gram-negative bacteria and staphylococci.

Adverse effects: Use limited by renal, cochlear and vestibular toxicity. Neuromuscular junction blockade may occur, particularly following rapid administration or when used in association with neuromuscular blocking drugs or anaesthetics.

Cautions: Almost all patients will demonstrate nephrotoxicity with prolonged use. Significant adverse effects are more likely with advancing age, preexisting renal impairment or hearing loss. Slow IV administration required.

Comments: Serum creatinine measurements should be made at the initiation of therapy and every 3–4 days during therapy. Monitoring is essential to minimise the effect of nephrotoxicity and reduce the risk of ototoxicity. Adjust dose according to serum aminoglycoside levels and renal function (as elimination of aminoglycosides is by renal excretion). Elderly patients should be given doses at the lowest end of the range. Once-daily IV dosing has replaced 8 h dosing for most indications. Shorter dosing intervals are required when used synergistically with penicillins in the treatment of endocarditis and Gram-positive infections.

Drug	Usual adult dose	Indications
Amikacin	20 mg/kg/day IV	Short-term treatment of serious infections with susceptible organisms. Active against many Gram-negative organisms resistant to other aminoglycosides. Used as second-line defence rather than initial therapy.
Gentamicin	4–7 mg/kg/day IV, or 1–2 mg/kg TDS IV as synergistic therapy for endocarditis	Initial antibacterial therapy for suspected or documented Gram-negative sepsis. Particularly useful for infection involving *Pseudomonas aeruginosa*, *Proteus* spp., *Escherichia coli*, *Klebsiella* and *Staphylococcus* spp.
Neomycin		Rarely used to suppress bowel flora preoperatively.
Tobramycin	As per gentamicin	Treatment of skin infection (including burns), bone infections, GI infections, CNS infections, LRTIs, recurrent and complicated UTIs.

Carbapenem antibiotics (B2, ertapenem/imipenem B3)

Indications: Broadest antimicrobial spectrum with good activity against Gram-negative and Gram-positive organisms and anaerobes.

Actions: Inhibit bacterial cell wall synthesis. Usually bactericidal–resistant to most beta-lactamases.

Adverse effects: Common–nausea, vomiting, diarrhoea, local injection site reactions (e.g. phlebitis).

Cautions: Hypersensitivity to other antibiotics, because of cross-reactions. Ertapenem and imipenem lower the seizure threshold.

Comments: Useful when single-agent treatment is required for complex mixed infections. Otherwise, use combinations of less expensive drugs to provide similar antimicrobial cover and clinical efficacy. Use is restricted to avoid emergence of bacterial resistance.

Drug	Usual adult dose	Indications
Ertapenem	1 g IV daily.	Useful for outpatient therapy. Not active against *Pseudomonas* or *Acinetobacter* spp.
Imipenem with cilastatin	500 mg IV 6-hourly. Max dose 4 g daily or 50 mg/kg/day, whichever is lower.	*Pseudomonas* and *Enterococcus* spp. infections. Empirical treatment of febrile neutropenic patient.
Meropenem	0.5–1.0 g IV 8-hourly. Max dose 2 g 8-hourly.	Used to treat a wide variety of infections, including meningitis, melioidosis and hospital-acquired pneumonia.

Cephalosporins (B1, cephalexin/cefalotin A)

Indications: Broad-spectrum antibiotics used for the treatment of septicaemia, pneumonia, meningitis, biliary tract infections, peritonitis and UTIs. Rarely first-line drugs, with the exception of ceftazidime or cefepime in febrile neutropenia, and cefotaxime or ceftriaxone with benzylpenicillin for the empirical treatment of bacterial meningitis.

Actions: Similar pharmacology to the penicillins: interfere with bacterial cell wall peptidoglycan synthesis. Renal excretion. First-generation are active against Gram-positive bacteria; second-generation are more active against Gram-negative; third- and fourth-generation are active against both with beta-lactamase stability. None are active against *Enterococcus* or *Listeria* spp.

Adverse effects: Common–diarrhoea, nausea, rash, electrolyte disturbances, pain and inflammation at injection site.

Cautions: Hypersensitivity to other antibiotics, because of cross-reactions.

Comments: All have a central beta-lactam ring structure, with the side chain determining the antibacterial, pharmacological and pharmacokinetic properties. Variable resistance to beta-lactamases.

Drug	Generation	Usual adult dose	Indications	Comments
Cephalexin	First	500 mg PO BD or TDS. Max dose 1.5 g TDS.	UTIs; respiratory tract infections, including otitis media, sinusitis; skin infections.	
Cefalotin	First	0.5–1.0 g IV 6-hourly or 2 g IV BD.	Predominantly for staphylococcal and streptococcal skin infections. Surgical prophylaxis.	Potentially nephrotoxic.
Cephazolin	First	0.5–1.0 g IV 6–8-hourly. Usual max dose 6 g daily.	Predominantly for staphylococcal and streptococcal skin infections. Surgical prophylaxis. UTIs caused by susceptible Gram-negative bacteria.	Useful for community IV treatment of cellulitis, as only needs to be administered BD.
Cefaclor	Second	250 mg PO TDS. Max dose 1.5 g daily.	UTIs, respiratory tract infections, including otitis media, sinusitis; skin infections. Good activity against *Haemophilus influenzae*.	
Cefuroxime	Second	250–500 mg PO BD. *Gonorrhoea:* 1 g single dose.	As for cefaclor. Surgical prophylaxis. Active against *H. influenzae*, *Neisseria gonorrhoeae* and *Staphylococcus aureus*.	Less susceptible to inactivation by beta-lactamases.
Cefoxitin	Second	1–2 g IV every 8 h.	Used for abdominal surgery prophylaxis. Higher anaerobic activity.	
Cefotaxime	Third	1–2 g IV 8–12-hourly. Max dose 6 g daily.	Empirical treatment of severe pneumonia (with a macrolide).	Less active than cefuroxime against Gram-positive bacteria, most notably *S. aureus*.

SECTION F – Formulary

Continued

Drug	Generation	Usual adult dose	Indications	Comments
Ceftriaxone	Third	1–2 g IM/IV once daily (or in 2 divided doses). Max dose 4 g daily.	Bacterial meningitis (sometimes with other antibiotics). Gonococcal infection, PID. Orbital cellulitis, epiglottitis, septicaemia. Acute cholecystitis (alternative to ampicillin with gentamicin). Acute peritonitis (with metronidazole).	Broad-spectrum activity may encourage superinfection with resistant bacteria or fungi.
Ceftazidime	Third	1–2 g IM/IV 8–12-hourly. Max dose 6 g daily.	Empirical treatment of neutropenic sepsis. Antipseudomonal activity.	
Cefepime	Fourth	1–2 g IV 12-hourly. Max dose 6 g daily.	*Pseudomonas aeruginosa* infections. Empirical treatment of neutropenic sepsis. Infections caused by organisms resistant to other cephalosporins.	Reserve for use in infections caused by multiresistant organisms (e.g. *P. aeruginosa*) and for empirical treatment of sepsis in patients with neutropenia.
Ceftaroline	Fourth	600 mg IV 12-hourly.	Complicated soft-tissue infections and community acquired pneumonia.	Broad spectrum with activity against MRSA but not *Pseudomonas*.

Clindamycin (A)

Indications: Gram-positive and anaerobic activity. No Gram-negative effect. Alternative in patients with severe allergy to penicillins and cephalosporins for endocarditis prophylaxis, aspiration pneumonia and dental, skin, soft-tissue and bone infections. Second-line agent for toxoplasmosis, bacterial vaginosis, pneumocystis pneumonia (PCP), malaria. Used topically for acne.

Actions: Bacteriostatic; inhibits protein synthesis by binding to the 50S ribosomal subunit.

Adverse effects: Limited use because of serious adverse effects including *Clostridium difficile*-associated diarrhoea (CDAD). Common—diarrhoea, nausea, vomiting, abdominal pain or cramps, metallic taste (with high IV doses), rash, itch, contact dermatitis (with topical use).

Cautions: Cautious use in the elderly and those with hepatic impairment—can cause build-up of toxic metabolites. Rapid development of resistance can occur.

Comments: Stop clindamycin immediately if patient develops diarrhoea and take faecal samples for detection of C. *difficile* toxin.

Dose: Available in 150 mg tablets and ampoules, topical gel/lotion. 150–450 mg PO 6–8-hourly. 600–2700 mg IV daily given in two-four equal doses, usually 600 mg 8-hourly. Maximum dose 4.8 g IV daily. *Acne:* Apply gel daily or lotion BD.

Doxycycline (D)

Indications: Broad-spectrum; usually used for respiratory infections, rickettsial infections, melioidosis, brucellosis, Q fever, chronic prostatitis, malaria prophylaxis and treatment, acne and genital tract infections.

Actions: Bacteriostatic—inhibits bacterial protein synthesis by reversibly binding to 30S subunit of the ribosome.

Adverse effects: Common—nausea, vomiting, epigastric burning, tooth discolouration, enamel dysplasia, reduced bone growth (in children <8 years), photosensitivity.

Cautions: Contraindicated in children <8 years. Avoid in patients with SLE.

Comments: Broad-spectrum antibiotic of decreasing value because of increasing bacterial resistance. Still the treatment of choice for infections caused by *Chlamydia*, *Rickettsia* (including Q fever), *Brucella* (with either streptomycin or rifampicin) and the spirochaete *Borrelia burgdorferi* (Lyme disease). Take with a large glass of water, and remain upright (do not lie down) for 1 hour afterwards to stop tablets or capsules sticking and causing mucosal ulceration. Avoid sun exposure, wear protective clothing and use sunscreen to avoid photosensitivity reactions.

Dose: Available in 50 mg and 100 mg tablets. Usual dose 200 mg PO on day 1 then 100 mg PO daily. *Acne:* 50 mg PO daily for at least 6 weeks with dose titrated to response.

Macrolides (erythromycin A, azithromycin/roxithromycin B1, clarithromycin B3)

Indications: Predominantly Gram-positive activity with effects on atypical respiratory pathogens (*Mycoplasma, Chlamydia, Bordetella* and *Legionella* spp.) and many causes of enteritis (*Campylobacter* spp. and *Salmonella* spp. [azithromycin]). Alternatives if allergy to penicillins and cephalosporins.

Actions: Inhibit bacterial protein synthesis by reversibly binding to the 50S subunit of the bacterial ribosome, thereby inhibiting translocation of peptidyl-tRNA. Mainly bacteriostatic, but can be bactericidal in high concentrations. Accumulate within leucocytes, so transported into the site of infection. Also have anti-inflammatory and immunomodulatory properties and reduce biofilm formation, so used in panbronchiolitis, cystic fibrosis.

Adverse effects: GI symptoms such as nausea, vomiting, abdominal cramps, diarrhoea, plus headache, dyspnoea, cough, *Candida* infections. Clarithromycin is associated with pulmonary infiltrates with eosinophilia. IV administration is associated with hearing loss and QT prolongation with possibility of torsades de pointes.

Cautions: In hepatic and renal impairment. QT prolongation.

Drug	Indications	Usual adult dose	Comments
Azithromycin	Treatment of choice for chlamydial infections. Used for streptococcal throat infections, community-acquired pneumonia, *Mycobacterium avium* complex, donovanosis, typhoid, paratyphoid.	500 mg PO or IV for 3 days for throat/ respiratory infections, traveller's diarrhoea. 500 mg PO for 7 days for donovanosis, typhoid, paratyphoid. 1 g PO as single dose for chlamydial genital infections.	Most effective for *Haemophilus influenzae*.

Drug	Indications	Usual adult dose	Comments
Clarithromycin	Respiratory tract infections, mild-to-moderate skin infections, otitis media, *Helicobacter pylori* eradication adjunct.	250–500 mg PO BD	Most effective for *Mycobacterium* spp.
Erythromycin	Upper and lower respiratory tract infections, rheumatic fever prophylaxis if penicillin allergy, coral cuts, *Campylobacter* enteritis.	250–500 mg PO QID	High rate of GI adverse effects.
Roxithromycin	Upper and lower respiratory tract infections, skin infections.	150 mg PO BD or 300 mg PO daily	

Metronidazole (B2)

Indications: Gram-positive and Gram-negative anaerobic bacterial infections such as *Bacteroides fragilis*. Protozoal infections such as giardiasis, trichomoniasis. Pseudomembranous colitis caused by *Clostridium difficile*. Dental infections, including acute gingivitis. Intra-abdominal infections. Aspiration pneumonia. Surgical prophylaxis. Topical cream also used for rosacea.

Actions: Metabolised to active metabolites, which bind to DNA, inhibiting DNA repair and synthesis. Bactericidal.

Adverse effects: Common—thrombophlebitis (IV), nausea, diarrhoea, metallic taste, 'Antabuse' effect with alcohol.

Cautions: Avoid alcohol during treatment and for 24 hours after finishing the course to prevent nausea, vomiting, flushing, headache and palpitations.

Comments: Oral bioavailability is 80%, so oral route is preferred to reduce costs. Take with food to reduce GI upset. The liquid is absorbed best if taken 1 hour before food.

Dose: Available in 200 mg and 400 mg tablets, 500 mg suppositories, 500 mg injection, topical cream and gel. PO 200–400 mg 8–12-hourly, up to 4 g daily. PR 1 g 8–12-hourly as a suppository. IV 500 mg 8–12-hourly as part of multidrug regimen. Maximum dose: 4 g IV daily. *C. difficile* infections: 400 mg PO 8-hourly. Apply gel or cream BD to malodorous fungating wounds.

Nitrofurantoin (A)

Indications: Uncomplicated UTIs; prophylaxis or long-term suppressive treatment in recurrent UTIs.

Actions: Inhibits bacterial protein, DNA, RNA and cell wall synthesis. Active against Gram-negative coliforms.

Adverse effects: Common—nausea and vomiting, anorexia, dyspepsia, allergic skin reactions, headache, drowsiness, vertigo, dizziness. Infrequent—intracranial hypertension, diarrhoea, abdominal pain, neonatal haemolytic anaemia.

Cautions: Monitor pulmonary, renal and hepatic functions during long-term treatment, as complications may be insiduous.

Comments: Antibacterial activity is lost if urine pH is >8; avoid excessive alkalinisation of urine. Can be used for vancomycin-resistant enterococcal and MRSA UTIs.

Dose: 50–100 mg PO QDS for 3–5 days for females, 7 days for males. UTI prophylaxis 50–100 mg PO at bedtime. Maximum dose 400 mg PO daily.

Penicillins (A; flucloxacillin, piperacillin, amoxycillin/clavulanate B1; dicloxacillin/ticarcillin with clavulanic acid B2)

Indications: Treatment or prevention of infection caused by susceptible, usually Gram-positive, bacteria.

Actions: Beta-lactam antibiotics inhibit the formation of peptidoglycan cross-links in the bacterial cell wall. Diffuse well into body tissues and fluids, but penetration into the CSF is poor except when the meninges are inflamed.

Adverse effects: Generally well tolerated. Common—diarrhoea, nausea, rash, urticaria, pain and inflammation at injection site (less common with benzylpenicillin), superinfection (including candidiasis) especially during prolonged treatment with broad-spectrum penicillins, allergy. Amoxycillin/clavulanate, flucloxacillin, ticarcillin, piperacillin can cause transient increases in liver enzymes and bilirubin, hepatitis.

Cautions: Allergic reactions to penicillins occur in 1–10% of exposed individuals. Anaphylactic reactions occur in less than 1 in 2000 treated patients. Patients with a history of atopy, such as asthma, eczema and hay fever, are at higher risk of severe anaphylaxis. Cross-reactivity with other antibiotics in 1–10% of patients truly allergic to penicillin.

Comments: Monitor renal and hepatic functions, and full blood count during prolonged high-dose treatment (>10 days).

Penicillins: narrow-spectrum

Drug	Indications	Usual adult dose	Comments
Benzylpenicillin or penicillin G	Bacterial endocarditis, meningitis, aspiration pneumonia, lung abscess, community-acquired pneumonia, syphilis, septicaemia in children.	0.6–1.2 g IV 4–6-hourly. Max dose 24 g IV daily (e.g. endocarditis, meningitis).	Inactivated by bacterial beta-lactamases. No longer first-line drug for pneumococcal meningitis.
Phenoxymethylpenicillin or penicillin V	Streptococcal tonsillitis/pharyngitis or skin infections, prophylaxis of rheumatic fever and against pneumococcal infections following splenectomy, moderate-to-severe gingivitis, with metronidazole.	250–500 mg PO 6–8-hourly. Max dose 3 g PO daily.	Similar antibacterial spectrum to benzylpenicillin, but less active. Suitable for PO administration, but should not be used for serious infections because absorption can be unpredictable and plasma concentrations vary.

SECTION F – Formulary

SECTION F – Formulary

Penicillins: broad-spectrum

Drug	Indications	Usual adult dose	Comments
Amoxycillin/ ampicillin	Exacerbation of chronic bronchitis; community-acquired pneumonia; acute bacterial otitis media; sinusitis; gonococcal infection; epididymo-orchitis, acute prostatitis, acute pyelonephritis, UTI; non-surgical prophylaxis of endocarditis; acute cholecystitis; peritonitis; eradication of *Helicobacter pylori* (with other agents).	250–500 mg PO 6-hourly. Usual max dose 3 g PO daily, 500 mg–1 g IV or IM 6-hourly.	Inactivated by penicillinases including those produced by *Staphylococcus aureus* and by common Gram-negative bacilli such as *Escherichia coli*. Almost all staphylococci, 50% of *E. coli* strains and 15% of *Haemophilus influenzae* strains are now resistant. Maculopapular rashes commonly occur with ampicillin (and amoxycillin) but are not usually related to true penicillin allergy. Ampicillin absorption affected by food, so amoxycillin used PO, IV use is similar.
Amoxycillin with clavulanic acid	Hospital-acquired pneumonia; epididymo-orchitis (urinary tract source); UTI; bites and clenched fist injuries; otitis media unresponsive to amoxycillin; acute bacterial sinusitis unresponsive to amoxycillin.	500–875 mg PO 12-hourly for 5–10 days.	Clavulanic acid inactivates beta-lactamases, so combination active against beta-lactamase-producing bacteria such as resistant strains of *S. aureus*, *E. coli*, and *H. influenzae*, as well as many *Bacteroides* and *Klebsiella* spp. Absorbed best if taken with food.
Flucloxacillin/ dicloxacillin	Staphylococcal skin infections including folliculitis, boils, carbuncles, bullous impetigo, mastitis, crush injuries, stab wounds, infected scabies; pneumonia; osteomyelitis, septic arthritis.	250–500 mg PO 6-hourly to a max of 1 g/day PO, 1–2 g IV 6-hourly. Max dose 4 g/day IV.	Is not inactivated by penicillinases and is thus effective in infections caused by penicillin-resistant staphylococci. Acid-stable, so can be given PO, as well as parenterally.

Penicillins: broad-spectrum antipseudomonals

Drug	Indications	Usual adult dose	Comments
Ticarcillin with clavulanic acid	Reserve for mixed aerobic and anaerobic, and *Pseudomonas aeruginosa* infections; febrile neutropenia.	3 g IV 4–6-hourly. Max dose 18 g IV daily.	Indicated for serious infections caused by *P. aeruginosa*. Also has activity against certain other Gram-negative bacilli including *Proteus* spp. and *Bacteroides fragilis*. Now available only in combination with clavulanic acid, so is active against beta-lactamase-producing bacteria. Used empirically with an aminoglycoside in moderate or severe Gram-negative infections.
Piperacillin with tazobactam	Serious infections caused by *P. aeruginosa* and other susceptible organisms; febrile neutropenia.	2–4 g IV 6–8-hourly. Max dose 24 g IV daily.	More active than ticarcillin against *P. aeruginosa*. Contains the ureidopenicillin, piperacillin, with the beta-lactamase inhibitor, tazobactam. Similar antibacterial spectrum to ticarcillin, but more active against some Gram-negative organisms and enterococci.

Quinolones (B3)

Indications: Predominantly Gram-negative with moxifloxacin having atypical respiratory organism, anerobic and some Gram-positive activity. Reserved for proven or suspected infections in which alternative agents are ineffective or contraindicated (e.g. complicated UTIs, bone or joint infections, epididymo-orchitis, prostatitis).

Actions: Bactericidal—inhibit bacterial DNA synthesis by blocking DNA gyrase and topo-isomerase, the enzymes responsible for developing double-stranded DNA.

Adverse effects: Common—rash, itch, nausea, vomiting, diarrhoea, abdominal pain, dyspepsia. Infrequent—headache, dizziness, insomnia, depression, restlessness, tremors, arthralgia, arthritis, myalgia, tendonitis, crystalluria, interstitial nephritis, raised liver enzymes.

Cautions: Serious allergic reactions. Increased risk of tendon damage in the elderly. Quinolones should be avoided in pregnancy because of potential for fetal arthropathy.

Comments: Have limited use in common infections unless caused by resistant organisms, or when other agents are contraindicated. Stop quinolone treatment at first sign of tendon pain or inflammation. Reduce dose in renal impairment.

Drug	Indications	Usual adult dose	Comments
Ciprofloxacin	Severe salmonella enteritis, including typhoid; complicated UTIs; bone or joint infections; epididymo-orchitis; meningococcal prophylaxis.	250–500 mg PO/IV BD. *Severe infections:* 300–400 mg PO/IV TDS.	Give IV infusion over minimum of 60 min. Well-absorbed orally; IV route necessary only when PO administration is not possible.
Moxifloxacin	Acute bacterial sinusitis or exacerbations of chronic bronchitis where other treatments have failed or are contraindicated; severe community-acquired pneumonia.	*Acute bacterial sinusitis:* 400 mg PO once daily. *Community-acquired pneumonia:* 400 mg PO/IV once daily for 7–14 days. *Acute bacterial exacerbation of chronic bronchitis:* 400 mg PO/IV once daily for 5 days.	Dosage remains the same when changing between IV and PO routes. No advantage over ciprofloxacin in the treatment of most Gram-negative infections.

Drug	Indications	Usual adult dose	Comments
Norfloxacin	UTIs caused by susceptible organisms; shigellosis; *Campylobacter* enteritis; traveller's diarrhoea.	*Uncomplicated UTIs:* 400 mg PO BD for 3 days. *Campylobacter:* 400 mg PO BD for 5 days. *Traveller's diarrhoea:* 400 mg PO BD for 3 days.	Take 1 h before, or 2 h after, meals for best absorption.

Trimethoprim (B3)

Indications: Empirical treatment for uncomplicated lower UTIs, epididymo-orchitis (non-STI source), acute and chronic prostatitis.

Actions: Bacteriostatic—competitively inhibits bacterial folate production essential for bacterial growth.

Adverse effects: Common—fever, itch, rash, GI disturbance, hyperkalaemia can occur with longer courses.

Cautions: Severe renal impairment; allergy.

Comments: Causes potassium retention in the same way as amiloride. Hyperkalaemia can occur with usual doses, but is more likely to be clinically significant as dose increases. Monitor FBC, potassium and folate status during prolonged or high-dose treatment. Give at night to maximise urinary concentration for UTI. Single-dose treatment for uncomplicated lower UTI in females may be considered; however, treatment for 3 days is more effective in preventing relapse. Not recommended as single agent in males.

Dose: Available in 300 mg tablets. *Acute cystitis:* 300 mg PO at night for 3 days. *Relapsing UTI:* 300 mg PO at night for 10–14 days.

Trimethoprim with sulfamethoxazole (co-trimoxazole) (C)

Indications: Drug of choice for treatment and prophylaxis of *Pneumocystis jiroveci* (*P. carinii*) pneumonia. Community-acquired MRSA skin and soft-tissue infections. Traveller's diarrhoea, melioidosis, shigellosis, pertussis. Primary prophylaxis of cerebral toxoplasmosis in HIV patients.

Actions: Sulfamethoxazole (sulfonamide) and trimethoprim competitively inhibit bacterial folate production.

Adverse effects: Incidence of some adverse effects (rash, fever, nausea, neutropenia, thrombocytopenia, raised hepatic transaminases) is substantially higher in patients with AIDS. Common—fever, nausea (with oral use), vomiting, diarrhoea, anorexia, rash, itch, sore mouth.

Cautions: Contraindicated in serious allergic reaction to sulfonamides and related drugs (sulfonylureas, acetazolamide, thiazide diuretics) or trimethoprim. Avoid in first trimester and in late pregnancy.

Comments: Ratio of trimethoprim to sulfamethoxazole is 1:5.

Dose: Available in 80/400 mg, 160/800 mg tablets, oral liquid and 80/400 mg ampoules. *Mild-to-moderate infections:* 160/800 mg PO BD. *Severe infections:* 160/800 mg IV BD to a maximum of 240/1200 mg BD.

Vancomycin (B2)

Indications: Gram-positive activity including MRSA. Vancomycin should be reserved for the following indications because of increasing resistance to vancomycin (e.g. VRE): serious infections caused by susceptible organisms resistant to penicillins (MRSA and MRSE) or in people with a serious allergy to penicillins. prophylaxis for endocarditis following certain procedures (e.g. some genitourinary and GI procedures) in penicillin-hypersensitive people at high risk. Surgical prophylaxis for major procedures involving implantation of prostheses (e.g. cardiac and vascular procedures) in institutions with a high rate of MRSA or MRSE. Pseudomembranous colitis unresponsive to metronidazole treatment or following relapse (PO).

Actions: Bactericidal—inhibits bacterial cell wall synthesis by preventing formation of peptidoglycan polymers.

Adverse effects: More common with rapid IV infusions. Common— itch, fever, chills, eosinophilia, pain, erythema (red man syndrome), thrombophlebitis. Infrequent—nephrotoxicity.

Comments: Avoid concomitant use of other nephrotoxic or ototoxic drugs (e.g. aminoglycosides). Modify dosing interval in renal impairment.

Dose: Available in 125 mg and 250 mg tablets, and 500 mg and 1000 mg ampoules. Slow IV infusion of 1–1.5 g 12-hourly (loading dose 25–30 mg/kg followed by 15–20 mg/kg 12-hourly) with serum concentration monitoring. Oral 125–500 mg QID for pseudomembranous colitis.

- **Aztreonam:** Monobactam with Gram-negative activity, used when other agents are not effective or not tolerated.
- **Benzathine penicillin:** Narrow-spectrum used as IM depot for acute treatment of streptococcal throat infections, prevention of rheumatic fever or treatment of syphilis. Duration of effect 2–4 weeks.
- **Chloramphenicol:** Used topically for ear and eye infections.

- **Colistin:** Used IV for acute or chronic infections with Gram-negative bacteria when other agents are unsuitable. Used inhaled for treatment of pseudomonal chest infections.
- **Daptomycin:** Used for treatment of MRSA infections when other agents unsuitable.
- **Fidaxomicin:** Used for *Clostridium difficile* infection. Poorly absorbed from GIT with limited activity against other bowel flora.
- **Framycetin:** Aminoglycoside used topically for otitis externa, chronic suppurative otitis media, ocular infections.
- **Fusidic acid:** Used for treatment of MRSA infections in conjunction with rifampicin when other agents unsuitable. Also used topically for staphylococcal skin infections if other agents unsuitable.
- **Hexamine hippurate:** Hydrolysed in urine to formaldehyde, used for treatment of urinary tract infections. Efficacy unclear.
- **Lincomycin:** Similar indications and action to clindamycin. Less potent so infrequently used. Available only as injection.
- **Linezolid:** Used for treatment of MRSA infections when other agents unsuitable.
- **Minocycline:** Tetracycline derivative, used for acne treatment.
- **Mupirocin:** Topical treatment of impetigo or infected skin wounds. Also used for eradication of nasal MRSA carriage.
- **Neomycin with bacitracin:** Aminoglycoside mixture used for otitis externa.
- **Nitrofurantoin:** Active against most urinary pathogens. Second-line agent for acute treatment or prophylaxis but can be effective against MRSA or VRE urinary infections.
- **Ofloxacin:** Topical eye drops for severe conjunctivitis.
- **Procaine penicillin:** Narrow-spectrum used as IM depot for acute treatment of streptococcal throat infections, prevention of rheumatic fever, or treatment of syphilis. Duration of effect 12–24 hours.
- **Rifabutin:** Treatment of mycobacterial infections if rifampicin is unsuitable.
- **Rifampicin:** Treatment of staphylococcal infections, meningitis prophylaxis, leprosy, *Mycobacterium* infections.
- **Rifaximin:** Treatment of hepatic encephalopathy, combined with lactulose.
- **Sulfadiazine:** Used as antibacterial for burns and leg ulcers as silver sulfadiazine. Tablets used for treatment of *Nocardia* and *Toxoplasma*.
- **Teicoplanin:** Alternative to vancomycin with similar indications, adverse reactions. Usual dose 10 mg/kg (up to 800 mg) 12-hourly

for three doses, then 6–12 mg once daily or less frequently depending on indication and renal function.

- **Tigecycline:** Broad-spectrum tetracycline derivative used for complex multi-organism infections.

Antifungals
Amphotericin (B3)

Indications: First-line agent for most fungal CNS infections, systemic fungal infections; cryptococcal meningitis, zygomycosis, histoplasmosis; second-line in oral and perioral candidiasis, aspergillosis. Also used for visceral leishmaniasis and amoebic meningitis.

Actions: Binds to sterols in susceptible fungal cell membranes causing leakage of cell contents.

Adverse effects: Infusion reactions common, esp with conventional preparation. Fever, chills, nausea, vomiting, diarrhoea, hypotension, nephrotoxicity, hypokalaemia, hypomagnesaemia, thrombophlebitis.

Cautions: Monitor renal function and potassium concentration (hypokalaemia). IV amphotericin affects renal function in all patients. Reduce the dose or consider alternative preparations if creatinine clearance falls. Avoid use with other nephrotoxic drugs.

Comments: Premedication with antipyretics, antihistamines, antiemetics and corticosteroids may reduce some of the adverse effects.

Dose: Available in 10 mg lozenges, 50 mg and 100 mg injection. Administer a test dose of 1 mg IV in 100 mL 5% dextrose over 2 hours. If tolerated, give another 10 mg on the first day. Increase dose by 5 mg every day to a desired dose of 0.5–1 mg/kg/day. Infuse over 4–6 hours. Liposomal or lipid complex preparations can be infused more quickly without a first-dose trial. *Oral candidiasis:* 1 lozenge dissolved in mouth QID.

Azoles (B3, fluconazole D)

Indications: Topical or systemic fungal infections.

Actions: Impairs ergosterol synthesis in fungal cell membranes causing membrane breakdown.

Adverse effects: Rash, headache, dizziness, GI disturbance.

Cautions: Monitor potassium, liver function, renal function.

Comments: Azoles interact with many commonly prescribed drugs. Check prior to commencing therapy.

Drug	Indications	Usual adult dose	Comments
Fluconazole	Candidiasis, cryptococcosis, coccidioidomycosis, histoplasmosis, fungal prophylaxis in immunocompromised patients. Resistant topical fungal infections.	*Oropharyngeal candidiasis:* 50–200 mg PO daily. *Systemic candidiasis:* 200–400 mg PO/IV daily. *Cryptococcal meningitis:* 800 mg IV loading dose, then 400 mg IV daily.	Max IV infusion rate 200 mg/h. Used as adjunct in fungal CNS infections.
Itraconazole	As per fluconazole, plus treatment of systemic fungal infections, prophylaxis of histoplasmosis.	*Oropharyngeal candidiasis:* 100–200 mg PO daily. *Recurrent vulvovaginal candidiasis:* 200 mg PO BD for 1 day. *Systemic fungal infections or secondary prevention in HIV:* 200 mg PO daily or BD.	
Posaconazole	Acute invasive fungal infections, prophylaxis of oropharyngeal or systemic fungal infections in immunocompromised patients.	*Invasive infections:* 400 mg PO BD. Prophylaxis 200 mg PO TDS.	Use if other treatments have failed. Alternative to amphotericin for zygomycosis.
Voriconazole	First-line for invasive aspergillosis, *Scedosporium.*	*Loading:* 6 mg/kg IV for 2 doses, followed by 3–4 mg/kg IV 12-hourly.	Multiple adverse reactions including thrombocytopenia.

Nystatin (A)

Indications: Oropharyngeal candidiasis (usually requires topical therapy only). Oesophageal candidiasis (requires systemic therapy). *Candida* infections of the skin, lungs, peritoneum and urinary tract. Prophylaxis against candidiasis in immunocompromised individuals.

Actions: Binds to ergosterol in fungal cell membranes, allowing leakage of intracellular components.

Adverse effects: GI intolerance.

Dose: Available in 500,000 unit tablets, oral liquid, cream. Usual dose 1–5 mL liquid PO QID, or 1–2 tablets PO QID, or topical cream TDS.

Pentamidine (B3)

Indications: *Pneumocystis juroveci* pneumonia (PCP).

Actions: Mode of action not fully understood. May include inhibition of protozoal DNA, RNA and protein synthesis, plus effects on folate metabolism.

Adverse effects: GI upset including nausea, vomiting, diarrhoea and taste disturbance. IV—reversible acute renal impairment, arrhythmias including prolonged QT interval, glucose abnormalities including hypoglycaemia, pancreatitis, hypotension (especially with rapid infusion). Inhalation—cough, bronchospasm (often reversible), eye discomfort.

Cautions: Risk of severe hypotension following administration. Administer with patient lying down and monitor BP closely during administration, and at regular intervals, until treatment concluded.

Comments: As effective as, but more toxic than, trimethoprim with sulfamethoxazole for the treatment of PCP. Used as an alternative for people who cannot tolerate or are allergic to trimethoprim with sulfamethoxazole. Use pentamidine IV to treat PCP, because the nebulised route is ineffective. Bronchospasm and cough from inhalation may be controlled by prior use of a bronchodilator.

Dose: Available as 300 mg injection. *Treatment:* 4 mg/kg IV infusion to a maximum of 300 mg daily for 21 days. *Prophylaxis:* 300 mg IV every 2–4 weeks.

- **Amorolfine:** Used topically for onychomycosis.
- **Anidulafungin:** Used for systemic candidiasis if other agents unsuitable.
- **Bifonazole:** Used topically for tinea, pityriasis and cutaneous candidiasis.
- **Caspofungin:** Second-line for invasive aspergillosis or candidiasis.
- **Ciclopirox:** Used topically for seborrhoeic dermatitis, onychomycoses.

- **Clotrimazole:** Used topically for tinea, pityriasis and cutaneous candidiasis.
- **Econazole:** Used topically for tinea, pityriasis and cutaneous candidiasis.
- **Flucytosine:** Used as adjunct with amphotericin for cryptococcosis.
- **Griseofulvin:** Used for resistant dermatophytosis and fungal nail infections.
- **Ketoconazole:** Used topically for tinea, pityriasis, seborrhoeic dermatitis and cutaneous candidiasis. Also available in tablets but uncommonly used due to adverse effects.
- **Micafungin:** Used for invasive candidiasis, oesophageal candidiasis and prophylaxis of *Candida* infection in patients with severe immunocompromise.
- **Miconazole:** Used topically for tinea, pityriasis, seborrhoeic dermatitis and oropharyngeal and cutaneous candidiasis.
- **Terbinafine:** Used for onychomycosis, or for dermatophyte infections when other agents not suitable.
- **Tolnaftate:** Used topically for dermatophytoses and pityriasis versicolor.

Anthelminthics
Albendazole (D)

Indications: Roundworm, threadworm, hookworm, whipworm, strongyloidiasis, neurocysticercosis, tapeworm, cutaneous larva migrans, liver fluke infection, hydatid disease. Drug of choice for mixed intestinal worm infestation.

Actions: Binds to beta tubulin and interferes with microtubule formation.

Adverse effects: Headache, GI disturbance, abdominal pain, dizziness, fever.

Cautions: Adverse effects more common in high-dose prolonged treatment. Contraindicated in ocular cysticercosis.

Comments: Taken on empty stomach to minimise absorption when used for intestinal infestations and vice versa for systemic infestations.

Dose: Available in 200 mg and 400 mg tablets. *Roundworm, threadworm, hookworm:* 400 mg PO single dose. *Strongyloidiasis, cutaneous larva migrans, whipworm, clonorchiasis:* 400 mg PO once daily for 3 days. Longer courses for other infestations.

- **Ivermectin:** Used for onchocerciasis and strongyloidiasis. Can also be used for resistant scabies, other intestinal nematode infections, cutaneous larva migrans and together with albendazole for lymphatic filariasis.

- **Mebendazole:** Similar mechanism of action as albendazole, but more narrow spectrum and higher rate of adverse reactions. Used for intestinal infestations.
- **Praziquantal:** Used for schistosomiasis and liver fluke infestation.
- **Pyrantal:** Depolarising neuromuscular blocker that paralyses intestinal worms.

Antiprotozoals
Artemether with lumefantrine (D)

Indications: First-line for acute *Plasmodium falciparum* malaria and for resistant *Plasmodium vivax*.

Actions: Interferes with the food vacuole of the parasite, leading to haem accumulation; also inhibits protein and nucleic acid synthesis.

Adverse effects: Headache, dizziness, sleep disturbance, GI disturbance, rash, arthralgia, myalgia.

Cautions: Caution in patients with prolonged ST syndrome.

Comments: Needs to be taken with food to improve absorption.

Dose: Available in 20 mg artemether/120 mg lumefantrine. Usually given as six-dose course with four tablets at 8, 24, 36, 48 and 60 hours after initial dose.

Quinine (D)

Indications: Severe *P. falciparum* malaria. (No longer recommended for leg cramps.)

Actions: Interferes with the malarial parasite's ability to break down and digest haemoglobin, thus starving the parasite and/or causing the build-up of toxic levels of partially degraded haemoglobin in the parasite.

Adverse effects: Usually occur only with higher doses (>1.8 g daily). Common—GI disturbances, CNS disturbances, reversible hearing loss, 'cinchonism' (tinnitus, headache, nausea, vertigo, visual disturbances), fever, rash, immune thrombocytopenia, hypoglycaemia, ECG changes.

Cautions: Overdosage may cause sudden blindness and fatal arrhythmias. Contraindicated in myasthenia gravis, optic neuritis, tinnitus.

Comments: IV infusions should be given over 4 hours. Omit loading dose if quinine or mefloquine taken within 24 hours.

Dose: Available in 300 mg tabs and 600 mg injections. Usual loading dose for severe infection 20 mg/kg (to max 1.4 g) IV followed by 10 mg/kg (to max 700 mg) IV 8-hourly. More rapid administration can be given in critical care areas.

- **Artesunate:** Used IV for severe malaria or for chloroquine-resistant malaria. First-line treatment if available (not marketed in Australia).

- **Atovaquone:** Used for treatment of mild–moderate PCP when other therapies unsuitable.
- **Atovaquone with proguanil:** Used for prophylaxis and second-line for treatment of *P. falciparum* malaria. Better tolerated than other drugs for prophylaxis.
- **Hydroxychloroquine:** Used for treatment of non-*P. falciparum* malaria.
- **Mefloquine:** Used for malaria prophylaxis in areas of chloroquine resistance, alternative to artemether for treatment of *P. falciparum* malaria and used to treat chloroquine-resistant *P. vivax* malaria.
- **Primaquine:** Used to eradicate latent phases in *P. vivax* and *P. ovale* malaria. Adjunctive therapy of *P. falciparum* gametocytaemia. Also used for malaria prophylaxis in certain areas.
- **Pyrimethamine:** Used for treament of toxoplasmosis in conjunction with sulfadiazine or clindamycin.
- **Tinidazole:** Similar action to metronidazole. Predominantly used for vaginal protozoal infections.

Antivirals
Guanine analogues

Indications: Herpes zoster, herpes simplex infection. Valaciclovir also for CMV. Ganciclovir and valganciclovir for CMV.

Actions: Prevents viral replication by inhibiting viral DNA polmerase and DNA synthesis.

Adverse effects: Nausea, vomiting, diarrhoea, headache, rash, paraesthesia. Encephalopathy if IV use.

Comments: Keep well hydrated to avoid renal damage. Drug of choice for herpes zoster. Alternatives: valaciclovir, ganciclovir in severe HIV-related infections.

Drug	Indications	Usual adult dose	Comments
Aciclovir	Herpes encephalitis, first-episode genital herpes, shingles, acute chickenpox if immunosuppressed, herpes labialis (topical).	*Genital herpes:* 400 mg PO TDS. *Herpes zoster infection:* 800 mg PO 5 times daily (every 4 waking hours) for 7 days. *Severe infections or encephalitis:* 10 mg/kg IV 8 hourly.	Use for varicella zoster disease within 72 h of rash onset. Reduce dose or frequency if renal impairment.

Continued

SECTION F – Formulary

Drug	Indications	Usual adult dose	Comments
Famciclovir	Treatment and prevention of herpes simplex infections; shingles.	*Herpes simplex:* 250 mg PO TDS or BD for prevention. Can also use 1500 mg as single dose for treatment of herpes labialis.	
Ganciclovir	CMV retinitis, pneumonitis, bone marrow disease in immunocompromised. Acute CMV colitis in AIDS.	5 mg/kg IV 12-hourly with dose changes for maintenance if required.	
Valaciclovir	Treatment of herpes simplex infections, shingles including herpes zoster ophthalmicus, CMV prevention.	500 mg PO BD for herpes simplex, 1 g TDS for shingles.	Alter dose if used for prevention, or if renal impairment.
Valganciclovir	CMV retinitis in AIDS, or prevention of CMV disease post-transplant.	*CMV retinitis:* 900 mg PO BD. *Prevention:* 900 mg PO daily.	

Oseltamivir (B1)

Indications: Treatment and prevention of influenza A and B.

Actions: Neuraminidase inhibitor, preventing release of new virus from cells.

Adverse effects: Nausea and vomiting, especially in first 48 hours, diarrhoea, headache. Neuropsychiatric symptoms can occur, especially in children, and can lead to self-harm.

Cautions: Decrease dose in renal impairment.

Comments: Higher risk of adverse reactions and resistance than zanamivir. Start treatment within 48 h of onset of illness.

Dose: Available in 30 mg, 45 mg and 75 mg tablets and oral liquid. Usual dose for prevention 75 mg PO daily, treatment 75 mg PO BD.

- **Adefovir:** Nucleotide analogue used for prevention of hepatitis B post-transplant.
- **Asunaprevir:** Used in combination with other antivirals for treatment of chronic hepatitis C in compensated liver disease.
- **Boceprevir:** Used in combination with other antivirals for treatment of chronic hepatitis C.

- **Cidofovir:** Second-line treatment for CMV retinitis in patients with AIDS.
- **Dalactasvir:** Used in combination with other antivirals for treatment of chronic hepatitis C in compensated liver disease.
- **Entecavir:** Guanosine analogue used for treatment of acute hepatitis B.
- **Foscarnet:** Pyrophosphate analogue used as second-line therapy for CMV retinitis in patients with AIDS, and aciclovir-resistant herpes infections in patients with HIV.
- **Ledipasvir with sofosbuvir:** Used in combination with other antivirals for treatment of chronic hepatitis C.
- **Palivizumab:** Monoclonal antibody used to prevent RSV disease in high-risk infants.
- **Paritaprevir with ritonavir, ombitasvir and dasabuvir:** Treatment of chronic hepatitis C.
- **Ribavirin:** Inhaled nucleoside analogue used for severe LRTI due to RSV. Oral preparation used for treatment of chronic hepatitis C in combination with other agents.
- **Ribavirin with peginterferon alfa:** Viral inhibitory and immunomodulatory effects used for treatment of hepatitis C.
- **Simeprevir:** Used in combination with other antivirals for treatment of chronic hepatitis C.
- **Sofosbuvir:** Used in combination with other antivirals for treatment of chronic hepatitis C.
- **Telbivudine:** Thymidine analogue used for acute hepatitis B.
- **Zanamivir:** Inhaled neuraminidase inhibitor used for treatment and prevention of influenza A and B.

Endocrine

Diabetes
Glucagon (B2)

Indications: Hypoglycaemia. Relaxes oesophageal smooth muscle, so used for food bolus obstruction. Also used as an inotrope in hypotension refractory to catecholamines.

Actions: Activates hepatic glucose production.

Adverse effects: Nausea, vomiting, hypokalaemia, hyperglycaemia.

Cautions: Contraindicated in pancreatic endocrine tumours. Ineffective if hypoglycaemia is due to inadeqaute body stores such as chronic malnutrition, hepatic failure, chronic alcoholism (use glucose).

Dose: Available in 1 mg injections. Usual dose 1 mg SC/IM/IV. May require larger doses when used as inotrope.

SECTION F – Formulary

Insulin (A)

Indications: Diabetes mellitus, hyperglycaemia and treatment of severe hyperkalaemia.

Actions: Enhances hepatic glycogen storage and the entry of glucose into cells, plus the entry of K^+ into cells. Inhibits the breakdown of protein and fat.

Adverse effects: Hypoglycaemia, local skin reactions, lipohypertrophy.

Cautions: Contraindicated in hypoglycaemia—do not give in undiagnosed coma without checking the BGL first.

Comments: Give SC or as IV infusion. Less immunogenicity with human insulin than with older insulins from animal sources.

Dose: Variable. Can use sliding scale or start with 0.15 units/kg SC 4–6-hourly. IV infusion at 0.05–0.1 unit/kg/h.

Action	Insulin type	Activity	Comments
Ultra-short-acting analogues	Insulin aspart Insulin lispro Insulin glulisine	Peak 1 h, duration 4–5 h	Given immediately before meals.
Short-acting	Neutral	Peak 2–3 h, duration 6–8 h	Given within 30 min of meals. Used for IV infusions for severe hyperglycaemia, diabetic ketoacidosis.
Long-acting	Isophane varieties Mixed or biphasic varieties	Peak 2–12 h, duration 16–24 h	Given once or twice daily. Biphasic varieties usually mixed with a short-acting insulin.
Long-acting analogues	Insulin detemir Insulin glargine	Duration 12–24 h	Usually given once daily to give a constant basal insulin level.

Metformin (C)

Indications: Type 2 diabetes as initial monotherapy, or combination therapy with glibenclamide, rosiglitazone or sitagliptin. Used particularly if patient is overweight.

Actions: Reduces hepatic glucose production and increases peripheral tissue glucose use.

Adverse effects: Malbsorption of vitamin B12, GI intolerance.

Cautions: Contraindicated in respiratory failure, dehydration, severe illness, alcohol misuse, ketoacidosis or type 1 diabetes. Decrease dose in renal or hepatic impairment—increased likelihood of lactic acidosis. Stop within 48 hours of use of intravascular iodinated contrast media as increased risk of renal damage and lactic acidosis.

Comments: Does not cause hypoglycaemia. Monitor renal function. May take 2 weeks to have effects.

Dose: Available in 500 mg, 850 mg, 1000 mg tablets and in combinations with glibenclamide. Usual dose of conventional tablet 500 mg PO BD or TDS up to maximal daily dose of 3 g. 500 mg PO once daily up to 2 g once daily of controlled-release tablet.

Sulfonylureas (C)

Indications: Type 2 diabetes as initial monotherapy, or combination therapy.

Actions: Increases pancreatic insulin secretion.

Adverse effects: Weight gain, hypoglycaemia (especially glibenclamide), rash, GI intolerance, metallic taste.

Cautions: Contraindicated in ketoacidosis or type 1 diabetes. Long duration of action, so hypoglycaemia usually prolonged if occurs. Decrease doses in renal impairment.

Drug	Usual adult dose	Comments
Glibenclamide	2.5–20 mg PO daily in 1 or 2 doses	Avoid in renal or hepatic impairment as increased likelihood of hypoglycaemia.
Gliclazide	30 mg PO daily for controlled-release agent, titrate weekly up to max 120 mg PO daily. 40–320 mg PO daily in 1 or 2 doses for regular product.	30 mg of the CR tablet is equivalent to 80 mg of the conventional preparation.
Glimepiride	1 mg PO daily titrate weekly up to 4 mg max	
Glipizide	2.5–40 mg PO daily	

- **Acarbose:** Used for type 2 diabetes. Delays intestinal absorption of carbohydrates, reduces post-prandial hyperglycaemia.
- **Alogliptin:** Similar to sitagliptin.
- **Canagliflozin:** Reduces glucose reabsorption in the kidney by inhibiting the sodium-glucose co-transporter. Used for type 2 diabetes, but avoid in renal impairment. Adverse effects include urogenital infections and euglycaemic ketoacidosis.
- **Dapagliflozin:** Similar to canagliflozin.
- **Empagliflozin:** Similar to canagliflozin.
- **Exenatide:** Injectable incretin mimetic used for combination therapy with metformin and/or a sulfonylurea for type 2 diabetes. Can be given as twice daily injections, or as a once-weekly

SECTION F – Formulary

injection as a slow-release preparation. The long-term harm–benefit profile is unclear.

- **Linagliptin:** Similar to sitagliptin.
- **Liraglutide:** Similar to exenatide.
- **Pioglitazone:** Used for type 2 diabetes as single therapy or with metformin and/or sulfonylurea, or insulin.
- **Rosiglitazone:** Used for type 2 diabetes as single therapy or with metformin or sulfonylurea. Associated with acute cardiac events and cardiac ischaemia.
- **Saxagliptin:** Similar to sitagliptin.
- **Sitagliptin:** Dipeptidyl peptidase-4 inhibitor for combination therapy with metformin or a sulfonylurea for type 2 diabetes. The long-term harm–benefit profile of gliptins is unclear.
- **Vildagliptin:** Similar to sitagliptin.

Thyroid
Thyroxine (T4) (A)
Indications: Hypothyroidism, suppression of thyroid cancer or euthyroid goitre.
Actions: Replaces endogenous thyroid hormone function.
Adverse effects: Tremor, tachycardia, palpitations, flushing, sweating, diarrhoea occur with excessive dosage.
Cautions: Gradual titration of dose required in elderly, in heart disease.
Dose: Available in 50, 75, 100 and 200 microgram tablets. Usual dose 100 microgram PO daily.

- **Carbimazole:** Blocks synthesis of thyroid hormone. Used for Grave's disease, preparation for thyroid surgery, thyroid storm.
- **Iodine:** Transiently inhibits thyroid hormone release. Used short term prior to thyroid surgery.
- **Liothyronine (T3):** Used for severe hypothyroidism, otherwise similar effects to thyroxine.
- **Propylthiouracil:** Similar to carbimazole but shorter duration of action. Also blocks peripheral conversion of T4 to T3.

Bone disease
Bisphosphonates (B3; tiludronate B2)
Indications: Paget's disease, prevention and treatment of osteoporosis, hypercalcaemia of malignancy, prevention of heterotopic calcification.
Actions: Inhibits osteoclasts, thus decreasing bone resorption.
Adverse effects: GI intolerance, headache, musculoskeletal pain, hypocalcaemia. IV administration may cause flu-like illness, hypotension, rarely osteonecrosis of the jaw.

Cautions: Ensure good dental hygeine to minimise osteonecrosis of the jaw. Avoid if renal impairment and ensure adequate hydration. Also ensure adequate intake of calcium and vitamin D.

Comments: Most oral preparations need to be taken on an empty stomach to ensure absorption.

Drug	Usual adult dose	Comments
Alendronate	*Paget's disease:* 40 mg PO daily. *Treatment of osteoporosis:* 10 mg PO daily or 70 mg PO weekly. *Prevention of osteoporosis:* 5 mg PO daily.	Associated with severe oesophageal erosions and ulcers.
Clodronate	2.4–3.2 g daily in divided doses.	Used in malignant hypercalcaemia or for some osteolytic bone metastases.
Ibandronic acid	2–6 mg IV every 4 weeks.	Used in malignant hypercalcaemia or for bone metastases from breast cancer.
Pamidronate	60 mg IV infusion for Paget's disease with dose repeated according to response. 30–90 mg IV infusion depending on level of hypercalcaemia.	Used in Paget's disease, malignant hypercalcaemia or for bone metastases from breast cancer or myeloma.
Risedronate	30 mg PO daily for Paget's disease. 5 mg PO daily, or 35 mg PO weekly or 150 mg PO monthly for osteoporosis.	
Tiludronate	400 mg PO daily.	Used for Paget's disease.
Zoledronic acid	4 mg IV once only for hypercalcaemia; 5 mg IV single dose for Paget's disease; 5 mg IV once a year for osteoporosis.	

Calcium (A) (see also *Cardiac arrest*)

Indications: Calcium deficiency, osteoporosis, osteomalacia, acute hypocalcaemia, hydrofluoric acid burns, calcium-channel toxicity, hyperkalaemia with cardiotoxicity.

Adverse effects: GI intolerance, infrequently can cause hypercalcaemia.

Cautions: Contraindicated in hypercalcaemia, hyperphosphataemia. Concurrent use with calcitriol increases risk of hypercalcaemia.

Dose: Available in multiple oral formulations, and calcium chloride and calcium gluconate injections. Usual dose 1000 mg daily for bone disease. Use higher dose of 1300 mg in men >70 years, adolescents aged 12–18 years and postmenopausal women.

Vitamin D (A; calcitriol B3; paricalcitol C)

Indications: Vitamin D deficiency, osteomalacia, rickets, hypocalcaemia, osteoporosis, secondary hyperparathyroidism, falls.

Actions: Regulates calcium homeostasis, increases intestinal absorption, increases renal reabsorption of calcium. Promotes bone mineralisation. Has immunomodulatory effects.

Adverse effects: Mostly due to causing hypercalcaemia.

Cautions: Contraindicated in hypercalcaemia, hyperphosphataemia.

Drug	Usual adult dose	Comments
Calcitriol	0.25 microgram PO BD. Can use 0.5 microgram IV 3 times weekly for dialysis patients.	Caution in renal impairment. Rapid onset and offset, so higher risk of hypercalcaemia.
Cholecalciferol	Usual dose 500–1000 U (12.5–25 microgram) PO daily.	May require larger doses (5000 units daily) for 6–12 weeks initially if severe vitamin D deficiency.
Ergocalciferol	200–600 U (5–15 microgram) PO daily.	Available over the counter for vitamin D deficiency.

- **Cinacalcet:** Reduces secretion of parathyroid hormone and reduces serum calcium concentration. Used for hyperparathyroidism and parathyroid carcinoma-associated hypercalcaemia.
- **Raloxifene:** Oestrogen agonist effect on bone used for treatment and prevention of postmenopausal osteoporosis, and oestrogen antagonist effect for primary prevention of breast cancer in high-risk patients.
- **Salcatonin:** Salmon calcitonin, inhibits bone resorption and increases urinary calcium excretion. Uncommonly used.
- **Strontium:** Increases bone formation, used for postmenopausal osteoporosis.
- **Teriparatide:** Active fragment of parathyroid hormone. Used for osteoporosis when other agents are unsuitable.

Other endocrine disorders
Desmopressin (DDAVP) (B2)

Indications: Pituitary diabetes insipidus, nocturnal enuresis, control of bleeding in haemophilia, type 1 von Willebrand's disease and certain platelet disorders (e.g. renal failure).

Actions: increases tubular reabsorption of water, increases factor VIII, von Willebrand factor and platelet coagulation activity.
Adverse effects: Headache, nausea, abdominal cramps, hyponatraemia.
Cautions: Avoid if renal impairment, heart failure, hyponatraemia.
Dose: Available in 200 microgram tablets, 120 microgram and 240 microgram wafers, 4 microgram and 15 microgram injections, and nasal spray. Usual dose for diabetes insipidus: 10–40 microgram daily intranasal, 1–4 microgram SC daily, 100–200 microgram PO TDS, or 60–180 microgram SL TDS.

- **Cortisone:** Steroid replacement in adrenal insufficiency. Not commonly used.
- **Fludrocortisone:** Mineralocorticoid replacement in adrenal insufficiency, also used for orthostatic hypotension.
- **Lanreotide:** Somatostatin analogue used for acromegaly when other treatment has been unsuccessful. Also used for symptomatic relief in carcinoid syndrome.
- **Octreotide:** Somatostatin analogue used for acromegaly, gastroenteropancreatic tumours, bleeding oesophageal varices and treatment of hypoglycaemia caused by sulfonylureas.
- **Orlistat:** Inhibits GIT lipases preventing some dietary fat absorption. Can cause oily stools or increased flatus. Contraindicated if pancreatic deficiency states, malabsorption syndromes.
- **Phentermine:** Central CNS stimulant increases activity and energy expenditure. Common adverse effects related to CNS stimulation. Multiple contraindications and drug interactions, subject to misuse.
- **Quinagolide:** Dopamine agonist used for hyperprolactinaemia.
- **Somatropin:** Growth hormone given for patients with deficiency.
- **Terlipressin:** Vasoconstrictor used for bleeding oesophageal varices and hepatorenal syndrome.
- **Testosterone:** Androgen replacement due to hypothalamic, pituitary or testicular disorder.
- **Vasopressin:** Vasoconstrictor used for pituitary diabetes insipidus. Also used as vasoconstrictor in cardiac arrest and in shock refractory to other agents.

Genitourinary

Drugs affecting bladder function
Alpha blockers

Indications: Relief of symptoms of benign prostatic hypertrophy.
Actions: Selective alpha-1 adrenergic blockade relaxing smooth muscle of bladder neck.
Adverse effects: Hypotension, particularly first-dose postural effect leading to syncope, nasal congestion, abnormal ejaculation.

Cautions: Avoid in elderly, dehydration. Alfuzosin contraindicated in hepatic impairment.

Drug	Usual adult dose
Alfuzosin	10 mg PO daily
Prazosin	0.5 mg PO BD initial dose, increase to 2 mg BD as tolerated
Tamsulosin	400 microgram PO daily
Terazosin	1 mg PO daily for 5 days, increase weekly up to 5–10 mg daily

Anticholinergics

Indications: Urinary urge incontinence.
Actions: Relax and increase capacity of the bladder.
Adverse effects: Dry mouth, blurred vision, constipation, confusion, urinary retention.
Cautions: Avoid in elderly.
Comments: Newer anticholinergics may have higher specificity for bladder muscarinic receptors, but clinical advantage is unclear.

Drug	Usual adult dose
Darifenacin	7.5 mg PO daily
Oxybutynin	2.5–5 mg PO BD or TDS
Propantheline	15–30 mg PO BD or TDS
Solifenacin	5 mg PO daily
Tolterodine	1–2 mg PO BD

- **Dutasteride:** 5-alpha-reductase inhibitor with reduction of dihydrotestosterone, thus reducing prostate size. Used for symptomatic treatment of benign prostatic hypertrophy.
- **Finasteride:** As per dutasteride.
- **Mirabegron:** Beta-3 agonist relaxes bladder muscle thus increasing capacity. Used for urge incontinence.

Erectile dysfunction
Phosphodiesterase-5 inhibitors

Indications: Erectile dysfunction.
Actions: Inhibit breakdown of cGMP, thus increasing blood flow to the corpus cavernosum.
Adverse effects: Headache, nasal congestion, rash, diarrhoea, dizziness and syncope. Associated with migraine.
Cautions: Contraindicated if nitrates used due to risk of profound hypotension. Hypotensive effect may be compounded by other vasodilators. Contraindicated if history of ischaemic optic neuropathy. Avoid if renal impariment.

Drug	Usual adult dose
Sildenafil	50 mg PO as initial dose. Can increase to 100 mg if necessary.
Tadalafil	2.5–5 mg once daily.
Vardenafil	5–20 mg once daily depending on response.

- **Alprostadil:** Prostaglandin E1, dilates cavernosal arteries.
- **Dapoxetin:** SSRI that modifies the ejaculatory reflex, used for premature ejaculation.
- **Papaverine:** Vascular dilation of the penile circulation, given by intracavernal injection.

Antidotes

Drug	Toxic agent
Acetylcysteine	Paracetamol
Atropine	Organophosphate poisoning
Calcium gluconate	Hydrofluoric acid, calcium-channel blockers
Deferasirox	Chronic iron overload
Deferiprone	Chronic iron overload
Desferrioxamine	Acute iron poisoning, chronic iron overload
Digoxin specific antibody	Acute or chronic digoxin toxicity
Ethanol	Acute ethylene glycol or methanol poisoning
Flumazenil	Reversal of benzodiazepine sedation
Fuller's earth	Acute paraquat ingestion
Glucagon	Refractory calcium-channel blocker or beta-blocker toxicity
Hydroxocobalamin	Cyanide
Idarucizumab	Full reversal of dabigatran in life-threatening bleeding or if patient needs emergency surgery
Insulin	Refractory calcium-channel blocker or beta-blocker toxicity
Naloxone	Opioid toxicity
Octreotide	Sulfonylurea-induced hypoglycaemia
Pralidoxime	Organophosphate poisoning
Pyridoxine	Isoniazid poisoning
Sodium bicarbonate	Sodium-channel blocker toxicity (tricyclics, antimalarials, some phenothiazines, some beta-blockers, some antiarrhythmics)
Vitamin K	Coumadins

Laboratory values

68

Normal laboratory ranges

Laboratory reference ranges

The ranges below are the approximate 95% confidence limits for laboratory reference values in healthy adult males and females.

As the test results can vary depending on measurement conditions and the laboratory methods utilised, always interpret results using your local testing laboratory's quoted reference ranges.

Seek senior doctor advice if in doubt.

Haematology

haemoglobin	females: 115–165 g/L
	males: 130–180 g/L
erythrocytes	females: $3.8–5.8 \times 10^{12}$/L
	males: $4.5–6.5 \times 10^{12}$/L
haematocrit (packed cell volume)	females: 0.37–0.47
	males: 0.4–0.54
mean corpuscular volume	80–100 fL
leucocytes (white cells)	$4–11 \times 10^9$/L
neutrophils	$2–7.5 \times 10^9$/L (40–75%)
lymphocytes	$1.5–4 \times 10^9$/L (20–40%)
monocytes	$0.2–0.8 \times 10^9$/L (2–10%)
eosinophils	$0.04–0.4 \times 10^9$/L (1–6%)
basophils	$<0.1 \times 10^9$/L (<1%)
platelets	$150–400 \times 10^9$/L
erythrocyte sedimentation rate (Westergren method)	females:
	under 50 years: <20 mm/h
	over 50 years: <30 mm/h
	males:
	under 50 years: <15 mm/h
	over 50 years: <20 mm/h
vitamin B12	120–680 picomol/L
folate	red cell: 360–1400 nanomol/L
	serum: 7–45 nanomol/L

iron	10–30 micromol/L
ferritin	females: 15–200 micrograms/L
	males: 30–300 micrograms/L
transferrin saturation	15–45%

Electrolytes, glucose

sodium	135–145 mmol/L
potassium	plasma: 3.4–4.5 mmol/L
	serum: 3.8–4.9 mmol/L
chloride	95–110 mmol/L
bicarbonate	22–32 mmol/L
urea	3–8 mmol/L
creatinine	females: 50–110 micromol/L
	males: 60–120 micromol/L
glucose	fasting: 3–5.4 mmol/L
	random: 3–7.7 mmol/L
calcium	ionised: 1.16–1.3 mmol/L
	total: 2.1–2.6 mmol/L
magnesium	0.8–1 mmol/L
phosphate	0.8–1.5 mmol/L
urate	females: 0.15–0.4 mmol/L
	males: 0.2–0.45 mmol/L
osmolality	280–300 mosmol/kg

Proteins

albumin	32–45 g/L (age variable)
protein (total)	62–80 g/L
bilirubin (total)	<20 micromol/L
bilirubin (conj)	<4 micromol/L

Enzymes

GGT	females: <30 units/L
	males: <50 units/L
ALP (non-pregnant)	25–100 units/L
ALT	<35 units/L
AST	<40 units/L
lactate dehydrogenase	110–230 units/L
creatine kinase	females: 30–180 units/L
	males: 60–220 units/L
lipase	<70 U/L
amylase	0–180 Somogyi U/dL

Lipids

triglycerides (fasting)	<1.7 mmol/L
cholesterol (total)	<5.5 mmol/L
HDL	males: 0.9–2.0 mmol/L
	females: 1–2.2 mmol/L
LDL	2–3.4 mmol/L

Arterial blood gases

pH	7.35–7.45
PaO_2	80–100 mmHg (10.6–13.3 kPa)
$PaCO_2$	35–45 mmHg (4.7–6.0 kPa)
bicarbonate	22–26 mmol/L
base excess	± 2 mmol/L
anion gap	8–16
A–a gradient	<10 torr

Miscellaneous

lactate	<2.0 mmol/L
CRP	<10 mg/L
free T_4	10–25 picomol/L
thyroid-stimulating hormone	0.4–5 mIU/L

Index

Page numbers followed by *f* indicate figures, *t* indicate tables and *b* indicate boxes.